ESSENTIAL MIDWIFERY

Edited by

CHRISTINE HENDERSON
MA (Warwick), DPHE (Surrey), MTD, DipN (Lond) RN, RM
Senior Research Fellow in Midwifery and Women's Health, Faculty of Health
and Community Care, University of Central England, Birmingham;
Editor of the British Journal of Midwifery

KATHLEEN JONES
BN, PGCE, DipN (Wales) RGN, RM
Midwife, Wrexham Maelor Hospital NHS Trust, Wrexham, Clwyd

Mosby
London Philadelphia St. Louis Sydney Tokyo

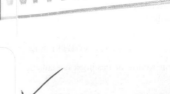

Project Manager:	Dave Burin
Publisher:	Nicola Horton
Development Editor:	Georgina Massy
Designer:	Lara Last
Layout Artist:	Jim Evoy
Cover Design:	Greg Smith
Illustration:	Mike Saiz
	Rob Dean
Production:	Hamish Adamson

Contents

Foreword

Midwives have attended upon women in childbirth since the beginning of time, but it was not until 1881 that attempts were made to regulate the training and practice of midwives. In response to the appalling levels of maternal and infant mortality and the subsequent lack of strong healthy men to fight in the wars, the first moves were made to begin the process of turning midwifery into a profession. It is now some 95 years since the first Registration of Midwives Act was passed and almost 110 years since the first publication of *Nursing Notes*, the journal of the Midwives Institute. Midwives or the 'handy women' were trained as apprentices and had a brief three-month training. The progress towards professional practice has been slow and influenced by changes in social policy and the medicalisation of childbirth.

For many midwives the transition from lay helper to academic professional midwife has not been easy. Many midwives express their concerns that the art of midwifery will be marginalised by what seems the current obsession with science and some are afraid that in the pursuit of scholarship and in striving for high academic standards, the essentials of midwifery, often defined only in terms of practical skills, will be lost.

These fears have some basis and those that care passionately about the traditions of midwifery are concerned and anxious. They search for evidence of a past 'golden age' where midwifery was an art handed down from midwife to midwife. Through rose-coloured spectacles they argue that in the past midwives had well-developed clinical skills and were fit for practice and by implication, those prepared in higher education today, somehow are not. However, for these midwives, the high mortality and morbidity rates of the past are conveniently forgotten, they are often hazy about the scientific basis of their decision making or vague about the advice they gave, based on ritual and routine.

Midwifery has come a long way in the past century; it has moved from a craft and a skill handed down from one generation to the next, to an art and a profession increasingly based on scientific evidence.

All courses leading to registration as a midwife, are at diploma level, with many more leading to degree qualifications. Midwifery education is now firmly part of the UK higher education system and tomorrow's midwives are likely to be much better equipped to deal with problems of clinical practice. In 1993 the Department of Health in England produced 'Changing Childbirth'; similarly in Scotland, Wales and Northern Ireland, government policy reflected the need to put women first. It became official policy that paternalism was to be replaced by partnerships and that women were no longer merely passive recipients of care. For the first time women's views were considered important enough to be heard and care was to be planned with women in mind. This is the context of midwifery care in today's rapidly changing National Health Service and it is out of these changes in priorities, that the need for a new core midwifery text has emerged.

For those midwives who value the art of the past and accept that well-informed, educated midwives are more likely to provide better care, then this book will be a valuable tool. It is a book to soothe the troubled mind and allay fears about the loss of the essence of midwifery. *Essential Midwifery* is just that: an essential for good midwifery practice and high quality care of women and their families. It has succeeded because each contributor has focused on what are the essentials of good midwifery care: this is care that is underpinned by the best possible evidence and continues to celebrate the increasingly complex art of professional practice.

Students studying for diplomas and degrees in midwifery will welcome this exciting publication. Each chapter will become essential reading for students and an invaluable resource for all practising midwives.

Professor Sheila C Hunt
Faculty of Health and Community Care
University of Central England in Birmingham

Preface

The need for a new approach to a textbook in midwifery arose against a background of momentous change taking place in practice and education. Common themes of the reviews of the maternity services in each country in the United Kingdom include the importance of choice, continuity and control for women using the services. The way in which maternity care is being provided has also been affected by the introduction of the market-led NHS.

The emphasis on a customer led, cost effective maternity service has brought change to the way in which midwives deliver care to their clients with the need, more than ever to provide evidence based practice.

Inevitably, there have also been changes to the way in which midwives are being prepared for practice and the way in which education is organized. Midwifery education has been re-located from the health service into institutions of higher education. Synonymous with this move has been the requirement to deliver midwifery programmes at a minimum of diploma level in Higher Education. There is also an increasing number of institutions providing post-registration degree and diploma programmes.

Customer orientated care and the emphasis to treat every client as an individual with holistic needs has led to changes within the curriculum for midwifery education. Greater emphasis is being placed on the psychological and sociological aspects of care as well as the physiological concepts that have always been fundamental to preparation for practice. All of these changes mean that there is a need for a new midwifery text which takes cognisance not only of the level of knowledge needed by the contemporary midwife, but also the changing knowledge base and skills required to effectively conduct their role within the modern health care arena. The diversity of background of the 29 contributors adds to the richness of the text which presents traditional and contemporary views from a variety of perspectives.

THE CONTENT OF THE BOOK

Essential Midwifery covers the whole spectrum of life events relating to reproduction, from puberty to parenthood. The approach taken is different from other midwifery texts in that it is from a stance of normality which includes those women who have special needs and therefore extends to areas not considered normal for others. It takes an integrated approach combining the social and behavioural sciences as they might be applied to midwifery. To be effective, midwives need to be aware of and understand the framework within which they practice, the importance of interpersonal skills, of finding out views of those they care for and the politics surrounding practice.

THE STRUCTURE OF THE BOOK

Unit 1, From One Family to Another, introduces students to the processes involved in the transition from girl to woman to motherhood, the period from puberty to pregnancy. Physiological changes are described, sociological differences discussed and physiological concepts expounded. Considerations regarding the planning of antenatal care are explored from screening to where, who and how care will be given. Women who require special needs including those experiencing loss are discussed under separate chapters.

Unit 2, From Birth to Health after Birth, describes the physiology and management of labour, what we know and what we do not know from the perspectives of an obstetrician and midwife. A comprehensive exploration of methods of pain relief during labour and the reality of the control of pain is dealt with and psychosocial support during labour is discussed. A midwifery and paediatric perspective is introduced in the chapters concerning the management of the newborn baby from resuscitation, to examination, to an explanation of some of the common problems experienced subsequent to birth. The importance of mother baby interactions is extensively explored. The knowledge and skills required for infant feeding are also dealt with in this unit. An important contribution to this unit, entitled Health after Birth, details the management of postnatal care, and the morbidity experienced by significant numbers of women. The chapter describes what those particular areas are, identified by recent research and discusses how they can be reduced. The unit concludes with a critical view of some of the key issues pertinent to expectant and new parents which includes men undergoing the transition to parenthood. The perspective taken is that the period surrounding birth is an important 'window of opportunity' for promoting a healthy family and parent child relationships. Various theoretical perspectives which have informed opinion and beliefs in the context of the family and parenting are also critically examined. Relevant psychological and sociological theories of importance to midwives are outlined and there are indications of how midwives may enhance the adaptation of families to parenthood.

Unit 3, Factors Influencing Midwifery Practice is an important section that covers the following: Regulation of Midwifery Practice includes discussion of women's rights and expectations, accountability of midwives, public protection and risk management. Maternity Policy and the Midwife outlines the influences on midwifery practice and policy and details their implications for midwives and women's choice and control from an historical and current viewpoint. The chapter entitled Consulting Consumers of the Maternity Services examines how close the link is between public policy and consumer wishes. It explores the activities, role and difficulties faced by consumer organisations and addresses the issue of who they do not serve. The potential of Maternity Service Liaison Committees is also addressed and concludes that a closer alliance between consumer and midwife is critical. Interpersonal Skills examines current theories that may assist the midwife to understand why sometimes her best intentions at communicating fails to produce the desired results. The importance of listening skills is highlighted. Developing Midwives for Practice examines the nature of professional knowledge and competence to practice and the paradoxes likely to be encountered during midwifery practice. Continued professional development following registration is explored with the final part outlining career pathways that midwives might pursue. The final chapter, entitled Women: The Focus of Care, explores the interactions and influences on the provision of a woman centred service and reflects on the implications of such a service to women, midwives and the organisation suggesting the way forward.

FORMAT OF THE CHAPTERS

The chapters are designed to aid effective student learning and to assist readers in quickly finding particular subjects.

Each chapter contains:

- Learning outcomes – the main concepts which can be learned from the chapter are outlined in order to reinforce student learning.
- Boxed highlights – to extract and emphasize important issues and points for the reader, pertinent to the chapter including boxed information in the form of case studies.
- Key concepts – located at the end of each chapter, these help the reader to summarize and assimilate key information.
- References – to give full citations of the literature and research on which the chapter is based in order to provide the reader with the opportunity to gather further information if required.
- Further reading – recommendations to explore further resources both general and related to specific conditions.

It is recognised, by the editors that any one book could never be sufficient to explore the concepts and issues in the depth necessary which is why each unit concludes with an annotated reading list, a useful resource for those needing or wishing to extend their knowledge further.

The overall purpose of the book is to identify research available, to share ideas, stimulate thought and debate; to encourage a spirit of enquiry, encouraging scholarship based on practice to benefit the women and families using the maternity services. It will undoubtedly raise many questions.

We hope you enjoy using *Essential Midwifery*. Should you have any comments about the book, please write to us care of the Publishers – we'll be pleased to hear from you.

Christine Henderson
Kathleen Jones

Contributors

Hazel Abbott
MSc, RN, RM, ADM, PGCE
Senior Lecturer in Midwifery
Faculty of Health Care and Social Studies
University of Luton
Luton
Chapter 14

Debra Bick
BA(Hons), MMedSci, RGN, RM, FPCert
Research Fellow in Midwifery
Department of Public Health and Epidemiology
University of Birmingham
Birmingham
Chapter 14

John M Delieu
BSc(Hons), CBiol, MIBiol, RGN, PGCE
Lecturer in Anatomy and Physiology
Faculty of Health Studies
School of Radiography
University of Wales, Bangor
Bangor
Chapter 4

Jenny Fonseca
MSc, BSc, MIBiol, CHBiol
Lecturer in Physiology
School of Nursing and Midwifery Studies
Faculty of Health Studies
University of Wales, Bangor
Bangor
Chapter 1

Diane M Fraser
MPhil, BEd, RM, RN, MTD
Head of Division of Midwifery
School of Nursing and Midwifery
Faculty of Medicine and Health Sciences
Queen's Medical Centre
University of Nottingham
Nottingham
Chapter 19

Harold Gee
MD, FRCOG
Consultant Obstetrician and
Director of Post-Graduate Education
Department of Fetal Maternal Medicine
Birmingham Women's Hospital
Birmingham
Chapter 9

Maureen Glynn
RGN, RM, ADM
Midwife
South Devon Healthcare Maternity Unit
Torbay Hospital
Torquay
Chapter 9

Ruth Hadikin
RGN, RM, ADM, Cert Ed (Adult)
Community Midwife
St Helen's and Knowsley Hospitals NHS Trust
Whiston
Preston
Merseyside
Chapter 6

Christine Henderson
MA (Warwick), DPHE (Surrey), MTD,
DipN (Lond), RN, RM
Senior Research Fellow in Midwifery
Faculty of Health and Community Care
University of Central England
Birmingham
Chapter 21

Lea Jamieson
MSc, BEd (Hons), RGN, RM, MTD
Head of Midwifery and Women's Health Studies
School of Life, Basic Medical and Health Sciences
The Nightingale Institute
King's College
London
Chapter 13

Rosemary Jenkins
MSc, RGN, RM, MTD, DMS, MBIM
Nursing Officer
Department of Health
London
Chapter 16

Kathleen Jones
BN, PGCE, DipN (Wales), RGN, RM
Midwife
Department of Midwifery
Maelor Hospital
Wrexham
Chapter 8

Linda Jones
PhD, MA, BA, PGCE
Senior Lecturer and Dean of the School of Health
and Social Welfare
School of Health and Social Welfare
The Open University
Chapter 1

Donna Kirwan
RGN, RM
Specialist Midwife and Coordinator
The Fetal Centre
Liverpool Women's Hospital
Liverpool
Chapter 6

Rosemary Mander
PhD, MSc, RGN, SCM, MTD
Senior Lecturer
Department of Nursing Studies
University of Edinburgh
Edinburgh
Chapter 10

Christine MacArthur
PhD, MSc, BSc, MIHE
Reader in Maternal and Child Epidemiology
Department of Public Health and Epidemiology
University of Birmingham
Birmingham
Chapter 14

Pam Miller
BA, SRN, SCM, DN
Senior Midwife
Neonatal Unit
Birmingham Women's Hospital
Birmingham
Chapter 12

Sue Moore
MSc, BA, RGN, RM, ADM, Cert Ed
Senior Lecturer
School of Women's Health Studies
Faculty of Health and Community Care
University of Central England
Birmingham
Chapters 1, 4 and 11

Imogen Morgan
MBChB, FRCP(G), FRCP, DCH
Consultant Neonatologist
Neonatal Unit
Birmingham Women's Hospital
Birmingham
Chapter 12

Fiona Murphy
MSc, HVcert, RGN, NDN, RCNT, PGCE (FE), BN
Lecturer in Nursing
Department of Nursing, Midwifery and Health
Care
University of Wales
Swansea
Chapter 8

Simon J Newell
MD, MRCPCH, FRCP
Consultant and Honorary Senior Lecturer in
Neonatal Medicine and Paediatrics
Department of Paediatrics
St James's University Hospital
Leeds
Chapter 12

Muriel O'Driscoll
RM, MTD, FPcert, MA
Senior Nurse/Psycho-sexual Therapist
Wirral Brook Advisory Centre
Birkenhead
Wirral
Chapter 20

Karl Olah
MBChB, FRCS, MRCOG
Consultant and Honorary Senior Lecturer in
Obstetrics and Gynaecology
Warwick Hospital
Warwick
Chapter 6

Lynne Pacanowski
BSc(Hons), RGN, RM, PGCEA, ENB 901
Principal Lecturer
Midwifery and Women's Health Studies
The Nightingale Institute
King's College
London
Chapters 2 and 3

Liz Paden
MSc, RN, RM, DAM, Cert Ed (FE)
Lecturer in Midwifery Studies
School of Nursing and Midwifery Studies
Faculty of Health
University of Wales, Bangor
Bangor
Chapter 15

Mel Parr
PhD, MA, BA(Hons), C Couns Psychol
Clinical and Research Director
Parents in Partnership-Parent Infant Network
Stevenage
Hertfordshire
Chapter 15

Margaret Reid
PhD, MA
Reader
Department of Public Health
University of Glasgow
Glasgow
Chapter 18

Ellena M Salariya
MPhil, RGN, RM
Freelance researcher/writer
Dundee
Scotland
Chapter 12

Jane Sandall
MSc, BSc, RN, RM, HV
Reader in Midwifery Studies
Department of Midwifery
St Bartholomew School of Nursing and Midwifery
City University
London
Chapter 17

Hilary Thomas
PhD, BA
Lecturer in Sociology
Department of Sociology
University of Surrey
Guildford
Chapter 7

Chris Warren
SRN, SCM, ADM
Independent Midwife
Cundall
Yorkshire
Chapter 5

Victoria Whittaker
BA, RGN, RM, HV Cert, Dip Ad Mid, PGCEA
Lecturer in Midwifery
Department of Nursing, Midwifery and Health
Care
University of Wales, Swansea
Swansea
Chapter 15

ACKNOWLEDGEMENTS

Christine Ager, Rose Allen, Tricia Anderson, Tricia Murphy-Black, Helen Caulfield, Helen Cheyne, Dr Nona Dawson, Mary Griffin, Sally Inch, Ruth Kirchmeier, Mavis Kirkham, Sheila Kitzinger, Jean Robinson, Heather Shaw, Dennis Walsh, Patricia Ward, Sandra Hollings, Jenny Clark, Janette Allotey.

unit 1

From One Family to Another

From Girl to Woman to Mother

CHAPTER OUTLINE

- Growth and development before puberty
- Changes in the physical characteristics of the body during puberty
- Maturation of reproductive functioning
- Factors that affect the onset and course of puberty
- Living in families
- Gender, race and social class
- Different ways of understanding society
- What is psychology?
- Gender differences
- Approaches to psychology
- Developmental psychology?
- Feminist psychology?

LEARNING OUTCOMES

After studying this chapter you should be able to:

- Describe the prenatal development of the sex organs.
- Identify the normal patterns of growth through childhood.
- Recognize the factors that effect the onset and course of puberty.
- Analyse the hormonal interactions that occur during the menstrual cycle, ovarian cycle and uterine cycle.
- Discuss the structure and social character of the contemporary family.
- Assess key features of the changing position of women within UK society.
- Explain the main differences between a structural and social action analysis of society.
- Outline the main features of quantitative and qualitative approaches to research.
- Discuss the relevance of psychology to midwifery practice.

(continued)

PHYSIOLOGICAL CHANGES

This section describes the general bodily changes and the development of the reproductive organs during adolescence in girls, and outlines the main factors affecting the timing and development of puberty.

The transition from childhood to adulthood encompasses profound changes in the physical appearance and the physiological characteristics of the body. These changes are brought about by complex, inter-related events and culminate in a physically mature individual, capable of reproduction. This biological transformation is known as puberty, and is accompanied by profound changes in the psychological state and the social outlook of the person, in preparation for the roles and responsibilities of adulthood.

The concept of adolescence as a stage of development in preparation for adulthood is well documented in history. The first references to adolescence were found on clay tablets from the Sumerian civilization, the first high civilization known to man, which flourished in the Middle East from the fifth to the second millennium BC. In the classical period, Greek philosophers speculated on the importance of the developmental stages in life and, in a essay on male youth, Aristotle described his observations on their sexual desires, sanguineness, recklessness, aspirations, sociability and many other aspects, in terms that are perfectly applicable to the youth of today.

In the Middle Ages, the distinctions between life stages were not de-emphasized, and the child was perceived as a small adult. Sperm cells, visible under the primitive microscopes available at the time, were believed to contain a miniature adult, or homunculus (**Figure 1.1**). This structure contained all the adult tissues in a preformed state and to develop into an adult required enlargement only.

Our understanding of the processes involved in the physiological development of both sexes has advanced considerably since then, especially over the past few decades. The structural changes which take place in the body before birth, during childhood and in puberty are now well characterized, as are the major hormonal changes. Other hormonal interactions and the factors affecting the timing of puberty are now being investigated.

Growth and Development before Puberty

The sex organs are formed and differentiate into recognizable structures before birth. They grow slowly during childbirth, but undergo no further development until the early stages of puberty.

Prenatal Development of the Sex Organs

The female sex organs (**Figure 1.2**) are the ovaries (which produce the female sex gametes or ova), the

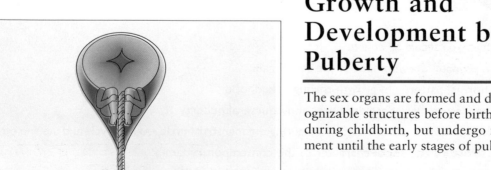

Figure 1.1 The homunculus: a sperm containing a miniature organism. (From Katchadourian, 1977.)

uterus (where the developing baby is protected and nourished) and the Fallopian tubes, vagina and breasts. Other structures associated with sexual functioning are the labia, vestibular glands and clitoris, generally known as the external genitalia.

All of the organs necessary for sexual functioning are present at the time a child is born. By weeks 8–10 of intrauterine life, the ovary is a well-defined structure that contains large numbers of primordial germ cells, some of which develop into ova after puberty. The primordial germ cells divide rapidly by mitosis until the fifth month of intrauterine life. They enter into the early

stages of meiosis and are called primary oocytes. Once surrounded by a single layer of stroma cells, they are known as primordial follicles. By the fifth month of gestation there are approximately seven million in the ovary. Small numbers of primordial follicles develop into primary and secondary follicles before birth or during childhood, and later degenerate in a process known as atresia. At birth, a girl has approximately two million primordial follicles, but by puberty less than half a million remain. Of these only about 400 to 500 will complete their development into ova.

Differentiation of the uterus and vagina is complete by 22 to 24 weeks of intrauterine life. Maternal and placental hormones stimulate development of the cervix and at birth the uterus is proportionally larger in relation to body weight than it is after puberty. In the first months after birth, the uterus decreases in size.

The external genitalia develop rapidly during week 7 or 8, and by week 10 or 11 are easily recognizable.

Growth during Childhood

During its development to adulthood, the body grows continuously. The overall growth rate is rapid before birth, during infancy and again at puberty (**Figure 1.3**). All tissues of the body grow simultaneously, but they do so at different rates. During the first year of

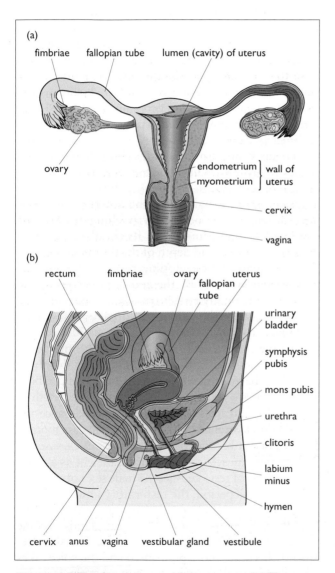

Figure I.2 The female reproductive system. (**a**) The vagina, uterus, fallopian tubes and ovaries, with sections cut away to show the continuity between the organs. (**b**) Section through the female pelvis.

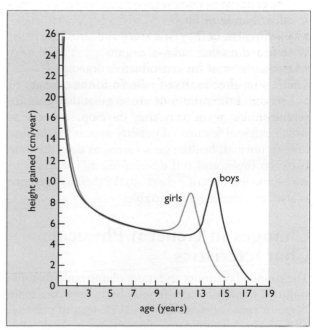

Figure I.3 Typical individual curves showing the velocity of growth in height for girls and boys. (Redrawn from Tanner *et al.*, 1966.)

life, growth is most rapid in the nervous system and lymphoid tissue. Growth of the nervous system slows down during the latter half of childhood, by which time the nervous system has almost reached its adult size. Lymphoid tissue, which is responsible for immunity to infection, continues to grow rapidly. Its growth peaks during the early teenage years and then declines with advancing age. Growth of the skeletal system during early childhood is greatest in the extremities, but afterwards continues more uniformly until adolescence. The reproductive organs grow slowly, but undergo little development until puberty.

Changes in the Physical Characteristics of the Body during Puberty

The physical changes of puberty start between 8 and 13 years of age in girls, some 2 years before the pubertal changes occur in boys. These changes can be divided into four categories.
- Acceleration and then deceleration of skeletal growth, i.e. the adolescent growth spurt.
- Altered body composition as a result of skeletal and muscular growth, and changes in the quantity and distribution of fat.
- Development of the respiratory and circulatory systems, and other internal organs.
- Development of the reproductive organs.

There is no precise, fixed pattern to the changes of puberty, and the variations are so great that girls are seldom alike in the way they develop. The age at which external features of puberty appear for the first time in normal, healthy girls varies, as does the time between onset and full development. The order in which the features of puberty make their appearance is also, to some extent, variable.

Changes in General Physical Characteristics

The rounded contours and more plump build that distinguish the adolescent female body from the male begin to appear before the sexual changes of puberty. Deposits of subcutaneous adipose tissue make the skin feel softer. Localized deposits begin to appear in the face, subclavian region, beneath the breasts, in the lower abdomen, the buttocks and the thighs. Less evident deposits of adipose tissue also accumulate on the upper arms, shoulders and calves. The rate of fat deposition reaches its maximum before the start of breast development or the growth spurt.

The pubertal growth spurt begins around the age of 10 or 11 years, some 2 years before the growth spurt in boys, and lasts for 2–3 years (Faust, 1983; Falkener and Tanner, 1978). During this period the rate of height increase is almost double that occuring in childhood – the most rapid growth occurs before the first menstruation or menarche. Once she has reached this stage, a girl usually grows little more in stature. Growth during puberty accounts, on average, for about one-sixth of the total adult body height, but there are enormous individual variations. Once the pubertal growth phase has finished, the epiphyseal plates (growing regions of the long bones) fuse to the main shaft of the bone and no further lengthening of the bone occurs. Once she is fully mature, a young woman is generally about 12–13 cm shorter than her male counterpart.

In early puberty, the limbs grow faster than the trunk. Limb growth later stops, but the trunk continues to grow well into adolescence. Trunk growth is usually greatest in the bony pelvis. The breadth increases more rapidly than the anterior–posterior measurement. The pelvic cavity elongates and the inlet widens, in keeping with its childbearing function. The breadth and depth of the thorax increase to accommodate the developing respiratory and cardiovascular systems. By the end of puberty, women have proportionally longer trunks, broader hips and shorter legs than they did as children.

Muscle mass increases in girls by about 70%, largely during the early years of adolescence. The muscles of women are less bulky than those of men, but their bodies tend to be more flexible than the male body. In both sexes, there is a progressive increase in the strength of the muscles, and an associated increase in endurance and coordination. Strength and endurance increase more in males, not just because of their greater muscle size, but also because muscle action is more efficient as a result of the effects of testosterone, the male sex hormone.

During this period, the respiratory and cardiovascular systems and most other internal organs grow rapidly. Sebaceous glands and sweat glands become more active, and axillary hair grows. The skin frequently becomes more pigmented and the voice takes on a deeper timbre owing to changes in the larynx.

Development of the Reproductive Organs

The reproductive organs undergo dramatic changes at puberty. Changes in the ovaries are followed by changes in other reproductive organs, and in the external genitalia. The structure of the reproductive system of a sexually mature woman is shown in **Figure 1.2**. Breast development is usually the first external sign of puberty. In the majority of cases, pubic hair appears in the early stages of breast development, although it may not appear until breast development is complete. Menarche is a late feature of puberty and does not usually happen until after the period of fastest body growth.

The ovaries

The ovaries (**Figure 1.2**) are the primary reproductive organs, or gonads. At sexual maturity, they produce the female germ cells, or ova. These develop within follicles which were established during gestation. The follicles produce sex steroid hormones, principally oestrogens, which induce most of the developmental changes at puberty. The sex steroids are also essential for the normal functioning of the menstrual cycle. The role of ovarian hormones in the menstrual cycle is described later.

The ovaries are the first sex organs to increase in size at puberty. They start to grow at around 8 years of age, and by late adolescence reach about six times their childhood weight. The follicles are present in the cortex of the ovary. Before puberty, primordial follicles and some primary and secondary follicles are present in the ovaries. After menarche, follicles begin to develop into mature ova, but several years usually elapse before ovulation is a regular feature of the menstrual cycle.

The breasts

The breasts of a sexually mature woman contain lobes of mammary tissue. These consist of ducts lined by epithelium. The ducts are embedded in adipose and connective tissue, and converge into larger ducts at the nipple. During childhood, the breasts contain little glandular tissue. With the onset of puberty, increased oestradiol levels cause a marked enhancement of duct growth and branching, and the deposition of fat. Much of breast enlargement at this time is due to fat deposition. During pregnancy and lactation, further development of mammary tissue occurs, and milk-producing alveoli are established along the ducts.

In most girls, breast development is the first external change in puberty. The external changes are usually divided into five stages.
- Stage 1: Pre-adolescent stage with elevation of the nipple only.
- Stage 2: Breast bud stage with elevation of the breast and nipple as a small mound, and enlargement of the areola diameter.
- Stage 3: Further enlargement and elevation of the breast and areola, with no separation of their contours.
- Stage 4: Enlargement of the areola and nipple to form a secondary mound above the level of the breast.
- Stage 5: Mature stage with projection of the nipple only, due to recession of the areola to the general contour of the breast.

The first sign of breast development may appear at 9 years of age, but by the age of 13 years most girls have some breast development. Most girls pass through all five stages of breast development, but some pass directly from stage 3 to stage 5, whereas others remain at stage 4 until their first pregnancy. **Figure 1.4** shows the age range and the mean age at which each stage of breast development is reached in British girls. One breast may enlarge earlier than

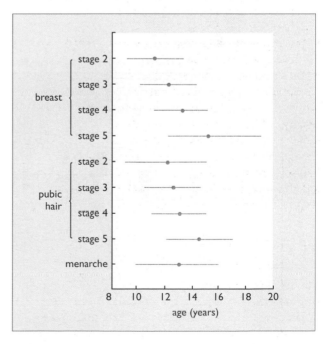

Figure 1.4 Graph indicating the age range and mean age at which the various stages of breast and pubic hair development are reached, and the age range and mean age at which menarche occurs. (From Edmonds, 1989.)

the other, but this inequality usually disappears as growth proceeds.

The uterus, vagina and external genitalia

The mature uterus (**Figure 1.2**) is a muscular organ enclosing a cavity, and is lined with a mucous membrane called the endometrium. Two Fallopian tubes lead from the uterus towards the ovaries. Each terminates in finger-like projections called fimbriae, which lie adjacent to the ovaries. They absorb the ovum when it is released from the surface of the ovary during ovulation, nourish it and transport it to the uterus.

During puberty, growth of the uterus starts approximately 2 years after that of the ovaries, and continues into the early 20s (Holm *et al.* 1995). The uterus becomes anteflexed (**Figure 1.5**) and the ligaments supporting it widen. Growth is faster in the body of the uterus than in the cervix, and occurs initially in the muscle or myometrial tissue. Approximately 2 years before menarche, the cervix begins to produce mucus. Later, the endometrium proliferates and the number of glands increases. Breakdown of the superficial layers of the endometrium occurs at menarche, and during subsequent menstrual periods. By late adolescence, the

uterus weighs more than 10 times its childhood value.

The vagina increases gradually in length during childhood, but at puberty grows rapidly (**Figure 1.5**). The vestibule and vagina become paler in colour, changing from red and shiny to pink and dull. The vaginal wall thickens and becomes increasingly pliable and elastic. Several months before menarche, the production of vaginal fluid increases. The fluid consists principally of desquamated, adult-type epithelial cells, and some mucoid secretion from the cervical and vestibular glands. Initially, the fluid is odourless, but after menarche it acquires the distinctive odour of the adult vagina. During childhood, the vaginal flora consists of a variety of nonpathogenic microorganisms. Before menarche, as the vaginal secretion increases and becomes richer in glycogen, the proportion of lactobacilli in the flora increases until they dominate the flora. The lactic acid that they produce creates an acid environment within the vagina and prevents the establishment of many types of potentially harmful microorganisms.

Before puberty, the hymen (which partially closes the entrance to the vagina) is a thin, semitransparent membrane. Towards puberty it becomes thickened, fleshy and covered with mucus. By the time puberty starts, its opening is about 1 cm in diameter.

During early puberty, the inner and outer folds of the labia enlarge, becoming rounder and fuller. By the time of the menarche, they touch each other and cover the vestibule.

The clitoris contains a large number of sensory neurones and is important in sexual arousal. It is responsive to tactile stimuli, even in childhood. During this time it grows slowly, but towards the end of puberty it grows rapidly and appears to continue growing, although more slowly, through adult life.

Menarche

Because of its sudden and unmistakable onset and because of its reproductive implications, the first menstrual period or menarche has been widely regarded in many cultures as the traditional step into womanhood. At menarche, the majority of girls have a bone age of 13–14 years (Tanner *et al.* 1975). Approximately 95% of girls in the UK and Western Europe will achieve the menarche between the chronological ages of 11 and 15 years (Marshall, 1974). The same is true for countries with similar cultures and living standards. Menarche usually occurs after the peak of the growth spurt (Faust, 1977; Tanner, 1970), and about 2 years after the start of breast development.

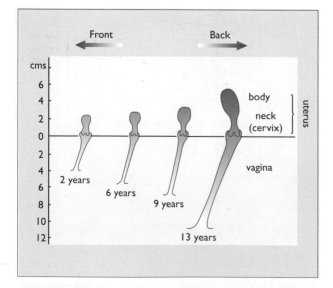

Figure 1.5 The growth of the vagina and uterus through childhood and at puberty. (From Buckler, 1987.)

Pubic hair

Pubic hair usually starts to appear around the time breast development begins. Its growth is also divided into five stages.
- Stage 1: No true pubic hair present.
- Stage 2: A little sparse, slightly pigmented hair appears first on the labia and then on the midline of the mons pubis.
- Stage 3: The hair spreads sparsely over the symphysis pubis and is darker in colour and more coarse.
- Stage 4: The hair has the typical adult texture. Growth is limited to the symphysis.
- Stage 5: The hair now has the typical triangular distribution of the adult female. Hair may also be present on the medial aspect of the thighs.

The age range and the mean age at which the various stages of pubic hair growth are evident in British girls is shown in **Figure 1.4**.

Maturation of Reproductive Functioning

The physical and functional developements in the body during puberty are orchestrated by hormonal changes. As the hormonal system matures, ovulatory menstrual cycles are established, and the adolescent girl is capable of reproduction.

The General Hormonal Changes during Puberty

The transition from childhood to sexual maturity requires development and maturation of the interacting hormonal systems of the hypothalamus, the pituitary gland and the ovaries. Early and midpuberty can be viewed as a cascade of increasing development of these systems.

The hormonal change which initiates the developmental changes of puberty is an increase in the circulating levels of luteinizing hormone (LH) and follicle-stimulating hormone (FSH) produced by the anterior pituitary gland. These hormones stimulate the ovary and are called gonadotrophins (**Figure 1.6**). Gonadotrophins are secreted in very small amounts during childhood, when FSH secretion exceeds LH

secretion. Their secretion before puberty appears to be necessary for an adequate rate of follicle growth throughout life.

At puberty, as the hypothalamus matures, gonadotrophins are secreted in pulses in a cyclical pattern, and LH levels exceed FSH levels. Gonadotrophins are released at first during sleep, and later also during daytime. The change in the LH/FSH ratio occurs at the same time as does breast budding.

The release of gonadotrophins in turn is stimulated by the secretion of gonadotrophin-releasing hormone (GnRH) from the hypothalamus. During childhood GnRH secretion is also low, but at puberty it increases and becomes pulsatile. The mechanism responsible for the increase in GnRH secretion and the maturation of the hypothalamic–pituitary–ovarian axis at puberty is not yet understood.

In early puberty, gonadotropins stimulate the initial stages of follicle development and oestrogen secretion. Oestrogens are a family of steroid hormones produced mainly by the granulosa cells of the ovary, but are also produced in small amounts by the adrenal

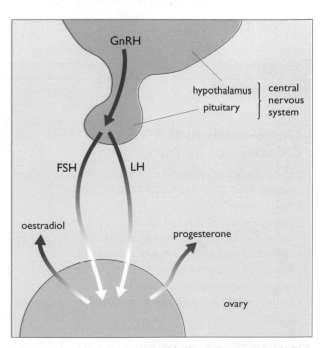

Figure 1.6 The principal hormones of the hypothalamic–pituitary–ovarian axis.

gland. Oestradiol is the most potent, and induces most of the somatic changes at puberty (**Box 1.1**). Changes in the amount of oestradiol secreted as puberty progresses and in the sensitivity of particular tissues to it appear to be important factors in determining the sequence of developmental changes of puberty.

Hormones and growth factors such as progesterone, thyroid hormone, growth hormone, insulin, insulin-like growth factor-I (IGF-I), cortisol, prolactin and epidermal growth factor have synergistic effects on the developmental actions of oestradiol.

Other steroid hormones are also involved in the changes of puberty. Androgens, responsible for development of the male sexual characteristics in boys, are released in small amounts in girls by the adrenal glands and by the ovaries. At puberty, their secretion increases. They stimulate pubic and axillary hair development, and may be involved in stimulating the growth spurt. They also stimulate sebum secretion, but when present in excess have been associated with acne. Androgens are responsible for the sex drive in women.

During the early and middle stages of puberty, increasing plasma levels of oestradiol generated by the follicles have a negative feedback effect on gonadotrophin secretion, i.e. they inhibit the release of gonadotrophins by the pituitary. In the later stages of puberty, the hypothalamic–pituitary–ovarian axis matures. Oestradiol is generated rapidly by the maturing follicle. The pituitary now responds to the high plasma oestradiol levels by positive feedback. LH secretion, in particular, increases extremely rapidly and this induces ovulation. The corpus luteum generated as a result of ovulation secretes progesterone.

The Menstrual Cycle

The mature menstrual cycle is a sequence of events involving the pituitary, hypothalamus, ovary and uterus. Hormonal interactions induce a cycle of follicle maturation in the ovary. At the same time, a complementary cycle of events is induced in the uterus, in preparation for receiving and nourishing a fertilized ovum.

The ovarian cycle

From the fifth month of gestation and throughout reproductive life, small numbers of primordial follicles spontaneously undergo development into primary follicles (**Figure 1.7**). The primordial follicles contain a primary oocyte, surrounded by a single layer of stroma cells and an outer basal lamina membrane. During the transformation into primary follicles, the spindle-shaped stroma cells develop into cuboidal granulosa cells.

Small numbers of primary follicles develop into secondary follicles, stimulated by FSH. The granulosa cells divide to form several layers around the oocyte, and secrete a halo of mucopolysaccharide, called the zona pellucida, between themselves and the oocyte. Cytoplasmic processes penetrating the zona pellucida provide nutrients and hormonal signals to the developing oocyte. The follicle recruits a further layer of stroma cells, called the theca interna, on the outside of the basal lamina.

No further development of follicles takes place before puberty. Secondary follicles are continually lost through atresia.

Once mature menstrual cycles have been established, each month approximately 20 secondary follicles begin a further stage of development (**Figure 1.7**). This stage may take almost three menstrual cycles to complete. The granulosa cells proliferate and secrete fluid which coalesces to form an antrum. The antrum grows and extends almost completely around the oocyte. The theca interna cells proliferate and become cuboidal. They secrete androgens which are then converted into oestradiol by the granulosa cells. Oestradiol entering plasma induces many of the developmental changes of

---

Box I.I

Developmental Effects of Oestradiol at Puberty

- Linear growth, acceleration and later closure of epiphyseal plates.
- Pelvic enlargement.
- Growth of the ovaries and follicles.
- Growth of lobular ducts and fat deposition in the breasts.
- Growth of the uterine myometrium and endometrium.
- Elongation of the vagina and thickening of the vaginal wall.
- Induction of vaginal and uterine secretions.
- Deposition of adipose tissue in the characteristic female pattern.
- Enlargement of the labia.
- Restriction of pubic hair to the female pattern.

puberty and contributes to the hormonal control of the menstrual cycle. Further stroma cells recruited on the outside of the structure, called the theca externa, provide vascularization to the follicle.

After this stage, one of the antral follicles, known as the dominant follicle, enters a 28-day cycle of events in the ovary. The cycle has three phases:

• Follicle development, which starts as menstruation starts and lasts about 10–12 days.
• Ovulation, which lasts 1–3 days.
• The luteal phase, which lasts about 14 days.

The remaining antral follicles degenerate.

By day 7 of the cycle the dominant follicle, also known as the graafian follicle, begins to grow exponentially as a result of cell growth of the granulosa and theca cells and fluid production. Oestradiol secretion increases rapidly and the thecal layer becomes more vascular. The follicle has a diameter of about 1.5 cm and bulges through the wall of the ovary. At this point, the oocyte completes its initial meiotic division and is known as a secondary oocyte. Part of the basal lamina close to the surface of the ovary is digested and the follicle ruptures. The secondary oocyte, surrounded by the zona pellucida and a crown of granulosa cells is released into the abdominal cavity. This process is called ovulation. The ovum is absorbed by the fimbriae, and passes down the Fallopian tubes towards the uterus.

During the final or luteal phase the remnants of the dominant follicle rapidly develop into the corpus luteum. The granulosa and theca cells enlarge, and blood vessels invade the area. The granulosa cells secrete progesterone and oestradiol. Progesterone optimizes the conditions of the endometrium for implantation of a fertilized ovum, and for maintaining the conceptus prior to the development of the placenta. The corpus luteum reaches its maximum development after 10 days, and degenerates rapidly after 14 days if pregnancy does not ensue, leaving an avascular scar called the corpus albicans.

Ovulation usually commences 3–12 months after menarche, but is not a regular feature of early menstrual cycles (Matsumoto *et al.* 1981; Vollman, 1977). This is because the hypothalamic–pituitary–ovarian hormone system is still immature. For this reason, early menstrual cycles tend to be less regular than they become later in life, and some girls may have 4, 5 or 6 months between cycles. By 2 years after menarche, about half the cycles are ovulatory and menstrual cycles are generally regular. By the early 20s, 98% of cycles are ovulatory.

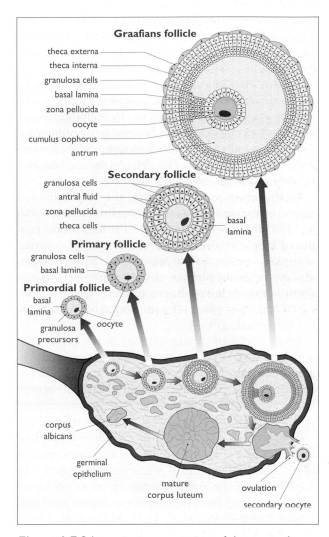

Figure 1.7 Schematic representation of the ovary showing the stages of follicle development, ovulation, the corpus luteum and the corpus albicans. (From Ham and Leeson, 1968.)

The uterine cycle

The uterine cycles taking place once ovulatory menstrual cycles have been established and can be divided into three phases (**Figure 1.8**).

The proliferative phase begins as menstruation finishes and continues until ovulation. At the end of menstruation, the endometrium is thin with sparse, straight glands. Rising levels of plasma oestradiol stimulate growth of the endometrium, increasing its thickness 3–5 fold. The glands grow, and the spiral arteries that supply the endometrium elongate. Oestradiol also affects the synthesis of cervical mucus, making it abundant, clear and nonviscous.

Shortly after ovulation, progesterone produced by the corpus luteum induces the secretory phase of the uterine cycle. Rapid growth of the endometrium is inhibited and blood vessels become more numerous. The glands coil and fill with glycogen, and their secretory activity increases. The cervical mucus becomes viscous and scant, plugging the cervix.

In the absence of pregnancy, the corpus luteum degenerates, oestradiol and progesterone levels fall and the menstrual phase ensues. Prostaglandins produced by the endometrium induce uterine contractions and constriction of the spiral arteries. Oxygen and nutrient supplies to the superficial layers are diminished. As a result, the tissue begins to break down and is sloughed off with clotted blood, to form the menstrual flow.

Some degree of dysmenorrhoea or pain associated with menstrual cycles is common, and may occur in about half of adolescents. Dysmenorrhoea appears to be more common with menstruation that follows ovulatory cycles, and appears to be related to an increased synthesis of prostaglandins by the endometrium.

When pregnancy occurs during adolescence, low birth weight and premature babies are more common than in sexually mature women. This appears to reflect general biological immaturity, and is exacerbated by social factors such as education level and prenatal care (Fraser *et al.* 1995; Miller *et al.* 1996).

Hormonal control of the menstrual cycle

The principal hormones controlling the mature menstrual cycle are oestradiol, progesterone, the gonadotrophins and GnRH (**Figure 1.8**).

FSH levels begin to rise slightly before the beginning of the follicular phase. FSH stimulates development of the follicles, particularly the antral follicles. The granulosa cells multiply and secrete oestradiol,

generating a slow increase in plasma levels over the first 6–8 days of the cycle.

The small increases in plasma oestradiol levels have a negative feedback effect on FSH secretion by the pituitary and on GnRH from the hypothalamus. FSH

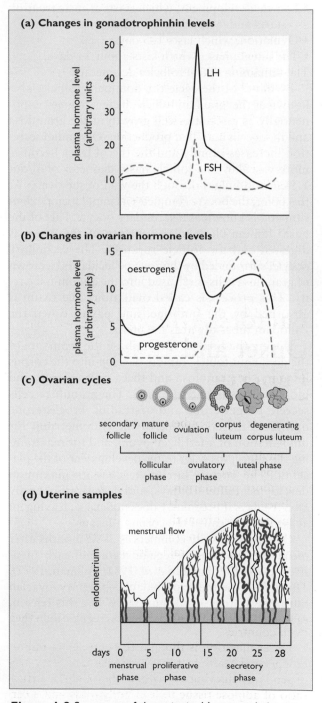

Figure 1.8 Summary of the principal hormonal changes and ovarian and uterine events of the menstrual cycle.

levels fall slightly over the second half of the follicular phase.

At the same time, LH levels rise slightly, increasing the synthesis of androgens by the theca cells, which are then used for the synthesis of oestradiol by the granulosa cells.

At the beginning of the second week, one follicle becomes dominant and the major producer of oestrogen. Plasma oestradiol levels rise rapidly. This has a positive feedback effect on gonadotropin secretion by the pituitary and on GnRH release from the hypothalamus, inducing a spike in LH levels and a smaller increase in FSH levels. The spike in LH levels induces ovulation about 18 hours later. As LH levels peak, oestradiol levels begin to fall.

LH and FSH levels initially decrease rapidly, then decline more slowly until just before the end of the cycle. LH induces the transformation of the granulosa cells and theca cells remaining in the follicle into the corpus luteum, and stimulates the synthesis of progesterone and oestrogen.

As the corpus luteum degenerates, the levels of oestrogen and progesterone decrease, and menstruation ensues.

Factors Affecting the Onset and Course of Puberty

The age at which puberty starts and its progression are affected by a variety of biological, psychosocial and environmental factors. The most important factor appears to be the general health of the individual.

In most populations, the age of menarche has declined over the past 100 years. In Western Europe, it has decreased from the age of 17 years in 1840 to around 13 years in 1980. This probably reflects improvements in general health, particularly improvements in nutrition, and the decrease in incidence and severity of infectious disease that occurred over the late eighteenth and early nineteenth centuries. It appears that this decrease has come to an end in developed countries.

Better nutrition is thought to be the most important general health factor. The timing of puberty may depend on achieving a critical body weight, a critical ratio of adipose tissue to lean body mass and a certain level of skeletal maturation. Chronic caloric deprivation lowers FSH and LH secretion. Where there is malnutrition, underweight or intense dieting, the onset of puberty is delayed or its progress slowed. Anorexic girls revert to the prepubertal stage and women may stop ovulating or become amenorrhoeic. In many cases, the pattern of LH release is similar to that of childhood. In moderately obese girls, menarche is earlier and the course of puberty is more rapid. Diabetes is also associated with earlier puberty.

Nutritional deficiency associated with significant chronic illness (e.g. inflammatory bowel disease or asthma) delays linear growth, skeletal maturation and pubertal onset (Albanese and Stanhope, 1995). Improvements in growth and the onset of puberty usually do not accompany the specific replacement of individual nutrients, but rather begin when body weight begins to normalize.

Menstrual dysfunction is common in athletes with very low body mass, such as long-distance runners and dancers, and is often associated with hypothalamic dysfunction.

Female athletes whose training begins before the usual age of menarche generally have delayed onset of menarche. They are more likely to show amenorrhoea or have irregular periods during intense physical training than do their peers who began training later. The associated ovarian dysfunction may be sufficiently serious to cause profound oestrogen deficiency with consequent osteoporosis.

Loss of cyclic gonadotropin secretion occurs with deprivation and severe emotional stress, with or without weight loss, delaying the onset and progression of puberty.

Genetic factors influence the age of menarche. Daughters of mothers who developed early or late are also likely to do so. The age of menarche is closest in identical twins, less close in nonidentical twin sisters, much less close in sisters of different pregnancies and least close in unrelated women.

Summary

- All the organs necessary for reproductive functioning are present by the end of the fifth month of gestation. Little further development takes place until puberty.
- Puberty starts between 9 and 13 years of age. The principal developmental features are the adolescent growth spurt, changes in the quantity and distribution of body fat and development of the reproductive organs.

- There is considerable variation in the age at which puberty starts and in the time taken between onset and maturity, but less variation in the sequence of pubertal change.
- The transition from childhood to sexual maturity is induced by maturation of the interacting hormone systems of the hypothalamus, pituitary and ovaries. Oestradiol is responsible for most of the somatic changes.
- The major factors affecting the time of onset and the rate of pubertal change are nutrition, genetics, chronic illness and stress. Intense physical training and low body weight associated with certain competitive sports also affect development at puberty.
- This section has identified changes to the body in the development of the female reproductive system. It has also referred to the main factors concerning pubery. At this time of bodily change , support from a sociological and psychological perspective is particulary important.

SOCIOLOGICAL PERSPECTIVES

Sociology is the systematic study of human society. It offers explanations of how society works, of people's social actions, of patterns of similarity and difference and of the distribution of social, economic and political power. Sociologists are interested in exploring what is going on under the surface of society as well as investigating the character of its visible structures. They are interested in how institutions within a society reflect particular types of social relationships. Their task is also to unravel and to interpret action through investigating not just what social actors consciously do, but also the hidden aspects of their actions and the unintended consequences. As Berger (1966) commented: 'The fascination of sociology lies in the fact that its perspective makes us see in a new light the very world in which we have lived all our lives.'

How can sociology help us to understand what it means to grow from 'girl to woman to mother to family'? First, it can illuminate difference. Growing up in a poor family, in which parents are unemployed and expectations are limited, represents a very different social experience from girlhood in a wealthy household in which opportunities are wide ranging. Second, sociology can highlight the patterns of such social differences, indicating, for example, how wealth and poverty or health and employment status reinforce each other. Third, it can draw attention to the contested nature of social experience. There is unlikely ever to be one generally accepted view of 'what society is' because, unlike a laboratory experiment, the study of society takes place under conditions that are inherently complex, unstable and dynamic.

This section explores how a sociological analysis can enhance midwives' understanding of both their clients and themselves. Different experiences of girls growing up in Britain today are examined in terms of the changing roles and positions of the family, gender, race and social class. To conclude, some different approaches that sociologists have used to understand the social world are highlighted.

Different Experiences: Growing up in the UK

Lets begin with the scenarios of two 15-year-old girls, Jane and Julia (**Case Studies 1.1** and **1.2**), which highlight some of the different experiences of growing from 'girl to woman to mother to family' in the UK today.

Jane has experienced the effects of poverty during her girlhood, through inadequate housing and a deprived local environment, whereas Julia has been comfortable and secure, probably being taken to school and leisure activities by car. Jane will have had a poorer diet and a greater risk of childhood illnesses than Julia. Although both have access to education, Jane will be under more pressure from family and peers to leave school than Julia. If the two girls left school at 16 years old Jane would find it far harder than Julia to find a job. If Julia fails her examinations she will be more likely to be given a second chance than Jane. Jane will probably start a family earlier than Julia and may see this as a way of gaining independence. Of course, they could end up with similar futures and careers. They might both go on to college and end up as midwives. But their experiences of growing up will have been very different.

The claims made about Jane and Julia are based partly on evidence gathered from reports such as the *Health Divide* (Townsend *et al.* 1988) and *Variations in Health* (Department of Health, 1995), which are

Jane

Jane is a girl of Afro-Caribbean background growing up in an inner suburb of Liverpool with her mother, grandmother and 17-year-old sister Marie. The unemployment rate in the area is 30%. Her mother does shift work as a care assistant in a private residential home for older people and the family lives in a 1960s high-rise flat which is damp and has mould on the bedroom walls. Marie works as a trainee hairdresser, having left school when 16 years old, and is engaged to Brian, an unemployed 20-year-old. Jane likes school and is doing well in her GCSE course. She would like to go to college and is thinking about applying for nursing, but would also like more independence and her own money coming in.

Julia

Julia is growing up in Tunbridge Wells, an affluent town with a low unemployment rate. Both her parents have professional careers – her father is a general practitioner and her mother is a health visitor. The family is white and they are members of the Church of England. They live on a private estate in a modern five-bedroom, detached house with a garden. Julia's brother, Richard, is studying medicine at London University and Julia expects to go on to college when she leaves school. She wants to become a midwife and is doing well in her 'A'-level courses in biology and politics at her local grant-maintained school.

---

based on surveys of the main differences in health status between occupational groups. For almost all diseases there is a 'social class gradient'; in other words, semiskilled and unskilled workers suffer more disease and higher death rates than those in professional and managerial jobs. In education, the rate at which children born into professional families stay on at school and take up university places is markedly higher than for those in manual workers' families.

Building on this we can also comment that Jane and Julia live in very different types of families. The two girls also have very different cultural backgrounds, beliefs and values. Jane may well have experienced racism as she grew up. She may have been discriminated against because she is black and other people judge her as 'different' and inferior. They are both girls and will have experienced the social and psychological state of 'being a girl' and learning what it means to be a woman and mother. However, their experience of being girls and learning what it means to be women and mothers will reflect the meanings attached to these states by parents, peers and other significant people in their lives. These scenarios lead us on to think about ways in which social class, race and gender influence and pattern people's experience and how this is expressed through family life.

Living in Families

Jane and Julia both live in families. A family represents, above all, a set of social relationships and the particular interest for sociologists lies in the dynamic interaction between social divisions, family structures and interpersonal relationships. The significant social and legal relationships that characterize families include residence, parenthood and marriage (Gittins, 1985). Increasingly, shared residence and housekeeping rather than marriage is the norm; over 30% of children are now born outside marriage and nonstandard family types, such one-parent families, are now more common (HMSO, 1994).

Family Structure and Roles

Families today are diverse, but a broad distinction can be made between the 'nuclear' family of two or less generations (like Julia's) and the 'extended' family of three generations and possibly other kin living together (like Jane's). Over 10% of British Asian households contain more than one family, compared with only 2% of Afro-Caribbean households and 1% of white households (Jackson, 1993). On the other hand, over four million people now live alone (HMSO, 1994).

Some conventional nuclear families have extensive local kinship ties (Graham and McKee, 1980) and black and minority ethnic groups also exhibit significant variation in family structure. Parmar (1988) warns against projecting damaging stereotypes of family life. Afro-Caribbean family structure, for example, ranges from 'Christian marriage' – based on the model of the Victorian family – to the 'common law' family of unmarried partners and the 'mother household' – in which a mother or grandmother is the sole household head and manager (Barrow, 1982). The 'cereal packet' family of advertising fame – breadwinner husband, dependent wife and two children – accounts for only 25% of British households today. An increasing number of women live alone with children, many in near poverty. Over 50% of fathers fail to keep up their maintenance payments to their children and ex-wives, and nearly 50% lose touch with their ex-families within 2 years (Department of Social Services, 1990).

Families also have social functions. They play a major part in maintaining and restoring the health of their members, as well as in taking on responsibilities for the care of dependent relatives (Graham, 1993). Families perform a vital economic role in supporting the present workforce and in its reproduction, although the pattern of household responsibilities has shifted. Until the 1950s, most women spent most of their married life in childbearing, but by the 1990s two-thirds were engaged in paid employment outside the home.

Many of the welfare benefits available today are targeted towards families (Jones, 1994). Child Benefit was developed in the 1970s to replace child tax allowances and give carers for children a small income that was independent of the breadwinner wage, and thus combat child poverty. Family Credit is a means-tested benefit designed to combat family poverty by supplementing family income. In addition, families may benefit from Income Support, Housing Benefit and a Community Care Allowance which is paid to people with disabilities to enable them to live independently in the community.

Socialization

Parenting involves the socialization of children; that is, the transmission of culture between generations through internalization of social norms and values. Primary socialization takes place in the first few years of life, whereas secondary socialization refers to the older child moving towards adulthood. In a classic text, Mead (1934) argued that the 'social self' is created by negotiation between the child, the immediate family and significant others. The child learns appropriate patterns of social action and begins to project selective images by observing and absorbing how other people act and respond in various situations.

In this view, children are social actors who can express and build their own individuality rather than merely model their behaviour upon the examples and responses of others. In secondary socialization, children play an increasingly larger number of different social roles negotiated in a complex sequence of interactions. They are exposed to generalized social ideologies (for example, femininity and masculinity), but what they make of these roles and how they choose to play them depends on how they 'write the script'.

In contrast to this, the constraining power of socialization has also been highlighted (Parsons, 1964). Social behaviour, norms, values and beliefs may be largely imposed, either with the consent of the individual or by coercive means. Ideological or material influences constrain individual behaviour, and the pattern and gender of family inequality derive from the wider society. The idea that each social actor is able to negotiate within society is viewed with scepticism. People have relatively little room for manoeuvre; most of their choices turn out to be predictable from their social background and upbringing.

Different Views of the Family

For some sociologists the family is an essential 'building block' and the modern nuclear family represents the effective adaptation of earlier family structures to meet the needs of industrial society (Parsons, 1964). This functional analysis emphasizes the efficiency of the nuclear family structure in meeting the needs of individuals for intimacy, security and sexual expression, as well as the needs of the wider economy and society. The New Right has viewed the decline of the conventional two-parent, two-child family as largely responsible for a wider moral crisis that involves increasing lawlessness, deviance and welfare dependency (Fitzgerald, 1985).

But this approach makes fundamental assumptions about what the family's roles and functions should be, without acknowledging how family life has been characterized by the subordination of women and children and the domination of men (Moore, 1988). For example, most sexual and physical violence towards women and most abuse of children still occurs within the home. Two facts, the rising divorce rate and the fact that 73% of diveroces being initiated by women, suggest that more and more women are escaping from marriages in which they do not feel valued (Jackson, 1993). Dalley (1988) drew attention to an ideology of familism: that is, an assumption that a gendered division of labour and caring is natural and normal.

Gender, Race and Social Class

Jane and Julia are girls growing up in the UK. To some extent they have experiences in common that arise from gender socialization. On the other hand, their shared experience of being female is counterbalanced by their experiences of class and race.

Sex and Gender

Sex is a biological term that refers to people's biologically given state. Gender refers to their socially acquired psychological and cultural characteristics, their learned masculinity or femininity. With a few exceptions, people are born as biological males or females. But the differences between men and women are small compared with the similarities between them, in terms of body plan, anatomy and function (Oakley, 1985). Some of the characteristics seen as biologically fixed, such as the sexual drive or maternal instinct, could instead be viewed as the product of social conditioning.

Gender Socialization

Children learn gender identity through their early social experiences. Parents, other adults and older children teach gender identity, often unconsciously.

Even at a very young age, girls and boys are treated and handled differently. Girl babies are called 'sweet' and 'pretty' by hospital staff whereas boys are 'tough' and 'handsome'. When young boys are hurt they are told to be brave, whereas it is much more acceptable for young girls to cry and show weakness. Women's greater use of health services may be partly attributed to the effects of this early gender socialization (Miles, 1991). Gender-specific advertising is used to sell toys; picture books and media images often project stereotypical masculine and feminine roles.

It is difficult to tease out the extent to which patterns of social conditioning influence children's behaviour, and to determine the contribution made by biology. Ginsburg and Miller (1982), for example, found that boys engaged in riskier types of play and had more frequent accidents than did girls, but this does not tell us how far such behaviours are learned or how much they are based in biology. Patterns of gender socialization produce systematic differences in the behaviour of the sexes that link to health status. Women with problems turn to tranquillizers added to which there has been an increase in the rate of smoking among young women. Men indulge in risk-taking behaviour: faster driving, higher rates of smoking and drinking and the greater use of dangerous drugs. This helps to explain their higher rates of accidents, cirrhosis of the liver, lung cancer and coronary heart disease (Miles, 1991).

Gendered Parental Roles

How widespread and significant is the gendering of roles in the UK? Women now form over 40% of the workforce; legislative change has promoted the equality of women in the workplace, enabled them to claim legal status as heads of households, reformed the bias in the tax system, made divorce easier and enforced the rights of women and children to property and personal choice. The emergence of a symmetrical family has been noted, nuclear in structure, with men and women workers sharing household tasks and taking joint responsibility for children (Wilmott and Young, 1975).

On the other hand, gendered parental roles are still a common feature of family life. In families with children the vast majority of housekeeping and child care is still undertaken by women. Men may do the supermarket shop, but women still do most of the shopping, cooking, washing, ironing and cleaning. Women take and fetch children from school, take time off work if children are sick, nurse children and care for dependants. In particular, they undertake most of the intimate and 'dirty' caring jobs (Graham, 1984; Popay, 1992). Most female work is either part-time or negotiated to enable women to combine housekeeping and mothering with paid labour.

Gender and Race

Jane is an Afro-Caribbean girl growing up in the UK where, despite antidiscrimination legislation, there is considerable evidence of racism (Jowell, 1986; National Association of Health Authorities, 1988; Jones, 1994). Although Jane and Julia have shared experiences because they are female, these are differentiated by race.

Race refers to physical and biological characteristics of population groups to which social meanings of superiority and inferiority have become attached, whereas ethnicity focuses on the shared cultural practices and values that differentiate a given population group. Racism refers to the prejudice and discrimination experienced by some social groups, in particular black and minority ethnic groups with skin colour other than white. Some sociologists are critical of a tendency to assume that all women share similar experiences of oppression and point out that black women have their own hidden histories of racism that have shaped their lives in very different ways (Stacey, 1993).

'Ethnic groups' has been the term in general use in health services, but this helps to disguise issues of race. Since the 1940s, the health sector has used black women as a reserve army of labour for the generally unskilled ancillary jobs or in lower levels of nursing (Doyal, 1979; Bryan *et al.* 1985). Black and minority ethnic groups today experience poorer health than white people as a result of the current and inherited effects of racism, which position them in disproportionately low paid work and poor housing (Smaje, 1995).

Gender and Social Class

Social class refers to groups that share a similar economic and social position in society with similar chances of social mobility. Jane and Julia have very different social backgrounds which influence their life chances. The Registrar-General classifies all occupations and hence all households according to five main categories, which over the years have produced a long run of relatively comparable statistics to analyze. As

an unskilled worker Jane's mother would be classified in social class V (unskilled manual) whereas Julia's father would appear in social class I (higher professional and managerial). As we noted earlier, there is a social class gradient in disease and death, with those in the lower classes experiencing higher rates than those in higher classes.

Extensive surveys of inequalities in health have concluded that occupational and environmental factors are the main influences on health status and that behaviour choices are heavily influenced by social factors (Townsend *et al.* 1988; Department of Health, 1995). The decisions that Jane makes about her lifestyle are influenced by her experience of living in an area of high unemployment, poor housing, racism and an unsupportive environment. In making her lifestyle choices Julia has very different social experience to draw on. Rates of smoking in professional groups, for example, have fallen dramatically over the past 20 years, so Julia may not have encountered much tobacco use, whereas they are still much higher among manual workers (Department of Health, 1995).

Different Ways of Understanding Society

The study of human society is such a complex task that it is not surprising to find conflicts of view among sociologists. Some of the main debates are between social action theorists and structural theorists.

Social Action

Social action theories explore the ways in which individuals and groups relate to society, and what meanings they themselves attach to events and situations. Interactionism, associated with the work of Mead, is one example of social action theory. It is concerned with the way in which people perceive and interpret different social situations and the role of the self, as in the study of socialization. The focus is on social actors who, by negotiating shared language and meanings, are able to coexist within society. Social action approaches are often used in gender research to explore the meanings which women themselves attach to their experiences of oppression, racism and social disadvantage (Jones, 1994).

Social Structure

Theories of social structure emphasize the way in which society shapes and constrains people by means of norms and values which are internalized as they grow up, and which direct and determine their behaviour. Both Durkheim (1858–1917) and Marx (1818–83) can be considered as structural sociologists. It is human social behaviour (responses to pre-set rules) that is stressed rather than action, which would suggest a greater freedom to choose what we do. People's social behaviour may be seen as the result of the types of social organization, processes and structures that exist in the society in which they live. Structural sociologists, although obviously they are not arguing that people's behaviour is totally determined, put much more emphasis on how people have their choices circumscribed by the norms and values of their social world.

In research on gender, for example, the concept of patriarchy (the domination by older men of women, children and younger men) has been used to focus attention on the wide range of oppressive and exploitative relations that exist in sexual divisions, parenting, economic power, civil rights and work (Walby, 1990). Although the character of patriarchy has changed, many feminist sociologists argue that women are still discriminated against in employment and through the state. Women often carry a double burden of paid and household labour, and media images of women tend to perpetuate stereotype ideas about female sexuality and women's work.

Structure and Agency

In practice, sociologists draw on structural and social action theories to make sense of the social world. Wright Mills (1970) commented that the essence of the sociological enterprise is the attempt to interpret the complex inter-relationship between social structures and human actions. 'The sociological imagination enables us to grasp history and biography and the relations between the two within society' (Wright Mills, 1970). In other words, the dilemmas and uncertainties of human action as well as the regularities of social structure must be kept in the frame. More recently, Giddens (1979) has attempted to reconcile these tensions by suggesting that neither human agents nor social institutions should be regarded as having primacy, but that each is influenced by the gradual and almost imperceptible shifts in the other. 'Each is constituted in and through recurrent practices. The notion

of human "action" presupposes that of "institution", and vice versa' (Giddens, 1982).

In relation to gender, it could be argued that 'woman' and 'man' are not fixed categories, but are socially constructed by both structural changes and social action. What we know and see as being female or male is constantly being reinterpreted because we ourselves are the subjects that occupy particular but changing positions (Stacey, 1993) and generate new social meanings. Ideas about fatherhood and motherhood, conception, birth and child-rearing have changed over time and across cultures (Moore, 1988; Stainton Rogers, 1993).

Quantitative and Qualitative Enquiry

Alongside these different approaches there are different emphases in sociological research. Quantitative research, associated with structural sociology, explores the patterned regularities that arise from shared social relationships and common experiences. In this view, the character of sociology is that of a science, analogous to natural science but with the social life of human beings as its object of study rather than, say, the human body or the nature of the universe. Both natural scientists and social scientists observe material phenomena; they develop hypotheses and collect data to test their soundness. In a similar way to natural scientists, it is suggested, sociologists can stand outside society and investigate it objectively.

Qualitative research is concerned to understand how people themselves see and interpret the social world; it is more descriptive and intuitive, relying on interviewing and observing people engaged in social action. The idea is to observe and carefully record the quality of human experience – people's ideas, thoughts and feelings – rather than imposing the researcher's own categories of meaning. Interpretative researchers reject a scientific model of sociology, or at least its abstract and quantitative treatment of human experience (Jones, 1994).

Summary

In this section, concepts of particular relevance to students of midwifery have been identified: gender, family, social class and race. Some different approaches to sociological enquiry which reflect distinctive preoccupations within sociology have also been sketched.

However, it has also been noted that distinctions between social action and structural approaches are not hard and fast, and that each offers important insights to illuminate the social world in which we live.

PSYCHOLOGICAL PERSPECTIVES AND MIDWIFERY

Psychology is a discipline which can appear complex to the uninitiated. Psychology textbooks tend to present a detailed introduction of the major theories and concepts that relate to the study of psychology from the perspective of a future psychology graduate. Student midwives and midwives themselves often have difficulty in seeing the relevance of some of the topics normally introduced in these texts. In this chapter an attempt is made to extrapolate some of the material relevant to midwifery practice, to the study of human behaviour in relation to female development and to a woman's potential role as a mother. Remember that each topic area is the focus of major psychological study, so the material presented here is a very basic introduction only.

What is Psychology?

Psychology is a major discipline, and is approached from a variety of perspectives. Fundamentally, it is about studying and understanding people, what they think and what they feel, and consequently how they behave. Psychology is therefore about understanding what goes on in a person's mind, and how that influences what the person does. The 'mind' may be considered as an abstract concept – there is no specific area of the brain that can be identified as the mind. However, the mind is usually perceived as the centre for human thought and emotion. Psychologists are interested in each individual, in contrast to sociologists, who study people within their society. However, as people exist and interact in a social context, both disciplines examine and explain similar concepts, and are often classified as the 'social' or 'behavioural' sciences.

Psychology is commonly perceived as the study and understanding of human emotion; it would, for example, be important for midwives to be aware of the emotional outcome of pregnancy and childbirth for women. Emotion, then, is about how a person feels; it encompass feelings such as happiness, plea-

sure, anxiety, fear, sadness and anger. Psychology is sometimes used synonymously with emotion, as aspects of experience and human thinking are encompassed. Emotion can also be influenced by individual components, such as personality and social context. However, referring purely to 'emotions' somewhat oversimplifies the many aspects of human behaviour and experience. Psychologists, consequently, are also interested in what makes a person behave in a particular way, i.e. what motivates that person. They also study processes within the mind, such as memory, attention, perception – the mental processes or cognition (cognitive psychology). Cognitive processes are those parts of the mind which enable humans to use imagination, make judgements and exercise reason. To summarize, psychology is a major discipline involved in the study of individual thought, feeling and behaviour, as well as of individual experience.

Psychology and Midwifery

Pregnancy and childbirth is a time of life which involves tremendous emotional readjustment. Midwifery care, generally, adopts an holistic approach, and frameworks for practice acknowledge the physical, social, educational, spiritual and, of course, the psychological needs of the mother and her infant. Midwives are currently involved in the implementation of woman-centred care. *Changing Childbirth* (Department of Health, 1993) presents many challenges, not least of all that of enabling women to have choice and control throughout their pregnancy and birth. Midwives therefore need to be aware of how women make choices, what factors influence decision making and what influences a woman's ability to be in control of a given situation. *Changing Childbirth*, by definition, has also involved midwives in change; changes in practice, changes in working environments and changes in beliefs and attitudes. A knowledge and understanding of psychology can therefore help not only to develop methods of managing change, but also to provide some insight into how people make decisions and choices relating to change, how change can be best managed and ways in which attitudes are formed. Psychology also provides the theoretical basis of many practical elements, such as the skills involved in counselling, or of approaches to education and strategies for managing people. Finally, psychology examines the changes that occur for a person at varying stages of childhood and adult life, identifying the factors that contribute towards development of personality, etc. In this section, however, a small area of psychology is concentrated upon and some of the differing explanations relating to female development and aspects of psychology associated with female identity and mothering are presented.

For most people, the first and closest relationship is with their mother. It is from that mother–infant relationship that children, particularly girls, begin to learn about being female and about 'loving' behaviour. Some psychologists concentrate on this area, examining the mothering role and the influence that mothering behaviour has on future emotional development. Chodorow (1978), for example, presents a view of a mother not only as the person who gives birth, but also as the person who in our society socializes and nurtures her child, and so is considered the primary parent. As fathers become more immediately involved in childrearing this view is being increasingly questioned; however, it is still usually the mother who is most closely involved in nurturing during the early weeks of life. The midwife must recognize the importance of understanding individual development in the neonatal period as she has a role in advising the new mother about aspects of normal infant behaviour. Perhaps one aspect of child development which has not typically been addressed in great detail within midwifery practice is the area of informing and advising parents about psychological (or emotional) development. In preparing women and their partners for their parental role, most midwives introduce aspects of care in pregnancy, advice about labour and some information about the immediate postnatal period, such as feeding or batheing the infant. The reality of becoming a parent is therefore seldom addressed. There is current evidence that parents need much more help, guidance and emotional support in adjusting to their new role in the postnatal period (Combes and Schonveld, 1992).

Gender Differences

The study of individual differences raises a fundamental issue – the debate as to whether women are psychologically different from men. The debate focuses on common perceptions of what characterizes masculinity or femininity, how such qualities are obtained and whether psychological differences between the sexes really exist. The topic often raises emotive discussion.

To understand the issues that relate to gender, it is helpful to introduce some terms associated with specific concepts of gender. *Sex* is a term that refers to a person's biological status, consisting of the physical features which distinguish males from females; i.e. genetic structure (sex chromosomes), sex hormones, the internal sex organs and external genitalia. *Gender identity* refers to how individuals see themselves – an awareness of themselves as male or female. Gender identity develops gradually, so most people do not remember when they were first aware of being male or female. *Gender (or sex) role* refers to how people behave in relation to their sex. A male gender role is to be masculine, i.e. to have a masculine attitude and to behave in a masculine way within society. A female gender role, therefore, is to behave in a feminine manner, conforming to beliefs about feminine behaviour. Some writers further distinguish between sex roles and *sex-role stereotypes*; sex roles being the behaviour patterns, whereas sex-role stereotypes are the beliefs that people hold about these patterns (Hargreaves, 1987).

Nature or Nurture?

From the moment of conception, females and males are different. The human genotype is made up of 23 pairs of chromosomes, one chromosome from every pair being inherited from each parent. It is the twenty-third pair of chromosomes that determine whether the individual will be a boy or a girl from the exact moment at which sperm and ovum unite. Females carry an XX pair of sex chromosomes and males an XY pair of chromosomes (*see* Chapter 3). There are some who would believe that aspects of every person's psychological makeup, such as their personality, level of intelligence and sex-role behaviour is determined by their genetic structure. The debate as to whether certain aspects of human behaviour are determined by genotype or are socially learned is usually termed the 'nature–nurture' debate. There are authors who currently argue that evolutionary factors and the process of natural selection predetermine how females and males ultimately behave. The question must be raised as to whether this biological factor predetermines each person's gender identity. Dawkins (1989) describes one of the fundamental differences 'which can be used to label males and females'; that is the sex cells (gametes) of males are much smaller and more numerous than the sex cells of females. This means that the male has the ability to produce a very much larger number of offspring than the female. As Dawkins rather wryly states 'female exploitation begins here!'

21

Women and Men

There can be no debate more likely to promote intense reaction than the question as to whether the male and female minds are different. A common-sense response would often be: 'of course, women are more sensitive than men, and men are more aggressive.' And yet, it could be argued that as women have become more emancipated, so too have they become more aggressive, and with the advent of the 'new man' men are now free to demonstrate their sensitivity. Psychologists therefore ask 'what aspects of male and female behaviour are biologically determined and what are socially learned?' Many studies have examined this very question. There is a suggestion that, as males are more susceptible to certain illnesses and genetically linked conditions they are biologically the weaker sex (Gross, 1992). Statistically males are more likely to be aborted, to be stillborn or suffer birth injury. Men are also more vulnerable to certain inherited disorders such as haemophilia. In addition, women are more likely to live longer than men; statistics have consistently shown that more women than men survive between the ages of 55 and 74 years (OPCS, 1994). However, the actual debate about male and female differences tends to focus on the differences in male and female behaviour, the way boys and girls are brought up and the potential for disadvantage related to gender.

There is no doubt that, despite the appearance of the 'new man', the task of caring for babies falls to women. The concept of maternal instinct presupposes that, based on some inherent drive, all women want to, and *should* want to, have children. However, the 'new woman' is increasingly achieving personal fulfilment through her career, so more women are choosing either to have their children later or, as is becoming increasingly common, to have no children at all. Society consequently imposes a form of 'emotional blackmail' and subsequent feelings of guilt on those women who choose not to have babies, or who have babies and also seek personal gain by continuing their careers. There are inevitably some women who are in a state of emotional insecurity, sometimes resulting in psychological illhealth, as the common perception that all women must naturally want to reproduce and raise families is perpetuated.

It has been shown that certain groups of women are more likely to return to work after the birth of a baby, particularly those who have their first baby over the age of 35 years (Robinson *et al*. 1988). One group showed a satisfactory level of adjustment to pregnancy and motherhood, and also demonstrated greater satisfaction with the mothering role (Ragozin *et al*. 1982). Women who have their first baby later may, however, also be susceptible to certain emotional difficulties. Berryman (1993) examined the level of maternal–fetal attachment in women over 35 years of age who were expecting a baby. Women in this age group are usually aware that there is an increased risk of their baby having certain genetically linked disorders, such as Downs syndrome. Berryman demonstrated some contradictory findings, in that there was a tendency for increased age to be associated with lower levels of fetal attachment for women who were expecting their first baby. There are, of course, many factors that influence anxiety levels for such women with respect to screening tests in pregnancy, but the implications of a positive result are especially important. Other factors may include the type of information given about the tests and how that information is conveyed. Berryman's findings do, however, raise the issue that certain factors relating to specific aspects of maternity care may potentially influence some mothers' relationships with their infants even before the birth.

Working Mothers

There are many women who choose to combine a career with having children. It is only in recent years that women have been provided with any form of encouragement or security for returning to work after the birth of a baby. Modern demands often necessitate that women return to work after having a baby – many families would not be able to cope financially without the extra income. Mothers therefore often feel tremendous guilt when returning to work, burdened with a common perception that they will cause the baby some sort of long-term emotional damage. There has rarely been any suggestion that a father's absence during normal working hours is likely to create problems. However, there seems to be a long-held view that a mother's absence is detrimental.

There is also a common misconception, based on the work of John Bowlby, that a child's mother is the only suitable person to provide care during its pre-school years. In fact, Bowlby and others involved in the development of attachment theory and the effects of maternal deprivation focused on the potential for emotional disturbance in a child who was in long-term institutionalized care. There has been little suggestion that a child in an emotionally secure mother–infant relationship is likely to be emotionally damaged by the mother returning to work. There is some suggestion however, that a child is more likely to suffer emotionally if the mother is stressed and guilt ridden (Randall, 1992), a factor which can be minimized by adopting a relaxed, planned approach to returning to work.

Approaches to Psychology

Psychological study is approached from a wide variety of perspectives. When exploring the various explanations for gender differences or the mothering role, it is helpful to consider the viewpoints that some of the major theoretical schools adopt. Each perspective is based on certain theoretical concepts or explanations relating to human behaviour and experience.

Everyone loves to be an 'amateur psychologist', examining the way people behave and the differences between individuals. In the first instance, most people adopt a common-sense explanation for the way humans behave; for example, adolescents become delinquents because of the way their parents bring them up, or teenage girls get pregnant because they want a baby to love. Common-sense perceptions, however, are not reliable or valid.

Psychology is traditionally approached objectively, and therefore, like midwifery, is research based. This introduces one of the areas of debate within the discipline of psychology – human experience, human emotion and what goes on in a person's mind are not easily studied quantitatively. There are many psychologists who believe that theories must be produced using objective, scientific evidence, adopting experimental methods of study; whereas others believe it is appropriate to study human behaviour and experience qualitatively, by means of observation and discourse. The psychological perspectives introduced here adopt differing views as to the ways in which theory is developed. However, it is important to recognize that the various approaches add to the knowledge which underpins any attempt to understand and explain the human mind. No single explanation is mutually exclusive; each perspective can help to inform midwifery which in turn can draw on the appropriate aspects to form a truly holistic approach for practice.

Psychodynamic or Psychoanalytical Psychology

Psychodynamics is a term which denotes a specific approach based on the belief that the mind (psyche) is mainly driven or motivated (dynamic) by unconscious forces. Psychodynamic theory originated with the work of Sigmund Freud. Freud's theory is therefore based on a belief that human behaviour is guided by the unconscious mind, and that nothing we do occurs purely by accident, i.e. psychological determinism.

Psychoanalysis is associated with Freud's original theory of the mind and also the form of therapy that developed, based on analysis of thoughts, dreams, mishaps and mistakes, and the interpretation of what occurs within the therapeutic relationship, focusing on unconscious interactions known as transference and counter-transference. Freud placed great emphasis on the stages of childhood development: humans like many other species are sexual beings from infancy. Central to psychoanalytic theory is that development of personality is based on sexuality; the human infant is born with innate sexual drives, such drives are as instinctual as feeding or sleeping.

Freud's theory has inevitably had a profound effect on psychology to this day, and never fails to raise intense debate. It can certainly be described as one of the most influential theories relating to the unconscious mind and emotional development of human beings. The debates has resulted in Freud's theory intruding into everyday language, with words such as ego, regression, denial or libido now part of most people's vocabulary.

Freud's model of the human mind comprises what is termed the 'psychic apparatus', i.e. the id, the ego and the superego (as when thinking about the 'mind' it is necessary to think of these 'components' as abstract, they are not anatomical features). Freud termed the unconscious part of the mind, which governs biological drives, the id. The id is therefore the part of the human psyche described as pleasure seeking. The ego is the part of the mind that directs reality, it is the rational, decision-making component. The superego represents what each person internalizes from the world around them. It can be seen as the conscience, it includes internalization of moral values and is generated by a person's culture initially given by their parents. Repression, denial, regression and projection are some of the unconscious 'defences' (defence mechanisms) that the ego uses to block the instinctual demands of the id.

Freud's theory relating to the development of sex roles focuses on psychosexual stages, and centres on the concept of what is known as the 'Oedipus complex'. It is based on a belief that a boy's intense love and unconscious desire for his mother (in Greek mythology Oedipus kills his father and marries his mother) results in the father being seen as a rival, so the boy develops what Freud termed a 'castration anxiety'. The boy eventually represses his desire for his mother and identifies with the father, taking on his male characteristics. Freud proposed that castration anxiety has a female equivalent whereby the girl has a belief that she has already been castrated, following her discovery of anatomical differences, and then develops a particular fascination for her father; Freud called this 'penis envy'. This female equivalent of the Oedipus complex has been termed the Electra complex. Freud's theory of the development of sex role in girls has consequently been the focus of much debate over the years, particularly among feminists.

There are some who suggest that Freud made a crucial error in not acknowledging what some of his female patients told him in therapy (Masson, 1990). Freud in his therapeutic practice treated women and girls who recounted histories of sexual abuse and incest, a fact which Freud then interpreted as 'hysteria'. The debate impinges on whether Freud, living in a virtuous, middle-class society, deliberately chose not to recognize the stories these women gave, or whether his own unconscious mind denied the possibility of something so terrible actually occurring. Freud's psychoanalytical theory has been developed and elaborated by psychologists such as Eric Erickson, Carl Jung and Alfred Adler. Carl Jung proposed that people have a 'collective unconscious' within which there are elements of both the feminine and masculine. The unconscious mind of a man therefore contains a complementary feminine element and a woman's unconscious mind contains a masculine element, what Jung called the 'anima' and 'animus'.

Object Relations Theory

The object in object relations theory is a 'human object' and therefore the theory reflects the significance of human relations with others. Object relations theory is founded in psychoanalysis, but it is based on a belief that human relationships arise from collusion, rather than from conflict as was Freud's belief. Melanie Klein, a psychoanalyst and a contemporary of Freud, developed her theory based on observations of the relationship between mothers and their babies. Fundamental to Klein's work was a belief that

development is inextricably linked to the infant's first relationship, the relationship with the mother. Donald Winnicott proposed that a child's initial relationship with the mother is symbiotic, i.e. that the newborn baby cannot exist on its own and that the baby is part of the 'nursing couple'. Many object relations theorists, however, acknowledge that the role of primary caretaker could be adopted by someone other than the infant's own mother. Object relations theory is detailed, complex and based in psychoanalytic work relating to the unconscious mind; and yet it should be meaningful to midwives.

Attachment Theory

The importance of not separating babies from their mothers is now an integral part of midwifery practice. However, this was not always the case, and there are some countries where even now babies are cared for by maternity nurses in a nursery. The significance of maintaining maternal links throughout childhood, even when the infant is placed in long-term care, is now acknowledged. John Bowlby, who first linked evolutionary principles of instinctual behaviour with psychoanalytical theory, undertook one of the first major investigations into the concept known as attachment theory. Bowlby believed that an attachment 'bond' must be successfully made between babies and their mothers in order to form the basis for healthy emotional development. Attachment theory has been interpreted in varying degrees of rigidity over the ensuing years. A belief that an infant must remain with its mother at all costs has been one area of criticism. Attachment theory was developed from observation of the natural behaviour of mother–infant interactions, demonstrating what is known as 'attachment behaviour'.

Although Bowlby believed that the mother is normally the attachment figure, he too acknowledged that in certain circumstances another person could fulfil that role. Attachment theorists believe that infants are genetically biased towards interaction with the people closest to them, from the moment of birth. Ainsworth *et al.* (1991) described how a child is preadapted to a social world, and examined how behaviour such as crying can elicit certain maternal responses. Ainsworth *et al.* (1978) first described certain types of attachment which are acquired in the early months of life, but can influence relationships and interaction later in life. Adams and Cotgrove (1995) identify the importance of understanding attachment theory and relate it to the role that professionals have in supporting and advising new parents.

Behaviourism

Some psychologists believe that theory can only be developed by a means of systematic, scientific study involving direct, experimentally based observation of behaviour. Behavioural theory attempts to identify laws (rather like physical laws) that demonstrate how behaviour is learned, thereby providing evidence founded on valid, reliable data. Behaviourists proposed that humans *learn* how to behave, through a process of conditioning. The original theory was developed from the work of a Russian physiologist, Ivan Pavlov (1849–1936), who demonstrated that animals can be conditioned to respond to certain stimuli, a process which has come to be known as classical conditioning. Burrhus F Skinner (1904–90) developed the concept of operant or instrumental conditioning, which demonstrates how behaviour can be modified through rewards and punishments. Behaviourists propose that children therefore learn by a process of positive or negative reinforcement. Many of these experiments were conducted with animals; the main area of interest was in behaviour which could be demonstrated and explained by direct observation.

It can be argued that traditional patterns of maternity care and parent education were often based on the behavioural approach to psychology. A generation of mothers were brought up to believe that good mothering was dependent on a rigid routine. Through a process of conditioning, babies could be 'trained' to feed every 4 hours; baby bath time, bedtime and playtime should be part of a regular daily routine; the 'reward' being a healthy, 'bouncing' baby. The 'bad mother' was therefore perceived as the mother who did not have a routine, who fed her baby 'on demand', who played with her baby rather than sticking to routines or (heaven forbid) who missed a bath time! Such views may seem laughable now, as modern childrearing takes a more relaxed approach, seeing the quality of the baby's relationship with its caregivers as most important for its emotional security. However, there is a generation of parents who may well argue that such routines provide children with some important 'boundaries' that also give security.

Social Learning Theory

A major psychological approach based on the principles of behaviourism is known as social learning theory, one of its first proponents being Albert Bandura (1977). Social learning theory, however, links the principles of learned behaviour through conditioning and reinforcement with cognitive processes. Bandura demonstrated that a child can learn certain forms of behaviour such as aggression through positive reinforcement. Bandura's studies demonstrated how children learned aggressive behaviour by modelling on aggression observed in adults.

Social learning theory therefore emphasizes that humans learn behaviour through observation of others on whom they model behaviour, and also the significance of reinforcement of behaviour. One of the most controversial areas in which social learning may play a significant part is the effect of the media on sex-role stereotyping. Films which portray aggressive, 'macho' behaviour are targeted by the general population as being one of the major influences on aggressive behaviour in young boys. There is a suggestion that boys model themselves on what they perceive as the ideal masculine stereotype. It can be argued, however, that even children are capable of rational thought and are able to identify appropriate, socially acceptable behaviour on which to model themselves, thus fitting into the everyday world around them.

Perhaps the most significant aspect of sex-role stereotyping relates to the images in the media surrounding pregnancy and motherhood. The idealized view of pregnancy in many women's magazines, portraying images of glamorous young women and glowing babies, would appear to contradict many women's experience of the realities of motherhood. There are some who now vociferously question media views which continue to represent a paradoxical image of the naked female breast as a sex object, openly displayed in magazines and films, and yet will not encourage the natural image of a breastfeeding mother.

Humanistic Psychology

Humanistic psychology focuses on development of the person at all stages of life; it acknowledges that humans are capable of conscious awareness, that they have personal agency (the ability to make choices) and that each person is a whole being. Humanistic psychology is often described as an orientation towards psychology rather than a theory. Its focus is on the subjective experience of the individual. Carl Rogers was one of the major proponents of humanistic psychology. Central to what Rogers eventually termed the person-centred approach to psychology were three elements which he described as 'genuineness, unconditional positive regard and empathic understanding'. Rogers (1980, p. 115) believed that 'individuals have within themselves vast resources for self understanding and for altering their self concepts, basic attitudes and self-directed behaviour; these resources can be tapped if a definable climate of facilitative psychological attitudes can be provided'.

Personal agency and an increased self-awareness leading to a process of personal growth underpin humanistic psychology. It can be argued that these are the principles which also underpin *Changing Childbirth* (Department of Health, 1993). Humanistic psychology popularized the principle of an 'holistic approach' to the person. The links between humanistic psychology and the philosophy of midwifery practice should therefore be apparent. Humanistic psychologists are more concerned with the conscious processes of the mind. Another well-known humanistic psychologist, with whom many are familiar, is Abraham Maslow. Maslow proposed that human motivation is based on a hierarchy of need, and his theory has become well known as a theory which explains human motivation. Again, it is possible to recognize the principles of many human needs based midwifery models of care. Maslow's theory suggests that people can only reach the level at which they have a need for self-actualization if their basic needs are first met, i.e. the need for physiological survival, safety, intimacy and self-respect.

These three major theoretical perspectives form the basis of many practical applications of psychology, e.g. counselling and education. Humans generally respond to unconscious processes, i.e. people aren't always consciously aware of why they do things (psychoanalysis); they learn to behave the way they do (behaviourism); and they are able to grow and develop, through a sense of self-awareness (humanism).

There are many areas of psychology which acknowledge aspects of any or all of the major theoretical schools. These include developmental psychology and feminist psychology, both of which encompass issues of value to midwifery knowledge and practice.

Developmental Psychology

Life can be seen as a series of stages, each of which influence psychological development and ultimately may influence a person's long term emotional well-being. Birth, childhood, adolescence, adulthood and old age represent some of the stages which characterize human growth and development. The question that developmental psychology poses is whether psychological growth occurs continuously throughout life or whether it occurs in stages, particularly in childhood. Developmental psychology has been described as an 'understanding of age-related changes in experience and behaviour ... to provide an account of development throughout the life span' (Butterworth and Harris, 1994, p. 3). Forming relationships, marriage, planning to have a family, childbirth and parenthood are events that take place at some of these stages of development. The stage of life at which these events occur may potentially have an impact on emotional adjustment to the event.

Adolescence, for example, is described as a time at which the person is seeking his or her own identity. To develop a healthy sense of self concept and role identity, adolescents seek independence from their parents. Erik Erikson, a psychoanalyst influenced by Freudian theory, presented what is known as a lifespan theory of human development. Unlike Freud's emphasis on psychosexual stages in childhood, Erikson (1968) focused on a series of psychosocial stages of human development which continue into adult life, identifying stages or life 'crises'. The adolescent may transcend the crisis favourably or unfavourably. Psychological well-being is therefore determined by the individual's success in dealing with the crisis. (It is important to remember that psychoanalytical psychology is focused on what happens in the unconscious mind.) Female adolescents who become pregnant may therefore be in increased emotional turmoil, apparently struggling with the dual transition of adolescence and young adulthood, together with the conscious realities of parenthood. There are some psychologists, on the other hand, who dispute that these stages are times of crisis and have found little evidence of such emotional turmoil in adolescence. Dusek and Flaherty (1981) reported that for most adolescents change occurs gradually and with little emotional difficulty.

Feminist Psychology

Feminist psychology has been generated in response to the male-dominated traditions of psychology. Oakley (1980, p. 264), while exploring whether a psychology of women actually exists, stated that 'through their intense attunement to the needs of others, women are likely to suffer from feelings of weakness, vulnerability and helplessness in far greater measures than men. These qualities are labelled disabilities by the male dominated culture (of men and the male-led psychoanalytic and psychiatric professions) and indeed they feel like disabilities to women who have internalized the dominant values.' In fact, Nicolson (1992, p. 24) questions that it is the motherhood role which is 'the key to women's oppression'. Motherhood is seen as central to all women's lives whether or not they become or want to become mothers themselves. Nicolson, in discussing women's health and health care, proposes that any normal female psychological experience is one of subordination and corresponds to what is perceived as 'socially desirable femininity' (Nicolson, 1992, p.6).

Ussher (1989), writing on the psychology of the female body, focuses on less obvious biological factors which differentiate males from females. She reflects on traditional views that women were often perceived as less intelligent then men, and even that female sanity (or insanity) was believed to be rooted in the female reproductive organs. Women who were independent and assertive were frequently labelled as 'hysterical'. Nineteenth century treatments for such 'conditions' included solitary confinement, rectal injections, ice and water in the vagina, leeching of the vulva and in some cases clitoridectomy. As Ussher (1989) suggests, modern diseases which relate to hysteria include premenstrual syndrome, postnatal depression and menopausal deficiency syndrome, and modern treatments that involve chemotherapy and hysterectomy would therefore appear to present a modern dilemma.

Women are therefore defined by their biology in contemporary times, and are 'socialized into looking at their body and sexuality for identity and self-definition' (Ussher, 1989, p. 10). Pregnancy, childbirth and motherhood are seen as intrinsic to women's experience, which has contributed towards the depersonalization of many women, particularly through the medicalization of childbirth. Like many feminist psychologists, Ussher challenges the prevalent ideologies surrounding reproductive issues. As she concludes, feminist psychology can contribute to a knowledge of women themselves, the female body and issues relating to women's reproductive and mothering abilities (Ussher, 1989, p. 142). Similarly, such a body of knowledge would inform midwifery practice. Psychology, from all approaches, is therefore of major significance to everyone studying midwifery and midwifery related topics.

Summary

People develop their gender identity through a process of internalization from others around them. Psychoanalytical psychology explores the unconscious processes of the mind. It emphasizes the influence of the person who is closest throughout childhood, i.e. the prime carer, usually the child's mother. Behavioural psychology examines the way people learn their behaviour from the environment, through a process of socialization. Humanistic psychology focuses on the importance of self and each person's ability to change throughout life through a process of personal growth. An awareness of the differing stances helps to appreciate the perspective from which various authors approach the topic in hand. Midwifery can adopt an approach which encompasses all the relevant areas of psychology to provide a unique and appropriate form of knowledge and practice for all, what Egan (1986) termed systematic eclecticism.

KEY CONCEPTS

- The transition from childhood to adulthood encompasses profound changes in the physical appearance and physiological characteristics of the body. This biological transformation is known as puberty.

- Complex interrelated events culminate in a physically mature individual capable of reproduction. It is essential for the midwife to know and understand these physiological changes

- Psychology is a major discipline which is viewed from many perspectives and therefore has developed differing theoretical bases:

- Feminine development can be viewed from any of these perspectives.

- Debates surrounding motherhood are an important aspect of psychology as this is often seen as the foundation of human emotional development.

- An understanding of psychology will help the midwife in many situations, including communication, counselling, human social interaction, implementation of change, education programmes, etc.

- Sociology is a systematic study of society, investigating patterned regularities and structural influences such as class, race, gender and the family.

- Sociologists investigate how people act in society, exploring socialization and social relationships in order to understand their intended and unintended consequences.

- Social action theory and structural theory represent distinctive approaches to sociological enquiry and each offer explanations of 'how society works'.

References

Adams L, Cotgrove A: Promoting secure attachment patterns in infancy and beyond, *Prof Care Mother Child* 5(6):158, 1995.

Ainsworth MDS, Blehar M, Waters E, Wall S: *Patterns of attachment*, Hillsdale NJ, 1978, Erlbaum.

Ainsworth MDS, Bell SM, Stayton DJ: Infant–mother attachment and social development: socialisation as a product of reciprocal responsiveness to signals. In Woodhead, Carr, Light, editors: *Becoming a person*, Buckingham, 1991, Routledge/Open University.

Albanese A, Stanhope R: Investigation of delayed puberty. *Clin Endocrinol* 43(1):105, 1995.

Bandura A: *Social learning theory*, Englewood Cliffs, NJ, 1977, Prentice-Hall.

Barrow J: West Indian families: an insider's perspective. In Rapoport RN, Fogarty MP, Rapoport R, editors: *Families in Britain*, London, 1982, RKP.

Berger P: *Invitation to sociology*, Harmondsworth, 1966, Penguin.

Berryman J: Pregnancy after 35: a preliminary report on maternal–fetal attachment, *J Reprod Infant Psychol*, 11:169, 1993.

Bowlby J: *A secure base: clinical applications of attachment theory*, London, 1988, Tavistock Routledge.

Bryan G, Dadzie S, Scafe S: *The heart of the race: black women's lives in Britain*, London, 1985, Virago.

Buckler J: Normal development in teenage girls. In *The adolescent years*, Ware, 1987, Castlemead Publications.

Butterworth G, Harris M: *Principles of developmental psychology*, 1994, Laurence Erlbaum Associates.

Chodorow N: *The reproduction of mothering: psychoanalysis and the sociology of gender*, London, 1978, University of California Press.

Combes G, Schonveld A: *Life will never be the same again: learning to be a first time parent*, London, 1992, Health Education Authority.

Dalley G: *Ideologies of caring: rethinking community and collectivism*, London, 1988, Macmillan.

Dawkins R: *The selfish gene*, Oxford, 1989, Oxford University Press.

Department of Health: *Changing childbirth, Part 1. Report of the Expert Maternity Group*, London, 1993, HMSO.

Department of Health: *Variations in health: what can the Department of Health and the NHS do?* London, 1995, Department of Health.

Department of Social Services: *Bulletin on Child Support Agency*, London, 1990, DSS.

Doyal L: *The political economy of health*, London, 1979, Pluto Press.

Duvek JB, Flaherty JF: The development of self concept during the adolescent years, *Monogr Soc Res Child Dev* 46:191, 1981.

Edmonds DK: *Dewhurst's practical and adolescent gynaecology*, 2nd Edn, London, 1989, Butterworths.

Egan G: The skilled helper, 1986, Brookes Cole.

Erikson E: *Identity: youth and crisis*, New York, 1968, Norton.

Falkener F, Tanner JM, editors: *Human growth: Volume 2. Postnatal growth*, New York, 1978, Plenum.

Faust MS: Alternative constructions of adolescence and growth. In Brooks-Gunn J, Petersen AC, editors: *Girls at puberty: biological, psychological and social perspectives*, New York, 1983, Plenum.

Faust, MS: Somatic development of adolescent girls, *Monogr Soc Res Child Dev* 42(1):1, 1977.

Fitzgerald T: The New Right and the family. In Loney M, Boswell D, Clarke J, editors: *Social policy and social welfare*, Buckingham, 1985, Open University Press.

Fraser AM, Brockert JE, Ward RH: Association of young maternal age with adverse reproductive outcomes, *New Engl J Med* 332(17):1113, 1995.

Giddens A: *Central problems in social theory: action, structure and contradiction in social analysis*, London, 1979, Macmillan.

Giddens A: *Profiles and critiques in social theory*, London, 1982, Macmillan.

Ginsburg H, Miller S: Sex differences in children's risk-taking behaviour, *Child Dev* 53:426, 1982.

Gittins D: *The family in question*, London, 1985, Macmillan.

Graham H, McKee L: *The first months of motherhood*, London, 1980, Health Education Council.

Graham H: *Hardship and health in women's lives*, Chichester, 1993, Wheatsheaf.

HMSO: *Social trends 24*, London, 1994, HMSO.

Gross RD: *Psychology: the science of mind and behaviour*, 2nd Edn, London, 1992, Hodder and Stoughton.

Ham AW, Leeson TS: *Histology*, Philadelphia, 1968, LB Lippincott.

Hargreaves DJ: Psychological theories of sex-role stereotyping. In Hargreaves DJ, Colley AM, editors: *The psychology of sex roles*, London, 1987, Harper and Row.

Holm K, Laursen EM, Brocks V, Muller J: Pubertal maturation of the internal genitalia: an ultrasound evaluation of 166 healthy girls, *Ultrasound Obstet Gynecol* 6(3):175, 1995.

Jackson S: *Family lives: a feminist sociology*, Oxford, 1993, Blackwell.

Jacobs M: *D.W. Winnicott*, London, 1995, Sage Publications.

Jones LJ: *The social context of health and health work*, London, 1994, Macmillan.

Jowell R: *British social attitudes*, Aldershot, 1986, Gower.

Katchadourian, H. *The biology of adolescence*, San Francisco, 1977, WH Freeman & Company.

Marshall WA: Growth and secondary sexual development and related disorders, *Clin Obstet Gynecol* 1(3):593, 1974.

Matsumoto S, Ishizuka J, Takenaka Y. Basal body temperature findings in girls aged 18 to 19 years, *Jpn J Adolesc Med* 4:7, 1981.

Masson JM: *Against therapy*, 1990, Fontana.

Mead GH: *Mind, self and society*, Chicago, 1934, University of Chicago Press.

Miles A: *Women, health and medicine*, Buckingham, 1991, Open University Press.

Miller HS, Lesser KB, Reed KL: Adolescence and very low birth weight infants: a disproportionate association, *Obstet Gynaecol* 87(1):83, 1996.

Moore H: *Feminism and anthropology*, Cambridge, 1988, Polity Press.

National Association of Health Authorities (NAHA, now NAHAT): *Action, not words*, Birmingham, 1988, NAHA.

Nicolson P: Towards a psychology of women's health and health care. In Nicolson P, Ussher J, editors: *The psychology of women's health and health care*, Basingstoke and London, 1992, The Macmillan Press.

Oakley A: *Women confined: towards a sociology of childbirth*, Oxford, 1980, Martin Robertson.

Oakley A: *Sex, gender and society*, London, 1985, Temple Smith.

OPCS: *Central Statistics Office: Annual abstract of statistics*, London, 1994, HMSO.

Parmar P: Gender, race and power: the challenge to youth work practice. In Cohen P, Baines HS, editors: *Multi-racist Britain*, London, 1988, Macmillan.

Parsons T: *The social system*, London, 1964, RKP.

Popay J: My health is all right, but I'm just tired all the time: Women's experience of ill health. In Roberts H, editor: *Women's health matters*, London, 1992, Routledge.

Randall P: Working mothers and the anxiety of separation, *Prof Care Mother Child* Vol 2 June:168–71, 1992.

Ragozin A, Basham R, Crnic K, Greenberg M, Robinson N: Effects of maternal age on parenting role, *Dev Psychol* 18:627, 1982.

Robinson G, Erlick OM, Garner D, Gare D: Transition to parenthood in elderly primiparas, *J Psychosom Obstet Gynaecol* 9(2):89, 1988.

Rogers C: *A way of being*, Boston, 1980, Houghton Mifflin Company.

Smaje C: *Health, race and ethnicity: making sense of the evidence*, London, 1995, Kings Fund.

Stacey J: Untangling feminist theory. In Richardson D, Robinson V, editors: *Introducing women's studies*, London, 1993, Macmillan.

Stainton Rogers R: The social construction of child-rearing. In Beattie A, Gott M, Jones LJ, Sidell M, editors: *Health and wellbeing: a reader*, London, 1993, Macmillan.

Tanner JM, Whitehouse RH, Marshall WA, Carter BS: Equations for the prediction of adult height from height and skeletal maturity at ages 4 to 16, *Arch Dis Child* 50:14, 1975.

Tanner JM: Physical growth. In Mussen PH, editor: *Carmichael's manual of child psychology*, Vol. 2, 3rd Edn, New York, 1970, Wiley.

Tanner JM: *Growth at adolescence*, 2nd Edn, Oxford, 1966, Blackwell Scientific Publications.

Townsend P, Whitehead M, Davidson N: *Inequalities in health: the Black Report and the health divide*, Harmondsworth, 1988, Penguin.

Segal H: *Introduction to the work of Melanie Klein*, London, 1988, Karnac Books and the Institute of Pyschoanalysis.

Ussher JM: *The psychology of the female body*, London and New York, 1989, Routledge.

Vollman RF: *The menstrual cycle*, Vol 7, Philadelphia, 1977, Saunders.

Walby S: *Theorising patriarchy*, Oxford, 1990, Blackwell.

Wilmott P, Young M: *The symmetrical family*, London, 1975, RKP.

Wright Mills C: *The sociological imagination*, Harmondsworth, 1970, Penguin.

Further Reading

Berne RM, Levy MN: *Principles of physiology*, 2nd Edn, St Louis, 1996, Mosby.

Buckler, J. *The adolescent years*, Ware, 1987, Castlemead Publications.

Combes G, Schonveld A: *Life will never be the same again: learning to be a first time parent*, London, 1992, Health Education Authority.

An essential book for all midwives to read. This is a review and survey undertaken for the Health Education Authority into the needs of parents; it includes some important information for anyone with a particular interest in psychological aspects of pregnancy.

DeRidder CM, Thijssen JHH, Bruning PF, *et al.* Body fat mass, body fat distribution and pubertal development: a longitudinal study of physical and hormonal sexual maturation of girls. *J Clin Endocrinol Metab* 75:442, 1992.

Flanagan C: *Applying psychology to early child development*, London, 1996, Hodder and Stoughton.

A very readable book which examines how psychology can be used to understand aspects of child development, from pre-natal through to puberty. A section on cultural influences on child development is particularly pertinent to an understanding of parenting.

Gross RD: *Psychology: the science of mind and behaviour*, 2nd Edn, London, 1992, Hodder and Stoughton.

This is one of the many psychology textbooks available. It does, however, present very clear explanations of some of the more complex theoretical concepts, particularly Freud's psycho-analytic theory.

Hopwood NJ, Kelch RP, Hale PM, *et al.* The onset of human puberty: biological and environmental factors. In Bancroft MD, Reinisch JM, editors: *Adolescence and puberty*, The Kinsey Institute Series, New York, 1990, Oxford University Press.

Jones LJ: *The social context of health and health work*, London, 1994, Macmillan.

This comprehensive textbook covers all aspects of sociology and social policy relating to health work. There are chapters on health policies and caring work as well as on gender, class, age and disability, race, and poverty.

Nicolson P, Ussher J, editors: The psychology of women's health and health care, Basingstoke and London, 1992, The Macmillan Press.

An interesting book which presents a feminist perspective of many aspects of women's health generally and includes chapters on pregnancy and related issues.

Saunders SA, Reinisch JM: Biological and social influences on the endocrinology of puberty: some additional considerations. In Bancroft MD, Reinisch JM, editors: *Adolescence and puberty*, The Kinsey Institute Series, New York, 1990, Oxford University Press.

Styne DM. Physiology of puberty, *Horm Res* 41(suppl 2):3, 1994.

Townsend P, Whitehead M, Davidson N: *Inequalities in health: the Black Report and the health divide*, Harmondsworth, 1988, Penguin.

This summary of research findings is still an important statistical source, providing a thorough explanation of health differences and inequalities. It can be supplemented by Benzeval M, Judge K, Whitehead M, editors: Tackling inequalities in health, an agenda for action, *London, 1995, King's Fund, which also discusses strategies for policy and behavioural change.*

Turner RT, Riggs BL, Spelsberg TC: Skeletal effects of oestrogen. *Endocrinol Rev* 15:275, 1994.

Wright Mills C: *The sociological imagination*, Harmondsworth, 1970, Penguin.

This classic statement of the sociological approach and understanding of the world is a good starting point for understanding the value of sociology in caring work.

2 Sexual Development and Preconception Health

CHAPTER OUTLINE

- Physiological maturity
- Health
- Health promotion
- Preconception

LEARNING OUTCOME

After studying this chapter you should be able to:

- Explain initial development of the reproductive organs.
- Compare the development of the anatomy of the female reproductive system with that of the male, up to and including puberty.
- Discuss the psychological effects of physiological changes during puberty.
- Define health, give examples of health norms and explore the consequences for the individual of deviating from these norms.
- Identify areas of midwifery practice where health promotion is indicated.
- Define and give a rationale for the provision of prepregnancy care.
- Empower women (and their partners) to adopt a healthy lifestyle prior to conception.

Physiological Maturity

When can a person be described as sexually mature? Of course there is no definitive answer, but in the first section of this chapter some of the factors which influence or contribute to sexual maturity are considered. Being physically able to reproduce may be regarded as confirmation of sexual maturity, so a description of the physiological changes that both females and males must undergo before reaching this state is given initially. However, it could be argued that to achieve sexual maturity, the individual must undergo more than just physiological change, so other influences, including psychosocial factors and gender differences, are also briefly considered. This section concludes with some examples of 'rites of passage' to adulthood.

A person's gender is determined at the moment the genetic content of the sperm combines with that of the ovum, although differentiation into the sexes does not become apparent until around the sixth week of gestation. The gonads of both males and females begin to develop from a mass of mesoderm, called the gonadal ridges, during the fifth week of gestation and at this stage the embryo is sexually indifferent. Primordial germ cells then migrate to the gonadal ridges and 'seed' them with stem cells, which will become either spermatogonia or oogonia. Once this has occurred, the primordial ridges differentiate and develop according to the genetic material; the testes of a male begin their development around the seventh week (**Figure 2.1**), the ovaries of a female begin to develop around the eighth week (**Figure 2.2**).

Physiological Maturity in the Female

The physiological development of the female is described in detail in Chapter 1. The following is a summary to underpin the reader's understanding of the concepts of sexual development and of preconception health.

Prenatal

From the eighth week of embryonic life, the female gonads begin to develop. At the same time, the external genitalia begin their development, as shown in **Figures 2.3** and **2.4**; the genital tubercle becomes the clitoris, the urethral folds become the labia minora and the labia majora are formed from the labioscrotal swellings. The urethral groove, which closes under the influence of testosterone in the male, remains open in the female.

Birth to puberty

At the moment of birth, the female has a lifetime supply (approximately 500,000) of primordial follicles in her ovaries, of which approximately 500 will develop as graafian follicles. Changes in the female reproductive organs are minimal until puberty, although there is some endocrine activity – at about 6 years of age a phase known as adrenarche (Bancroft, 1989) occurs, when the level of certain adrenal steroids begins to rise. It is thought that this change in adrenal function may initiate changes that lead to

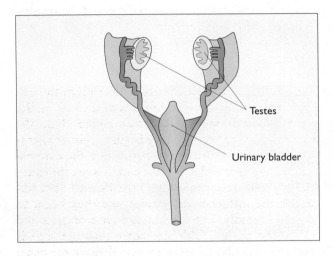

Figure 2.1 The development of the testes in the male embryo at 7 weeks.

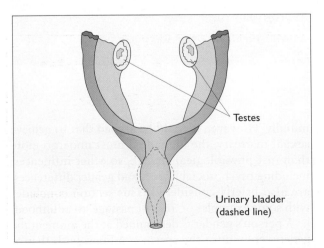

Figure 2.2 The development of the ovaries in the female embryo at 8 weeks.

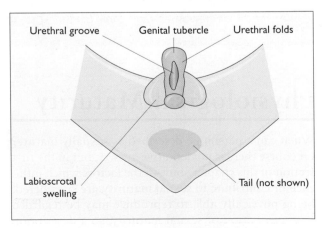

Figure 2.3 External genitalia in the embryo at 5 weeks.

puberty. Also, between 6 and 10 years of age there is a very gradual rise in the levels of follicle-stimulating hormone (FSH) and luteinizing hormone (LH).

Puberty

Puberty is often seen as being synonymous with sexual maturity, as it is during this life stage that the individual acquires the ability to procreate. In the female, the first sign of puberty is an enlargement of the breasts which occurs at a mean age of 10.5 years (Wu, 1988) in response to the oestrogen secreted by the developing follicles in the ovary. Oestrogen also initiates a growth spurt which continues throughout puberty and then stops, by which time the girl reaches her maximum height. A third result of the increase in oestrogen is enlargement of the uterus and proliferation of the endometrium. Other characteristic changes include the development of pubic and axillary hair, which occurs in response to the androgens secreted by the ovaries and adrenal glands, and a rounding of the hips. Less obvious are the changes of the vagina, labia and clitoris, which all develop at this time.

Although all these gradual changes contribute to the girls transition to womanhood, it is the onset of menstruation (menarche) that is often used to determine the age of sexual maturity, even though it is very unlikely (although not impossible) that the girl would be able to conceive at this time. In fact, most girls have irregular, anovulatory cycles for the first 12–18 months following menarche, after which time LH surges occur and the regular (ovulatory) menstrual cycles commence (Wu, 1988). The average age of menarche in the UK is 13 years (Llewellyn-Jones, 1986), which is 2 years earlier than it was a century ago. This may reflect the improved nutritional status of the population, which has resulted in girls reaching a critical level of body fat at a younger age than previously; a suggestion supported by research results which show that secondary amenorrhoea can be successfully treated if the weight loss due to conditions such as anorexia nervosa, bulimia, simple dieting, involuntary starvation and excessive exercise is restored.

Physiological Maturity in the Male

The physiological changes that lead to sexual maturity in the male can be categorized into three stages – prenatal, birth and puberty.

Prenatal

The gonads of the male begin to develop in the seventh week of embryonic life, about a week earlier than the development of the female gonads. Once the testes have been formed, they begin to release testosterone and it is in response to this that the external genitalia are formed. Up to the eighth week the external reproductive organs are undifferentiated, but under the influence of testosterone they begin to develop rapidly. The urethral groove elongates and closes, the urethral folds become the shaft of the penis and the labioscrotal swellings develop, as the name suggests, into the scrotum (**Figures 2.3** and **2.5**).

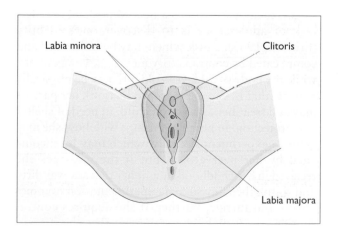

Figure 2.4 External genitalia in the female fetus near term.

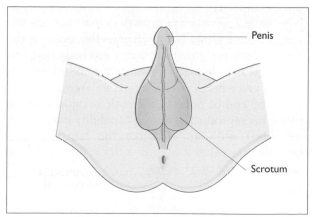

Figure 2.5 External genitalia in the male fetus near term.

Birth to puberty

Descent of the testes has normally occurred by the time a boy is born. The process begins at around the seventh month of gestation, when each testis, accompanied by a peritoneal extension known as the vaginal process, descends into the scrotum through the inguinal canal. From birth to puberty there are only minimal changes, although (as in the female) there is an adrenarche from around the age of 6 years, when the levels of certain adrenal steroids increase.

Puberty

Unlike the female, the male has no dramatic moment such as the menarche to announce the onset of puberty. Development of secondary sex characteristics is initiated by increasing levels of testosterone, which happens at about 12 years of age. Levels of FSH and LH also increase during puberty. The first physical change to occur is accelerated growth of the testes and scrotum, followed by the appearance of pubic hair. About a year later (at an average age of 12.5 years), the penis starts to grow and the internal structures, seminal vesicles and prostate begin to develop. Approximately a year after this the male experiences his first ejaculation, usually at night. These nocturnal emissions (known as 'wet dreams') usually contain infertile semen. It is only after several more months, following further development of the penis, scrotum and testes, that the semen contains mature sperm, this being considered a sign of sexual maturity.

The growth spurt in boys begins approximately 2 years later than the growth spurt in girls, and it has been postulated (Prader, 1984) that this accounts for the 13 cm difference in stature between the sexes (as boys have 2 years extra growth before their growth spurt begins). Other bodily changes that occur at this time include the growth of facial and body hair, and increased muscle mass. Towards the end of puberty a boy's voice breaks as his larynx enlarges.

By the end of puberty, the male is capable of fulfilling his reproductive role, a capability that continues until old age – unlike the female whose reproductive capability ends with the menopause, at an average age of 51 years.

Psychosocial Factors and Gender Differences

Although the physiological changes that occur during puberty follow the same sequence for everyone (Marieb, 1989), there are wide variations in the age at which these begin. This results in comparison and competition among both boys and girls – penile size is a major concern for boys (as many people erroneously believe that size affects performance), whereas the development of breasts and onset of menarche are areas of concern for girls. Another challenge for individuals in this age group is to learn to cope with their emerging adult sexuality, which may be particularly difficult for anyone whose development deviates from the norm (that is, the early and late developers).

How an individual copes with the changes of puberty depends on several factors, including their childhood experience, the existence of role models, their peer group and, to a certain extent, their understanding of anatomy and physiology. For example, the first menses may be alarming if the girl had not discussed menstruation either with her mother (who perhaps found it too embarrassing to mention) or at school because it was not part of the curriculum!

In Britain, as in countries such as the USA, the teenage years, when the pubertal changes occur, is a period termed adolescence and has been described in various psychological terms. G Stanley Hall (1881) viewed adolescence as a time of 'storm and stress', implying that it is a turbulent time for everyone; this extreme theory has been criticized and a more individualistic approach proposed. Erik Erikson, a psychoanalyst who carried out much research on adolescents, proposed a theory of human development in which the lifespan is divided into distinct stages, each of which has a task to be achieved. The task of adolescence is to discover one's identity (Erikson, 1963), a task which may be influenced and complicated by contradictory messages. For example, while the body of a 15-year-old girl may be physically mature (that is, capable of reproduction), her parents may still treat her as a young child, in need of shelter and protection. In her relationships with boys she may want to experiment sexually, which may be encouraged by her peer group, but if the messages she received in her childhood taught her that sex was dirty and sinful, then any sexual experimentation becomes covert and furtive. Further, if she acquires contraception, she is making a statement that she is sexually active. Although she is actually behaving responsibly by protecting herself from pregnancy (and sexually transmitted diseases if she a uses barrier method), she is viewed by society as promiscuous and irresponsible. This double standard affects girls more than boys, as society considers it acceptable, or even desirable, for adolescent boys to be sexually active. (*See* Chapter 1 for greater detail on sexual identity, gender roles, gender differences and body image.)

In many cultures, the prolonged state of 'adolescence' does not exist; rather, the transition to adulthood is identified by a single ritual, a rite of passage. For women, it is often menarche that denotes the transition to adulthood: 'In rural societies the menarche was a mark that the girl was now a woman, and could take up the duties and obligations of womanhood' (Llewellyn-Jones, 1986, p. 36). Among the Apaches of North America and the Brahmins of India, menarche is accompanied by ritual scarring, rubbing of the vulva with nettles and then isolation from the community, followed by a celebratory feast (Ussher, 1989).

As men do not experience such a dramatic and well-defined physiological change, a traditional ritual may be observed at a certain age. For example, in Mangaia, an island in the South Pacific, boys are initiated into manhood at 13 years of age (Marshall, 1971). The initiation involves superincision (whereby a slit is made on the top of the penis, along its entire length) performed by a male elder, who also instructs the boy on how to sexually satisfy women. Two weeks after the operation the boy has intercourse with an experienced woman who gives him practical instruction on how to satisfy his partner. The boy is then likely to have intercourse at least once a night, and both boys and girls are encouraged to have several different sexual partners before marriage.

The Mangaian attitude to sexual behaviour was described by Messenger (1971) as being in stark contrast to that of the inhabitants of Inis Beag, a small island off the coast of Ireland. Inis Beag was considered to be naiive and sexually repressive; sex education was nonexistent, parents never discussed sex with their children, premarital sex was virtually unknown and even nudity was abhorred. Through ignorance, both menstruation and the menopause were feared – menstruation because it was thought to make the woman dangerous and the menopause because it was believed to cause insanity. The comparison between the beliefs and expectations of these two societies serves to illustrate the influence of a person's culture in defining sexual maturity.

The issue of sexual maturity has implications for midwifery practice. For instance, if a woman has been taught that exposing her genital area (even to her hus-

band) is sinful, she will be extremely reluctant to do so in front of a total stranger. This situation can be helped if the same midwife cares for the woman throughout her childbearing, as the woman's fears (such as physical examination in labour) can be discussed during the antenatal period, and an acceptable strategy devised. Labour is also the time when the results of traditions such as female circumcision affect midwifery care and, once again, continuity of carer is recommended.

Health

To promote health or to provide health education there needs to be an agreed understanding of what 'health' actually means (**Table 2.1**). Many attempts have been made to define health, so this section begins with some examples of these definitions. Health norms and the consequences of deviating from them, using obesity as an example, are then considered. The section concludes with a discussion on various aspects of sexual health.

In Western society traditionally there has been an emphasis on medical health (that is, freedom from illness); however, there are several other dimensions of health which should be considered if a holistic picture of an individual's 'health status' is to be described. These can be divided into individual dimensions (physical, emotional, spiritual, mental, social and sexual) and the broader dimensions of societal and environmental health (Ewles and Simnett, 1995). To understand what constitutes health, some of these dimensions are considered in greater detail below.

Several of the individual aspects of health can be seen as inextricably linked – for a person to feel healthy in the spiritual dimension (that is, they have peace of mind), they also need mental health (the ability to think clearly) and emotional health (which includes the ability to cope with stress). Similarly, for a person to be able to make and maintain relationships (social health), they need to be able to recognize emotions and express them appropriately (emotional health). This implies that to achieve health within a society, the individual must understand and exhibit acceptable (appropriate) behaviour. Every society has its norms and mores: 'ill health', or the inability to achieve one's potential, can arise when there is deviation from these norms.

Table 2.1 What is Health?		
Reference	**Definition**	**Comment**
World Health Organization (WHO, 1946)	'Health is a state of complete physical, mental and social well-being, and not merely the absence of disease and infirmity'	Criticized as being utopian, for implying that health is the same for everyone, and for being static
Dubois (1960)	Health is 'a process of adaptation to the changing demands of living and the changing meanings we give to life'	Viewed health as dynamic
WHO (1984)	Health is 'the extent to which an individual or group is able to realize and satisfy needs'	Recognized the idea of the fulfilment of individual potential
Seedhouse (1986)	'A person's optimum state of health is equivalent to the state of the set of conditions which fulfil or enable a person to work or fulfil his or her realistic chosen and biological potentials'	Individual potential is placed within a wider social context
Your definition?		

Health Norms

One of the norms in British society applies to an individual's weight: although being extremely underweight or overweight can result in physical illhealth, it is often the societal pressure to conform to a defined size which causes an individual to experience 'disease' (that is, not at peace with oneself), and consequently feel 'unhealthy'. In countries such as the UK and the USA, society's message to women in particular is that thin is beautiful (ergo, fat is ugly, unattractive, undesirable), and that obese women are deviant. In an attempt to conform to societal expectations (to become a 'better' person), the woman may actually put her physical health at risk. This is perfectly illustrated by adolescent girls who starve themselves, literally to death in some cases, to become what they believe society demands them to be.

In the 1990s, because their role models (fashion models, pop stars, film stars) are thin, the message to adolescent girls is that thinness equates with success, popularity and acceptability. Unfortunately, during adolescence the normal physiological changes, such as the deposition of fat around the hips and breasts, are regarded as gross and unacceptable by as many as 10% of women (Llewellyn-Jones, 1986), and they embark on a regime which may involve severe restriction of food intake and excessive exercise (anorexia nervosa), or bingeing and purging (bulimia). Orbach (1986) explains the behaviour of the anorexic girl as being a way for her to regain control over her body. For sufferers of bulimia this feeling of control is gained by purging which is achieved by induced vomiting and excessive use of laxatives (up to 200 per week – Marieb, 1989). The actual ingestion of food, which can be as much as 55,000 calories per hour (Marieb, 1989), is viewed by the individual as disgusting, and serves to perpetuate their belief that they are an ugly, deviant, 'sick' individual.

In extreme cases, the ultimate consequence of anorexia is death caused by starvation; in less severe cases, physical problems can include long-term damage to the gastrointestinal tract, renal failure, muscle wasting and endocrine disturbance. Secondary amenorrhoea, or delayed onset of menarche, is common, and the woman becomes temporarily infertile. Paradoxically, although a woman suffering from bulimia may appear 'healthy' (that is, she is an appropriate and societally acceptable weight for height), she may actually have many physical disorders including pancreatitis, liver and gall-bladder problems, damage to the stomach and oesophagus, and kidney damage. She is also at risk of potentially fatal heart failure because of electrolyte imbalance, which occurs as a result of potassium loss. Thus, sufferers of both anorexia and bulimia put their lives at risk in their attempts to achieve what they perceive as a desirable 'healthy' body.

Aspects of Sexual Health

Few (1994) proposed that three significant policies directly affected the sexual health of British society. First, the Children Act (1989) was passed to make the social services aware of the needs of young people. In particular, it emphasized access to information and confidential services concerning sexual health, thus empowering adolescents to build and maintain fulfilling relationships with others. Second, the Community Care Act (1990) promoted the recognition of individual needs through cooperative work between the various health professionals. Third, in 1992 the Government issued a document entitled *The Health of the Nation: A Strategy for Health in England* (Department of Health, 1992a) within which five aspects of health were identified as priorities for action. Sexual health, together with human immunodeficiency virus (HIV) and autoimmune deficiency syndrome (AIDS), was identified as one of these key areas, the others being coronary heart disease and stroke, cancers (lung, skin, breast and cervical), mental illness and accidents. A total of 27 targets were set concerning reduction in mortality and morbidity rates, and changes in health behaviour.

It is suggested in the document that the responsibilities for actions to achieve these targets is widely spread from individuals to government (Department of Health, 1992a). However, it has been suggested (Smith, 1991) that strategies such as that in *The Health of the Nation* place the onus of responsibility solely on the individual, in the same way as previous documents did. In 1976, for example, the Government document *Prevention and Health: Everybody's Business* contained the following statement: 'To a large extent ... it is clear that the weight of responsibility for his own health lies on the shoulders of the individual himself' (Department of Health

and Social Security, 1976).

The two main objectives set in *The Health of the Nation* regarding sexual health were (Department of Health, 1992a):

- To reduce the incidence of gonorrhoea by at least 25% by 1995 (using the figure for 1990 as a baseline), as an indicator of HIV and/or AIDS trends.
- To reduce by at least 50% the rate of conceptions among under-16-year-olds by the year 2000 (using the figure from 1989 as the baseline).

Clearly, both conception among the under-16-year-olds (referred to hereafter as teenage pregnancy, for convenience) and gonorrhoea are considered by the government as 'unhealthy', although there may be incongruence between the government's and the individual's definitions of what constitutes illhealth. For example, from an individual's perspective, being a pregnant teenager may be absolutely normal, a healthy behaviour. Indeed, Phoenix (1991) reported on a growing body of studies in which both mother and child do well, thus refuting the popular notion that teenage pregnancies present difficulties. To understand why incongruity may arise, it is worth considering first gonorrhoea and then teenage pregnancy using the health dimension model.

Gonorrhoea can certainly affect the individual's physical health: men are likely to complain of a green, purulent discharge, and of frequency of micturition and dysuria caused by urethritis. Although women may be asymptomatic (Emens, 1983), they may still suffer physical consequences and, as **Table 2.2** illustrates, other health dimensions may also be affected. Physical effects of teenage pregnancy include an

Table 2.2 Gonorrhoea				
Condition	Physical health	Emotional health	Social health	Societal health
Woman with untreated gonorrhoea	Bilateral salpingitis and formation of scar tissue	Infertility may cause anger, guilt	Relationships (for example with a partner) may be adversely affected	The woman may be seen as deserving of the consequences of 'deviant' behaviour (Hogan, 1980)
	Increased risk of obstruction of Fallopian tubes			
	Increased risk of infertility			
Pregnant woman with untreated gonorrhoea	Infection passed on to baby causing ophthalmia neonatorum (Fong, 1987)	Guilt	(as above)	(as above)
				The woman may also be blamed by society

increased risk of anaemia and postpartum haemorrhage; also, if the teenager actually suffers from any medical conditions, then she can be described as physically unhealthy. However, pregnancy in itself is not a physical illness, and even among teenagers it is usually medically uncomplicated. It could be argued, therefore, that teenage pregnancy has been targeted by the government as an area for change because it is considered to be societally unacceptable. It could be further argued that it is the attitude of society which accounts for the teenage pregnancy rate: for example, the rate in the UK is seven times greater than that in the Netherlands, where it is acknowledged that teenagers are sexually active and where contraception and advice are widely available. Few (1994) identified three essential components of sexual health, the first two of which are control of fertility and avoidance of both unwanted pregnancy and sexually transmitted diseases (including HIV). It would appear that the third component, 'sexual expression and enjoyment without exploitation, suppression or abuse', is recognized in the Netherlands but not in the UK.

In conclusion, it can be seen that health is defined in many ways, and that to be an effective promoter of health (which midwives should be), one must first determine how an individual perceives 'good health'. Having ascertained this, the health promoter can then offer appropriate health promotion.

Health Promotion

In Britain during the past decade there has been increasing pressure on people of all ages to become more health conscious. Alarming data warning the public of the perils of drinking too much alcohol, eating saturated fats, taking inadequate exercise, sunbathing and smoking appear regularly in the media. These data are often taken from research commissioned by the Government, and the way in which the information is presented implies that each individual has a responsibility to society to lead a healthy lifestyle. Indeed, those who choose not to conform may be punished – for example, a surgeon may refuse to operate on someone who smokes heavily. Frightening people with alarming statistics is just one method of inducing a change in their behaviour. In this section, alternative (and usually more effective) approaches to health promotion are described briefly. Smoking cessation in pregnancy, an area of health

promotion in which midwives have a major part to play, is then discussed.

Approaches to Health Promotion

Health promotion, which encompasses more than just health education, has been defined by the World Health Organization (WHO, 1984) as 'the process of enabling people to increase control over, and to improve, their health.' Five main approaches to the facilitation of this process have been identified (Ewles and Simnett, 1995), each of which employs different activities to achieve a slightly different aim within the overall objective of health promotion.

- The medical approach, like the medical model of health care, focuses on disease and disability that it aims to eliminate through medical intervention.
- The behaviour change approach, which is more individualized, aims to change the individual's attitude towards a certain health behaviour, and promote a change.
- The educational approach is often used by health professionals – knowledge is 'passed on' to clients with the intention of enabling them to make choices about their health.
- In the client-centred approach, however, the agenda is set by the client who is seen as an equal, in contrast to the educational programmes in which the content is usually defined by the health promoter. This client centred approach encourages self-empowerment and allows the client to focus on those aspects of health which they identify as being of importance.
- The fifth approach to health promotion involves societal change – activities such as political action are undertaken with the aim of making the physical or social environment conducive to the choice of healthier lifestyles.

Smoking Cessation in Pregnancy

When encouraging smoking cessation, the midwife obviously prefers to use the most effective approach. Numerous smoking cessation programmes that employ various health promotion approaches can be found. By evaluating the outcome of these programmes, the midwife can adopt an approach which has been shown to be effective, but which is also realistic and appropriate to her situation. For example, widespread campaigns (such as the *Quit Campaign* launched in 1992 in the state of Victoria, Australia, which involved massive distribution of materials such as brochures and posters), have been shown to be highly effective, but are obviously beyond the scope of an individual midwife because of the resources required.

In a major review of more than 20 smoking cessation programmes, Walsh and Redman (1993) made several recommendations regarding the components of a successful programme. They recommended a combination of health promotion approaches – effective programmes needed to have an educational focus whereby knowledge was passed on by the health promoter to the client (educational approach), but the agenda for imparting this information needed be set by the client (client-centred approach). Further, the programme that aim to facilitate smoking cessation by giving information in a persuasive, individualized manner (behaviour change approach). Programmes which offered ongoing support, advice and encouragement from the health professional most closely involved with the other aspects of the client's care appeared to be the most effective (Power *et al.* 1989, for example). Obviously the midwife is ideally placed to undertake this role, so to facilitate smoking cessation successfully she has to have knowledge (of the health hazards of smoking, for example), the ability to impart this knowledge (which requires effective communication skills), realistic expectations regarding the outcome of the health promotion activity and access to necessary resources.

There is incontrovertible evidence that smoking is hazardous to health, so when a pregnant woman smokes she is putting not only her own health at risk, but also that of her unborn child (*see* 'Lifestyle' in the 'Preconception' section below). Given this knowledge, it should be part of midwives' role to inform women of the consequences of smoking, and to help them to quit. However, many midwives may feel that they are in danger of jeopardizing their relationship with women if they raise the issue of smoking (HEA, 1994). Midwives could feel that women may view her as being judgemental and critical, and so do not discuss women's smoking behaviour or offer them any help in quitting. Midwives may also feel that they have inadequate knowledge and skills to be able to facilitate smoking cessation.

In 1994, having evaluated several smoking cessation pilot projects, the Health Education Authority (HEA) published a training pack entitled *Helping Pregnant Smokers Quit: Training for Health Professionals* (HEA, 1994), in which they aimed to equip health professionals (for example, midwives) with the required knowledge. In the pack, the readers are challenged to examine their own attitude to smoking (particularly the readers who are smokers) and exercises are provided to enable readers to practice questioning women about their smoking behaviour in a positive, unthreatening manner. The pack also offers advice on smoking cessation interventions – for example, a regularly updated smoking cessation 'contract' (agreed by the woman and the health professional), showing the woman's progress, could be used. The recommendation is for a client-centred, individualized, ongoing, supportive and encouraging approach; as this is how midwives should be functioning in all aspects of their work, they should hopefully feel confident to take on the challenge of facilitating smoking cessation during pregnancy.

Preconception

'Thou art barren and bearest not, but thou shalt conceive and bear a son. Now therefore beware, I pray thee, and drink not wine nor strong drink and eat not any unclean thing' (Judges 13:3–4). This early example of preconception care, taken from the *Old Testament*, was apparently effective – the recipient of the advice was the mother of Samson!

Although the benefits of prepregnancy advice have been suspected for centuries, it is only in the past few years that sufficient research has been undertaken to prove these beliefs. Using the results from this research, prospective parents can now be given care and advice which aims to achieve three objectives. The first objective is that the couple actually conceive; second, that they conceive a healthy baby; and third that the couple, particularly the woman, remain healthy after conception to reduce the factors which may cause prematurity, low birth weight and congenital abnormality (the three main causes of perinatal morbidity and mortality). In this section, the advice and treatment needed to meet these objectives are presented under five main headings.

- Lifestyle.
- Environment.
- General health.
- Obstetric history.
- Existing medical disorders.

Availability of preconception care is then mentioned briefly, and the section concludes with a discussion on the role of the midwife.

Lifestyle

The four aspects of the couple's lifestyle to be considered are diet, exercise, stress and drugs.

Diet

Before embarking on a pregnancy, the woman should ensure that her weight is within normal parameters. A measure known as the Quetelet (or Q) Index, in which body weight-to-height ratio is calculated, is generally accepted as an indication of what these normal parameters are. **Table 2.3** (Pickard, 1984) shows the type of health effects which result from being underweight, of a normal weight and overweight, as defined by the Quetelet Index, plus an example of a body weight-to-height ratio using this measure.

Example: For a person who weighs 58.5 kg and is 1.62 m tall, the calculation is as in the following equation:

$$\frac{\text{(Weight in kilograms)}}{\text{(Height in metres squared)}} \quad \frac{58.5}{1.62 \times 1.62} = 22.3$$

As 22.3 falls within the desirable weight range, this person is classed as being of normal weight.

There is a considerable body of evidence to suggest that severe food deprivation has a direct influence on both fertility and pregnancy outcome. Stein and Susser (1974), in their studies of the Dutch population, found a 50% reduction in the conception rate during the Dutch famines of 1944, plus a significant increase in abnormalities of the central nervous system, in particular, among the babies who were conceived at this time. A similar trend was reported by Mosley (1979), who studied the population of Bangladesh following the floods and famines of 1974–75. Stein and Susser (1974) also noted that the reduction in conception rate persisted for 4 months after the food shortages, suggesting that it took this length of time for the population to recover.

Although the UK as a whole does not suffer famines, a significant proportion of the population is malnourished either through poverty, ignorance or strict dieting. One effect of malnourishment on women of childbearing age is amenorrhoea; it has been suggested that this is due to a reduction in the proportion of body fat to lean body mass.

If the woman presenting for preconception advice is amenorrhoeic and underweight, dietary advice to increase her calorific intake is indicated: conversely, if she is obese, then she should be advised to reduce her calorific intake in order that her weight falls within the normal range at the time of conception, as obesity during pregnancy increases the risk of pre-eclampsia and thromboembolic disorders.

General dietary advice for all women prior to pregnancy should be for a well-balanced diet which includes sufficient quantities of the four main food groups:

• Bread and cereals.
• Fruit and vegetables.
• Dairy products.
• Meat, fish, beans and nuts.

Specific information should be given regarding vitamin

Table 2.3 Quetelet index measure indicating weight-to-height ratio and health effects		
Q Index	**Effect**	**Weight-to-height ratio**
<20 Underweight	Increased risk of amenorrhoea	19.5 = 51 kg
	Infertility	
	Long-term health hazard	
20–25 Desirable	Ideal range for pregnancy and long-term health	22.3 =58 kg
26–30 Moderate obesity	Slight risk to health	27.7 = 72 kg
	May lead to severe obesity	
>30 Severe obesity	Increased risk of menstrual problems and pregnancy complications	30.3 = 80 kg
	Long-term health hazard	

B$_6$ (a deficiency of which is associated with low birth weight in babies), zinc (a deficiency of which is also associated with low birth weight as well as reduced sperm motility) and folate. There is clear evidence that a deficiency of folic acid and folates at the time of conception and during the first trimester of pregnancy increases the risk of neural tube defects (Department of Health 1992b; Czeizel, 1993). Therefore women should be advised to increase their folic acid and folate intake by 400 µg a day, either by eating more folate-rich foods (lightly boiled green vegetables, oranges), by eating foods fortified with folic acid (cornflakes, wholemeal bread) or by taking folic acid supplements.

Exercise

Although a total lack of exercise is often associated with obesity (*see above*) and vigorous exercise may result in menstrual irregularities, such as delay in menarche or secondary amenorrhoea (Wu, 1988), it is generally accepted that a moderate amount of exercise is good for everyone and before pregnancy the advice is the same. If a woman normally takes very little exercise, she should be advised to begin exercising regularly before conception in order to increase her ability to cope with the extra demands that pregnancy and labour put on her body.

Stress

It has been suggested that psychological stress was a contributory factor in the reduction in the birth rate following the Dutch Winter of Hunger (Stein *et al.* 1975). Nucholls *et al.* (1972) have also demonstrated a link between stress and infertility, and Laukaran and van den Berg (1980) suggested an association between stress and pregnancy complications such as accidental injury, psychological disorders, perinatal mortality and postpartum infection and haemorrhage. Psychological health is as important as physical health preconception, and if the psychological health of either of the couple is negatively affected by stress, the cause needs to be identified and advice or treatment offered. For example, if there is a psychological disorder or relationship problem, counselling may be appropriate.

Drugs

Unlike the complications caused by existing disorders, such as epilepsy and hypertension, the problems caused by tobacco, alcohol and recreational drugs can be eliminated. The couple should therefore be advised that to stop smoking will make a positive contribution to the outcome of their planned pregnancy, as will reducing their alcohol consumption to an acceptably safe level and not using recreational drugs. Ideally, both partners should be involved, partly because both tobacco and alcohol adversely affect men and women, even though in different ways, and partly because it is easier to change a lifestyle behaviour if those closest to you are doing the same.

The evidence for the adverse effects of smoking is overwhelming – in addition to the effects on the individual's general health (increased risk of coronary heart disease, chronic bronchitis and emphysema, cardiovascular accident, atherosclerotic peripheral vascular disease), all stages of the childbearing process are implicated. Howe *et al.* (1985) found a lower fertility rate among smokers, the risk of spontaneous abortion was shown to be increased by 27% (Royal College of Physicians, 1992), the average birth weight was estimated as being 170–200 g lower (Brooke *et al.* 1989) and premature birth was twice as likely – as a result of these and other adverse effects, the incidence of perinatal mortality was increased by one-third (Royal College of Physicians, 1992). Following delivery, there is an increased risk of sudden infant death syndrome (Action on Smoking and Health, 1988), slower rate of growth and reduced mental aptitude (Fogelman and Manor, 1988) and a higher morbidity and mortality in the first year of life (Rantakallio, 1979). In light of all this evidence and given the fact that many couples consider pregnancy as the motivation they need, every effort should be made to help them to quit smoking before they try to conceive. (For further information on smoking cessation, *see* Smoking Cessation in Pregnancy above.)

Evidence to show the adverse effects of alcohol on pregnancy outcome is less conclusive than the evidence against smoking, although there are several complications that may arise from drinking before and during pregnancy. In addition to the possibility that sperm motility may be adversely affected, there is also the more fundamental problem of impotence caused by alcohol; as Shakespeare observed in 1606, drink provokes the desire but it takes away the performance! (from *Macbeth*, Act 2 Scene 3). During pregnancy, the most severe consequence of heavy drinking is fetal alcohol syndrome, common features of which are antenatal and postnatal growth deficiency, microcephaly and developmental delay or mental retardation (Jones and Smith, 1973). Even moderate drinking (more than 10 units of alcohol per week) has been related to prematurity and small head

(Wright *et al.* 1983). The best precon-
e for the couple who are moderate to
rs is therefore to change their drinking
habits and reduce overall alcohol intake.

The use of recreational drugs is another activity which should ideally be tackled before pregnancy as there may be adverse effects both before and after conception. For example, marijuana has been shown to affect reproductive functioning (Petersen, 1980) and to increase the chance of preterm labour, abruptio placentae and low birth weight (Hingson *et al.* 1982). The effects of opiates on pregnancy include an increased risk of anaemia, multiple pregnancy, haemorrhage and intrauterine growth retardation. In addition, neonatal withdrawal symptoms occur in 60--90% of infants born to drug-dependent mothers. Because the effects of opiates are so significant and because pregnancy is a far from ideal time to try 'breaking the habit', this problem should be addressed (for example by referral to a drug dependency clinic) before conception occurs.

Environment

There is a certain amount of controversy surrounding the extent to which various environmental hazards affect the outcome of pregnancy – for example, although the results of some research suggest an association between the regular use of visual display units (VDUs) and a higher than average miscarriage rate, the small sample numbers have cast doubt on the validity of these findings.

However, there are some environmental hazards that the couple should be advised to avoid in the preconception period and during early pregnancy, as teratogenic effects can cause very significant damage. Although this may be difficult if the hazards are occupational, the couple should be encouraged to discuss the problem with their employer and try to reach a compromise. An example of this is when one of the couple is an anaesthetic nurse because an association has been suggested between exposure to waste anaesthetic agents and an increased risk of miscarriage (Vessey and Nunn, 1980); the nurse could ask to be transferred to a general ward during the first 3 months of pregnancy, when the person is at greatest risk of complications. With forward planning this should be possible. Other areas of employment associated with an increased risk of miscarriage are in metal and electrical factory work, sales and services (McDonald *et al*, 1988), so again the woman should be encouraged to request a transfer for the first trimester.

In some areas of employment, where there is a substantial body of evidence regarding the effects of a particular substance, legislation exists to protect the individual, so the person receiving prepregnancy advice should be encouraged to ascertain whether this applies to them. An example of such a substance is lead – in the UK, in the *Control of Lead at Work Regulations* (HMSO, 1985), it is stated that 'a woman of reproductive capacity' should be withdrawn from work that exposes her to lead at a defined level of 40 µg/100 ml and for pregnant women to be suspended from working with lead.

Unfortunately, the risk of some occupations (such as that involving men working at nuclear power plants) has yet to be properly acknowledged and more research is needed in such areas of potential risk.

General Health

Several aspects of general health can be checked before conception through careful history taking and screening procedures. Baseline measurements can be recorded and preventive measures taken against certain infections, particularly rubella.

Blood pressure

One of the major complications of pregnancy is preeclampsia – if a pregnant woman has raised blood pressure during pregnancy, it is helpful to have a baseline reading to know how far the pregnancy reading deviates from her usual blood pressure. This baseline reading is normally recorded at the antenatal booking visit, but there is an obvious advantage in recording the blood pressure before the woman is actually pregnant.

Urinalysis

Urinalysis can be performed to exclude proteinuria (which may indicate pyelonephritis or chronic renal disease) and glycosuria (which may be associated with diabetes mellitus). If any abnormality is detected, further investigations can be undertaken to diagnose the cause and treatment given accordingly.

Blood tests

A blood test to ascertain haemoglobin should be offered; if the level is low, the cause should be ascertained and appropriate treatment given. Haemoglobinopathies can also be detected from a blood sample – both partners should be screened and genetic counselling offered if there is a risk of the baby being affected.

Rubella

Screening for rubella antibodies is a vital element of prepregnancy care. The devastating teratogenic effects of rubella are entirely preventable by checking the woman's rubella status before pregnancy, and immunizing her if she is susceptible. If the rubella vaccination is given, pregnancy must be avoided for 3 months (Horstmann, 1982) so effective contraception such as, an injectable hormonal method, should be prescribed. It is also recommended that the woman has a second blood test following rubella vaccination to confirm immunity (Banatvala, 1982).

Other infections that can be screened for and that may require treatment include sexually transmitted diseases and hepatitis.

Child spacing

Family spacing is an important consideration as there is an increased risk of prematurity and intrauterine growth retardation if the interval between children is too short (Wynn and Wynn, 1991).

Contraception

Advice on ceasing the use of contraception depends on the method being used. There is some evidence of lowered blood zinc levels and an interference with vitamin-A metabolism in users of the combined oral contraceptive pill; it is therefore recommended that an alternative method (such as a barrier method) be used for 3 months before conception (Pickard, 1984). A similar time lapse is also recommended following removal of the intrauterine contraceptive device, to enable the endometrium to become healthy and vascular.

Obstetric History

The relevance of previous pregnancies with relation to morbidity and other problems is significant and needs careful exploration to produce an accurate history before conceptual advice.

Previous problems

Couples commonly seek prepregnancy advice following a previous obstetric problem. For example,

the woman may have suffered previous miscarriages and need investigation to establish whether there is any treatment available that could improve her chances of a normal pregnancy. Alternatively, she may have had a stillbirth or neonatal death, or a child with an anomaly caused by hereditary factors. In all these cases, she and her partner should be referred to the appropriate health professional – an obstetrician, a geneticist or a counsellor, as necessary.

Existing Medical Disorders

There are several medical disorders, for example hypertension, diabetes mellitus and epilepsy, that are affected by or that affect pregnancy. By reviewing and perhaps revising management of these disorders before conception, pregnancy outcome may be much improved. Preconception advice and ongoing treatment should involve all the relevant members of the multiprofessional team.

Hypertensive disease

Hypertensive disease is associated with an increased risk of premature labour and intrauterine growth retardation and a higher incidence of perinatal mortality; it is also one of the most common causes of maternal death. Blood pressure should be stabilized before conception and then closely monitored throughout pregnancy.

Diabetes mellitus

A link has been shown between hyperglycaemia around the time of conception and abnormality of organ formation, particularly the neural tube, heart and kidneys (Burden, 1985). Complications that may arise during pregnancy include pre-eclampsia, polyhydramnios and preterm labour; also, there is a higher incidence of congenital abnormalities. It is therefore essential that a woman who has diabetes mellitus be properly counselled and her diabetes be controlled carefully both preconception and throughout childbearing.

Epilepsy

If either partner has epilepsy, there is an increased chance of congenital malformations, particularly cleft lip, cleft palate and congenital heart disease (de Swiet, 1986). Because the degree of abnormality is more severe if the epilepsy is controlled with anticonvulsant therapy, this should be reduced or, if possible, discontinued before conception. In addition, the couple should be counselled and informed of the possibility of their child having a congenital malformation or of developing epilepsy.

Availability of Prepregnancy Care

Prepregnancy advice can be given in either a formal or informal setting. Informal education should begin in childhood, both at home and in school. Formal sessions in schools, focusing on relationships, sexuality and parenting, could be part of the curriculum. The mass media play an important role, particularly among young people for whom magazines, newspapers, films and TV soap operas are all important sources of information. Issues raised in the mass media could be used as discussion points in the classroom.

Prepregnancy care is traditionally associated with family planning clinics where advice is available on conception as well as on contraception. Investigations such as blood pressure monitoring, urinalysis and screening for sexually transmitted diseases and rubella status can also be offered at the family planning clinic. Well-woman clinics offer a similar service, as do health centres and some occupational health departments. Education on lifestyle behaviours, such as smoking, weight control, alcohol and exercise, should also be available.

Organizations like Foresight provide a variety of resources, such as books and videos, which address all aspects of prepregnancy care (*see* Barnes and Bradley, 1990), whereas other organizations provide help and advice on specific aspects (the British Diabetic Association, for instance). Other sources of information are telephone helplines and mobile 'health buses'.

The Role of the Midwife

We need to see that the profession is properly represented in [prepregnancy care] and takes its correct place in looking after the health and mental welfare of future mothers and fathers... to improve the results of their pregnancies.

In this statement Professor Geoffrey Chamberlain (Chamberlain, 1986) is referring to the medical profession. However, it could also be applied to midwives, who have a vital role to play in preconception care as their involvement at this stage could lead to continuity of carer during pregnancy and more effective health promotion, thus enabling them to offer realistic choices for women and their families. The midwife's role extends beyond pregnancy, labour and the puerperium, as is reflected in the definition of a midwife formulated by the World Health Organization: 'She has an important task in health counselling and education, not only for the patients but also within the family and community' (UKCC, 1991).

Several of the activities of a midwife also suggest involvement in preconception care – for example, to provide sound family planning information and advice, to diagnose pregnancies, to prescribe or advise on the examinations necessary for the earliest possible diagnosis of pregnancies at risk and even to provide a programme of parenthood preparation (UKCC, 1991). Although the midwife is most likely to be giving prepregnancy advice in the postnatal period (in preparation for the next pregnancy!), she may also be working in or alongside a family planning clinic, well-woman clinic or a health centre. She may be involved in teaching in the local school, she may offer a 'drop-in' facility in a shopping centre or she may be invited to attend a 'health fair'. As a health professional whose work revolves around childbearing, she is seen as the expert on all matters relating to childbirth, including prepregnancy care. Therefore she has a responsibility, not only to the women in her care, but also within the wider community, to ensure that her knowledge is up to date and that she can give relevant, helpful information to anyone who needs advice regarding the preconception period.

Summary

The overall aim of this chapter is to provide the reader with an understanding of an individual's sexual, physical and psychological development from the moment of conception up to the point when the individual can reproduce. For the midwife to provide successful effective individualized and holistic care it is important for her to remember that each woman she cares for has an individual personal history.

This individual history has been influenced by biological, psychological and cultural factors and an understanding of all three dimensions and how they ineract with each other is of paramount importance, as is an understanding of the concept of health and the different ways this may be defined and viewed by individuals. In the western world health has traditionally adopted a medical focus and has been seen to be defined as 'freedom from illness'; however, more recently, a more holistic view has been adopted with an emphasis on the physical, emotional, spiritual, mental, social and sexual health of the 'whole' person. The broader dimensions of societal and environmental health should also be considered. Midwives are an important resource in promoting the health of the mother and her family. To do this she must have an understanding of the different modes of health promotion, she should be familiar with their assets and their limitations for the selection of the most appropriate model is of prime importance if she/he is to empower women and their partners to create healthier lifestyles for themselves and their family. Crucial to the empowering process is the ability to distinguish between those aspects of health behaviour that are under the individuals control and those that are not. This is an important distinction, as by focusing on those behaviours which can be changed the midwife will give the most effective advice.

KEY CONCEPTS

- The midwife needs to have a knowledge of each woman's personal, sexual history if she is to effectively plan and provide individualized and holistic care.
- Adaptation to the physiological and psychological changes that occur during puberty is influenced by social and cultural norms and mores.
- There are several different approaches to health education, so the midwife needs an understanding of the advantages and limitations of each of these approaches if she is to be a successful educator.
- Health promotion is one of the key roles of the midwife.
- By empowering women and their partners to adopt healthy lifestyles before conception, the midwife can help to reduce maternal and infant morbidity and mortality rates.

References

Action on Smoking and Health: *Smoking and reproduction*, Fact Sheet No. 8, London, 1988, ASH.

Banatvala JE: Rubella vaccination – remaining problems, *Br Med J* 284(1 May): 1285, 1982.

Bancroft J: *Human sexuality and its problems*, 2nd edn, Edinburgh, 1989, Churchill Livingstone.

Barnes B, Bradley SG: *Planning for a healthy baby*, London, 1990, Vermilion.

Brooke DG, Anderson HR, Bland JM, *et al.*: Effects on birth weight of smoking, alcohol, caffeine, socio-economic factors, and psycho-social stress, *Br Med J* 298(25 March):795, 1989.

Burden AC: Diabetic control during pregnancy, *Pract Diabetes* 2(5):16, 1985.

Chamberlain G: Prepregnancy Care. In Chamberlain G, Lumley J, editors: *Prepregnancy care: a manual for practice*, Chichester, 1986, John Wiley and Son.

Czeizel AE: Prevention of congenital abnormalities by periconceptual vitamin supplementation, *Br Med J* 306(19 June):1645, 1993.

Department of Health: *The health of the nation: a strategy for health in England*, London, 1992a, HMSO.

Department of Health: *Folic acid and the prevention of neural tube defects*, Report from an Expert Advisory Group, London, 1992b, HMSO.

Department of Health and Social Security: *Prevention and health: everybody's business*, London, 1976, HMSO.

de Swiet M: Pre-existing medical disorders. In Chamberlain G, Lumley J, editors: *Prepregnancy care: a manual for practice*, Chichester, 1986, John Wiley and Son.

Dubois R: *Mirage of health*, London, 1960, Allen and Unwin.

Emens M: The diagnosis and treatment of vaginitis and vaginal discharge, in Studd J, editor: *Progress in obstetrics and gynaecology* Vol. 3, Ch 17, Edinburgh, 1983, Churchill Livingstone.

Erikson EH: *Childhood and society*, New York, 1963, Norton.

Ewles L, Simnett I: *Promoting health. A practical guide* 3rd edn, London, 1995, Scutari Press.

Few C: Promoting sexual health, *Community Outlook* 4(2):29, 1994.

Fogelman KR, Manor O: Smoking in pregnancy and development into early adulthood, *Br Med J* 297(30 April): 1233, 1988.

Fong R: Present trends in the treatment of gonorrhoea and syphilis, *Maternal Child Health* 12(4):103, 1987.

Hall GS: The content of children's minds on entering school, *Ped Semi* 1;139–73:1891.

HEA: *Helping pregnant smokers quit: training for health professionals*, London, 1994, Health Education Authority.

Hingson R, Alpert JJ, Day N, *et al.*: Effects of maternal drinking and marijuana use on fetal growth and development, Pediatrics 70(4):539, 1982.

HMSO: *Control of lead at work regulations 1980: approved code of practice – control of lead at work, Revised June 1985*, London, 1985, HMSO.

Hogan RM: *Human sexuality. A nursing perspective*, Connecticut, 1980, Appleton-Century-Crofts.

Horstmann DM: Viral infections. In Burrow GN, Ferris TF, editors: *Medical complications during pregnancy* 2nd edn, Philadelphia, 1982, Saunders.

Howe G, Westoff C, Vessey M, *et al.*: Effects of age, cigarette smoking and other factors on fertility: findings of a large prospective study, *Br Med J* 290(8 June): 1697, 1985.

Jones KL Smith DW: Recognition of the fetal alcohol syndrome in early infancy, *Lancet* ii(3 Nov): 999, 1973.

Laukaran VH, van den Berg BJ: The relationship of material attitude to pregnancy outcomes and obstetric complications, *Am J Obstet Gynecol* 136;374–79:1980.

Llewellyn-Jones D: *Everywoman. A gynaecological guide for life* 4th edition, London, 1986, Faber and Faber.

Marieb EN: *Human anatomy and physiology*, California, 1989, The Benjamin/Cummings Publishing Co. Inc.

Marshall DS: Sexual behaviour on Mangaia. In Marshall DS, Suggs RC, editors: *Human sexual behaviour*, New York, 1971, Basic Books.

McDonald AD, McDonald JC, Armstrong B, *et al.*: Fetal death and work in pregnancy, *Br J Ind Med* 45(3): 145, 1988.

Messenger JC: Sex and repression in an Irish folk community. In Marshall DS, Suggs RC, editors: *Human sexual behaviour*, New York, 1971, Basic Books.

Mosley WH: The effects of nutrition on natural fertility. In Menken JA, Leridon H, editors: *Patterns and determinants of natural fertility*, Liege, 1979, Ordina.

Nucholls KB, Cassel J, Kaplan BH: Psychiosocial assests, life assests, life crisis and the prognosis of pregnancy. *Am J Epid* 95;431–44:1972.

Orbach S: *Hunger strike*, London, 1986, Faber and Faber.

Peterson RC: Marijuana and health. In *Marijuana research findings*, Maryland, 1980, NIDA Research Monograph.

Phoenix A: Mothers under twenty. Outsider and insider views. In Phoenix A, Wollitt A, Lloyd E, editors: *Motherhood*, London, 1991, Sage.

Pickard B: *Eating well for a healthy pregnancy*, London, 1984, Sheldon Press.

Power FL, Gillies PA, Madeley RJ, Abbot M: Research in an antenatal clinic – the experience of the Nottingham Mothers Stop Smoking Project, *Midwifery* 5(3):106, 1989.

Prader A: Biomedical and endocrinological aspects of normal growth and development. In Borms J, Hauspie R, editors: *Human growth and development*, New York, 1984, Plenum Press.

Rantakallio P: Social backgrounds of mothers who smoke during pregnancy and influence of these factors on offspring. Soc Sci Med 13A;423–49:1979.

Royal College of Physicians: *Smoking and the young*, A Report of the Working Party of the RCP, London, 1992, RCP.

Smith R: First steps towards a strategy for health, *Br Med J* 303(2 Feb):297, 1991.

Stein Z, Susser M: Famine and fertility, in Mosley WH, editor: *Nutrition and human reproduction*, New York, 1978, Plenum Press.

Stein ZA, Susser M, Saeger G, Marolla F, *Famine and human development: The Dutch hunger winter of 1944–45*. New York, 1975, Oxford University Press.

UKCC: *A midwife's code of practice*, 1991, United Kingdom Central Council for Nursing, Midwifery and Health Visiting, London.

Ussher JM: *The psychology of the female body*, London, 1989, Routledge.

Vessey MP, Nunn JF: Occupational hazards of anaesthesia, *Br Med J* 281:696, 1980.

Walsh R, Redman S: Smoking cessation in pregnancy: do effective programmes exist? *Health Promotion Int* 8(2):111, 1993.

WHO: *Constitution*, Geneva, 1946, World Health Organization.

WHO: *Health promotion: a discussion document on the concept and principles*, Copenhagen, 1984, WHO Regional Office for Europe.

Wright JT, Waterson FJ, Barrison IG, *et al.*: Alcohol consumption, pregnancy and low birthweight, *Lancet* i(26 March):663, 1983.

Wu FCW: The biology of puberty. In Diggory P, Potts M, Teper S, editors: *Natural human fertility. Social and biological determinants*, Basingstoke, 1988, Macmillan Press.

Wynn M, Wynn A: *The case for preconception care of men and women*, Oxon, 1991, AC Academic Publishers.

Further Reading

Naidoo J, Wills J: *Health promotion. Foundations for practice*, London, 1994, Ballière Tindall.

This readable and informative text is organized into three sections: The Theory of Health Promotion, *which looks at concepts, models and measurements of health;* Dilemmas in Practice, *which covers such areas as ethical issues and politics of health; and* Working for Health Promotion, *which focuses on implementing health promotion.*

Bradley SG, Bennett N: *Preparation for pregancy: An essential guide*, London, 1995, Argyll Publishing.

This useful reference book is designed for both health professionals and prosepective parents, and gives detailed infomation on all aspects of preparation for pregnancy.

3 Conception

LEARNING OUTCOMES

After studying this chapter you should be able to:

- Explain the physiology of reproduction.
- Discuss the influence of psychological factors on the reproductive process.
- Define subfertility and infertility and discuss the major causes, investigations and treatment of these.
- Demonstrate an understanding of the ethical implications of assisted conception and other reproductive technologies.
- Empower women to make an informed choice regarding infertility treatment and to take control of their fertility.
- Explain the physiological basis of all methods of contraception.
- Discuss the physiological, social and cultural factors which influence the choice of contraception.

Reproduction

It was estimated that in mid-1994 the world population was approximately 5.7 billion (**Box 3.1**; Central Statistical Office, 1995) – yet of all these people, every single one is unique. In this section, the process is discussed whereby a new human life is created. An understanding of this process is essential for the midwife, as it is only with this fundamental knowledge that the appropriate care, advice and treatment can be given on related issues such as preconception, contraception and infertility. The male reproductive system is described (*see* Chapter 1 for the female system). After a brief discussion of the male hormones involved in reproduction and of spermatogenesis, physiological and psychological aspects of sexual arousal are considered. Events that lead up to the moment of conception are then explained.

Male Reproductive System

The primary sex organs of the male are the testes, or male gonads – the scrotum, ducts, glands and penis are accessory reproductive organs. **Figure 3.1** illustrates the anatomy of the male reproductive organs.

The scrotum

The scrotum is a pouch of skin and superficial fascia that lies below the symphysis pubis and between the upper parts of the thighs behind the penis. The superficial fascia, which contains a layer of smooth muscle (the dartos muscle, responsible for scrotal wrinkling), forms an incomplete septum that divides the scrotum into right and left halves, one compartment for each testis. The function of the scrotum is to provide an environment for the testes that is conducive to the production of sperm.

The testes

Each of the two testes is approximately 4.5 cm long and 2.5 cm wide, and comprise three layers:
- Tunica vasculosa, an inner layer of connective tissue containing a fine network of capillaries.
- Tunica albuginea (literally 'white coat'), a fibrous connective tissue capsule which divides each testis into 250–300 wedge-shaped compartments or lobules in which there are between one and four seminiferous tubules.
- Tunica vaginalis testis, the outer layer, which is derived from peritoneum brought down with the descending testis.

Blood supply is from the testicular arteries which arise from the abdominal aorta; venous drainage is through the testicular veins which form a vine-like network called the pampiniform plexus around the testicular artery. Scrotal structures are served by both divisions of the autonomic nervous system, and the nerve fibres, together with the blood vessels and lymphatics, are enclosed in a connective-tissue sheath known as the spermatic cord.

The function of the testes is to produce spermatozoa and testosterone. The actual production of sperm (spermatogenesis) takes place in the seminiferous tubules – the sperm is then conveyed to the epididymis

---

Box 1.1

World population

Population Figures
- In mid-1994 the world population was estimated as 5.7 billion.
- By 1998 the world population is predicted to rise to 6.6 billion.
- By 2025 the world population is predicted to rise to 8.5 billion.
- By 2050 the world population is predicted to rise to 10 billion.

(As compiled by the United Nations, cited in CSO, 1995, p. 15.)

Population Growth Areas
Africa and South Asia are projected to account for half of the growth in the world's population between 1997 and 2020. The current growth rate in Africa is 2.9%, which compares with the much slower growth rate of 0.3% in Europe (CSO, 1995, p. 26).

Total Period Fertility Rates
There are significant variations worldwide in the total period fertility rates (TPFR) – that is, the average number of children that would be born per woman if women experienced the age-specific fertility rates of the period in question throughout their childbearing span. In the period 1990–1995, the TPFRs were (CSO, 1995, p 26):
- 6.0 for African women.
- 3.9 for Indian women.
- 1.7 for European women.

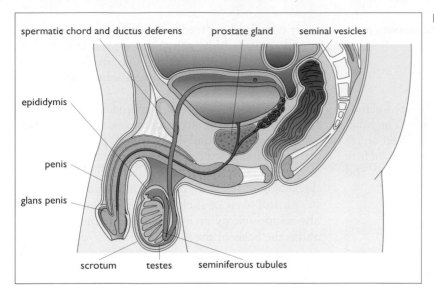

spermatic chord and ductus deferens   prostate gland   seminal vesicles

epididymis

penis

glans penis

scrotum   testes   seminiferous tubules

Figure 3.1 Male reproductive organs.

through the tubulus rectus (a straight tubule formed by the convergence of the seminiferous tubules within each lobule), the rete testis (a tubular network) and through the efferent ductules. Testosterone is produced in the interstitial (Leydig) cells which lie in the soft connective tissue surrounding the seminiferous tubules.

The epididymis

The epididymis is a comma shaped, coiled tube of about 6 m in length. The head of the epididymis caps the superior aspect of the testis whereas its body and tail regions lie on the posterolateral aspect of the testis. The function of the epididymis is to store and transport sperm – the immature sperm enter the epididymis from the testis, are stored temporarily and are then transported to the tail section, becoming motile and fertile during their 20-day journey. During ejaculation, the smooth muscle in the walls of the epididymis contracts and the sperm are expelled into the ductus deferens.

The ductus deferens

The ductus (vas) deferens, which is approximately 45 cm in length, runs upwards from the epididymis through the inguinal canal into the pelvic cavity, over the ureter and along the posterior aspect of the bladder. It then joins with the duct of the seminal vesicle to form the ejaculatory duct, which passes through the prostate gland and merges with the urethra. The function of the ductus deferens is to propel sperm from storage sites to the urethra.

The spermatic cord

The spermatic cord, which comprises the ductus deferens, the testicular blood vessels, lymph vessel and nerves, is a sheath of connective tissue which runs upwards through the inguinal canal. The main function of the spermatic cord is to transmit the ductus deferens up into the body.

Seminal vesicles

There are two seminal vesicles, each of which is 5 cm in length and pyramid shaped. They are composed of columnar epithelium, muscular tissue and fibrous tissue, and are situated at the base of the bladder. The duct of each seminal vesicle joins that of the ductus deferens on the same side to form the ejaculatory duct. The function of the seminal vesicles is to produce a viscous secretion, containing fructose sugar, ascorbic acid, amino acids and prostaglandins, which keeps the sperm alive and motile.

The prostate gland

The prostate gland, a single gland measuring approximately 4 cm in length, 3 cm in width and 2 cm in depth, encircles the upper part of the urethra just below the bladder, and lies between the rectum and the symphysis pubis. It is composed of columnar epithelium, smooth muscle and an outer fibrous layer. The main function of the prostate gland is to produce a milky, alkaline secretion that facilitates sperm activation. The prostatic gland secretion, which accounts for one-third of the semen volume, enters the urethra through several ducts when the prostatic smooth muscle contracts during ejaculation.

Bulbourethral glands

The two pea-sized bulbourethral (Cowper's) glands are situated inferior to the prostate gland. The function of these glands is to produce a thick, clear secretion which is released into the urethra before ejaculation to neutralize any acidity from urine and to increase lubrication during intercourse.

The penis

Together the penis and the scrotum make up the external genitalia of the male. The penis consists of an attached root, which lies in the perineum, and a free shaft (accounting for approximately two-thirds of the total length), which is outside the body. The shaft ends in an enlarged tip known as the glans penis. The skin covering the penis is loose and is able to slide distally to form the prepuce (foreskin) around the proximal end of the glans. Internally the penis contains part of the urethra and three columns of erectile tissue, which comprise connective tissue and smooth muscle, interspersed with numerous vascular spaces. The two dorsal columns, the columnar cavernosa (cavernous bodies), lie on either side and in front of the urethra. The middle column, the columnar spongiosum (spongy body), surrounds the urethra and expands distally to form the glans. The proximal end is also enlarged, to form the bulb of the penis.

The penis functions as a carrier for the urethra, through which passes urine and semen – as a reproductive organ, the penis is penetrative, designed to deliver the sperm into the female reproductive tract.

Male Hormones

Spermatogenesis and the production of testosterone are regulated by an inter-relationship between the hypothalamus, anterior pituitary gland and testes, which is similar to the control of the female gonads; however, unlike in the female, control of the male gonads is not cyclical. In response to the release of gonadotrophin-releasing hormone (GnRH) from the hypothalamus, the anterior pituitary gland releases follicle-stimulating hormone (FSH) and luteinizing hormone (LH). The FSH stimulates spermatogenesis in the testes, whereas LH binds to the interstitial cells and stimulates them to secrete testosterone. The sperm count and the level of testosterone are kept fairly constant by a feedback mechanism – when the sperm count is high, release of a protein hormone called inhibin is increased (this inhibits the release of FSH) and, conversely, when the sperm count is low inhibin secretion decreases.

Testosterone is vital for spermatogenesis and is also responsible for the secondary sex characteristics which appear around the time of puberty. These pubertal changes include the appearance of pubic, axillary, facial and chest hair, a deepening of the voice, thickening of the skin, bone growth and an increase in size and mass of skeletal muscles. Testosterone is also responsible for an increase in basal metabolic rate and is the basis of the sex drive.

Spermatogenesis

Spermatogenesis begins at puberty and continues throughout the man's adult life. It occurs in the seminiferous tubules within the testes under the influence of FSH and testosterone. In response to FSH, the sustentacular (Sertoli) cells within the seminiferous tubules release androgen-binding protein, which enables the spermatogenic cells to bind and concentrate testosterone, which in turn stimulates spermatogenesis.

The entire process of spermatogenesis takes approximately 68 days, during which time each sperm goes through several stages; from primary to secondary spermatocyte, to spermatid and finally to spermatozoon, by which time it has a head, body and tail.

At the end of the process, when the sperm are released into the lumen, they are still immature, so maturation continues as they progress through the tubular system of the testes into the epididymis.

A mature spermatozoon consists of a head which contains the deoxyribonucleic acid (DNA), a body which provides the energy required for the propulsion of the sperm and a tail which whips around in order to propel the sperm forward at a rate of 1–4 mm per minute. The head also has a helmet-like covering called an acrosome which enables the sperm to penetrate the ovum.

Normal Sexual Response

Although they received much criticism regarding the methodological approach and subjects used (some of them were prostitutes), the research undertaken by Masters and Johnson in the 1960s (Masters and Johnson, 1966) provided the first comprehensive explanation of the human sexual response; much research around this subject carried out since the publication of their work used their findings as a starting point.

Masters and Johnson (1966) suggested that the normal sexual response involves four overlapping phases:
• Excitement phase.
• Plateau phase.
• Orgasmic phase.
• Resolution.

The physiological factors involved in each of these phases are described below, and although these are necessarily different in the female and the male, the overall response was described by Masters and Johnson as being fundamentally the same in both sexes. The excitement phase is initiated by whatever the individual finds stimulating and continues as sexual tension increases until the plateau phase is reached. The plateau phase ends as the individual reaches a climax, this being the orgasmic phase which involves an involuntary response. Resolution, when sexual tension decreases and the individual returns to the unstimulated state, marks the completion of the response cycle.

Female physiological response

During the excitement phase the clitoris, vaginal mucosa and breasts become engorged with blood. Vaginal lubrication occurs, the labia minora, labia majora and clitoris increase in size, the uterus elevates away from the bladder and vagina, and the nipples become erect. As the woman reaches the plateau phase, the outer third of the vagina becomes engorged with blood and distends, the clitoris retracts and the 'sex flush' (Masters and Johnson, 1966), a measles-like rash, may spread from the breasts to all parts of the body. During the orgasmic phase there is a peak and then a release of muscle tension as blood is forced out of the engorged blood vessels. The woman's pulse, respiration rate and blood pressure all rise, and rhythmic contractions of the uterus occur. Orgasm is accompanied by an intense sensation of pleasure. Unless the woman is stimulated to reach another orgasm, she is then in a phase of resolution during which time all the organs return to their normal size and state.

Male physiological response

The main male response during the excitement phase is erection of the penis, which is caused by engorge-ment of the vascular spaces of the corpora cavernosa. Shortening of the spermatic cords, causing the testes to be drawn up further into the scrotal sac, begins during the excitement phase and continues into the plateau phase, when it is accompanied by a marked rise in pulse and respiration rates, and in blood pressure. The orgasmic phase is chiefly characterized by ejaculation. This occurs as a result of the emptying of the contents of the reproductive ducts and glands into the urethra (caused by peristaltic contractions) and propulsion of semen from the urethra, caused by rapid contractions of the bulbospongiosus muscles of the penis. During orgasm there is also a further increase in pulse, respiration rate and blood pressure. Once orgasm has been reached the male enters the resolution period, when there is muscular relaxation, vasoconstriction of the arterioles serving the penis (causing the penis to return to a flaccid state) and a gradual return to normal levels of the vital signs. In the male, resolution is followed by a latent period when the man is unable to achieve another erection.

Psychological Aspects of Sexual Arousal

Although the human sexual response can be explained in physiological terms, there are many psychological factors that can influence the process. For both partners to achieve all phases of the sexual response there needs to be an initial attraction which leads to sexual stimulation. This attraction may in part be triggered by sensory mechanisms such as smell, visual signals or tactile stimuli. Although humans, unlike most mammals, do not have the dual olfactory system which makes the sense of smell so important, there is evidence that the human olfactory system has some influence on reproductive behaviour; for example, the results of research by Hassett (1978) suggest that smelling the substances found in vaginal secretions may stimulate the desire for intercourse in some couples. There is also an enormous market for scents, perfumes and deodorants although, as Bancroft (1989) observed, 'this may be as much concerned with masking unattractive odours as exploiting attractive ones'!

Visual stimuli vary from person to person; whereas some people may be aroused by photographs of the opposite sex naked or by pictures of couples engaged in sexual activity, others may view this with disgust and therefore not be aroused at all. Tactile stimulation plays an important role in all phases of sexual response – before and during the excitement phase touching the other person's body, particularly the breasts and genitals (Kinsey *et al.* 1965), kissing and stroking may all enhance feelings of arousal. During the plateau and orgasmic phases arousal is maintained by bodily contact and during resolution many couples enjoy a feeling of warmth and closeness as their bodies relax.

Human emotions play a vital part in sexual arousal; although desire increases sexual arousal, feelings such as shame, guilt, disgust and fear inhibit the sexual response. These negative emotions may be caused by many different factors:

- A traumatic past experience such as sexual abuse may cause shame and anger.
- Guilt at the enjoyment of sex may be felt by someone brought up to believe that sex is sinful.
- Fear may be caused by ignorance (for example, an individual with little knowledge of basic human anatomy may believe that certain sexual practices are harmful), by feelings of low self esteem or by a lack of trust in their partner.

Finally, for both partners to be able to enjoy a sexual experience the 'mood' needs to be right – for example, some couples need total privacy and complete darkness before they feel able to enjoy any form of sexual activity. There is a need for each partner to understand and respect the feelings and preferences of the other in order for sex to be mutually satisfying.

Conception

For conception to occur several criteria need to be met:

- Sexual intercourse must occur during the appropriate part of the female reproductive cycle.
- The woman must release a healthy ovum at ovulation.
- The man must release sufficient normal, healthy sperm at ejaculation.
- There must be no barriers or obstructions that prevent the sperm from reaching, penetrating and ultimately fertilizing the ovum.

Conception is most likely to be successful if sexual intercourse occurs just before ovulation – sperm can live for 3–4 days in the female genital tract and should ideally be in the Fallopian tubes when ovulation occurs, as the ovum can only live for 12–24 hours. The woman can predict ovulation by monitoring changes in her body; for example, around the time of ovulation the cervix shortens, softens and dilates slightly. One of the most accurate indicators of ovulation is the state of the cervical mucus, which becomes transparent, slippery and copious (Flynn,

1992). The mucus can also be stretched, a property known as spinnbarkeit. Following ovulation the mucus again becomes thick, sticky and decreases in quantity (Norman, 1986). One further observation which the woman can make is of her basal body temperature, which rises by approximately 0.2°C immediately following ovulation.

Although approximately 300 million sperm are deposited in the posterior fornix of the vagina at intercourse, it is estimated that only a few thousand reach the Fallopian tubes. The majority fail to survive the journey as they leak out of the vagina, are unable to pass through the cervical mucus or are destroyed by the acid medium of the vagina or by the phagocytic leucocytes within the uterus. As there is such an enormous wastage of sperm, to maximize the chance of conception the number of healthy, motile sperm contained in the ejaculate needs to be high.

Before a sperm is capable of penetrating and fertilizing an ovum, it must undergo a process known as capacitation (lasting approximately 7 hours), whereby the sperm membrane becomes fragile and the release of hydrolytic enzymes from the acrosome (the helmet-like covering on the sperms head) is made possible. These enzymes (hyaluronidase, and proteinases) must digest the corona radiata and the zona pellucida before the membrane of the ovum can be reached; although numerous sperm are involved in this digestive process, only one single sperm is allowed to penetrate the ovum. As soon as one sperm enters the ovum, chemical changes occur that initially prevent any further sperm from fusing with the ovum membrane and subsequently detach all remaining sperm from the ovum.

Once the sperm has entered the ovum, it remains temporarily in the peripheral cytoplasm while the female nucleus matures and the female chromosome number reduces from 46 to 23. The ovum and sperm nuclei swell and move towards one another as female and male pronuclei while a 'spindle' develops between them. The pronuclei membranes then rupture and the released chromosomes combine to form the zygote, this being the actual moment of fertilization.

Infertility

Although it should be the right of all individuals to choose whether and when to have children, for some people having a child is difficult or even impossible. The causes of this 'involuntary childlessness' are usually physiological, although social and psychological factors may also be influential. If a person is described as being infertile, it is implied that it has been proved medically that pregnancy is impossible; the term subfertile is used until absolute infertility is proved. In 1988 the World Health Organization (WHO) defined subfertility as the inability to achieve a pregnancy after 1 year of unprotected intercourse (WHO, 1988); this definition has been used as the basis for advice to couples as to when to seek medical help. However, it causes just one of the many dilemmas surrounding subfertility and its treatment – namely, as the trend for delaying childbearing continues (Central Statistical Office, 1995) and as fertility rates decline with increasing age (van Noord-Zaadstra *et al.* 1991), should a couple in their late 30s delay seeking help for a whole year even though, biologically, the time for childbearing is running out? In this section, some of the causes of infertility, plus the usual investigations performed and treatment available, are described. Assisted conception is then considered and some of the ethical implications using reproductive technology are discussed briefly. Having explored the midwife's role in helping women and their partners with fertility problems, the section concludes with one woman's account of her experience of fertility treatment.

Causes, Investigations and Treatment

Causes of infertility can be divided into three approximately equal groups: one-third of problems relate to the woman, one-third to the man and one-third are either caused by a combination of both male and female factors or by unexplained causes.

Female infertility

To become pregnant, the woman needs to be ovulating regularly, her ova need to be normal and there should be no obstruction to the passage of sperm or implantation of the fertilized ovum. Causes of female infertility, which can be physical, psychosocial or a combination of both, can therefore be divided between ovulatory problems or a blockage or abnormality in the reproductive tract.

Ovulatory problems
Causes
As normal ovulation is under hormonal control, certain irregularities within the endocrine system could

affect fertility. By revisiting the sequence of events that result in ovulation, the pertinent areas of the endocrine system become apparent. First, the hypothalamus needs to release gonadotrophin releasing factors which act on the pituitary gland, causing the release of FSH and LH. The FSH stimulates a follicle to ripen and causes the production of oestrogen, and the LH stimulates the release of the ovum and the production of progesterone. Production of oestrogen and progesterone is also influenced by the levels of circulating prolactin from the pituitary gland.

Ovulatory problems can therefore be caused by dysfunction of the hypothalamus, pituitary gland or thyroid gland (as raised prolactin levels may be caused by a problem with either the pituitary or thyroid glands). From a psychological perspective, a correlation has also been demonstrated (among couples attending an infertility clinic) between hyperprolactinaemia and high levels of stress, although there is a need for more research into the effects of stress on fertility (Edelmann and Golombok, 1989). Systemic diseases including diabetes mellitus, coeliac disease and renal failure, which affect endocrine function and may also interfere with the normal cycle.

Even though there may be normal hormonal function, disorders of the ovary may influence ovulation. For example, ovarian cysts or tumours, polycystic ovary disease or damage to the ovaries as a result of endometriosis or previous surgery could interfere with the ovarian cycle and thus influence fertility. Further, there could be problems with the production and release of ova; for example, the ova that are produced may be released before they are fully mature, or they may be persistently defective (they may have chromosomal abnormalities, for instance). Another problem could be that the ova reach maturity but are not released and therefore cannot be fertilized.

Finally, ovulatory function may be affected by women being underweight (those suffering from anorexia nervosa are often amenorrhoeic), by being overweight [severe obesity has been found to cause menstrual difficulties (Pickard, 1984)] or by over-exercising [for example, the rigorous training undertaken by professional athletes has been shown to delay the onset of menarche in young girls, and to cause secondary amenorrhoea in older women (Marieb, 1989)].

Investigations
By taking a full and thorough history some causes can be identified or excluded; for example, if the woman has an existing disorder, such as diabetes, or if she is

severely underweight, then these existing conditions need to be considered as the cause of infertility.

In the absence of any obvious cause, certain investigations can be performed. To ascertain the levels of circulating oestrogen, progesterone, LH and FSH, a series of blood tests can be taken throughout the menstrual cycle. Ovulation can be confirmed by the use of a predictor test which measures the amount of LH in the urine. This test can be done by the woman, who can also examine her cervical mucus to detect the anticipated changes throughout the menstrual cycle. Finally, an ultrasonographic scan can be performed to visualize a ripening follicle and release of an ovum.

Treatment

If existing disorders are thought to be the cause of infertility, then management of the underlying condition may need to be revised; if diabetes, this would be done in consultation with an endocrinologist. Severe weight problems need to be addressed – an appropriate diet needs to be worked out and the woman should be offered help to maintain it.

Hormone imbalances can be corrected with the use of drugs, the most common of which are clomiphene, human chorionic gonadotrophin, human menopausal gonadotrophin and bromocriptine. Clomiphene, a synthetic compound, is taken orally and induces ovulation by stimulating the pituitary (via the hypothalamus) to release FSH. It may be used in conjunction with human chorionic gonadotrophin, which acts in the same way as LH. Human menopausal gonadotrophin is an injectable substance used when clomiphene has been tried and failed. Bromocriptine is used to correct hyperprolactinaemia, which may be suppressing ovulation. These drugs can also be used to stimulate ovulation as part of an assisted conception regime (*see below*).

Reproductive tract problems
Causes

Problems within the female reproductive tract may inhibit the movement of the ova to the uterus, prevent the passage of sperm or inhibit implantation of the fertilized ovum.

Blockage of the fallopian tubes is one of the more common causes of subfertility; it may occur as a result of infection or tubal surgery, or be due to adhesions caused by endometriosis or inflammation (Hall *et al.* 1974). Although *Escherichia coli*, among others, has been found to cause pelvic inflammatory disease (PID), the most common organisms that can lead to PID are *Neisseria gonorrhoeae*, *Mycoplasma hominis*

and *Chlamydia trachomatis*, 50–75% of which are sexually transmitted (Austin, 1989). Other causes of PID include medical procedures, such as vacuum aspiration, dilatation and curettage, or it may follow peritonitis. PID is also more common among women who use the intrauterine contraceptive device, particularly young nulliparous women (Kaufman et al. 1983).

If the passage of sperm is blocked for some reason, then fertilization will obviously not occur. One cause of obstruction is cervical mucus that remains 'hostile' to the sperm even during the fertile phase (before and during ovulation), preventing sperm from reaching the uterus. The woman's body could also be producing antibodies that appear in the cervical mucus and attack the sperm, which are seen as foreign bodies. Some structural abnormalities of the female reproductive system (either congenital or caused by trauma or surgery) may block the passage of sperm, and other structural anomalies may prevent implantation. For example, the uterus may be congenitally abnormal or may contain fibroids which are either very large or situated so as to cause a blockage.

Investigations

Again, all investigations should begin with a thorough history, which may reveal a past history of PID, for example, or a known structural abnormality of the uterus. A general physical examination may then be performed. Specific investigations include laparoscopy, hysterosalpingography and a postcoital test:

- Laparoscopy, which is carried out under general anaesthesia, allows the Fallopian tubes to be examined for patency and evidence of PID or endometriosis. Abnormalities of the ovaries can also be ascertained.
- During a hysterosalpingography, opaque dye is injected through the cervix and radiography is then performed to determine the patency of the tubes and shape of the uterine cavity.
- In the postcoital test, the cervical mucus is examined approximately 6 hours following intercourse, ideally around the time of ovulation. Unsuccessful penetration of the mucus by the sperm is indicative of either hostile sperm or poor quality sperm (or both).

Treatment

Surgery may be indicated to correct some reproductive tract problems – for example, myomectomy (fibroids in the uterine cavity or large ovarian cysts may need to be surgically removed) or ovarian cystectomy. Laser surgery may also be used in an attempt to unblock the Fallopian tubes, although this technique has limited success. To reduce hostility of the cervical mucus, hormonal treatment can be used.

Male infertility

Causes of male infertility can be divided into defective spermatogenesis and problems associated with transport or delivery of the sperm to the ovum.

Defective spermatogenesis
Causes

The two main problems of spermatogenesis are that too few sperm are produced or that the motility of the sperm is poor. Low sperm production (oligospermia – defined as fewer than 20×10^6 per ml) or failure to produce any sperm (azoospermia) may be due to several different factors. For sperm to be produced normally, the amount of testosterone needs to be kept at a reasonable level, and as the production of testosterone is dependent on the levels of FSH and LH, any dysfunction of the hypothalamus or pituitary gland, which control the levels of these hormones, ultimately affects spermatogenesis. (Of less significance are the functions of the thyroid and adrenal glands, although disturbance in the functions of either of these endocrine glands could affect fertility.) As spermatogenesis occurs in the testes, any testicular disorder also affects fertility to some extent. Sperm production may be affected by congenital disorders, such as hydrocele or undescended testes (cryptorchidism), or by acquired problems, such as varicocele or following mumps. Also, as the temperature for optimal sperm production is below body temperature, spermatogenesis is assumed to be less efficient in men in certain occupations (furnacemen, long-distance lorry drivers), or among men who wear tight underpants. Other environmental threats, such as excessive alcohol, smoking, recreational drugs, radiation, lead and certain antibiotics (penicillin and tetracycline, for instance) may also affect spermatogenesis.

Investigations

As for the woman, a thorough history and general physical examination of the man should precede any specific tests as these may reveal existing conditions (an endocrine disorder, for example, or undescended testicles).

The initial specific test to be carried out is semen analysis – volume of semen, total sperm count and quality of sperm (motility and percentage of abnormal sperm) are assessed by performing the postcoital test (*see above*). Other investigations include blood tests, which may reveal hormonal imbalances, and testicular biopsy, which could be performed to confirm sperm production.

Treatment

Hormonal treatment may be indicated if the sperm count is low or if the sperm is of poor quality; for example, clomiphene, human chorionic gonadtrophin, bromocryptine or testosterone may be prescribed. If a varicocele is present then this can be surgically ligated – although varicocele is the cause of infertility in only a small percentage of men, the operation is usually worthwhile as it has been shown to double the chance of pregnancy (Pfeffer and Woollett, 1983). Surgery to rectify undescended testicles needs to be performed during childhood, so if a man presents with this problem it cannot be rectified.

Health education is indicated if the problem is thought to be associated with the man's lifestyle – this advice may range from a change in occupation to avoiding tight clothing.

Sperm Transport and Delivery Problems
Causes

Before they reach the ovum, the sperm need to be transported from the testes to the penis. Problems with this part of the process could be a blockage in the vas deferens, or an obstruction (or even absence) of the seminal vesicles.

The second part of the process is the delivery of the sperm to the vagina; for this to occur the man must be able to achieve and maintain an erection, and then to ejaculate.

Erection occurs when the blood vessels of the corpora cavernosa of the penis dilate and become engorged with blood, thus causing rigidity. The man needs to be able to maintain this stiffness for sufficient time to achieve coitus. If a man has never been able to achieve this, he is described as suffering from primary impotence; if the problem arises even though coitus has been achieved in the past, it is termed secondary impotence.

Causes of impotence may be physiological or psychological. Physical causes include such problems as neuromuscular disease or certain endocrine disorders, which may prevent transmission of impulses from the spinal cord to the penis. Psychologically, impotence may be caused by a fear of failure, which may originate in the person's upbringing or may be a result of a previous unsatisfactory sexual experience. Secondary impotence may also be caused by excessive alcohol consumption or be drug-induced.

Investigations

Specific physical tests that may be performed, having taken a history and performed a general examination, include vasography and certain blood tests. Vasography involves the use of opaque dye and radiography, and is used to check normality of the vas deferens. Blood tests may be undertaken to exclude endocrine disorders.

If impotence of a psychological origin is thought to be the cause of infertility, this should become apparent during the initial interview – the specific problem can then be identified through further questioning.

Treatment

If the vas deferens are blocked, then surgery may be successful in removing the obstruction. If the problem is psychological in origin, then psychosexual counselling could be offered to the man alone, or to the couple together.

Female and male infertility

Occasionally infertility is the result of a combination of causes and both the woman and man need to undergo investigations and treatment.

Note: Ideally, even though the cause can be identified as affecting either the woman or the man, both partners should be involved in the investigations and treatment, in order to try and minimize the chance of blame being apportioned.

Combined causes

Infertility may be caused by a combination of some of the problems stated above – for example, if the woman has partially blocked Fallopian tubes *and* the motility of her partners sperm is poor, then fertilization is unlikely. The problem could also be associated with the couple's sexual behaviour; if sexual intercourse occurs very infrequently and never around the time of ovulation, then conception will not occur. Finally, there could be stress felt by both partners if, for instance, there is pressure on them from relatives to produce a child; this could adversely affect both the act of intercourse (the man may not be able to achieve an erection) and the hormonal balance (there may be hyperprolactinaemia).

Investigations

A fundamental investigation is to ascertain the couple's pattern of sexual activity, to ensure that intercourse is taking place at the optimal time for conception. It is also vital to assess the psychological state of both partners. Therefore, the history needs to be taken from the couple with great sensitivity, in a suitable environment and by an appropriate health professional. Physical tests (such as laparoscopy, postcoital test, blood tests) should be performed where indicated.

Treatment

Appropriate treatment is offered to either or both partners, depending on the problems identified.

Assisted Conception

Once a diagnosis has been made, appropriate treatment can be advised – as described above, initial treatment may involve surgery, drugs or counselling. However, for many couples either no cause for their infertility can be identified or they need further assistance in their attempt to conceive. Several methods of assisted conception are now considered; each technique is described and indications for its use mentioned. Each section concludes with information regarding regulations, legal requirements and/or ethical considerations pertaining to the particular technique. One woman's experience of infertility is described on page 59 (case study 3.1). The regulations and legal requirements are taken from the Human Fertilisation and Embryology Act 1990, an Act which came about as a result of the findings of the Warnock Committee Report of 1984, which was itself commissioned by the Government following the birth of the first 'test-tube' baby in 1978.

Artificial insemination by husband (AIH)

This procedure involes the use of the sperm from the husband and the woman's ova.

Technique

Artificial insemination by either 'husband' (the term 'husband' is used although the couple do not have to be married) or donor involves placing semen inside a woman's vagina or uterus by means other than sexual intercourse. Around the time his partner is due to ovulate, the husband is required to provide a semen sample through masturbation. The sperm are separated from the remainder of the ejaculate and then injected into the vagina or uterus – the technique for placing the sperm in the uterus is more complex, but is more likely to be successful as the cervix, which may be producing hostile mucus, is by-passed.

Indications

This technique is appropriate when the man's sperm count is low (oligospermia), when there are cervical problems such as hostile mucus, when the man is unable to ejaculate during intercourse or if he is unable to achieve intercourse because of physical disability. This method may also be used if the man is to undergo treatment which may render him sterile (chemotherapy or radiotherapy for example); in this instance the man's sperm is frozen before treatment, stored and then used at a later time.

Additional information
If the man's sperm are to be stored, he has to sign a consent form to allow their use at a later date.

Artificial insemination by donor (DIH)

The DIH procedure like AIH involves the use of the woman's ova but in this case insemination is with donor sperm.

Technique
The technique for artifical insemination by a donor is similar to that of insemination by the husband, except that the sperm from a donor are used. Donors are often students or men who have already had children. They undergo careful screening to ensure that they are fit, healthy and of reasonable intelligence; that there is no family history of genetic disorders; and that they are free of any sexually transmitted diseases including human immunodeficiency virus (HIV). As far as possible, donors are also matched for physical characteristics such as height, skin, hair and eye colouring and even blood group. The donated sperm is stored for at least 3 months, after which time it is retested for HIV.

Indications
If the husband has azoospermia or if the sperm quality is very poor, if there is a need to avoid inherited disorders or if there is no male partner, then donor sperm should be used.

Additional information
A register was set up on August 1, 1991, to monitor information concerning both the individuals undergoing licensed fertility treatments and the donors. The register is kept by the Human Fertilisation and Embryology Authority (HFEA), which was created in response to the Human Fertilisation and Embryology Act 1990. The duty of the HFEA is to 'monitor treatment and research, both in general and at particular centres. In time it will also have a legal duty to tell adults who ask whether they were born as a result of treatment using donated eggs or sperm. People aged 16 and over, who ask, will be told whether the register shows they are related to someone they want to marry' (HFEA, 1992). To be able to provide this information, all centres offering artifical insemination by a donoar must be licensed by the HFEA, who also stipulate that there should be a maximum of 10 paternities from any sperm donor. The sperm donor is not considered to be the legal father of any resulting child.

In-vitro fertilization/embryo transfer (IVF/ET)

In-vitro (literally 'in glass') fertilization involves collecting sperm and ova, 'mixing' them outside the body and then returning any fertilized eggs to the woman's uterus.

Technique
There are several stages which the couple have to go through: first they are given information and counselling, after which they must give consent regarding the use and storage of their sperm and ova, consent to treatment and consent to disclosure of identifying information.

The first part of the actual procedure is induction of ovulation, which is achieved with the use of drugs such as buserelin (which suppresses the woman's own hormones), human menopausal gonadotrophin, which stimulates the production of a number of ova in the ovaries, and human chorionic gonadotrophin, which ripens the ova in order that they can be fertilized. Ovulation is monitored with the use of ultrasonography.

Ovum collection, the second stage, is normally performed transvaginally under the guidance of an ultrasound scan. Before the procedure, which normally takes between 5 and 20 minutes, the woman is given a tranquillizer and pain killer. She is then advised to rest for about 1 hour after the procedure, before returning home. Occasionally ovum collection has to be performed via laparoscopy under local or general anaesthesia. At the same time as the ovum collection, the husband needs to provide a semen sample to be prepared for fertilization. Once both the ovum or ova and the sperm have been prepared, they are placed together in a dish in an incubator where fertilization occurs and the ova becomes known as a zygote (embryo).

The third stage of the procedure is the transfer of embryos into the uterus. This normally takes place 48 hours after the egg collection and is achieved by passing a catheter through the cervix and depositing up to three embryos in the uterine cavity.

Indications

In-vitro fertilization/embryo transfer is suitable for women who have tubal damage, cervical problems or endometriosis; for men whose sperm quality may be poor; and for couples in whom no cause for infertility can be found. It may be the first treatment of choice or may follow artifical insemination using the husband's or donor's sperm.

Additional information

All centres offering IVF/ET must be licensed by the HFEA and all relevant consent forms completed prior to treatment. There may be variations on the procedure described above – for example, donated sperm and/or ova may be used. In this case, the couple undergoing treatment are considered the legal parents of any child born (not the donor). Also, a technique known as intracytoplasmic sperm injection (ICSI) may be used, whereby the sperm is actually injected into the egg.

The chances of success for IVF/ET can be measured in terms of the percentage of treatment cycles resulting in a pregnancy [estimated as 16.9% in 1992 (HFEA, 1995)], or as the percentage of treatment cycles resulting in a baby [estimated as 12.7% in 1992 (HFEA, 1995)]. Although these success rates are gradually improving, many couples remain childless even after undergoing several cycles of treatment; it is the issue of 'when to stop trying' that has caused much debate. Several factors influence this decision – the cost of treatment shows wide variations throughout the country, as does availability; some centres restrict the number of attempts, others may not offer treatment to women over a certain age (usually 40 years old) or to single women. If the couple has to be treated privately, then the number of attempts they undergo obviously depends on what they can afford. Other couples find that their relationship suffers as a result of the constant focus on the quest for a child (see **Case Study 3.1**). Unfortunately, many couples feel unsupported and isolated, and are unable to make an informed choice about whether to continue with treatment.

Gamete intrafallopian transfer and zygote intrafallopian transfer

Each of these procedures is similar to in-vitro fertilization in that ovulation is induced and ova are collected.

Technique

In gamete intrafallopian transfer (GIFT) the ova are added to the prepared sperm immediately after col-lection and then placed in the distal end of a patent fallopian tube where fertilization takes place. During zygote intrafallopian transfer (ZIFT) the ova are also returned to the fallopian tube, but they are fertilized *in vitro* and then returned as zygotes.

Indications

Both GIFT and ZIFT are suitable for women who have patent, healthy fallopian tubes, but who have a cervical problem such as hostile mucus.

Additional information

Donated sperm and/or ova can be used in both GIFT and ZIFT, in which case the regulations as defined by the HFEA apply.

Surrogacy

Surrogacy can be defined as 'the practice whereby one woman carries a child for another with the intention that the child should be handed over at birth' (DHSS, 1984). There are several variations regarding surrogacy. The commissioning mother may or may not be the genetic mother, and the genetic father may be the husband of the commissioning mother, or of the carrying mother, or he may be an anonymous donor. Also, the egg could have been donated by a relative (for example, a sister) of the commissioning mother, although extra counselling for all members of the family is recommended in this case. Surrogacy is legal in the UK as long as it is not done for financial gain. When the child is born, the carrying mother is the legal mother – the commissioning parents must apply to the court within 6 months of birth to become the legal parents. Surrogacy is probably the most controversial of all fertility treatments but at present is not common.

The Role of the Midwife

Unless she/he is working in a specialized area, such as an Assisted Conception Unit or an Ultrasound Scanning Department, the midwife is unlikely to have much direct contact with women who are undergoing fertility treatment. However, to give optimal care, the midwife needs sufficient knowledge of the current fertility treatments available to be able to advise women who have a history of fertility problems. The midwife also needs to understand not only of the procedures involved, but also the sort of pressure that couples undergoing fertility treatment may be experiencing. As for all women, if the midwife offers individualized care and continuity of carer she will be able to identify and hopefully meet the needs of women for whom conception is not straightforward.

Family Planning

There are a number of methods that can be used for family planning. Some are more reliable than others and some have greater advantages than others with varying degrees of risk. **Tables 3.1–3.5** summarize methods, advantages and disadvantages identifying medical contraindications. The most important thing is the acceptability of the method used by the couple. Effective family planning implies that an individual can control when and whether they have children; that is, that they can exercise free choice. In many instances this choice and ultimately the individual's control over their own fertility is restricted, whether by physiological, social or cultural factors. In this section several aspects of family planning are addressed – having discussed the methods of contraception available, some of the factors which influence choice of method are considered. Family planning around the time of childbearing is then discussed with a particular emphasis on the midwife's role.

Case study 3.1

One woman's experience of fertility treatment

I became an infertility treatment addict in November 1988 when I attempted my first GIFT. My husband and I both wanted children very much. We had married in March 1986 and I had my IUCD removed a couple of months before. We ran a transport business together, but the financial and mental pressures were quite intense. In May 1988 we separated for a month. When we reunited we decided to seek medical help regarding our childless state. I had been a nurse and was lucky enough to get an appointment in July with a gynaecology consultant I knew. He booked me in for a laparoscopy at the local National Health Service (NHS) hospital in October, which showed no abnormalities and which was the most painful and unpleasant of any treatments I was to undergo.

The consultant then referred us to a fertility consultant, a colleague of his at a private hospital; as it was private we commenced as soon as the blood tests were completed. The staff were tremendously helpful and kind. After the stress of organizing the regular injections of Pergonal, remembering to sniff the buserelin spray and swallowing gallons of water for the frequent scans, it was almost a relief to reach the operation stage.

Unfortunately, the first attempt failed. We were both upset but determined to persevere. We already knew my husband had a low sperm count. He saw a consultant in andrology and had a ligation of left varicocele in February 1989. By this time, to complicate matters, my husband was having an affair and we separated again (for a few months). We had another attempt at GIFT in September 1989. This failed and they found that one of my Fallopian tubes was not patent and the other one was twisted. My consultant recommended IVF. I was on a 'rollercoaster' now and proceeded to have six attempts at IVF during the next 9 months (even though) I was living apart from my husband. Proceeding with each next attempt gave me the strength to overcome the devastation I felt after each failure. It was a hard time emotionally, especially with the lack of a happy marriage.

My eighth attempt in August 1990 was the long awaited success – I was PREGNANT with TWINS! To say I was ecstatic would be an understatement. However, at 7 weeks I had a slight bleed and have never been so terrified in all my life. I was told to rest, but unfortunately I lost one of the twins. I was disappointed, especially after the initial scans had shown both heartbeats, but I was so concerned for the baby I still carried that I brainwashed myself with the advantages of a single and hopefully uncomplicated birth. During this scariest part of the ride on my fertility 'rollercoaster' my mother became ill and, sadly, died.

Happily, there were no more pregnancy complications and my daughter was born well and hungry on 22nd May 1991. My husband was present at the birth, but more for his own benefit. We made another attempt at mending our marriage, but unfortunately it was not to be.

I'll never forget the first night there with my daughter. It was the moment I had awaited for so long. I watched and held her all night, just unbelievably happy and so relieved that she was all right. She is my little miracle.

Table 3.1 Natural Methods of Family Planning

Method	Advantages	Disadvantages	Medical contraindications
Natural family planning – general	Under woman's control Not related to sexual intercourse (SI) No hormones or mechanical devices involved No side effects No follow up needed Cheap	Need high level of motivation Need thorough explanation (which may not be available)	None
Temperature method	(as above)	Restricts SI to postovulatory phase of the cycle	Temperature may be affected by illness or medication
Cervical mucus	(as above)	Woman must feel comfortable touching her genitals	None
Coitus interruptus	May enhance sexuality as it develops the couple's skills (Mosse and Heaton, 1990)	Reliant on man's control Semen leakage before withdrawal (before ejaculation)	None
Breast feeding	Vital in developing countries to maintain birth intervals (Thapa et al., 1988). Effectiveness rates of up to 98% (Kennedy, et al., 1989)	Woman must breastfeed only	None

Table 3.2 Barrier Methods

Method	Advantages	Disadvantages	Medical contraindications
Diaphragm and cap	Reduced risk of sexually transmitted diseases (STDs) Reduced risk of pelvic inflammatory disease (Kelaghan et al., 1982) Possible protection against cervical cancer No health risks No side effects Woman is in control Allows spontaneity in love-making	Perceived as messy, premeditated, inconvenient and causing reduced sensation for the woman and the man Woman needs to feel comfortable touching her genitals Needs to be fitted Teaching on care of cap required	Diaphragms require good muscle tone
Female condom	Lubricated with spermicide Protection against STDs and HIV Possible protection against cervical cancer (Belfield, 1993) No fitting required Readily available	Perceived as indiscreet Difficult to dispose of Expensive [not supplied free at all family planning clinics (FPCs)]	None
Male condom	(Usually) lubricated with spermicide Protection for both partners against STDs and HIV (Hicks et al., 1985) Widely available Free of charge (from FPCs) No side effects No medical supervision required	Related to sexual intercourse Cannot be used with oil-based products	May cause an allergic reaction

Table 3.3 Hormonal Contraception

Method	Advantages	Disadvantages	Medical contraindications
Combined oral contraceptive pill (COC)	Reliable, reversible, convenient	Unsuitable for breastfeeding women	Medically contraindicated for women who have a history of cardiovascular disease, thrombosis, disorders of lipid metabolism, focal or crescendo migraine, markedly impaired liver function, malignancy of the breast, liver or genital tract, psychosis or severe depression
	Not related to SI	Increased risk of hypertension, arterial and venous disease among some women	Potential drug interactions
	Reduced risk of iron-deficiency anaemia, fibroids, ovarian cysts, ectopic pregnancy and benign breast disease	Possible increased risk of breast and cervical cancer (McEwan, 1985a, 1985b).	Unsuitable for women over 35 years of age who are obese (particularly if they smoke)
	May relieve dysmenorrhoea and premenstrual symptoms	No protection against STDs/HIV Possible pregnancy (Nicholas, 1987)	
	Protection against ovarian and endometrial cancer (Loudon, 1985) and against pelvic inflammatory disease	Side effects include weight gain, nausea, altered libido, mild depression	
Progesterone only pill	Suitable for women who want oral contraception, but who are unable to use the COC pill because of the oestrogenic effects, e.g. breastfeeding women	Maximum time allowed for a forgotten pill is only 3 hours	Possible pregnancy, abnormal vaginal or uterine bleeding of unknown cause, previous ectopic pregnancy, acute liver disease, any serious side effects from the use of the COC pill not attributed to oestrogen
Injectable contraceptive	Reliable, safe and discreet	May cause irregular menstrual bleeding, weight gain, depression	Possible pregnancy, cancer of the breast or genital tract, undiagnosed vaginal or uterine bleeding, past arterial disease
	Not SI related Minimal metabolic effects	Delay in return of fertility (of up to a year)	
	Can be used by breastfeeding women Gives most of the non-contraceptive benefits of the COC pill	Not reversible (until the next injection is due)	
Implant	Highly effective, long term, reversible Requires little supervision	Needs operative procedure (for insertion and removal) Increased risk of functional ovarian cysts and ectopic pregnancy	Possible pregnancy Women who have active thromboembolic disorders, known or suspected cancer of the reproductive organs, acute liver disease
	Not related to SI		
	Does not affect future fertility	May cause intermenstrual bleeding	

Table 3.4 Intrauterine Contraceptive Devices			
Method	**Advantages**	**Disadvantages**	**Medical contraindications**
IUCD (copper coated)	Effective, easily reversible	Side effects include menorrhagia, dysmenorrhoea, intermenstrual bleeding and spotting	Contraindicated among women with a history of pelvic inflammatory disease (Salih, 1987), menorrhagia, undiagnosed abnormal uterine or vaginal bleeding, nulliparous women and women with a distorted uterine cavity
	Associated with low morbidity and mortality Requires little attention (apart from checking the threads) Not related to SI	Increased risk of pelvic infection and ectopic pregnancy	
Hormone-releasing IUCD	(as above) plus a reduced risk of ectopic pregnancy (as compared with the copper IUCD)	(as above)	(as above)

Table 3.5 Sterilization			
Method	**Advantages**	**Disadvantages**	**Medical contraindications**
Female sterilization	Immediately effective, permanent, very effective	Considered irreversible	Relatively contraindicated for women with severe psychiatric disorder, immediately post-Caesarean section or termination, or for women under 20 years of age
		Woman usually needs general anaesthesia	
Male sterilization	Performed under local anaesthesia and is safer and simpler than female sterilization	Not immediately effective	None
		Considered irreversible	

Factors which Influence Choice of Contraception

Factors that influence choice of contraception fall into three main categories – physiological, social and cultural (**Tables 3.1–3.5**).

Physiological

For many women the choice of contraception is necessarily restricted by a history of or an existing medical condition – for example, the combined oral contraceptive pill is contraindicated for a woman with a history of thrombosis, the diaphragm is unsuitable for a woman with an allergy to spermicides or latex, the intrauterine contraceptive device (IUCD) is contraindicated for a woman with a history of PID and all hormonal methods are contraindicated for women with known malignancy of the breast. There are many contraindications to each of the methods (*see above*), which need to be discussed fully before a choice of method is made.

Social

There are many social factors that need to be considered when choosing a method of contraception. Age is important as fertility declines over the age of 31 years (van Noord-Zaadstra *et al.* 1991), making the less effective methods more acceptable to the older woman for whom a permanent method may be more appropriate. Whether contraception is being used to prevent pregnancy completely or for family spacing is also an issue, as effectiveness is obviously more important in the former instance.

If a woman has more than one partner her choice of contraception will be affected, as she may require protection from sexually transmitted diseases in addition to prevention of pregnancy.

The woman's home circumstances need to be considered – if she is living in a bed-sit, sharing washing and toilet facilities, barrier methods such as the diaphragm are inadvisable. Further, if access to family planning services is restricted in any way, then a long-lasting form of contraception, such as an IUCD or subdermal implant, may be the method of choice. A woman's feelings about her body also influence her choice – for example, she may not wish to use anything 'unnatural' and so would choose a natural method. If she feels uncomfortable touching her own genitals, female barrier methods, natural methods and even the IUCD may be contraindicated. Motivation to use any method will improve its effectiveness, so the woman's choice should always be respected and supported despite what may be construed as difficulties, such as a language barrier or low educational attainment.

Cultural

Although culture and religion may have a general influence on choice of contraception, it should never be assumed that the individual woman will conform to the anticipated norm. For example, for a woman from a society which views women who are menstruating as unclean, the IUCD, which prolongs menstrual bleeding and would normally be considered unsuitable, may be the ideal choice. Similarly, many couples who belong to religions where semen is regarded as sacred feel comfortable in their use of chemical barriers, which actually destroy sperm. To give the most effective advice and support, the health professional needs to have a knowledge of religious and cultural restrictions and recommendations, but should also acknowledge and respect the choice of the individual.

Family Planning, Childbearing and the Midwife's Role

The first activity of a midwife as defined in *A Midwife's Code of Practice* (UKCC, 1991) is 'to provide sound family planning information and advice' – within the midwife's sphere of practice there are several opportunities to fulfil this role. The midwife may give advice on family spacing or information regarding availability of services, she may advise a woman on contraceptive options or she may be involved in facilitating the use of a particular method of contraception.

Some examples of the midwife's role in family planning are:
- Preconception: recommending a highly effective method of contraception following a rubella vaccination; advising on stopping the use of contraception; helping a woman who is trying to conceive to predict the time of ovulation.
- During pregnancy: with continuity of carer, it may be appropriate during an antenatal consultation to discuss aspects of postnatal contraception, such as the options available, and when and where to obtain contraception.
- Postpartum: advising on the most appropriate method (taking account of all physical, social and cultural factors); ensuring that the woman has access to family planning facilities; informing the woman of the optimum time to commence the use of her contraceptive method of choice.

Summary

This chapter has addressed several aspects of childbearing which could be considered peripheral to 'mainstream' midwifery, but in which all midwives have some involvement, whether directly or indirectly. It has covered the male reproductive system, the physiological sequence of events from sexual arousal to sexual response, to sexual intercourse and finally to conception. Psychological factors that may hinder this process have also been discussed, and this theme was continued in the second section, which focused on infertility. Having discussed the causes, investigations and treatments available, the reader is challenged to consider the ethical issues that arise from the use of reproductive technology. A case study of one woman's experiences of fertility treatment is included to illustrate how a woman's life may be affected by infertility. In the final section, entitled

Family Planning, the focus is on how control over one's fertility can be achieved with the use of contraception. Although the midwife may feel that her role in this area is limited, she needs to understand the mode of action, advantages, disadvantages, contraindications and efficacy rates of all methods of contraception so that the women in her care can make an informed choice.

KEY CONCEPTS

- It is vital for the midwife to remember that each individual is unique – and to treat them as such.

- Although the human sexual response can be explained in physiological terms, there are many psychological factors which affect this process.

- Although infertility is usually caused by physiological problems, psychological and social factors may also be influential.

- Causes of infertility can be divided into three approximately equal groups – one-third of problems relate to the woman, one-third to the man and one-third are either caused by a combination of both female and male factors or by unexplained causes.

- Many women remain involuntarily childless as, despite rapid progress in reproductive technologies, infertility treatment is often unsuccessful.

- There are numerous moral and ethical issues surrounding infertility treatment – the midwife needs to examine and acknowledge her own personal beliefs and opinions and ensure that they do not compromise her professionalism.

- By facilitating informed choice about contraception, the midwife can enhance an individual's control over their own fertility.

References

Austin CR: *The debate on assisted reproduction*, Oxford, 1989, Oxford University Press.

Bancroft J: *Human sexuality and its problems* 2nd edn, Edinburgh, 1989, Churchill Livingstone.

Belfield T: *FPA contraceptive handbook*, London, 1993, FPA.

CSO: *Social trends*, 1995 edn, London, HMSO.

DHSS: *Report of the Committee of Inquiry into Human Fertilisation and Embryology*, London, 1984, HMSO.

Edelmann RJ, Golombok S: Stress and reproductive failure, *J Reprod Infant Psychol* 7(2):79, 1989.

Flynn AM: Natural methods of family planning control I, *Postgrad Update* 1st July 1992:39, 1992.

Hall R, Anderson J, Smart GA, Besser GM: *Clinical endocrinology* 2nd edn, Philadelphia, 1974, Lippincott.

Hassett J. Sex and smell. *Psychol Today* 11(10):40, 1978.

Hicks DR, Martin LS, Getchell JP: Inactivation of HTLV-III/LAV infected cultures of normal human lymphocytes with nonoxyl-9 *in vitro*, *Lancet* ii(16 Nov):1422, 1985.

HFEA: *The role of the HFEA*, London, 1992, Human Fertilisation and Embryology Authority.

HFEA: *In vitro fertilisation*, London, 1995, Human Fertilization and Embryology Authority.

Kaufman DW, Watson J, Rosenberg L *et al.*, The effect of different types of intrauterine devices on the risk of pelvic inflammatory disease, *JAMA* 250(6):759, 1983.

Kelaghan J, Rubin GL, Ory HW, Layde PM: Barrier method contraceptives and pelvic inflammatory disease, *JAMA* 248(2): 184, 1982.

Kennedy KI, Rivera R, McNeilly AS: Consensus statement on the use of breastfeeding as a family planning method, *Contraception* 39:477, 1989.

Kinsey AC, Pomeroy WB, Martin CE, Gebhard P: *Sexual behaviour in the human female*, New York, 1965, Pocket Books.

Loudon N, editor: *Handbook of family planning*, Edinburgh, 1985, Churchill Livingstone.

Marieb EN: *Human anatomy and physiology*, California, 1989, The Benjamin/Cummings Publishing Co.

Masters WH, Johnson VE: *Human sexual response*, Boston, 1966, Little Brown.

McEwan J: Hormonal contraception methods, *Practitioner* 229(1403): 415, 1985a.

McEwan J: Hormonal methods of contraception and their adverse effects. In Studd J, editor: *Progress in obstetrics and gynaecology* Vol. 5, Part 2(17):259, Edinburgh, 1985b, Churchill Livingstone.

Mosse J, Heaton J: *The fertility and contraception book*, London, 1990, Faber and Faber.

Nicholas NS: What pill? *Maternal Child Health* 8(12):468, 1987.

Norman C: *Charting the fertility cycle*, Birmingham, 1986, Natural Family Planning Centre.

Pfeffer N, Woollett A: *The experience of infertility*, London, 1983, Virago Press.

Pickard B: *Eating well for a healthy pregnancy*, London, 1984, Sheldon Press.

Salih D: Complications of intra-uterine contraceptive devices, *Maternal Child Health* 12(12): 355, 1987.

Thapa S, Short RV, Potts M: Breastfeeding, child spacing and their effects on child survival, *Nature* 335(10):679, 1988.

UKCC: *A midwife's code of practice*, London, 1991, United Kingdom Central Council for Nursing, Midwifery and Health Visiting.

van Noord-Zaadstra BM, Looman CWN, Alsbach H, *et al.*: Delaying childbearing: effect of age on fecundity and outcome of pregnancy, *Br Med J* 302(8 June): 1361, 1991.

WHO: *Laboratory recommendations*, Geneva, 1988, World Health Organization.

Further Reading

Re: Infertility texts. As the information of infertility treatment and issues is in a constant state of flux, it is difficult to recommend any particular book. However, two texts of interest are: Stanworth M (ed.): *Reproductive technologies, gender, motherhood and medicine*. Cambridge, 1987, Polity Press. Mack S, Tucker J: *Fertility counselling*. London, 1996, Bailliere Tindall.

Andrews G (ed): *Women's sexual health*. London, 1996, Bailliere Tindall.

This comprehensive text is written from a woman-centred perspective. It is divided into three sections: Women today, Family planning and Women's health issues, and encompasses the full range of women's sexual health issues.

Cowper A, Young C: *Family planning. Fundamentals for health professionals* 2nd edn, London, 1989, Chapman and Hall.

As the name implies, this book aims to address the fundamentals of family planning; areas including 'Cervical cytology', 'Special needs' and 'Fertility problems' in addition to chapters on all methods of contraception.

Niven CA, Walker A: *Reproductive potential and fertility control*, 1996, Butterworth Heinmann.

Covers current approaches to reproductive issues and questions common assumptions.

4 *Adaptation to Pregnancy*

LEARNING OUTCOMES

After studying this chapter you should be able to:

- Identify some of the factors influencing psychological well-being in pregnancy.
- Discuss the concepts and the psychological effects of anxiety, stress and psychological illhealth in pregnancy.
- Consider the skills used by the midwife in reducing psychological distress.
- Describe the anatomical changes that occur and how these structural changes determine the physiological response of the woman.
- Recognise how the total body water and blood volume increase dramatically in response to the fetal demands.
- Discuss how fertilization and implantation occur.
- Describe how the placenta acts as an interface between the maternal and fetal circulations.
- Identify how progesterone has a dramatic effect on other organs/systems.

PSYCHOLOGICAL ADAPTATION IN PREGNANCY

As well as maintaining optimum physiological health in pregnancy, one of the main aims of midwifery care is to facilitate healthy psychological adjustment of the woman to pregnancy and motherhood. There are many factors that contribute towards a woman's ability to adapt to her pregnancy and mothering role – for example, social circumstances, social support, the type of professional care and support she receives, as well as her personal characteristics, and conscious and unconscious psychological processes.

It is possible to make many assumptions about how a woman (Jane, for example), might adjust to her new role. If Jane has a demanding job, she will have a new responsibility with the baby as well as a need to consider and organize childcare when she returns to work. A midwife meeting Jane for the first time is aware of how these factors may influence a woman during pregnancy. The stresses relating to the pregnancy itself, the demands of her job and the pressures of arranging childcare are likely to contribute to Jane's anxiety in early pregnancy. The type of support available from her partner and family, and the influences on her expectations and perceptions of pregnancy from her own childhood and upbringing also affect her anxiety levels and coping mechanisms. However, her confidence and pleasure in being pregnant doubtless bring about enjoyment in the preparation and planning for the forthcoming baby. In this chapter some of the factors that may influence a woman's attitude towards her pregnancy and future role are identified; also some of the psychological evidence surrounding adaptation to pregnancy and motherhood is examined.

Pregnancy: Crisis or Normal Life Event?

Pregnancy is traditionally viewed by some psychologists as a time of emotional crisis. This often relates to Erikson's theory of developmental crises. Erikson (1963) proposed that all humans move through a number of life stages or life events each of which marks a transition throughout the lifespan. Erikson believed that progression from one stage to the next is dependent on psychological negotiation of each event or 'crisis' before moving successfully on to the next. The life crisis of 'intimacy versus isolation' in young adulthood, for example, marks the stage at which people develop a need to love another person and make some commitment to that person. As the 'crisis' resolves, the individuals begin to face the next 'crisis' of 'generativity versus stagnation'. Generativity is in turn frequently resolved by having a family. This applies as much to males as females, as a need to contribute to a future generation is then fulfilled.

There are other examples from psychology which suggest, for example, that adjustment to parenthood is one of life's most stressful events. Dohrenwend *et al.* (1978) identified that the birth of the first infant is one of the most stressful events a person can experience in life. Holmes and Rahe (1967) rated pregnancy as the twelfth most stressful life event in the development of their well-known 'Social Readjustment Rating Scale', which has been recognized as a means of quantifying the stresses in daily life. This scale provides a measure for assessing the degree of cumulative stress contributing towards what might be considered as a mild, moderate or severe life crisis, and which in turn may potentially lead to psychological illhealth.

However, such views of pregnancy as a period of crisis are seen by some as perpetuating the maladaptive view, which focused on the 'pathology' of pregnancy and thus emphasized the negativity of pregnancy. Many feminist psychologists paradoxically also identify pregnancy as a potential negative event, but their view is from a different perspective. Oakley (1980) and Ussher (1993) see women's experiences of pregnancy and childbirth as being the consequences of a patriarchal society that denies women the possibility of personal fulfilment. Ussher describes pregnancy and childbirth as 'an intrinsic part of women's experience, regardless of whether or not we decide to give birth to children. These experiences need to be seen in the context of the whole life cycle and of the dominant beliefs surrounding the female body...' (Ussher, 1993, p. 76). Smith argues that many psychological studies view pregnancy from a positivistic perspective and therefore he presents an alternative viewpoint of pregnancy as a period of 'practical and symbolic preparation for motherhood' (Smith, 1992, p. 192). This study draws on the personal experiences of women during pregnancy, and focuses on pregnancy as a normal life transition rather than a medical event or illness.

Discussion within much of the psychological literature therefore relates to whether anxiety in pregnancy presents as psychological distress to the woman and at what level this may become detrimental to health. Bibring was one of the earliest psychologists to describe pregnancy and its outcomes from a psycho-analytic perspective. Her views that pregnancy 'involves intense upheaval of psychological processes... and the possible effects this may have on the attitude of mothers towards their infants' (Bibring, 1959, p. 117) reflected the literature at that time. The focus was then, as it often is now, on the disturbance of the mother–infant relationship, the 'vicious circle' of negative reactions finally resulting in long-term adverse consequences of the relationship. It is, however, important not to lose sight of the fact that for a large proportion of women adaptation to pregnancy and motherhood takes place effectively. This is particularly so when certain factors are acknowledged that make the transition and adaptation easier, such as adequate professional and social support and appropriate advice and information, which facilitate a positive emotional environment. For some women, however, pregnancy outcome is not always positive; this is addressed in later sections.

Psychological Well-Being

Psychological health may be described as an absence of anxiety, depression or the symptoms which people who suffer from different forms of psychological ill-health display (Argyle, 1992). However, there are times when most people inevitably feel some degree of anxiety or stress. In fact, stress may be seen as a normal reaction to adverse conditions which everyone experiences at intervals throughout life. There is, therefore, a need to distinguish between what may be perceived as 'normal', and anxiety and stress that is 'pathological', i.e. detrimental to health or quality of life. Anxiety is often associated with adjustment to pregnancy. Combes and Schonveld (1992), in a major research review commissioned by the Health Education Authority, explored women's experiences, feelings and concerns at different stages of pregnancy. During the first 3 months of pregnancy women were found to express certain anxieties, particularly about labour, being a parent, the baby's health, conflicting advice (especially about diet) and worries about miscarriage. Many of these anxieties disappear during the middle trimester of pregnancy; however, in the last 3 months

anxieties return about labour, as well as worries about body image appearing for the first time.

The majority of women approach pregnancy with an outward feeling of pleasure; nevertheless an underlying anxiety may well exist. Psychologists examine the balance of psychological well-being and psychological illhealth in an attempt to identify predisposing factors and potential outcomes, especially emotional disturbances such as antenatal or postnatal unhappiness and depression. In most situations women are consciously aware of the circumstances which create increased anxiety and distress in pregnancy and childbirth. Midwives are also aware of the degree of immediate emotional distress caused by factors that include obstetric complications in pregnancy, as the majority of women expect a normal healthy pregnancy and are usually devastated if things go wrong. The concern of every midwife is to help a woman to adjust to such events in the most effective way, utilizing the necessary skills to the full.

Unfortunately, pregnancy occasionally ends in tragedy, such as miscarriage, stillbirth or perinatal death. At such times, the effect on the woman and her family is apparent as they deal with their inevitable grief and loss. The long-term psychological effects are, however, not always so clear. Most people have the resources to deal with emotional crises when given the necessary understanding and support from both social networks and health care professionals. However, the human mind copes with and confronts such situations in many ways. The ability to express and work through grief openly comes readily to most people given the right environment. Coping emotionally with tragic events involves conscious and *unconscious* processes, including the psychological 'defence mechanisms' such as repression, denial and splitting.

Severe psychological trauma experienced by some women during pregnancy may include physical and emotional abuse, sexual abuse or relationship problems, any of which are inevitably associated with negative emotional consequences. The midwife needs to be aware of the possible depth of emotion and the potential for negative psychological repercussions when such events are not dealt with adequately at the time they occur. The way that people react in some situations may consequently be influenced even by events that occurred in the distant past. For example, victims and survivors of sexual abuse and sexual assault can have the experience revived by events in pregnancy and childbirth. One woman's very graphic description of her birthing experience, which she could only describe as 'birth rape' (Christensen, 1992), provides some evidence of the emotional and physical trauma of what was for her an unnecessary forceps delivery. Kitzinger (1992) studied the long term effects of sexual abuse – 39 women who had experienced childhood sexual abuse were interviewed and it was found that more than half were reminded of the abuse by events in pregnancy and childbirth, including vaginal examinations, cervical smears, patronizing treatment, being surrounded by medical students and lack of eye contact during medical procedures (reviving 'voyeuristic elements' of sexual abuse).

Coping Behaviour

Worry and anxiety in pregnancy appear to be relatively common, and it seems that the things pregnant women are anxious about are often realistic concerns. In fact, a degree of anxiety may act as a motivational factor towards preparing for imminent parenthood. Niven (1992) refers to this as anticipatory anxiety and identifies how realistic expectations of labour, for example, may reduce levels of pain perception for some women.

In times of increased anxiety and distress individuals adopt certain behaviours or techniques for coping with the event. Pearlin and Schooler referred to coping as the 'things people do to avoid being harmed by life-strains' (Pearlin and Schooler, 1978, p. 2). Psychological research into the responses to stressful situations was undertaken by Lazarus and colleagues (Lazarus, 1966; Lazarus and Folkman, 1984). Using a series of experimental studies Lazarus and his associates identified different cognitive processes that people use when experiencing stress, i.e. anticipatory action, attack, avoidance and inaction. These processes or coping mechanisms can be further divided, first into 'appraisal' of the situation and second into the responses adopted. Coping behaviour is therefore typically 'anticipatory' when planning and preparation for the stressful event is undertaken. Midwives are aware of women who can plan and prepare for the events throughout pregnancy which normally cause anxiety and stress, and who are therefore able to cope more effectively. Early antenatal support (through pregnancy and childbirth preparation classes) and receipt of adequate information are ways to help achieve such planning and preparation. Psychological coping mechanisms frequently involve some form of 'attack' (taking positive action to confront the stress), such as gaining control over the situation. Women who can be assertive and maintain control, or who are empowered by others to have control over the situation, are adopting this aspect of coping behaviour.

Coping responses such as 'avoidance' behaviour may, for example, be demonstrated by a woman who is very anxious and therefore ignores advice or avoids contact with professional support through antenatal clinics and classes. There may even be a degree of denial that the pregnancy exists, the 'burying your head in the sand' phenomenon. Such denial may be at an unconscious level, whereby in extreme situations some women may even totally deny the possibility that they are pregnant, resulting in the inevitable 'undiagnosed' or 'concealed' pregnancy. Continuing anxiety and stress may therefore eventually lead to 'inaction'. The stressed person reaches a stage at which they are just not able to cope with the situation and motivation declines. An image can be conjured up of the pregnant woman who 'finds it all too much', 'doesn't make the effort' or feels that 'everything is hopeless'. It is at this stage that symptoms characteristic of psychological illhealth may become apparent.

Some Factors Influencing Emotional Response to Pregnancy

There are inevitably many factors that are likely to influence a woman's emotional response to pregnancy, and consequently how well she adapts. Some of these factors, together with relevant theoretical concepts, are introduced in the following text.

Planned or Unplanned?

There are many potential causes of increased anxiety in pregnancy, many of which effective midwifery care can help to alleviate. Anxiety concerning the pregnancy itself may be exacerbated, particularly when it is unplanned. Although an unplanned pregnancy appears at first to result in an increased level of stress, studies indicate that this decreases over time. Najman *et al.* (1991) conducted a relatively large prospective study and found that depressed mood in pregnancy diminished over a 6 month period following birth. Although it is possible to distinguish between pregnancy which is unplanned and one which is unwanted, in most cases there appears to be little difference in the long-term emotional outcome. Most women seem to be able to adjust eventually to the infant and experience little psychological illhealth; however, they may need more support and encouragement in order to make the transition effectively. Nevertheless, the potential problems which occur during any period of increased anxiety and stress and the possible 'knock-on' effects should be considered also. The immediate effect of stress on marital and family relationships may have profound long-term consequences. For example, it has been demonstrated that marital happiness reaches a peak low period at the time of childbirth (Argyle, 1992, p. 62). Although information that identifies the proportion of marriages that break down as a result of childbirth is not readily available, it is worth considering that in 1990 alone there were over 106,000 divorces where one or more children were under the age of 16 years (Central Statistics Office, 1994). Although it is not possible to associate marriage breakdown with childbirth from these statistics, there is nevertheless some suggestion that further investigation is necessary.

Many pregnant women become aware of the reality of the baby, particularly when fetal movements are first felt. Wolkind and Zajicek (1981) demonstrated that some women adopt a more positive attitude to their pregnancy at this time. Antenatal care that provides the woman with an opportunity to get to know her baby before its arrival may therefore help to minimize distress. Antenatally, in contrast to listening with the Pinard stethoscope many prefer the Sonicaid 'doppler'. This may be a situation when the use of a Sonicaid to listen to the fetal heart is appropriate, enabling the mother to experience hearing her own baby. An ultrasound scan provides her with an opportunity to visualize the baby. Sympathetic scanning techniques may therefore have a place in helping women adjust positively to their pregnancy and, in addition, may help the father to adapt more easily. May (1981) suggests that fathers adapt more readily to parenthood in the immediate postnatal period, again when the baby is a reality. It is possible, therefore, that fathers may also feel more positive towards the developing pregnancy when the baby is visualized on a scan. Most midwives are aware of the positive reaction of the majority of parents on seeing their baby moving or its heart beating, and maybe even sucking its thumb *in utero*.

There is, however, a view that routine ultrasound scanning should be used with caution (Laurence Beech and Robinson, 1993), suggesting that more research

in this area is required as long-term consequences of ultrasound on the fetus are still somewhat uncertain. In this context, there is a need for research into the psychological consequences for women undergoing scans. Although scanning has been shown to reduce anxiety (Reading and Cox, 1982), Statham *et al.* identify one woman's experience of not being able to see the baby's legs on the scan, '...the picture doesn't show the legs and I have been worried about deformities' (Statham *et al.* 1992, p. 60). The unnecessary distress for this particular woman highlights an aspect of which all those undertaking scanning in pregnancy should be aware. A sensitive approach, along with adequate explanation and information, reduces the possibility of such an event occurring and also provides an opportunity for the woman and her partner to ask questions so that they are not left with the profound emotional distress of such a misunderstanding.

Effect of Obstetric Risk Factors

Other pregnancy-related factors likely to increase anxiety understandably include the experience associated with complications of pregnancy, such as pregnancy-induced hypertension, multiple pregnancy, antepartum haemorrhage, fetal growth retardation or predisposing medical conditions such as diabetes. Spirito *et al.* (1992), for example, examined the stability of mood state in women with diabetes mellitus in pregnancy. This study indicated that women with diabetes were more anxious than nondiabetic women and there was a trend for the diabetic women to be more depressed. Worries and anxieties around pre-existing medical conditions, such as diabetes, epilepsy or asthma, often focus on concerns about whether medication may affect the baby. Combes and Schonveld reported that women with conditions such as asthma worry about whether they can take advantage of the drugs used when in labour and the possible effects of medication during the pregnancy (Combes and Schonveld, 1992, p. 13). This particular review and survey also emphasized that many women would have welcomed more information and advice as well as support, but were either uncertain about where they could obtain such help or did not feel confident about asking for help.

Although there appear to be few research results as to the emotional consequences of a complicated pregnancy, there can be little doubt that the need for more visits to the General Practitioner (GP) and hospital consultant, the possible intervention in pregnancy and potential hospitalization are likely to create distress and disruption for the woman and her family. Centralized maternity services often mean that women have to travel long distances on a regular basis to access such care. Implementation of the Changing Childbirth policy (Department of Health, 1993), which is aimed at reducing emotional, social and practical distress by reducing the number of hospital visits and transferring care to community clinics, will almost certainly help to minimize some of the stress and fear:

> Antenatal care should be provided so as to maximize the use of resources. It should also ensure that the woman and her partner feel supported and fully informed throughout the pregnancy, and are prepared for the birth and care of their baby.
> (Department of Health, 1993, p. 22.)

Anxiety and Age

Spirito *et al.* (1992) also found that younger women and unmarried women are more likely to be at risk of increased emotional distress. It is difficult to identify the source of anxiety for these groups of women, as there are many other potential factors that influence their emotional state. Some of the elements identified as having varying effects on how they adjust to pregnancy are education and employment issues, financial security, level of social support and other social factors, as well as the type of maternity care received.

Teenage pregnancy is therefore commonly associated with adverse psychological outcomes because of the potential long-term effect on education and future career, financial implications of caring for a child, lack of knowledge about childrearing and the psychological struggle at a time of one's own identity formation. There is evidence that pregnancy rates are increased among teenagers in lower socioeconomic groups, which is often associated with poor school attendance before the pregnancy (Ineichen and Hudson, 1994). The opportunity for schoolgirl mothers to continue their education has been somewhat erratic over the years, despite a statutory requirement that children should continue education up to the age of 16 years. Although there are many teenage mothers who adapt well to their mothering role, this group are often in need of psychological and practical support in order to prevent ongoing disadvantage to themselves and, potentially, their infants. Hudson and Ineichen (1991) found that 46% of a sample group of 102 pregnant teenagers had neither planned their pregnancy nor were pleased about it. However, the work of Phoenix (1991) suggests that young women

between the ages of 16 and 19 years are satisfied with motherhood and believe that they cope well; however, the young women in this particular group were well supported by their family.

At the opposite end of the childbearing age spectrum there is an equally common perception that the more mature woman may be influenced by factors which affect her ability to adapt well to pregnancy. The proportion of women who become pregnant for the first time at 35 years of age and over is steadily increasing (Registrar General, 1994). The risk of fetal congenital abnormality, such as Down's syndrome, is known to be increased for this age group. There may be a possible subfertility factor, if the woman has been attempting to conceive for any length of time. Windridge and Berryman (1996) suggest that these women are therefore more likely to be offered antenatal screening tests which 'differ in nature and quality' from those offered to women in a younger age group. There is also evidence that women over 35 years are more likely to be offered a Caesarean section for delivery, demonstrating the increased concern of health professionals. The management of antenatal screening tests, the advice given and the attitudes of health care professionals may therefore influence the potential emotional outcome for this group of women. The use of effective interactive skills and careful use of appropriate language when offering antenatal tests is paramount. It is not helpful to use phrases such as 'don't worry' or 'the chance of having a positive result is very low', especially if the woman goes on to become the one who eventually *does* have a positive diagnosis of fetal abnormality.

The Leicester Motherhood Project (Windridge and Berryman, 1996) examined the experiences of women older than 35 years giving birth compared with those of women in the age range 20–30 years. The study utilized a standardized questionnaire for measuring maternal adjustment and maternal attitudes (MAMA; Kumar *et al.* 1984), which incorporates five subscales:

- Exploring aspects of body image.
- Somatic symptoms.
- Marital relationship.
- Attitudes to sex.
- Attitudes to pregnancy.

The findings of this study showed that women over 35 reported fewer somatic symptoms and had more positive perceptions of their bodies than did the younger women in late pregnancy. However, there was some suggestion that women in the older age group were slightly less positive about their marital relationship and attitude towards sex 1 year after the birth of the baby. This study therefore identifies an aspect of adjustment to pregnancy for which women may need more constructive help and support than previously realized by health professionals; yet again, the potential effect of childbirth on the marital relationship is recognized.

Substance Use and Abuse

There is little doubt that cigarette smoking, alcohol and drug abuse have a negative effect on health, as well as the addictive component. Women who smoke, or who have alcohol dependency or drug dependency in pregnancy, may experience increased anxiety about the developing baby. The pregnant woman herself is almost certainly aware of the potential problems and may feel extreme guilt and emotional turmoil during pregnancy, which may in turn prevent her from attending for antenatal care, often fearing censure by health professionals. In addition, pregnant women who are dependent on drugs or alcohol may fear possible intervention by agencies, such as the social services, and the possibility of their baby being placed in care, in turn imposing even more emotional pressure. The popular stereotype of the female who is dependent on alcohol or drugs as irresponsible, homeless and making a living through crime or prostitution is often far from the truth. For example, in the recent past many people, especially women, became dependent on drugs such as the benzodiazepines, which were frequently prescribed by GPs for anxiety states. Negative attitudes displayed by some health professionals towards these women may prevent them from seeking professional help at a time when they are in most need. It is perhaps worth considering that there is some suggestion that only a small proportion of drug users are actually identified to the health services (Institute for the Study of Drug Dependency, 1992). Many areas now run highly specialized support services for pregnant women who have a drug or alcohol dependency – information is available through the Institute for the Study of Drug Dependency.

Psychological Effect of the Pregnancy – a Psychoanalytic Explanation

Raphael-Leff (1991) identified three 'maturational phases' throughout pregnancy, which are influenced by the woman's individual experience at the time, which in turn often relating to physical processes and body changes. As a psychoanalyst with a particular interest in the psychology of childbearing, Raphael-Leff has explored the unconscious, as well as conscious, psychological processes of women in pregnancy. She distinguishes three psychological phases, which equate to each trimester of pregnancy. The first phase is associated with the first trimester and ends when fetal movements are first felt. The second phase ends and the third begins when women become increasingly preoccupied with the forthcoming labour (Raphael-Leff, 1991, p. 61).

Raphael-Leff elaborates on some of the common psychological experiences associated with each phase. In true psychoanalytic tradition, the emphasis is on the unconscious psychological processes experienced by women in pregnancy, such as fantasies, unconscious conflicts and parapraxis (commonly known as 'Freudian slip', i.e. forgetting, making mistakes, slips of the tongue and losing things). Such occurrences are often associated with physiological processes, as hormonal and metabolic changes take place. Many women are aware of having lost things, misplaced objects and suffered mood changes, particularly in early pregnancy, and attributed such events to their 'changing hormones'. As Raphael-Leff points out, a growing awareness in the third phase of pregnancy can, in turn, make some women 'confident of their own expertise, their own intimate knowledge of this one particular pregnancy', which many health-care professionals acknowledge, accepting that women are good judges of what goes on in their bodies (Raphael-Leff, 1991, p. 77). However, as she suggests, there have been times when some professionals were reluctant to believe that many women are able to recognize the subtle changes which alert them to possible problems – for example, changes in fetal movement patterns or the changing position of the baby *in utero*.

Body Image

Anderson *et al.* (1994) examined mood changes that women experienced as a result of pregnancy and parenthood. This study suggested that there was some association between a positive mood in both pregnancy and postnatal period and happiness within the marital relationship. In addition, Anderson *et al.* found that women who experienced more 'dysphoric moods' perceived that they had a lower tolerance to pain (i.e. they thought that they would not be able to cope with labour pain) and were more dissatisfied with their body image, believing that they were unattractive in pregnancy. As Anderson *et al.* point out, factors relating to 'media images and cultural stereotypes of what is considered to be an attractive female body' are likely to add to negative feelings. Combes and Schonveld (1992) also identified the worries that women have about how they will cope with labour pain, as well as worries about body image, particularly whether they will get their shape back after the birth.

Several studies have highlighted that many women are dissatisfied with their body image in pregnancy. Change in body shape during pregnancy may lead some women to experience 'altered body image'. Price defines altered body image as 'a state of personal distress, defined by the individual, which indicates that the body no longer supports self-esteem, and which is dysfunctional, limiting the individual's social engagement with others' (Price, 1996, p. 12). Price suggests that for the majority of women pregnancy does not cause altered body image, as it is relatively temporary. Ussher suggests that changes in body shape during pregnancy have a 'considerable effect on personal identity and image of self' (Ussher, 1993, p. 98). In modern society, where women's expectations are to be slim and to achieve happiness through physical appearance, pregnancy is, however, the one occasion when they are 'permitted to be large'. Although a large proportion of women are happy with their changing shape, many women express a feeling of unhappiness about their body shape and size in pregnancy, as some of the studies identified previously have illustrated. Price (1996) suggests that this is only temporary, and normal body image resumes following the birth of the baby. However, as Raphael-Leff suggests, even the most assured woman has uncertainties which 'entail revision of her feminine identity... and the emotional and relational changes it brings about' (Raphael-Leff, 1991, p. 48).

Price (1996) also reported that the women in his study were concerned about regaining their prepregnancy figure 3 months after the birth, which was in turn influenced by the discomfort associated with perineal sutures, a perceived need to exercise and the attitudes of their partners regarding a return to what was seen as an 'attractive shape'. It is important to consider that body image is part of 'self-image' and self-concept. There may be some women for whom personal distress associated with body image, even of a temporary nature, may reinforce their poor self-image. Feeling attractive or having a positive body image is needed to maintain confidence and self-esteem. In turn, a negative body image may create a negative self-image, which can ultimately lead to longer term psychological problems or illhealth.

Fathers and Changing Childbirth

Although the emphasis has been on the woman during pregnancy, it must be remembered that anxieties and stresses are also experienced by her partner. The consequences of anxiety and ineffective coping behaviour can therefore have similar unfavourable psychological effects on him. Midwifery practice is currently focused on 'woman-centred care', as the philosophy of *Changing Childbirth* is implemented. Although the significance of this policy is recognized, midwives must continue to be aware of the potential psychological effects of pregnancy and childbirth on the couple and their relationship (**Case Study 4.1**). The father also needs to prepare and plan, and be acknowledged and involved throughout the pregnancy. Men are often at work when antenatal clinics and classes are provided and therefore are denied the opportunities for the same degree of involvement by the way maternity services are organized. Combes and Schonveld (1992) identify the need for increased knowledge and understanding of pregnancy and parenthood by the father to provide support for his partner and to prepare himself for the fathering role. In some instances this has been effected by the provision of father's preparation classes, organized and presented by men for men.

Wolkind and Zajicek (1981) demonstrated the changing attitudes to pregnancy that women displayed as their pregnancy progressed. This longitudinal study, which examined the psychological and social effects of pregnancy, found that women who experienced emotional distress in early pregnancy were able to resolve their conflicts and react more positively by 7 months. Wolkind and Zajicek's findings associated the anxieties in pregnancy to women's concerns about a lack of preparation for the birth and the potential problems that a baby would create in their lives.

Applications of Attachment Theory

One of the most influential psychological theories relating to mother–infant interaction is attachment theory. Attachments patterns formed in childhood are influential in forming and maintaining relationships even in adult life. Marris describes attachment as:

Case study 4.1

Gemma

Gemma met her husband, Bob, while they were both at university. They had decided that when they got married they did not want to have children until they were well established in their respective careers. Gemma's childhood had been unsettled, with an overprotective mother who also imposed a lot of discipline. Bob's parents were more open and liberal. Gemma's plans were totally disrupted when she discovered that she was pregnant just as she graduated. She was devastated at first, but in the later stages of her pregnancy she began to feel more excited and to respond more positively to the baby. Bob was also fairly devastated at first; it was not until after Jenny was born that he began to take a real 'fatherly' interest.

Gemma and Bob's experience of pregnancy and birth under such circumstances may appear to be fairly typical and illustrates many of the issues presented so far: an unplanned pregnancy leading to shattered plans for the future, Gemma's eventual adjustment in late pregnancy and Bob's adjustment to parenthood on arrival of the baby.

Following Jenny's birth, Gemma unfortunately developed post-natal depression. She considered herself to be as far from an 'ideal' mother and never felt a strong sense of attachment to Jenny, although she provided for her material needs and gave her all the care and attention she needed. As the months went by, Gemma began to respond angrily to her daughter. It was not until some months after the birth that her Health Visitor eventually realized the extent of Gemma's anger and aggression towards Jenny.

---

neither an emotion nor a purpose. Rather, like falling in love, it is the condition from which emotions and purposes arise. It is a predisposition to become attached, realized by the availability of an appropriate figure which generates feelings of comfort, anxiety, anger and joy.

(Marris, 1986, p. viii.)

If the 'appropriate figure' or, in terms of attachment theory, the 'primary caregiver' is not available, an infant may grow to fear close intimate relationships or separation from the 'attachment figure'. Being 'available' does not mean merely being present for the child, but includes an emotional presence and availability that is reliable, in body and in mind. The fears surrounding intimacy and separation pervade adult life and apply to adult relationships, yet are based on the type of attachments made in infancy. Adams and Cotgrove (1995) illustrate forms of attachment behaviour, based on the work of Ainsworth *et al.* (1978).

Gemma's childhood experience (**Case Study 4.1**) of an extremely strict and overprotective mother may have resulted in an 'insecure ambivalent' or 'insecure avoidant' attachment pattern in subsequent relationships, patterns that could even be perpetuated with her own infants. A woman's emotional experiences in her own childhood may have a profound effect on her own mothering style and responses.

Attachment theory has been the subject of potential misunderstanding and misinterpretation since the work of Bowlby was first published. The idea of a 'bond' between infant and mother which represents some sort of invisible 'gluing' together of the pair is an image often created when the term 'bonding' is used. As Bowlby points out, central to parenting is:

the provision of a secure base from which a child... can make sorties into the outside world and to which he can return knowing for sure that he will be welcome when he gets there, nourished physically and emotionally, comforted if distressed, reassured if frightened.

(Bowlby, 1988, p. 11.)

Helping parents to adjust to their roles was a factor Bowlby identified, acknowledging that one of the most effective ways of teaching parenting is not just through education, but through example. Bowlby identified the potential for parent's self-help groups in providing opportunities to meet and discuss the mistakes and successes that the vast majority of parents encounter and overcome. As Adams and Cotgrove (1995) point out, insecure attachments may increase the 'internalized feelings of helplessness and low self-esteem' which in turn are associated with depressive illness. Gemma may therefore have an increased predisposition to postnatal depression.

The association between insecure attachments in infancy and psychological illhealth in later life has been the concern of psychologists and psychiatrists for many years. Condon (1993) investigated the attachment made during pregnancy between mother and fetus. Condon (1993) suggests that understanding attachments that begin even in the antenatal period is of great help in understanding and managing many of the psychological problems associated with pregnancy and the postnatal period, such as reactions to loss and bereavement, as with miscarriage, neonatal death or parting with a baby through adoption.

Separation Anxiety, Loss and Mourning

Children spend their early years forming attachments with the primary caregiver. Ainsworth *et al.* (1978) suggested that infants are clearly attached by the age of 6 months, and then begin to demonstrate a fear of strangers. Bowlby (1971, 1975) used the term 'separation anxiety' to describe the anxiety that children feel when they lose or become separated from someone they love. Separation anxiety is seen as a basic human response to situations that signal an increased risk of danger. Bowlby suggests that understanding separation anxiety helps in understanding 'why threats to abandon a child, often used as a means of control, are so very terrifying' (Bowlby, 1981, p. 30). Parenting therefore involves helping a child to grow up, to accept separations without fear of abandonment. The child is then able to form new relationships and yet is also able to cope with being separate when appropriate. Adolescents, for example, undergo a process of separating from their parents and then form new attachments as they eventually prepare to settle with a permanent partner in adulthood.

The type of attachment experienced in childhood influences an individual's sense of security and subsequently their resilience to loss experienced at other times of life. There are certain factors which influence the process of recovery from loss, including the meaning of the loss itself, the ability to prepare for the loss and circumstances that occur after the loss. Loss is associated with many emotionally alarming situations, including the loss of a relationship, through separation or death, the loss of a community when people are rehoused [as occurred with many slum clearance policies (Marris, 1986)] and also loss of identity or status. Gemma experienced a loss of future career opportunities that for her had significant meaning; in turn, motherhood was for her something which she felt inexperienced and ill-prepared for, which undermined her confidence.

Individual Differences

The way each person experiences events throughout life and the way in which each views the world around them may be associated with their individual characteristics. Midwives believe that they treat every woman as an individual, and provide individualized, or personalized, care. To do this, it is necessary to know and understand some of the psychological characteristics of that particular person, and how these might influence the way she behaves. It is suggested that this calls for a great deal of skill in getting to know the woman, her partner and her family, her personal and social circumstances and subsequently her individual needs in relation to her pregnancy. To provide individualized care when the midwife meets the woman for the first time on admission in labour would be extremely difficult. A knowledge of some of the characteristics, traits and qualities that differentiate people or, alternatively, the similarities between individuals is therefore likely to complement the skills a midwife utilizes in practice. In psychological terms, individual characteristics are often typified as those characteristics which contribute towards personality.

Stereotypes

There are many facets to an individual's personality – other people can view the same person's personality in different ways or, adding to the complexity, aspects of human personality may appear to be different on separate occasions. There are many situations in which people are classified in terms of their personal characteristics, particularly if that person is not known, and generalizations are subsequently made. In everyday terms this system of classification is known as stereotyping – for example, 'people with red hair have fiery tempers' (or 'bleed freely!'), or plump people are jolly. These stereotypical views can be adopted easily in health care environments, when care is provided on a nonindividualized basis. It is easy to make assumptions about women who fall into such stereotypes and to make generalizations about their individual needs, thus forming a particular attitude towards, or belief about, certain women.

It is not unusual for certain groups of women to be referred to in a stereotypical way by many health care professionals, such as the 'typical teacher' or 'nurses get all the complications'. Such views are formed subjectively and therefore can prove unreliable and can often be derogatory. Stereotypes which are associated with prejudicial thinking can, of course, lead to discrimination (prejudicial behaviour). Human behaviour is often based on everyday assessments that people make of one another, judgements are based on observations made and assumptions are made on which actions are then based. These assessments, judgements, beliefs and assumptions contribute to and make up attitudes. In exploring concepts and theories of personality, it is therefore important to remember that prejudicial assumptions can be made, if not considered objectively.

Green *et al.* (1990) examined two of the stereotypes frequently adopted by midwives working in the labour ward environment, those of the 'well-educated, middle-class NCT type' and the 'uneducated working-class woman'. As Green and colleagues suggest, once such stereotypes have been formed assumptions can then easily be made about what the women who fit the stereotype need, particularly in terms of the care provided, which in turn can be both inappropriate and misleading. The assumptions made about the 'well-educated NCT type' tend to focus on her having 'high expectations' of the birth, or a 'rigid approach' to labour and a belief that, to her, childbirth must be a positive experience. Alternatively, the stereotype can be more positive, someone who is 'well-informed, reasonable and rational' (Green *et al.* 1990, p.126). On the other hand, the 'uneducated working class type' is often perceived as 'wilfully ignorant', 'unconcerned with emotional fulfilment', admitted in labour 'thoroughly unprepared' and 'abdicates all responsibility to the staff'. Green *et al.* examined the evidence for these stereotypes and concluded that the stereotypes were not supported, particularly in relation to a number of important aspects:

- Women of different educational backgrounds were equally likely to want a natural, drug-free labour.
- The less-educated women had higher expectations.
- Less-educated women did not want to hand control over to the staff.

Such evidence supports the need for individualized care whereby the midwife is able to get to know the woman over a longer period of time, thus providing opportunity to identify and meet her psychological as well as her physical needs.

Personality

Personality has been defined as 'those relatively stable and enduring aspects of individuals which distinguish them from other people, making them unique, but which at the same time permit a comparison between individuals' (Gross, 1992). It can be said that in attempting to study and explain personality differences, psychologists are trying to identify the fundamental psychological differences between people. There are many theorists, some of whom present well-known views of personality and personality development, such as Freud, Eysenck and Maslow (*see* Chapter 2). Health psychologists have examined the links between personality and health behaviour – for example, certain personality 'types' may be more susceptible to anxiety or stress, depression or certain diseases, such as coronary heart disease. To make assumptions about a person's health-related behaviour, it is important to identify personality in a way that is accurate and reliable, and which does not lead health-care professionals into the trap of making negative stereotypes or 'labelling' the individual. It is equally important to remember that there are circumstances, such as illness or certain social situations, that may have an effect on personality; for instance, the long-term effect of chronic pain, permanent physical disability or social deprivation.

It is not uncommon to classify people in terms of their personality 'traits', such as a midwife is caring, reliable, ambitious or committed. Allport (1937, 1961) was one of the early psychologists to produce a theory of personality based on the concept of personality traits. Allport developed his theory as a reaction to the preceding psychodynamic theory which focused on unconscious processes. He emphasized that personality should be considered as being embodied within each person, it should be consistent and should not be considered to be influenced by social events and roles. Eysenck (1953), on the other hand, adopted a different view of personality and produced a theory of personality based on a belief that it is inherited and has a biological basis. Eysenck's 'type theory' of personality is founded on the existence of three personality dimensions, i.e. extraversion–introversion, neuroticism–stability and psychoticism.

Eysenck conducted a great deal of experimental research to support his theory, and eventually developed methods of testing and measuring personality dimensions of extraversion and introversion. These 'psychometric' tests have been utilized in many areas, such as interviewing and assessing for specific jobs (e.g., fighter-pilots, when the ability to perform the skill of flying at the same time as being able to remain calm and cool under extreme conditions may be very important). The technique has been extended to many other areas, such as employment selection, where it is anticipated that the required characteristics of a prospective employee can be assessed for her or his suitability for the job.

Some studies examined the possible association between personality and emotional well-being around childbirth. Ball (1994) explored the emotional outcome for women experiencing childbirth. From the available literature she identified certain factors associated with postnatal depression:

- The personality of the mother.
- Whether the mother had been separated from her own mother before the age of 11 years.
- Certain life crises.
- The time of first holding her baby after it was born.
- Her self-image.
- Her reported feelings following the birth.

This study did not find any relationship between personality traits, as measured using the Eysenck Personality Inventory (EPI), and emotional outcome of childbirth generally. However, it did find that women who had been separated from their own mothers before the age of 11 years were more likely to have difficulty in adjusting to motherhood. In turn, this group of women demonstrated a significant difference on the anxiety–neuroticism dimension of the EPI, suggesting that the separation had had an effect on their personality development. Brown and Harris's well-known study (1978) had previously found that certain vulnerability factors were associated with depression in women, which included loss of the woman's own mother during childhood, as well as other sociological factors. These included lack of a supportive relationship from her husband, unemployment and other children at home.

Facilitator–Reciprocator–Regulator

Raphael-Leff (1983) proposed a specific model of mothering, which originally identified two distinct styles or 'orientations': these were the **facilitator** and the **regulator**. Each orientation is associated with particular attributes and patterns of behaviour that are evident throughout pregnancy and which, in turn, point to and attempt to predict the type of mother–infant interaction after birth. Raphael-Leff's model has developed over recent years and now extends to a third orientation termed the **reciprocator** (Raphael-Leff, 1993). As she suggests, there are many ways in which women respond to pregnancy – 'some blossom and feel enriched others fade and feel depleted'. However, she was able to discern certain trends which 'may make sense of seemingly contra-

dictory approaches to pregnancy, birth and motherhood' (Raphael-Leff, 1993, p. 65). This model is therefore a theory specific to pregnant women and individual differences in pregnancy, and may help in predicting emotional disturbances such as the incidence of postnatal depression.

Raphael-Leff developed her model from psychoanalytical and object relations theory, proposing that 'maternal responses are not restricted to the domain of psychoanalytic theorists but are inherent in the unconscious views of mothers to their babies' (Raphael-Leff, 1983, p. 377). The facilitator mother, then, 'regards her baby as an intimate from birth or pregnancy', she trusts the baby to convey its needs to her and *facilitates* these needs by adapting to the baby. On the other hand, the regulator mother sees the baby as a 'bundle of needs', which she must *regulate*, through training the baby and making it adapt to reality. Raphael-Leff recognizes that there are few women who are pure types and, rather than the original dimension first presented, the model is now represented as being circular, including the intermediary reciprocators (Raphael-Leff, 1993, p. 66).

The reciprocator, then, is ambivalent about pregnancy, being both overjoyed and regretful about the changes to her life, yet able to maintain a balance of awareness of her ambivalence and her 'internal contradictions'. The facilitator responds to her pregnancy as a fulfilment and realization of all her wishes, fantasizing about idealized conception, wanting to show off her 'bump' and often wearing maternity clothes from early pregnancy. The regulator sees her pregnancy as tedious, keeping her pregnancy news to herself until it is obviously apparent, determined to maintain her way of life and not be changed by the developing baby.

Orientations also exist in expectant fathers, identified as **participators** and **renouncers** (Raphael-Leff, 1985). The participator is the man 'passionately involved in pregnancy' and takes a great interest in caring for the infant. The renouncer, on the other hand, resists involvement in the pregnancy, may be reluctant to attend the birth and prefers to become more involved with the baby when it is a year or two in age.

Raphael-Leff in developing her model recognized the importance of examining parenthood from the 'perspective of the participants' (Raphael-Leff, 1985, p. 170). As women and their partners seek more involvement in, and information about, pregnancy and childbirth there is an increased potential for emotional conflicts to be created by the 'clash between the budding freedom of choice and simultaneous conflicting pressures of both child-centred experts and personal fulfilment advocates' (Raphael-Leff, 1985, p. 171). In turn, midwives and other health-care professionals who are knowledgeable and informed about the psychological effects of pregnancy and childbirth on each individual are in a better position to provide effective individualized support, facilitating choice and encouraging the expectant couple's involvement in events, consequently increasing the possibility of a positive adaptation to pregnancy.

Psychological Distress and Illhealth

Psychological illhealth associated with childbirth is perhaps most often typified by postnatal depression. The debate encountered in areas of the psychological and sociological literature relates to whether depression in the postnatal period is a medical condition or a consequence of negative social circumstances that influence the emotional outcomes of pregnancy and childbirth. From a psychological perspective, there can be no doubt that there are a significant number of women for whom pregnancy leads to a form of emotional distress that influences the quality of their lives. The prevalence of postnatal depression has been cited as being between 11% and 17% (Pitt, 1968; Paykel *et al.* 1980; Kumar and Robson, 1984). A study undertaken in general practice, where women are routinely seen by their own GP in the postnatal period, however, found that 24% of young mothers experienced depression between 3 months and 1 year after childbirth (Blacker, 1989).

Postnatal depression has been defined as a 'nonpsychotic, depressive disorder arising during the first year of childbirth' (Levy and Kline, 1994, p. 154). Depression associated with childbirth can be viewed on a dimension similar to that associated with many other forms of psychological illhealth, ranging from the anxiety and mood instability often termed 'the blues', to postpartum psychotic disorder usually requiring admission to hospital. Depression is therefore often categorized as either a minor or major disorder. Depression in the general population has an average duration of approximately 8 months; postnatal depression, on the other hand, lasts on average 14 months (Blacker, 1989). The term 'dysphoria' ('fed-up', irritability, listlessness) is frequently used to distinguish between the milder forms of depression and major depressive illness, when individuals experience symptoms such as persistent low mood, a loss of interest (sometimes in life itself), feelings of worthlessness, lack of motivation and drive.

Green (1995) warns of the constraints placed on ways of thinking about postnatal depression, as well as research undertaken in this area, when the terms 'postnatal' and 'depression' are used routinely. Postnatal (or puerperal) implies that the symptoms only present following childbirth. Green found that data obtained from 1272 women suggest that dysphoria is as prevalent in the antenatal period as it is postnatally. Anderson *et al.* (1994) identified that women who experienced depressive symptoms during the postnatal period were also more likely to have had depressive symptoms during their pregnancy. In addition, they found that women who experienced depressive mood tended to have more negative attitudes and perceptions, particularly towards body image and pain tolerance.

The potential effect of postnatal depression on the interaction and developing relationship between the mother and her baby also needs to be considered. It has been demonstrated that normal mother–infant interaction can be disrupted by an expressionless or 'still' face. Interaction normally involves exchanges of baby talk, smiling, cooing and playful signals. A study in which mothers were asked to act in a depressed manner, with less smiling and the interaction less lively, showed that the babies also reacted in a depressed manner (Field *et al.* 1988). Although such findings are not accepted by all psychologists, there is some suggestion that the children of mothers who suffer from depression may also experience emotional problems.

Explanations for psychological illhealth or depressive illnesses are many and varied, as are the debates surrounding such explanations. Depression can be explained physiologically by an imbalance in the individual's neurochemical and hormonal make-up, and is therefore treated by drugs which attempt to correct this. Alternatively, many people experience severe emotional distress because of social factors such as poverty and deprivation. Treating such problems imposes greater demands on support services and forms the basis of much sociological and political debate. Midwives in some areas of the community have been involved in specific schemes set up to help relieve the distress experienced by certain groups of women and their families. Davies and Evans (1990) demonstrated the effectiveness of 'enhanced community midwifery', which ultimately helped in improving diet for women and their families living within a deprived area; it also helped in reducing the amount of cigarette smoking and in improving access to antenatal education. In addition, the women involved in this study emphasized the importance of having adequate support and a one-to-one relationship, which in turn improved their overall levels of satisfaction. Such initiatives often incorporate support from a team of professionals, including social workers, health visitors and other representatives from various benefits agencies.

Social Support

The effectiveness of adequate support and a supportive environment in relieving anxiety and depression is a theme that runs throughout this chapter. Support during pregnancy can be provided by the woman's partner or her family and friends, as well as the specialist support provided by midwives and other healthcare professionals. Voluntary organizations also have a role in providing various forms of support, particularly at times of crisis. Organizations such as the Citizen's Advice Bureau, may provide help and advice in relation to financial and legal issues, Samaritans provide support in times of crisis and despair and Relate can help with difficulties in relationships.

Effective support has been defined in various ways. Social support can be what people do for each other or it can be the 'caring culture provided by society and its care services' (Ball, 1994, p. 23). One longitudinal study examined the effect of social support and its effect on family health in the longer term. Oakley *et al*. (1996) undertook a randomized controlled trial to investigate the effect of pregnancy support on the health of women and their children. This study examined the results of a 7-year follow-up of families who initially participated in a programme in which a research midwife provided home visits and a 24-hour contact service (Oakley *et al*. 1990). These midwives did not carry out clinical care, but provided a 'listening ear' for any issues the women wanted to talk about. The support was restricted to pregnancy and one brief postnatal visit, and involved referral to social services and health agencies when appropriate, as well as practical advice, information and help as requested by the mothers. The study hypothesized that women who receive support in pregnancy would have better health outcomes (as would their children) than those who were not offered support. The results of this study supported the trends of the previous

studies, i.e. the women who received support during pregnancy demonstrated significant differences in their health and in the developmental outcomes of their children. The health-promoting effects of support in pregnancy not only improved women's experiences, but also benefited their children's health and development in childhood.

Ball, drawing on the work of Caplan (1969), describes effective support:

> *as that which enables the stressed individual to accept the helper as an ally, and which assures her that the helper's skill, time and understanding are available for as long as needed. The secret of success in being such a helper lies in the relationship which develops between the individual and the caregiver.*
>
> (Ball, 1994, p. 108.)

Ball and Oakley, therefore, acknowledge some key factors which are important for the provision of midwifery care and the role of the midwife in maintaining and improving psychological well-being.

The Midwife's Role and Skills in Psychological Support

The roles of the midwife in helping a woman to adjust to pregnancy, providing emotional support, informing and advising, detecting psychological illhealth, reducing anxiety, relieving stress and identifying the factors which may lead to psychological illhealth involve the skills of being 'with woman'. Such skills encompass the ability to promote a helping relationship between midwife and woman, to communicate effectively, to provide empathic support and an ability to listen at times of need.

Listening involves more than hearing the words of another person. Listening, in counselling terms, is usually referred to as active listening – that is, that the other person is being heard and also feels he or she is being heard. The counselling process involves exploration and understanding of a client's situation, an ability to relate and respond to the client and to help that person find a way of resolving their problems, drawing on their own resources. Rogers (1980) identified three basic elements to a person-centred approach to counselling – warmth, genuineness and empathic understanding:

- Warmth involves being approachable and open, treating the other person with equal worth, being nonjudgemental.
- Genuineness is about showing genuine interest in the other.
- Empathy is a response which demonstrates that the counsellor (or midwife) has perceived *accurately* the feelings of the other person and communicates this understanding to them.

These skills have been identified by the British Association of Counselling (1989) as the skills which are used to enhance the performance of many professionals, including midwives, in their role. The skills of counselling can therefore be considered as an integral part of midwifery practice – they are the skills of helping and supporting other people to adjust to changes that affect their lives.

Clement (1995) examined the effectiveness of 'listening visits' in pregnancy as a strategy for preventing postnatal depression. Although there are inherent difficulties, such as the timing of such visits and the methods of identifying those women who are to be approached, this research review suggests that psychological interventions in pregnancy can have a beneficial effect on emotional well-being postnatally. It is proposed that 'psychological interventions' should involve a form of psychological screening to detect low emotional well-being, followed by approximately eight antenatal 'listening visits'. As Clement (1995) suggests, there is a need to consider and evaluate the expanded counselling role of the midwife. However, it must also be considered that by providing women with psychological support in times of increased anxiety or depressed mood, it may be possible to encourage and help women to adapt to their maternal role and improve psychological well-being. It is therefore only through implementation and evaluation that such strategies can be thoroughly examined. There is growing evidence of the value of postnatal listening services for women who encounter emotional distress arising from the birth experience (Charles and Curtis, 1994). It is therefore apparent that such interventions could also be invaluable in the antenatal period.

Midwives are not psychiatric nurses and therefore are not prepared to deal with severe emotional disturbances and psychological illness. However, knowing the risk factors and influencing factors for psychological illhealth, understanding the importance of there being a person that can be trusted and available for the woman to talk to, having an awareness of their own limitations and knowing what facilities are available for referral when those limitations are reached, are all part of the midwife's professional role. Working closely with other members of the health care team, including community psychiatric nurses, health visitors, social workers and medical colleagues, can only enhance the opportunities for identifying and dealing with such problems at an early stage.

PHYSIOLOGICAL RESPONSES OF THE MOTHER TO PREGNANCY

The relationship of the mother and fetus is not simply as host and parasite, but is a joint relationship in which the mother provides an adequate environment for the developing fetus. Whether it is harmonious is debatable, as there are many stresses exerted on the mother, many of which are potentially harmful to both the mother and child.

In this section the normal physiological responses of the mother to the fetus are discussed, not the abnormal pathophysiology. These normal physiological responses are, of course, adaptive measures by the mother's body to the developing fetus.

Fertilization and Implantation

Before embarking on the physiological changes incurred by the mother in response to fetal demands, there is a need to have some knowledge of the implantation of the zygote and its early nurturing by the corpus luteum.

Fertilization normally takes place in the dilated part of the ampulla of the fallopian tube. There is a short delay before the zygote starts dividing and forms a morula (ball of cells). A fluid-filled cavity is formed inside, called a blastocoele, which is surrounded by a single layer of cells, called the trophoblast. The trophoblast cells form the placenta and embryonic membranes. The whole structure is called a blastocyst (**Figure 4.1a**).

At one end of the blastocoele there is an accumulation of cells that will form the fetus. The embryo is now called a blastocyst. This takes approximately 2–4 days, during which time the zygote traverses from the ampulla and comes to rest on the posterior wall of the uterus. The trophoblast cells invade this area to form a double layer. The outer layer is called the syncytiotrophoblast and the inner is called the cytotrophoblast (**Figure 4.1b**). The trophoblast layer forms the chorion (**Figure 4.1c**). The chorion therefore consists of the trophoblast plus the supporting vascular mesenchyme.

The embryo–maternal relationship is biologically alien to a parasite–host relationship; normally there is a balance between the invasiveness of the trophoblast and the protective reaction of the endometrium. It is necessary to overcome the problems of menstrual loss and therefore abortion. Progesterone is necessary to maintain the uterine lining. The corpus luteum has to be maintained for it to continue to secrete progesterone and oestrogen. The corpus luteum is probably maintained by two protein hormones from the trophoblast of the blastocyst. These hormones are known as human chorionic gonadotrophin (HCG) and human chorionic somatomammotrophin (HCS). After 6 weeks the placenta takes over the role of the corpus luteum by producing progesterone and oestrogen. In a way the placenta takes over the role of the pituitary gland. The embryo is immunologically different from the mother and might be expected to be rejected, as would be a graft from an incompatible donor – HCG may be involved in this (*see* Human Chorionic Gonadotrophin, p. 92).

The ovary is able to synthesize progesterone from acetate, which is the starting point of all steroids (**Figure 4.2**), and then can convert this into oestrogens. The placenta does not have the necessary enzymes to convert the acetate into progesterone and then to oestrogens, so it is reliant on cholesterol from the maternal blood. This cholesterol is then converted into progesterone.

When the conceptus implants into the endometrium, the continued secretion of progesterone causes the endometrial cells to swell still more and therefore to store more nutrients. The endometrial lining is greatly modified during pregnancy, the cells are now called decidual cells and the total mass of cells is called the decidua. After implantation and until about the fourth month of gestation, three parts of the decidua can be identified (**Figure 4.3**):

• Decidua basalis, which forms the base of the developing placenta.

• Decidua capsularis, which encapsulates the surface of the implanted embryo.

• Decidua parietalis, which lines the rest of the uterus. For the first few days after implantation, nutrients reach the embryo by diffusion, but as the embryo grows the development of a simple circulatory system becomes a necessity. When the chorion is differentiating and growing vigorously, 9–10 days after fertilization, the villous characteristics of the future placenta are established. These villi originate from what are called trophoblastic trabeculae. At about 1 month of gestation, when most of the organ systems are present, the embryo's outer surface of the chorionic sac is thickly clothed by villi. These have an outer covering of trophoblast and a central core of extraembryonic mesoderm, containing blood vessels through which circulates embryonic blood.

The chorionic villi are bathed in circulating **extravasated** maternal blood and here the exchanges of nutritive and waste material and of respiratory gases take place between the two blood streams. This type of nutrition is called haemotrophic, as opposed to the histotrophic nutrition of the early conceptus.

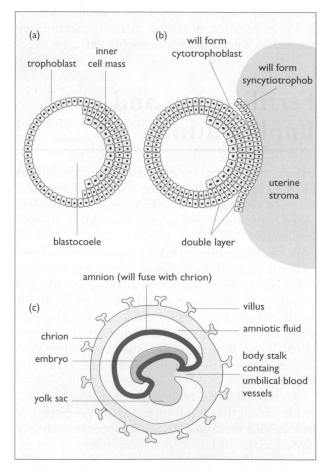

Figure 4.1 Stages in the development of the embryo.

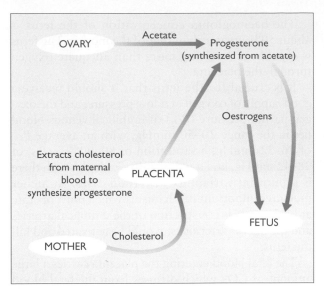

Figure 4.2 Syntheses of oestrogens and progesterone.

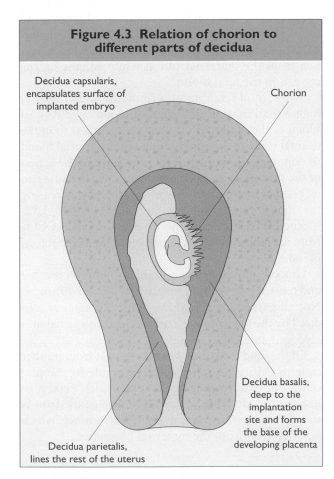

Figure 4.3 Relation of chorion to different parts of decidua

Decidua capsularis, encapsulates surface of implanted embryo

Chorion

Decidua basalis, deep to the implantation site and forms the base of the developing placenta

Decidua parietalis, lines the rest of the uterus

Figure 4.3 Relationship of the chorion to different parts of the decidua.

The embryo is suspended from the inner surface of the chorion by the body stalk (**Figure 4.1c**), which contains the umbilical blood vessels. The amnion encloses the embryo and contains amniotic fluid. A yolk sac is present which nourishes the embryo in the early stages.

The Placenta

The placenta weighs approximately 500–600 g. The ratio of the neonatal weight to that of the placenta is about 6:1. One umbilical vein distributes the blood, rich in nutrients and requirements for the growing fetus. Two umbilical arteries return the deoxygenated blood back to the placenta. The placenta can be thought of as an interface between the maternal and fetal circulations, in which the fetus derives its oxygen, amino acids, minerals and vitamins from the mother. The fetus must discharge carbon dioxide (CO_2) and other waste products into the maternal circulation. These are all transferred across the membranes by transport mechanisms, namely simple and facilitated diffusion.

The placenta consists of several lobes that are, of course, variable. It grows, keeping pace with the growing fetus.

The placenta is described as having a fetal component, the chorion (which is the outermost membrane of the conceptus), and a maternal component, formed by the decidua basalis and by maternal blood circulating in intimate contact with the chorion.

Fetal blood is conveyed to the placenta through two umbilical arteries. These anastomose as they approach the placenta and their branches then ramify over the surface of the chorion. These branches then pierce the chorion and form the main stem vessels for the placental villi. Each stem branch vascularizes a discrete group of villi. These so-called villous units are known as fetal cotyledons, of which there are approximately 200. The villi have a root-like structure and at the terminal villi there are arterio–capillary–venous systems whereby the capillaries come into close proximity with the villous membrane. The veins drain back along the course taken by the arteries to then emerge as the umbilical vein, which carries the oxygenated blood back to the fetus.

Placental membrane

The placental membrane is the structure that is interposed between the maternal and fetal blood. The transfer of substances between mother and fetus is controlled by this membrane, which is often called the placental barrier.

Amniotic fluid

Amniotic fluid provides the fetus with a favourable environment, absorbing mechanical pressures and yet allowing freedom of movement. The volume of amniotic fluid increases from about 30 ml at the tenth week of pregnancy to a maximum of about 1000 ml at 36–37 weeks of gestation. Thereafter it falls by approximately 150 ml per week, so that if pregnancy is prolonged until 42 weeks very little fluid remains. There is a wide variation in these values between individuals. In the first half of pregnancy, the volume is closely related to fetal weight.

Amniotic fluid resembles a dialysate of fetal plasma. Because the fetal skin is permeable at this stage, the amniotic fluid probably forms an extension of fetal extracellular fluid. Beyond midpregnancy, when the fetal skin keratinizes and becomes impermeable, the amniotic fluid volume is a balance between that added by fetal urine and that taken away by fetal swallowing.

The fluid therefore increasingly reflects urinary characteristics, becoming hypotonic, with increasing concentrations of urea and creatinine. It is now realized that the amniotic fluid also serves an important purpose in preparing the fetus for when it is born (Uvnas-Moberg, 1989).

Functions of the placenta

As stated before, the placenta is an interface between fetal and maternal blood, but it is also a fetal organ. The term fetoplacental unit is often used to describe this inter-relationship. Anatomically the placenta is simply an extension of the fetal capillary bed, covered by a layer of trophoblast, in which it provides a large surface area of approximately $10 m^2$ that is in intimate contact with the maternal blood.

The newborn infant acquires nutrients from and excretes waste products into its environment at a number of specialized sites, namely, the lungs, kidneys, liver and gut. In contrast, the only effective environment of the fetus is its mother's blood and the placenta is the principle site for the exchange of all materials. The placental villi is analogous to many of the functions of the lung alveoli, renal glomeruli and tubules, and intestinal epithelium; in addition to this the villi also produce protein and steroid hormones.

The haemoglobin concentration of the fetus is about 50% greater than that of the mother. The fetus is capable of receiving more than adequate oxygen through the placenta.

It is crucial for the fetus that it should receive a good supply of oxygen at a low pressure, and the oxygen partial pressure (P_{O_2}) of umbilical venous blood lies in the range 20–50 mmHg, with an average P_{O_2} of 26–32 mmHg, a saturation of 80–90%, a P_{O_2} of 38–42 mmHg, and a pH of 7.30–7.35, although there is significant variability in certain cases. At higher pressures important mechanisms which must operate at birth, such as constriction of the umbilical arteries and the ductus arteriosus, would be activated and kill the fetus.

The fetal blood entering the placenta carries a large amount of CO_2 which diffuses from the fetal blood into the maternal blood. Loss of the CO_2 makes the fetal blood more alkaline, whereas the increased CO_2 in the maternal blood makes this more acidic. These changes cause the combining capacity of fetal blood for oxygen to become increased and that of the maternal blood to become decreased. This forces more oxygen from the maternal blood while enhancing the oxygen in the fetal blood.

The P_{CO_2} of fetal blood is found to be 2–3 mmHg higher than that of the maternal blood. The P_{CO_2} of blood in the maternal sinuses is usually less than the normal value of 40 mmHg found in the arterial blood of nonpregnant women. This is because of the action of the oestrogen and progesterones, which causes an increase of the mother's breathing, thereby increasing the minute ventilation (minute volume) by 40–50% (Branch, 1992), causing her to blow off excess CO_2 from the lungs. This, of course, keeps the P_{CO_2} of fetal blood low.

Glucose moves down a gradient between mother and fetus at a very rapid rate, by facilitated diffusion. Not all passes directly to the fetus, but some is oxidized by the placenta itself and some is converted into glycogen and lipid.

Of the lipids only free fatty acids pass from mother to fetus. More complex lipids are made by the placenta and fetus from maternal precursors. Fetal proteins are made from maternal amino acids. Iron is transferred by transferrin in the villous surface, which takes up iron from the maternal plasma.

Maternal Physiological Changes

At the end of the first trimester, the uterus occupies most of the pelvic cavity. Towards the end of full-term pregnancy, the uterus fills nearly all of the abdominal cavity. The weight of the uterus increases from about 50 g to approximately 1100 g. This increase results in the maternal viscera being displaced. The liver, intestines and stomach move in an upwards direction. In the third trimester of pregnancy the stomach is inevitably displaced towards a horizontal position and its ability to fill is considerably restricted. Pressure on the stomach may force the food contents up into the oesophagus, resulting in the common symptom of heartburn. The pelvic compartment also undergoes a directional stress on its viscera, with compression of the ureters and urinary bladder. Also, the breasts approximately double in size. At the same time the vagina enlarges and the introitus opens more widely.

The above can be considered as anatomical changes, but there are also physiological changes. These changes include weight gain caused by the fetus, amniotic fluid, placenta, uterine enlargement and increased total body water. All the various hormones that have substantially increased in concentration can cause marked changes in the appearance of the mother, sometimes resulting in the development of oedema, acne and various skin pigmentations.

Volume Homeostasis

Volume homeostasis is the 'continuous adjustment of blood volume to the changing size of the vascular bed so that at all times an adequate fullness of the blood stream is available to the left ventricle' (Gauer and Henry, 1976). Achieving this aim in normal pregnancy is somewhat difficult in view of the multitude of rapidly changing factors which influence the vascular bed and blood volume. Normal pregnancy is characterized by arteriolar and venous dilatation as well as by increasing the need for volume accumulation in the fetal and placental tissues. Therefore, volume homeostatic mechanisms must be repeatedly readjusted throughout pregnancy.

Extracellular fluid volume

Extracellular fluid volume (ECFV) is primarily dependent on sodium content, and therefore regulation of renal sodium excretion is critical to maintenance.

Changes in ECFV are sensed by stretch receptors in the atria and arterial baroreceptors. It has been found that stretching of the atrial wall stimulates the secretion of a peptide hormone called atrial natriuretic peptide (ANP). This acts upon vascular smooth muscle, especially on vessels precontracted with angiotensin II, thereby acting as a vasodilator in pregnancy. Thereby one can say the increased blood volume stimulates ANP release and that the increased ANP concentration is one of the factors responsible for the peripheral vasodilatation and fall in the sensitivity for angiotensin II (Thomsen *et al.* 1993). Changes in solute concentrations are sensed by osmoreceptors in the hypothalamus. In pregnancy, which is not a steady state, there is progressive weight gain, of which 6–8 kg represents expansion of the ECFV (Brown and Gallery, 1994), both interstitial and plasma volumes being increased.

Volume and composition of the blood

There is an increase in the total red-cell volume during pregnancy, but the plasma volume is proportionately much higher. The size and haemoglobin content of the cells show little change, so the haemoglobin concentration and haematocrit fall in parallel with the red-cell count. **Table 4.1** shows the variations incurred with pregnancy.

Most estimates of the increase in blood volume during pregnancy are in the range 1–2 litres with an average being 1100 ml, or a 42% increase over the nonpregnant state. The red blood cell volume also increases by about 24%, or 350 ml (Mashburn *et al.* 1992). Again, this is only an average and is, of course, variable, depending on what literature is accessed. Duffy (1991, p. 1707) writing in what one can call the haematologist's bible, *Haematology: Basic Principles and Practice*, states that expectant mother's blood volume consists of an increase in plasma volume (40–60%) that is approximately twice the simultaneous expansion in red blood cells (20–30%).

Haemoglobin

In healthy nonpregnant women the haemoglobin concentration, on average, is 13.7–14.0 g/100 ml (**Table 4.1**). In the first 3 months of pregnancy the haemoglobin concentration falls by about 0.5 g/100 ml. The minimum concentration is reached at about 30–32 weeks.

Approximately 65% of the iron in the body is present as haemoglobin. The rest of the stored iron in

Table 4.1. Plasma Volume, Red Cell Volume, Total Blood Volume and Haemoglobin Concentration (adapted from Hytten and Leitch)

	Non-pregnant	Weeks of pregnancy			
		20	30	34	40
Plasma volume (ml)	2600	3150	3750	3830	3600
Red-cell volume (ml)	1400	1450	1550	1600	1650
Total blood volume (ml)	4000	4600	5200	5430	5250
Haematocrit (%)	35.0	31.5	29.8	29.5	31.5
Haemoglobin (g/100 ml)	13.7–14.0	12.8.0–13.0	12.4–12.9	12.7–12.9	12.7

the body is divided between ferritin and haemosiderin (accounting for 30%), myoglobin (3.5%), haem enzymes (0.5%) and transferrin-bound iron at 0.1% (Hoffbrand and Pettit, 1995, p. 38).

The physiological changes in the iron compartments during pregnancy mimic those in iron deficiency. Serum iron and ferritin decrease because of the demands of the increasing red-cell mass and the growth needs of the fetus. Transferrin increases, probably because of oestrogen stimulation. A nonpregnant woman has about 2.6 g of iron, of which 1.7 g (65%) is contained in haemoglobin. The daily iron loss for menstruating women averages about 2 mg. During pregnancy, this loss or requirement increases to 3–4 mg/day, because of the demands of the fetus. The average Western diet supplies 15–20 mg of iron, of which 5–30% is absorbed (Mashburn *et al.* 1992). The usual intake and absorption of dietary iron does not meet the average daily requirement in pregnancy, which usually has to be supplemented by taking oral medication.

The fetus requires iron for the synthesis of fetal haemoglobin, so 1 g of additional iron is needed during the course of the pregnancy; this leads to a drain on the mother's iron reserves. Another requirement of the fetus is folate, which is used for the synthesis of nucleic acids.

The changes in plasma and red-cell volume that occur in pregnancy are caused by the necessary internal environmental adaptations for correct perfusion of the placenta and growth and protection of the fetus. The flow of maternal blood depends on the available volume in the space of the uterine vascular compartment. The expanded blood pool of the mother compensates for the increased metabolic and perfusion needs of the fetus together with its placenta. There is

also the added bonus that this acts as a reservoir to compensate for any blood loss at time of delivery.

Thus the competence of the fetus to adapt to independent life is significantly affected by the haemodynamic state of the mother at birth; if the fetus is considered a parasite it can be seen that this excess burden on the mother has to be adequately compensated by a correct blood composition.

In the first 6 weeks of pregnancy, the plasma, red-cell and total circulatory blood volumes are comparable to those of the normal nonpregnant woman. Around about the eighth week of gestation, the plasma volume steadily increases and by the 20th week it has increased to 21%. In other words there is, in effect, a haemodilution as the red-cell volume does not increase to any appreciable degree. Up to this period the volume is at the same level as that of a nonpregnant woman, that is 26–27 ml/kg. This uniform red-cell volume, on the basis of body weight, emphasizes how the maternal marrow responds to the vigorous demands of the fetus. After the 24th week of pregnancy, the maternal plasma volume stabilizes to about 67–68 ml/kg and is fairly constant throughout the rest of the pregnancy. The red cell volume also remains constant at 27 ml/kg. The total plasma volume increases by about 50% and the total red cells by about 20% in the gestation period. This consistency of the plasma and red cell volumes, keeping in step with the growth of the fetus, is necessary for the correct conveyance of an adequate oxygenated blood supply.

The maintenance of an adequate red-cell volume is also influenced by iron intake during pregnancy. The fetus is totally dependent on the mother in extracting the nutritional requirements from her.

The change in the concentration of red cells affects

the viscosity of the blood. Hamilton (1950) demonstrated that relative blood viscosity fell from 4.61 in nonpregnant women to 4.20 in early pregnancy and then to 3.84 at 22–28 weeks when the mean haemoglobin concentration was at its lowest. Because of the reduced viscosity the load on the heart is reduced, which is therefore able to cope with an increased cardiac output. As an analogy, this is like comparing oil with water. Oil has a high viscosity compared to that of water. If the water in a domestic central heating supply was replaced by oil, the pump would have to be very substantial to move the oil around the heating system. Also, a larger amount of energy would be required to meet these needs. Iron medication presumably reduces this advantage as the blood viscosity would not fall as much.

As plasma volume changes, so to does the composition. There is a decrease in the electrolytes and plasma protein concentrations. There is a decreased serum albumin concentration in normal pregnancy, associated with the rise in plasma volume. The reduced concentration in the circulation is usually a dilutional effect from the increase in plasma volume (Whittaker and Lind, 1993). Besides the reduced serum albumin concentration and a rise in plasma volume, there is also an increase in the intravascular albumin mass (IVM). An increased rate of albumin synthesis explains the higher IVM during pregnancy, as the turnover of albumin is relatively rapid compared to the rate of change in plasma volume. Factors that increase albumin synthesis may include the low serum albumin concentration and reduced oncotic pressure, as well as the nutritional and hormonal changes of pregnancy.

There is an increase in the concentration of clotting factors and a decrement in the body's fibrinolytic capacity. The rise in plasma fibrinogen is evident by the 3rd month of pregnancy, and the level increases to 4.0–6.5 g/litre in late pregnancy (Hathaway and Bonnar, 1978). Prothrombin (factor II) has been shown to be affected only slightly by pregnancy. Both factor VII and factor X undergo marked elevation in pregnancy. The notable change in the ratio between fibrinogen and fibrin-stabilizing factor (factor XIII) may have some influence on the process of clot stabilization and subsequent lysis in pregnancy.

Cardiovascular Dynamics

As already discussed in the previous section, during pregnancy there is a rise in cardiac output; because the cardiac rate and stroke volume increase, so the vascular resistance falls (Branch, 1992). A study by Robson *et al.* (1989) showed that cardiac output rose from 4.88 l/min before conception to 7.34 l/min (66% increase) in the 34th week. It is accepted that an increase in the order of 1.5 l/min is probably reached before midpregnancy. This increase in output is achieved by an increase in both heart rate and stroke volume. Remember that:

Cardiac Output = Heart Rate × Stroke Volume
and that:

Blood Pressure = Cardiac Output × Peripheral Resistance
It was accepted for many years that cardiac output falls in late pregnancy, but it now seems certain that these observations reflect that most measurements of cardiac output were with the patient in the supine position. A 50% rise in cardiac output certainly meets the requirements necessitated by the fetus for an adequate blood supply to nourish its development. There is not always consistency between these figures and those of other researchers, but the general consensus is that there is a tendency towards a higher cardiac output in the second trimester compared with the first trimester, and a lower cardiac output in the third trimester compared with the second trimester (van Oppen *et al.* 1996). It is probably better to state that there is an increase in cardiac output which begins during the eighth week of pregnancy and is 30–50% above normal near term (Elkus and Popovich, 1992). The change in cardiac output is secondary to increases in heart rate and stroke volume and a decrease in peripheral vascular resistance. During labour and delivery the cardiac output increases by an additional 10–15% in response to endogenous catecholamines and the increased venous return that occurs during uterine contractions (Elkus and Popovich, 1992).

During pregnancy, total blood volume increases by up to 35%, which in turn causes the previously mentioned haemodilution, with decreased red blood cell volume, haemoglobin, haematocrit and serum protein levels. Extracellular water also increases by 1–2 litres and, in addition to mechanical compression of the inferior vena cava by the fetus, contributes to the development of peripheral oedema seen in 50–80% of normal pregnancies. At the same time there is venous distensibility, especially in the third trimester when the plasma volume is maximal. In normal pregnancy, this venous distensibility reflects adaptation to the changes in circulation, as already mentioned. Hormonal changes may be responsible because it has been demonstrated that there was an increase of venous distensibility during oral contraceptive therapy and that the venous distensibility curve parallels the steroid curve of pregnancy (Sakai *et al.* 1994)

There are two theories regarding the aetiology of expansion of blood volume in pregnancy. The 'overfill' hypothesis suggests that there is a primary mineralocorticoid excess that stimulates sodium and water retention; consequently, there is an increase in blood volume. The second hypothesis, the 'underfill' theory, claims that sodium and water retention is spurred by hormonally mediated vasodilatation, produced by vasodilating prostaglandins E_2 and I_2 (PGE_2, PGI_2), oestrogen and progesterone, and placental arteriovenous shunting. The 'underfill' theory is supported by research (Phippard *et al.* 1986) and the fact that blood pressure, especially the diastolic component, is lower in the gravid women.

Pregnant women are susceptible to profound positional hypotension. In the supine position, the uterus compresses the inferior vena cava, thereby reducing venous return, stroke volume and, consequently, cardiac output and blood pressure. The normal maternal compensatory response is tachycardia and lower extremity vasoconstriction. Hypotension from aortocaval compression can be minimized with uterine displacement achieved by right or left tilt of the pelvis.

A fall in cardiac output during the last trimester of pregnancy is probably caused by compression of the inferior vena cava by the uterus with subsequent reduction of venous return and hence a reduced stroke volume. Variation in the development of collateral venous channels may influence variations of cardiac output in individuals.

This extra 1.5 litres is distributed to the various sites; blood flow to the uterus rises throughout pregnancy to a mean maximum of about 500 ml/min. Renal blood flow increases in early pregnancy by about 400 ml/min. It is said to decline in late pregnancy, but as for cardiac output this may be caused by the mother's position when taking measurements. Blood flow through the skin is greatly increased. It may amount to 500 ml/min. The kidneys and skin serve elimination, the kidney of soluble waste and the skin of heat. Both processes require plasma rather than whole blood, which gives point to the disproportionate increase of plasma volume in the expansion of blood volume.

Most of the increased cardiac output is balanced by a reduction in the peripheral resistance of the blood vessels and also by a reduced sensitivity to the vasoconstrictive effects of angiotensin II (*see above*, Extracellular Fluid Volume). This is caused by the effect of oestrogen and progesterone. As already mentioned the increase in plasma volume causes haemodilution because the red-cell volume does not increase in line with the plasma volume. The haemoglobin value falls, giving rise to physiological anaemia. This is different from true anaemia in that it is purely related to the haemodilution of pregnancy and is not a consequence of an underlying pathological condition.

Blood pressure is dependent on cardiac output and the peripheral resistance of the blood vessels. The increased cardiac output (stroke volume multiplied by the heart rate) tends to raise blood pressure, whereas peripheral resistance of the blood vessels decreases blood pressure. Because progesterone dilates the vessels the peripheral resistance is reduced and so blood pressure is maintained within a correct range.

Respiration

The resting minute volume (or minute ventilation) increases throughout pregnancy by about 40%. Branch (1992) states that it begins to increase in the first trimester by 40–50%. This is achieved by an increase in tidal volume rather than respiratory rate. There is a decrease in the functional residual capacity (FRC). Oxygen uptake increases by only 15% so overbreathing results. Alveolar $P\text{co}_2$ falls from about 5.1 kPa in nonpregnant women to about 4.0 kPa in late pregnancy.

Increased progesterone levels increase the resting minute ventilation so there are changes in alveolar $P\text{co}_2$. The mother in effect blows off this excess CO_2 by hyperventilating. There is an arterial CO_2 tension of less than 30 mmHg, resulting in chronic respiratory alkalosis (Branch, 1992). This sets the maternal arterial pH in a typical range of 7.40–7.45. One can conclude that progesterone is responsible for the chronic hyperventilation of pregnancy, either by changing the sensitivity of the respiratory centres to $P\text{co}_2$, or by acting as a primary respiratory stimulant. Oestrogen may additionally cause increased stimulation of the respiratory centre, which would also cause an increase in respiratory rate.

The airways, thoracic cage, respiratory muscles and cardiovascular system are all affected by normal pregnancy.

Within the upper respiratory tract there are mucosal changes consisting of hyperaemia, hypersecretion and mucosal oedema. These are most pronounced in the third trimester. These changes frequently cause nasal obstruction, epistaxis, sneezing spells and a change in vocalization. The obstructive symptoms are often made worse by an upper tract infection.

Oestrogen is responsible for the nasal mucous membrane changes. They cause a change in the composition of the tissue whereby hydration occurs and hence oedema. This in effect reduces the diameter of the tract, so causing the obstructive symptoms. Oestrogen also cause the capillaries to become congested and hypersecretion of the mucous glands (Elkus and Popovich, 1992).

Prostaglandins can affect the bronchial mucosa. $PGF_{2\alpha}$, a uterine smooth muscle stimulant, constricts bronchial mucosa, whereas PGE_1 and PGE_2 have a bronchodilatory effect.

During pregnancy, the enlarging uterus causes up to 4 cm elevation in the level of the diaphragm. Despite this upwards displacement, diaphragmatic function is not impaired. Breathing generally tends to be more diaphragmatic than costal. This also explains why the abdominal muscles have less tone and are less active during pregnancy, serving to counterbalance the effects of upwards physical displacement by the gravid uterus. There is a 2 cm increase in the anteroposterior and transverse diameters of the thoracic cage, which counterbalances the rise of the diaphragm. There is an increase of 50% in the subcostal angle, which changes from 68.5° to 103.5° (Elkus and Popovich, 1992). Thus there is a 5–7 cm increase in chest circumference. The relaxation of the ligaments, again caused by hormonal effects, cause this change.

One question remains: 'How do the lung volumes change?' Studies have shown that the expiratory reserve volume decreases by 8–40% and the residual volume by 7–22% throughout pregnancy. As a result, there is a 10–25% decrease in FRC after the fifth or sixth month of pregnancy. Because of flaring of the lower ribs, widening of the rib cage and also musculatory changes, the inspiratory capacity increases. The vital capacity and total lung capacity are not substantially changed. Because the residual volume decreases progressively and the total lung capacity remains unchanged, the residual volume to total lung capacity ratio is low in the third trimester.

The tidal volume increases markedly, from 450–600 ml and is largely due to increased respiratory drive and rib cage volume displacement. Maximum breathing capacity is not significantly affected by pregnancy; also, vital capacity, forced vital capacity, peak flow rates, maximum flow rates and velocity index are not appreciably altered during pregnancy.

Total pulmonary resistance, consisting of both airway and tissue resistance, has been shown to be significantly reduced in pregnancy.

Because pregnant women usually have a reduced FRC and hypocapnia, which would tend to increase airway resistance, other mechanisms must be in play. These may be caused by relaxation of the bronchial smooth muscle because of an increase in levels of cortisol, relaxin or progesterone and improved compliance secondary to pulmonary ventilation.

As the enlarging uterus encroaches on the diaphragm, chest wall compliance and therefore total respiratory compliance are reduced in late pregnancy.

FRC is reduced in pregnant women because of a decrease in the residual volume and expiratory reserve volume. The FRC decreases even further in the supine position. These changes may result in airway closure during normal tidal volume breathing in pregnancy, and partially account for supine hypoxaemia. Oxygen consumption is elevated during pregnancy as a result of fetal and maternal tissue mass growth and a small increase in cardiac and respiratory work.

Because the FRC is reduced and the oxygen consumption increased in a normal pregnancy, there is a concomitant lowering of the oxygen reserve. If not properly compensated, exercise could result in further depletion of the oxygen reserve and detrimentally affect the fetus.

Of normal healthy gravidas with no history of cardiorespiratory disease 60–70% complain of dyspnoea during pregnancy (Tenholder and South-Paul, 1989).

Renal Function

Glomerular filtration rate increases by as much as 50% (Resnick and Laragh, 1983). The usual glomerular filtration rate is about 90 ml/min in nonpregnant women, rising to 150 ml/min in the first trimester which is maintained throughout pregnancy. The albumin concentration may be important here, as there is a fall in serum albumin concentration which naturally reflects a fall in oncotic pressure. This may increase the fragility of the red cells and enhance glomerular filtration; also, because of this reduced serum albumin concentration, the binding of hormones is reduced (Whittaker and Lind, 1993). This reduced concentration is due to the dilutional affects brought about by the increased plasma volume, described earlier (*see above*, Volume and Composition of the Blood).

The rise leads to changes in blood composition. Urea, uric acid and creatinine are cleared more efficiently and hence the plasma concentration of these are reduced. Glucose may be excreted in large quantities in a normal pregnancy and up to 3 g of amino acids may be lost daily. Folate is excreted at 4–5 times the usual rate and the loss of other water soluble vitamins also occurs.

Nutritional Requirements of Pregnancy and Metabolism

The greatest growth of the fetus occurs during the last trimester when its weight almost doubles during the final 2 months of pregnancy. In this period the mother does not absorb sufficient protein, calcium, phosphates and iron from the gastrointestinal tract to supply the fetus with the appropriate amounts. This is not a problem as at the beginning of pregnancy the mother's body stored these substances.

Nutritional status can also affect albumin metabolism and studies suggest a role for albumin as a source of placental and hence fetal amino acids, thus providing an important reserve pool of nitrogen for the mother and the growing fetus. Recent work also shows that insulin has a stimulatory effect on albumin synthesis, perhaps to capture essential amino acids (Whittaker and Lind, 1993).

During a normal pregnancy, the developing fetus imposes a significant demand on maternal calcium homeostasis, particularly in late gestation. Approximately 200 mg/day of calcium are deposited in the fetal skeleton during the third trimester, with a net accumulation of 25–30 g of calcium (Hojo and August, 1995). There is also an increased loss of calcium in the urine, with levels in late pregnancy that are on average double the usual urinary calcium excretion of nonpregnant women. The hypocalcuria in pregnancy is most probably caused by a combination of increased gastrointestinal absorption of calcium and the increased glomerular filtration rate. Despite the increased transfer of calcium to the fetal skeleton and the increased urinary calcium excretion, there is surprisingly little evidence that pregnant women suffer from skeletal demineralization.

The maternal adjustments in calcium metabolism that occur during pregnancy, compensate at least in part for the fetal calcium demands and the urinary losses. Despite the increased gastrointestinal tract absorption of calcium, total serum calcium levels decrease during pregnancy. This is caused by a decrease in the serum albumin which, as mentioned earlier, acts as a carrier protein that binds to the calcium. However, serum ionized calcium levels remain unchanged. There is considerable controversy regarding levels of parathyroid hormone (PTH) during pregnancy, with reports of increased, unchanged or decreased levels. PTH levels have recently been found to be slightly lower than those measured in nonpregnant women. These suppressed levels of PTH may be a consequence of the increase in vitamin D.

Energy Requirements

Traditional estimates of the energy requirements for pregnancy have been approximately 300 cal/day or 80,000 cal for a full-term pregnancy (Catalano and Hollenbeck, 1992).

Protein accumulation increases steadily during pregnancy and oxygen consumption progressively increases during gestation. Maternal fat accumulation increases primarily between 10 and 30 weeks gestation.

Weight Gain in Pregnancy

The mother may gain something like 12.5 kg, or in the case of a Swedish study about 15 kg (Uvnas-Moberg, 1989), during pregnancy. On average the weight increases at a rate of about 0.5 kg/week during the second trimester of pregnancy, the most rapid rise occurring between the 16th and 24th weeks.

The average weight gain during pregnancy stated in Guyton (1991) is 10.9 kg (24 lb) but this varies in the literature. Using the 10.9 kg weight, this can be broken down into approximately 3.2 kg (7 lb) for the fetus and 1.8 kg (4 lb) for amniotic fluid, placenta and fetal membranes. The uterus increases by approximately 0.9 kg (2 lb) and the breasts another 0.9 kg (2 lb), still leaving an average increase in weight of the mother's body of 4.1 kg (9 lb). About 2.7 kg (6 lb) of this is fluid in the blood and extracellular fluid that is excreted in the urine during the first days after birth (that is, after loss of the fluid-retaining hormones of the placenta).

Often during pregnancy a mother has a greatly increased desire to intake food, partly as a result of fetal removal of food substrates from the mother's blood and partly because of hormonal factors. Without appropriate prenatal care weight gain may be as great as 34.0 kg (75 lbs) or more.

Musculoskeletal Changes

There are numerous musculoskeletal changes during normal pregnancy. These are caused by hormonal changes that affect the ligaments and connective tissue. The sacroiliac joints loosen and the gravid uterus results in a posture of lumbar lordosis. It is for this reason that, often, pregnant women complain of some degree of lower back pain (Branch, 1992). There may be mild ankle, knee and hip pain due to the increasing weight on the skeletal framework. There is also a marked widening of the symphysis pubis.

Neurological Changes

A brief mention is in keeping here as childbirth is a psychological milestone. The mother grows emotionally during the process by adaptive mechanisms. A psychotic or potentially psychotic individual lacks the resilient psyche needed to handle either pregnancy or the subsequent presence of a child. Hormonal changes probably play a role. Unresolved conflicts and other psychological factors have been identified in pregnant and puerperal women who develop mental illness. These factors are operable in situations where no hormonal changes can be implicated (Donaldson, 1989, p. 325).

Endocrinological Changes

These are numerous and so the remainder of this chapter is dedicated to the endocrine system and the changes that occur within a normal pregnancy.

Thyroid Gland

A number of changes in thyroid function occur during pregnancy, a major one being the mother appearing to have a hyperthyroid state. Before the fetal thyroid gland is able to synthesize thyroxine its requirements are drawn from the mother across the placental barrier.

There is enlargement of the thyroid by about 50% during pregnancy to meet the increased demands of of the fetus for thyroxine. The increased thyroxine production is caused at least partly by a thyrotrophic effect of HCG and also by small amounts of a specific thyroid-stimulating hormone, human chorionic thyrotrophin, secreted by the placenta.

The normal thyroid gland accumulates dietary iodide at a fairly constant rate; this is incorporated into the thyroid hormone or its precursors. The remainder of the ingested iodide is excreted by the kidneys. The thyroid hormones are either stored in the gland or released into the circulation. The secreted thyroid hormones, thyroxine and triiodothyronine, are transported in the blood and extracellular fluid to the cells. The primary hormone binding proteins in the serum are thyroxine-binding globulin (TBG), thyroxine-binding prealbumin (TBPA) and albumin. The binding capacity of TBG increases, during pregnancy, from 25 µg/dl to about 50 µg/dl (Furth, 1983). This accounts for the increase in measured circulating thyroxine during pregnancy. Once the circulating thyroid hormones reach the cell, the unbound fraction is free to enter the cell. The thyroid hormone synthesis and release is regulated by a negative feedback mechanism involving the pituitary gland and the hypothalamus. Thyrotrophin-releasing hormone (TRH) is released by the hypothalamus and stimulates the pituitary to release thyroid-stimulating hormone (TSH). TSH stimulates the trapping of iodide into the thyroid.

The enlarged thyroid gland together with an increased oxygen consumption, raised pulse rate, heat intolerance and a rise in protein bound iodine (PBI) has in the past been interpreted as evidence of hyperthyroidism.

Various changes occur to the physiology of the thyroid during pregnancy. There is an increase in the concentration and binding capacity of TBG, although TBPA remains constant. This rise is due to oestrogen stimulation. Besides this there is also an increase in iodide turnover by the thyroid gland and often an increase in the size of the gland, but there is no evidence of increased thyroid activity as the enlargement is mainly caused by colloid deposition. The basal metabolic rate increases in pregnancy, probably as a result of an increase in net oxygen consumption of mother and fetus. Also there is some alteration in hypothalamic pituitary function.

Parathyroid Glands

Normal calcium homeostasis is maintained by the parathyroid glands. This involves the interchange of calcium in bone and other body tissues and its regulation by vitamin D, parathormone and calcitonin. To meet the needs of the fetus, mechanisms that can facilitate these demands must be available. Maternal calcium intake has to be increased to accommodate the fetal needs. Maternal vitamin D increases so as to promote the absorption of calcium and hence its transport to the fetus.

Renin–Angiotensin–Aldosterone System in Normal Pregnancy

The blood pressure in a normal pregnancy shows an early fall in diastolic value, beginning as early as the eighth week of pregnancy. The lowest point is reached by about the 28th week. Pressures then increase, but even at 38 weeks these are reduced compared with those of nonpregnant women. The renin system responds in normal pregnancy to correctly perceived relative volume depletion and hence is protective and compensatory to further haemodynamic compromise. Also the ANP, already discussed under Extracellular Fluid Volume, causes a fall in sensitivity for angiotensin II. Therefore, in summary, because of the increased cardiac output but a reduced vasoconstriction and a relative salt depletion, the renin–angiotensin–aldosterone system provides adequate compensation under the circumstances of a normal pregnancy.

Prostaglandins

Prostaglandins can be considered as modulators of autonomic nervous activity (Fuchs and Klopper, 1983) and have been briefly mentioned under Respiration. They are responsible for such activities as increased platelet activity and constriction of vascular smooth muscle. They are too numerous to go into any detail here – see the recommended reading list at the end of this chapter for further information.

Human Chorionic Gonadotrophin

Its role is in the maintenance of the corpus luteum in secretion of progesterone. After 6 weeks of pregnancy the placenta becomes the main site of progesterone production. Evidence (Fuchs and Klopper, 1983) suggests that HCG secreted by the trophoblast may also contribute to the immunoregulatory processes that operate during pregnancy. Being associated with the microvillous border of the syncytial trophoblast, HCG is in direct contact with the maternal blood. Because the trophoblast produces organ-specific antigens, HCG may be involved in the modulation of their expression.

It is now thought that there is an important thyrotrophic role of HCG in regulating the thyroid gland during normal pregnancy (Glinoer *et al.* 1993).

Progesterone

In conjunction with oestrogen, progesterone stimulates the growth of the uterus, differentiates the endometrium into a secretory tissue with an increased accumulation of glycogen, stimulates the decidualization of the endometrium required for implantation and inhibits myometrial contraction. Progesterone enters the cell by diffusion across the cell membrane and interacts with its specific receptor. This steroid–receptor complex then interacts with the nucleus, which results in an increase in the rate of protein synthesis (Fuchs and Klopper, 1983).

The ability of progesterone in converting the endometrium from a proliferative into a secretory type is by means of signals orchestrated by the deoxyribonucleic acid (DNA) within the nucleus of the cells in response to the progesterone. Progesterone has an inhibitory effect on smooth-muscle contraction, namely on the ureters, stomach and gut. This accounts for the ureteric dilatation and reduced intestinal peristaltic activity which occur in pregnancy (Llewellyn-Jones, 1990, p. 34).

Progesterone also regulates the storage of body fat, which leads to a rise in temperature of 0.5–1°C. Its action on brain cells may be responsible for the placid response commonly found in pregnant women. It is implicated in the hyperventilation of pregnant women. A small amount of placental progesterone enters the fetal circulation, where it is carried to the adrenal glands to act as a precursor for fetal corticosteroids.

Effects on the mammary gland

Progesterone, in conjunction with oestrogen and other hormones, stimulates breast growth during pregnancy, making them ready for lactation and effecting acinar growth. When progesterone and oestrogen fall abruptly following delivery, in the presence of the elevated prolactin, milk secretion begins. In summary the prerequisites for milk production are:

- A rise in prolactin.
- A fall in progesterone and oestrogen.
- Involvement of insulin, and adrenal and thyroid hormones.

From a physiological point of view, lactation is a continuation of pregnancy. The mother's endocrine and digestive system continues to provide nourishment for the child. The major differences are that the mother now stores energy in a special depot, the breast, and the baby now receives its nourishment in the form of milk rather than from the passage of nutrients through the umbilical cord. A mother's need for calories is even higher during lactation than in pregnancy. It has been calculated that a lactating mother should increase her intake of calories by 25% above her normal intake. Suckling on the breast enhances the mother's food intake, as it stimulates the vagal nerve and also increases maternal prolactin and oxytocin levels therefore promoting milk production and flow.

In summary, suckling by the baby triggers a vagally mediated gut-hormone response in both the baby and mother. The frequency and intensity of suckling regulates gastrointestinal function in both and therefore synchronizes their metabolisms. The mother and baby are rendered symbiotic not only psychologically but also physiologically.

Effects on the kidney

Aldosterone affects the renal tubules in terms of the absorption of sodium. Progesterone inhibits aldosterone by blocking the sodium uptake; on the other hand, progesterone, by way of relaxing smooth muscle, may produce vasodilatation and favour natriuresis through a blood flow effect. Progesterone maintains potassium homeostasis in normal pregnancy.

Effects on the brain

The behavioural changes that occur in pregnancy are well documented. Some of these effects may be caused by the high levels of progesterone acting on neurones. The administration of progesterone to humans and small animals is known to anaesthetize and put to sleep at high dosage (Merryman *et al.* 1954).

Cortisol

Oestrogens affect cortisol metabolism. The plasma levels of cortisol and aldosterone increase progressively throughout gestation. As stated before, the progesterone levels inhibit aldosterone actions. The oestrogen increases the unbound plasma cortisol levels.

Adrenal Gland

The total corticosteroids increase progressively in pregnancy. This accounts for the tendency to develop abdominal striae, glycosuria and hypertension, and also for the heavier morphological features commonly seen.

Pituitary Gland

The hormones oxytocin and vasopressin are secreted by the posterior lobe of the pituitary gland and are often called neurohypophyseal hormones. Oxytocin stimulates smooth muscle contraction by a direct effect on the cell membrane. Vasopressin increases permeability and diffusion of water through the cells of the distal tubules in the kidneys.

Oxytocin is found in maternal plasma from 6 weeks, increasing significantly with gestational age because of the rise in circulating oestrogen levels. Of course, it is the increased oestrogen levels that eventually initiate the uterine contractions and start the labour process. The mother's oxytocin levels also play a role by determining the precise time of day that the baby is born (Nathanielsz, 1994). Studies conducted primarily in sheep have demonstrated that the fetal brain provides the signal to start the birth process. Some 3–4 weeks before giving birth, the fetal hypothalamus stimulates the fetal pituitary to secrete more adrenocorticotrophic hormone (ACTH) and, as a result, fetal adrenocortical glucocorticoid secretion increases. The adrenal steroids play a key role in the maturation of many vital organ systems as they are prepared for independent life.

The anterior lobe of the pituitary gland secretes melanocyte-stimulating hormone (MSH) which is produced in increasing amounts and is probably responsible for the characteristic skin pigmentation of pregnancy. Darkening of the vulva may also occur and a dark line, the linea nigra, is often seen. In nonpregnant women this is referred to as the linea alba, which extends from the symphysis pubis to the umbilicus. Pigmentation is of course variable and affects individuals in different ways. In some women, particularly brunettes, there is an increase in pigmentation during pregnancy. In some, a mask-like area of pigmentation covers the forehead and upper part of the cheeks; this disappears after delivery.

There is a progressively reduced tolerance to a glucose load in spite of increasing amounts of circulating insulin.

Effects on the Gastrointestinal Tract

Beginning early in pregnancy, a woman gains weight, storing energy as fat against the demands of the fetus and in preparation for the heavy demands that come with lactation and breast feeding. Therefore, the normal activity of the gastrointestinal tract changes in response to the pregnancy, this being an important factor in the characteristic weight gain.

Much emphasis has been made of the fact that the musculature of the gastrointestinal tract is relaxed, which cause of many uncomfortable symptoms of pregnancy. The cardiac sphincter is relaxed and allows oesophageal reflux, which causes heartburn. There appears to be some controversy over the secretion of gastrin and therefore gastric juice secretion. Uvnas-

Moberg (1989) showed that there is an increase in gastric secretion which enhances the digestion of food.

Because increased nutrition is a prerequisite for growth and because food is digested in the gastrointestinal tract, the stomach and intestines need to function optimally during periods of reproduction and intense growth. This depends on the activity of the various gastrointestinal hormones that play a part. Gastrin, produced in the lower part of the stomach, enhances digestion by stimulating both gastric motility and secretion of gastric acid. Cholecystokinin, secreted from the upper part of the small intestine, inhibits movement of food out of the stomach, therefore enhancing digestion and absorption of nutrients into the circulation. It also stimulates the release of bile from the gall bladder. The hormone secretin, also secreted from the small intestines, stimulates secretion by the pancreas of bicarbonate.

It has been shown that these polypeptide hormones also stimulate the growth of organs they affect; in particular, there is increased thickening of the mucosa. In other words they are acting on the gut as if they were growth hormones (Uvnas-Moberg, 1989). Somatostatin does not have the same role as the other hormones; instead it exerts an inhibitory effect on the gut. Its release is inhibited by vagal activity and stimulated by splanchnic activity. The splanchnic nerve is a division of the sympathetic part of the autonomic system.

As previously mentioned, women may put on an average of 12.5–15 kg during their pregnancy. Part of the gain reflects the weight of the fetus itself, the growth of the uterus and an increase in the blood volume, but at least 4 kg represents the deposition of fat. Changes in the hormone activity of the gastrointestinal tract play a leading role here.

The postprandial release of cholecystokinin increases in pregnant women. This increase and a decrease in the inhibitory effects of somatostatin work to optimize the digestive process. Anabolic metabolism is prominent, which entails the building up from small molecules of larger molecules that contribute to growth or are stored in the body for future use. Therefore weight gain is favoured because the levels of the hormones that potentiate the glucose-induced release of insulin rise and the somatostatin level drops. The postprandial rise in cholecystokinin is probably responsible, by way of vagal signals to the brain, for the sleepiness and tiredness, particularly after meals. This is characteristic of early pregnancy. This fatigue has an adaptive effect in that it tends to reduce physical activity, so energy is saved and stored.

Anabolic metabolism dominates after the ingestion of food, when resources required for the fetus are deposited in the liver and fat tissue. This storage of future requirements is by the facilitated glucose uptake promoted by the hormone insulin. Insulin is secreted by the β-cells of the Islets of Langerhans found in the pancreas. When the blood glucose levels rise in response to the digestion of food, insulin is secreted. Eating also increases the activity of the parasympathetic nervous system and thus the endocrine system of the gastrointestinal tract. The parasympathetic vagus nerve inhibits the release of somatostatin, therefore favouring the growth-promoting effects of the hormones gastrin, cholecystokinin and secretin. These hormones in turn enhance the release of insulin, therefore further stimulating anabolic metabolism. Somatostatin inhibits the uptake of nutrients and their deposition into the liver and as fat.

Early pregnancy is characterized with the symptoms of intense hunger, nausea, hypotension and vertigo. The hunger and vertigo may be related to a fall in blood glucose level and also due to the insulin-releasing effect of cholecystokinin, gastrin and secretin. There may be excessive salivation due to the influence of parasympathetic stimulation.

The nausea is more than likely caused by the delayed emptying of the stomach brought about by the high levels of cholecystokinin. This is particularly marked during labour, when food can remain in the stomach for up to 24 hours (Llewellyn-Jones, 1990, p. 40). The changes are probably brought about by the hyperactivity of the vagus nerve. This in turn increases the secretion of cholecystokinin. Vagal stimulation can be brought about by the hormone oxytocin, which is produced by the paraventricular nuclei contained within the hypothalamus. As already mentioned in discussing the pituitary gland, oxytocin fibres project to the posterior lobe of the pituitary. Here it is stored until it needs to be secreted into the circulation. Besides this route there is also a direct link to the vagus nerve itself, by fibres, again from the hypothalamus, that project to the vagal motor nucleus in the brain stem. This then stimulates the vagus directly. The increased levels of the oestrogens further stimulate the hypothalamus to produce more oxytocin. The gastrointestinal hormone release may be affected locally by both oestrogen and progesterone.

Due to evolutionary, genetic and environmental effects, modern humans have inherited the genetic material and physiological aspects of their ancestors. Any physiological mechanisms that made more energy available during pregnancy must have been very important for the gestation and development of healthy offspring when food was sparse. This is no longer the case in today's advanced societies, characterized (by most people) as having an abundance of food, but the inherent ability of the female to cut down on energy expenditure during pregnancy is still being genetically expressed. The problem is now that the effects are negative, that is resulting in the unpleasant symptoms already mentioned and the risk of overweight. The ease with which most women put on weight and the higher frequency of obesity in women than men may reflect women's latent and life-giving ability to store energy, an ability that is fully expressed during periods of active reproduction.

Amniotic fluid ingestion is important to the development of the fetal gastrointestinal tract in preparation of the fetus to be born. The periods of ingestion of amniotic fluid are followed by secretion of fetal gastrin, somatostatin and gastric acid. There is a high gastrin level in the newborn, in fact levels are 5–10 times more than those in adults. These high gastrin levels in the newborn are not secondary to a large intake of nutrients, as the baby ingests very little milk during the first few days of breastfeeding; in other words, the high gastrin levels precede the high food intake that comes later in infancy. The high gastrin levels can be explained on the grounds that the baby's gastrointestinal function has been prestimulated during fetal life when amniotic fluid ingestion occurs. The amniotic fluid contains various substances, including epidermal growth factor and gastrin, that stimulate gastrointestinal maturation.

Summary

The woman undergoes considerable physiological changes during pregnancy with all systems of her body affected. These changes are adaptive measures by the body to the developing fetus. The midwife needs to be aware of these changes to adequately monitor and determine that fetal and maternal health are being maintained.

KEY CONCEPTS

- The consequences of psychological illhealth in pregnancy may be far-reaching for the woman, her partner and her family.
- The factors that pre-dispose to psychological ill health in pregnancy and motherhood are diverse, but these may be identified and appropriate support given by the knowledgeable and caring midwife.
- Effective use of appropriate midwifery skills can help to reduce long-term psychological illhealth and facilitate support for women and their children.
- The relationship of the mother and fetus is not simply as host and parasite, but as a joint relationship in which the mother provides an adequate environment for the developing fetus. This environment may not always be harmonious as there are many stresses exerted on the mother.

References

Adams L, Cotgrove A: Promoting secure attachment patterns in infancy and beyond, *Professional Care Mother Child* 5(6):158, 1995.

Ainsworth MDS, Blehar M, Waters E, Wall S: *Patterns of attachment*, Hillsdale, 1978, Erlbaum,.

Allport GW: *Personality: a psychological interpretation*, New York, 1937, Rinehart and Winston.

Allport GW: *Patterns and growth in personality*, New York, 1961, Holt, Rinehart and Winston.

Anderson VN, Fleming AS, Steiner M: Mood and the transition to motherhood, *J Reprod Infant Psychol* 12:69, 1994.

Argyle M: *The social psychology of everyday life*, London, 1992, Routledge.

Ball JA: *Reactions to motherhood: the role of postnatal care*, Hale, 1994, Books for Midwives Press.

Bibring GL, Some considerations of the psychological processes in pregnancy. *Psychoanalytic study of the child* 14:113–21, 1959.

Blacker CVR: *Depression in general practice*, MD Thesis, London, 1989, University of London.

Bowlby J: *Attachment and loss, Vol. 1, Attachment*, Harmondsworth, 1971, Penguin.

Bowlby J: *Attachment and loss, Vol. 2, Separation: anxiety and anger*, Harmondsworth, 1975, Penguin.

Bowlby J: *A secure base, clinical applications of attachment theory*, London, 1988, Tavistock Routledge.

Branch DW: Physiologic adaptations of pregnancy, *Am J Reprod Immunol* 28:120, 1992.

British Association of Counselling: *Code of ethics and practice for counselling skills*, Rugby, 1989, British Association for Counselling.

Brown B, Harris T: *Social origins of depression,*

Brown MA, Gallery EDM: Volume homeostasis in normal pregnancy and pre-eclampsia: physiology and clinical implications. *Bailliere's Clin Obstet Gynaecol* 8:2:287, 1994.

Caplan G: *An approach to community mental health*, London, 1969, Tavistock.

Catalano PM, Hollenbeck C: Energy requirements in pregnancy: A review. *Obstet Gynecol Survey* 47(6):368, 1992.

Central Statistics Office: *Annual abstract of statistics*, London, 1994, HMSO.

Charles J, Curtis L: Birth afterthoughts: a listening and information service, *Br J Midwifery* 2(7):331, 1994.

Christensen M: Birth rape, *Midwifery Today* 22:34, 1992.

Clement S: 'Listening visits' in pregnancy: a strategy for preventing postnatal depression? *Midwifery* 11:75, 1995.

Combes G, Schonveld A: *Life will never be the same again: Learning to be a first time parent*, London, 1992, Health Education Authority.

Condon JT: The assessment of antenatal emotional attachment: Development of questionnaire instrument, *Br J Med Psychol* 66:167, 1993.

Davies J, Evans F: Care in the community. In Faulkner T, Murphy-Black T, editors: *Excellence in nursing, the research route: midwifery*, London, 1990, Scutari Press, p. 69.

Department of Health: *Changing childbirth: Report of the Expert Maternity Group*, London, 1993, HMSO.

Dohrenwend B, Krasnoff L, Askenasy A, Dohrewend B: Exemplification of a method for scaling life events, *J Health Soc Behav* 19:205, 1978.

Donaldson JO, editor: *Neurology of pregnancy*, 2nd edn, Vol. 19, London, 1989, WB Saunders.

Duffy TP: Hematologic aspects of pregnancy. In: Hoffman R, Benz EJ, Shattil SJ, Furie B, Cohen HJ, editors: *Hematology: Basic principles and practice*, New York, 1991, Churchill Livingstone, p. 1707.

Elkus R, Popovich J: Respiratory physiology in pregnancy, *Clin Chest Med* 13(4):555, 1992.

Erikson EH: *Childhood and society*, New York, 1963, Norton.

Eysenck HJ: *The structure of human personality*, London, 1953, Methuen.

Fuchs F, Klopper A, editors: *Endocrinology of pregnancy*, 3rd edn, Philadelphia, 1983, Harper and Row.

Furth ED: Thyroid and parathyroid hormone function in pregnancy. In: Fuchs F, Klopper A, editors: *Endocrinology of pregnancy*, 3rd edn, Philadelphia, 1983, Harper and Row, p. 176.

Gauer OH, Henry JP: Neurohormonal control of plasma volume. In: Guyton AC, Cowley AW, editors: *Cardiovascular physiology 2. International Review of Physiology* Vol. 9, Baltimore, 1976, University Park Press, p. 145.

Glinoer D, De Nayer P, Robyn C, Lejeune B, Kinthaert J, Meuris S: Serum levels of intact human chorionic gonadotropin (hCG) and its free alpha and beta subunits, in relation to maternal thyroid stimulation during normal pregnancy. *J Endocrinol Invest.* 16(11):881, 1993.

Green JM, Kitzinger JV, Coupland VA: Stereotypes of childbearing women: a look at some evidence, *Midwifery* 6: 125, 1990.

Green J: Postnatal depression: Is it postnatal, is it depression? A paper presented at the Society for Reproductive and Infant Psychology 15th Annual Conference, 1995, University of Leicester.

Gross RD: *Psychology: the science of mind and behaviour*, 2nd Edn, London, 1992, Hodder and Stoughton.

Guyton AC: Pregnancy and lactation. In: Wonsiewicz MJ, editor: *Textbook of medical physiology*, 8th edn, Philadelphia, 1991, WB Saunders, Ch 82, p. 915.

Harris P: *Loss and change*, London, 1986, Routledge and Keegan.

Hamilton HFH: Blood viscosity in pregnancy, *J Obstet Gynaecol.* 56:548, 1950.

Hathaway WE, Bonnar J, editors: *Perinatal coagulation*, New York, 1978, Grune and Stratton.

Hoffbrand AV, Pettit JE, editors: *Essential haematology*, 3rd edn, Oxford, 1995, Blackwell Science.

Hojo M, August P: Calcium metabolism in normal and hypertensive pregnancy, *Semin Nephrol* 15(6):504, 1995.

Holmes TH, Rahe RH: The social readjustment rating scale, *J Psychosom Res* 11:213, 1967.

Hudson F, Ineichen B: *Taking it lying down: sexuality and teenage motherhood*, London, 1991, Macmillan.

Hytten FE, Leitch I, editors: *The physiology of human pregnancy*, Oxford, 1964, Blackwell Scientific Publications.

Ineichen B, Hudson F: *Teenage pregnancy*, London, 1994, National Children's Bureau.

Institute for the Study of Drug Dependency: *Drug misuse in Britain: National audit of drug misuse statistics*, Institute for the Study of Drug Dependency, 1992.

Kitzinger JV: Counteracting, not re-enacting the violation of women's bodies: The challenge for perinatal caregivers, *Birth* 19(4):219, 1992.

Kumar R, Robson KM: A prospective study of emotional disorders in childbearing women, *Br J Psychiatry* 144:35, 1984.

Kumar R, Robson KM, Smith AMR: Development of a self-administered questionnaire to measure maternal adjustment and maternal attitudes during pregnancy and after delivery, *J Psychosom Res* 28:43, 1984.

Lamb JF, Ingram CG, Johnston IA, Pitman RM: Reproductive physiology. In: Lamb JF, Ingram CG, Johnston IA, Pitman RM, editors: *Essentials of physiology*, 2nd edn, Oxford, 1988, Blackwell Scientific Publications, Ch 12, p. 379.

Laurence Beech B, Robinson J: Ultrasound scanning, *AIMS J* 5:1, 1993.

Lazarus RL: *Psychological stress and the coping process*, New York, 1966, McGraw Hill.

Lazarus RL, Folkman R: *Stress, appraisal and coping*, New York, 1984, Springer.

Levy V, Kline P: Perinatal depression: a factor analysis, *Br J Midwifery* 2(4):154, 1994.

Llewellyn-Jones D, editor: *Fundamentals of obstetrics and gynaecology, Vol. 1, Obstetrics*, 6th edn, London, 1996, Mosby.

Marris P: *Loss and change*, London, 1986, Routledge and Keegan and Page.

Mashburn J, Graves BW, Gillmor-Kahn M: Hematocrit values during pregnancy in a nurse-midwifery caseload, *J Nurse-Midwifery* 37(6):404, 1992.

Matthews KA: Coronary heart disease and Type A behaviours: update on and alternative to the Booth-Kewley and Friedman (1987) quantitative review, *Psychol Bull* 104:373, 1988.

May KA: Three phases of father involvement in pregnancy, *Nurs Res* 31:337, 1981.

Merryman M, Boiman R, Barnes L, Rothchild I: Progesterone 'anesthesia' in human subjects, *J Clin Endocrinol Metab* 14:1567, 1954.

Najman J, Morrison J, Williams G, Andersen M: The mental health of women six months after they give birth to an unwanted baby: a longitudinal study, *Social Sci Med* 32(3): 241, 1991.

Nathanielsz PW: A time to be born: Implications of animal studies in maternal–fetal medicine, *Birth* 21(3):163, 1994.

Newton RW: Psychosocial aspects of pregnancy: the scope for intervention, *J Reprod Infant Psychol* 6:23, 1988.

Niven CA: *Psychological care for families: Before, during and after birth*, Oxford, 1992, Butterworth Heinemann.

Oakley A: *Women confined: Towards a sociology of childbirth*, Oxford, 1980, Martin Robertson.

Oakley A, Rajan L, Grant A: Social support and pregnancy outcome: report of a randomised controlled trial, *Br J Obstet Gynaecol* 97(155), 1990.

Oakley A, Hickey D, Rajan L, Rigby AS: Social support in pregnancy: does it have long-term effects? *J Reprod Infant Psychol* 14:7, 1996.

Passmore R, Robson JS: Reproduction. In: Passmore R, Robson JS, editors: *A companion to medical studies*, 2nd edn, Vol. 1, Oxford, 1976, Blackwell Scientific, Ch 38, p. 1.

Paykel ES, Emms EM, Fletcher J, Rassaby ES: Life events and social support in puerperal depression, *Br J Psychiatry* 136: 339, 1980.

Pearlin LI, Schooler C: The structure of coping. *J Health Soc Behaviour* 19:2–21, 1978.

Phippard AF, Horvath JS, Glynn EM: Circulatory adaptation to pregnancy: Serial studies of hemodynamics, blood volume, renin and aldosterone in the baboon (*Papio hamadryas*), *J Hypertens* 4:773, 1989.

Phoenix A: Mothers under twenty. Outsider and insider views. In Phoenix A, Willet A, Lloyd E (eds)), London, 1991, Sage.

Pitt B: Atypical depression following childbirth, *Br J Psychiatry* 114:1325, 1968.

Price B: Changing body image, *Modern Midwife*, 6(4):12–15, 1996.

Raphael-Leff J: Facilitators and regulators: Two approaches to mothering, *Br J Med Psychol* 56:376, 1983.

Raphael-Leff J: Facilitators and regulators; participators and renouncers: mothers and fathers orientations towards pregnancy and parenthood, *J Psychosom Obstet Gynaecol* 4:169, 1985.

Raphael-Leff J: *Psychological processes of childbearing*, London, 1991, Chapman and Hall.

Raphael-Leff J: *Pregnancy: the inside story*, London, 1993, Sheldon Press.

Registrar General: *Birth statistics 1992*. Review of the Registrar Generals birth and patterns of family birthing in England and Wales, Series FM 1 No. 16, London, 1994, HMSO.

Resnick LM, Laragh JH: The renin–angiotensin–aldosterone system in pregnancy. In: Fuchs F, Klopper A, editors: *Endocrinology of pregnancy*, 3rd edn, Philadelphia, 1983, Harper and Row, p. 197.

Reading A, Cox D: The effects of ultrasound examination on maternal anxiety levels, *J Behav Med* 5:237, 1982.

Robertson J, Bowlby J: Responses of young children to separation from their mothers, *Courrier Centre Int Enfance* 2:131, 1952.

Robson SC, Hunter S, Boys RJ, Dunlop W: Serial study of factors influencing changes in cardiac output during human pregnancy, *Am J Physiol* 256:1061, 1989.

Rogers CR: *A way of being*, Boston, 1980, Houghton Mifflin Company.

Sakai K, Imaizumi T, Maeda H, *et al.*: Venous distensibility during pregnancy: Comparisons between normal pregnancy and preeclampsia, *Hypertension* 24(4):461, 1994.

Sharp HM, Cooper SA: Mothering orientations – ideal expectations versus outcome characteristics within a representative population of primiparous women. Paper presented at the sixth International Conference of the Marce Society, Scotland, 1992.

Smith J, Pregnancy and the transition to motherhood. In (eds) Nicolson P, Ussher J, *The psychology of womens health care*, 1992.

Spirito A, Ruggerio L, Coustan D, McGarvey S, Bond A, Mood states of women with diabetes during pregnancy, *J Reprod Infant Psychol* 10:29, 1992.

Statham H, Green J, Snowdon C: Psychological and social aspects of screening for fetal abnormality during routine antenatal care, Research and the Midwife Conference Proceedings, p. 44, 1992.

Tenholder MF, South-Paul J: Dyspnoea in pregnancy. *Chest* 196:381, 1989.

Thomsen JK, Fogh-Anderson N, Jaszczak P, Giese J: Atrial natriuretic peptide (ΛNP) decrease during normal pregnancy as related to hemodynamic changes and volume regulation. *Acta Obstet Gynecol Scand* 72(2):103, 1993.

Uvnas-Moberg K: The gastrointestinal tract in growth and reproduction. *Sci Am* 261(1):60, 1989.

Ussher J: *The psychology of the female body*, London, 1993, Routledge.

van Oppen ACC, Stigter RH, Bruinse HW: Cardiac output in normal pregnancy: A critical review, *Obstet Gynecol* 87(2):310, 1996.

Whittaker PG, Lind T: The intravascular mass of albumin during human pregnancy: a serial study in normal and diabetic women, *Br J Obstet Gynaecol* 100:587, 1993.

Windridge KC, Berryman JC: Maternal adjustment and maternal attitudes during pregnancy and early motherhood in women of 35 and over, *J Reprod Infant Psychol* 14:45, 1996.

Wolkind S, Zajicek E, editors: *Pregnancy: a psychological and social study*, London, 1981, Academic Press.

Further Reading

Ball JA: *Reactions to motherhood: the role of postnatal care*, Books for Midwives Press, 1994, Hale.

This book is an account of research into the reactions of women to pregnancy and the first 6 weeks of motherhood. It looks specifically at the emotional response and support systems and identifies some of the mismatches between women's needs and support systems.

Burrow GN: The thyroid gland in pregnancy. In: Friedman EA, editor: *Major problems in obstetrics and gynecology*, Vol. 3, Philadelphia, 1972, WB Saunders.

Although this is fairly old it is not out of date and has some relevant and interesting information.

de Alvarez RM, editor: *The kidney in pregnancy*, New York, 1976, John Wiley & Sons.

An interesting reader for those requiring more information.

Guyton AC: Pregnancy and lactation. In: Wonsiewicz MJ, editor: *Textbook of medical physiology*, 8th edn, Philadelphia, 1991, WB Saunders, p. 915.

Those requiring more information will find this is a very useful and palatable textbook.

Kalkhoff RK, Kim H-J: The influence of hormonal changes of pregnancy on maternal metabolism. In: Beard RW, Hoet JJ, editors: *Pregnancy: metabolism, diabetes and the fetus*, Ciba Foundation Symposium 63, Amsterdam, 1979, Excerpta Medica, p. 29.

More for the specialist but never the less has some interesting information.

Niven CA: *Psychological care for families: Before, during and after birth*, Oxford, 1992, Butterworth Heineman.

A very readable book that introduces many of the major psychological concepts and areas of particular importance and interest for midwifery practice.

Raphael-Leff J: *Psychological processes of childbearing*, London, 1991, Chapman and Hall.

This book draws on the clinical work of the author in psychotherapeutic practice with women in pregnancy and childbirth. It includes comprehensive discussion of the conscious and unconscious psychological processes relating to pregnancy.

Torrora GU, Grabowski SR: *Principles of anatomy and physiology*, 8th edn, New York, 1996, Harper Collins College Publications.

An easy to follow and informative textbook. Has a glossary of common terms used and would be of use for those with a limited knowledge of anatomy and physiology.

Ussher J: *The psychology of the female body*, London, 1993, Routledge.

A book that presents a feminist critique of psychological issues surrounding women's health. The content is approached in terms of the life cycle: from menarche to menopause.

5 *Planning Antenatal Care*

Care should be Centred on the Individual

A missed period is always significant. Planned or not, a woman's reaction will vary. The management of her pregnancy, birth and subsequent care is of enormous importance. Interactions with health-care professionals will affect her mothering, how she views herself and rates her abilities as a woman and mother. The policy of the UK government to a 'user-oriented' service is reiterated in the report of the Expert Maternity Group:

> *The woman must be the focus of maternity care. She should be able to feel that she is in control of what is happening to her and able to make decisions about her care, based on her needs, having discussed matters fully with the professionals involved.*
>
> (Department of Health, 1993.)

Flexibility and adaptability are needed to respond to the needs of individual childbearing women and their families. Women need to be the centre of care and assured of support before they can confidently plan for the pregnancy and birth.

Effective Antenatal Care

Ideally preconception care and advice should be sought and optimum health and well-being achieved before procreative sex. This is seldom the case. It is estimated that 50% of pregnancies are not planned (Whyte, 1995), so the importance of maintaining a healthy lifestyle cannot be stressed enough.

There are physical, spiritual, social and psychological aspects to antenatal care. The main aim of the carers is not simply to ensure a live healthy mother and baby at the end of the pregnancy. Greater emphasis needs to be placed on the psychological effects of childbirth. Pregnancy may lead to conditions in which life is at risk. In such situations, the aim is to minimize any potential harmful effects to the woman and her baby – termination of the pregnancy may be appropriate if the woman's life is threatened. Psychological support may also be the most important aspect of antenatal care for a woman known to be carrying a baby with an abnormality, i.e. anencephaly or trisomy 18. Antenatal care can and should be empowering. This can only occur when information is shared, given honestly and sensitively, thus allowing the woman to explore her choices and feel supported regardless of the outcome (Chitty *et al.* 1996).

Once pregnancy occurs, one of the endeavours of antenatal care is to detect any potential problems early enough to be able to prevent or correct them. Childbirth is uncomplicated for the majority but, even in the UK, mothers and babies still die. In nearly one-half of the 325 maternal deaths reported between 1988 and 1990, care was considered to be substandard. Antenatal care can contribute to reducing mortality, but it is not foolproof. Even the best care cannot detect all life-threatening diseases. In 5 of the 13 women who suffered a pulmonary embolism and died antenatally there were no signs, symptoms or any other indication of problems (Department of Health, 1994).

It is not known how many deaths are prevented or how much morbidity is reduced by women attending for antenatal care. But for care to be effective, women need information and need to be involved in care. Shielding them from worrying facts may result in them failing to appreciate and report signs and symptoms or from understanding the possible benefits of antenatal care. Recently, The Action on Pre-Eclampsia (APEC) group produced a leaflet to help women understand the importance of checking their blood pressure, with instructions as to when to seek medical or midwife referral (**Box 5.1**; APEC, 1996).

Formal risk scoring using protocols and guidelines aims to identify women at high risk, so that extra attention can be given to them. The usefulness of these systems has not been proved, so some woman may be exposed to an increased risk from unnecessary interventions (Enkin *et al.* 1995). From an international perspective, Yuster (1995) demonstrates the fallibility of formalized risk scoring and states that antenatal care is more effective when used to detect

---

Box 5.1

Treating Women as Partners – Advice on Symptoms which may Herald Pre-Eclampsia

- Bad headache.
- Blurred vision or flashes before eyes.
- Severe pain below ribs.
- Vomiting.
- Sudden swelling of your face, hands or feet.

Source: APEC, 1996.

complications and to educate and advise women of obstetric danger signs. For woman-centred care, individuals need to be involved in all decisions about their care. Women need information to plan who to book with, how often to be seen and where to go for help and advice. With the full knowledge of what to expect and of the limitations of antenatal care, women can properly plan ahead.

What do Women Want?

The Winterton report made history by acknowledging and accepting women's views as valid. This review of the maternity services along with the Expert Group's recommendations in the *Changing Childbirth* report (Department of Health, 1993) has led to many changes, including a focus on woman-centred care. Women have consistently said that they want continuity, choice and control. They want safe care, organized so they can get to know those who provide the care. They want care that is flexible and responsive to their needs. Purchasers and providers have a responsibility to find out what sort of service women want, including those groups who are under-represented in the locality. However, this is not always easy to establish. Information is available from surveys, research studies and listening to individuals and members of pressure and support groups.

Surveys

Good surveys include qualitative and quantitative questions (**Box 5.2**) and focus sessions with under-represented groups. If asked general questions soon after the birth, most women report satisfaction. They are on an emotional high. It is important to look critically at surveys to be sure that they have been conducted in an open manner and that the interpretation of the results is correct. Women on a postnatal ward may be reluctant to be critical of their carers as it might jeopardize their future care. If, antenatally, women ranked the qualities wanted in their midwives as follows:
• provides safe and competent care,
• involves you in choices,
• is known to you,
it could be said that safe care was more important to the women than knowing the midwife, but this does not show that women do not want choice or how important knowing the midwife is to women. Jacoby and Cartwright (1990) give an overview of the advan-

---

> ## Box 5.2
>
> ### Examples of Well-Constructed Survey Questions
>
> • During your pregnancy, how involved were you in decisions about your care?
> • Would you have liked to have been more or less involved?
> • Had you met any of the midwives and/or doctors who were with you in labour before you gave birth?
> • Would you have liked to have know them more before you gave birth?
>
> *Source: Gready et al. 1995.*

---

tages and disadvantages of the different ways of finding out women's views of the maternity services.

Other Ways of Ascertaining Women's Views

Work done postnatally with a small group of new mothers used collages to help them express feelings and emotions. The women described and explained their collages to the group and talked of the anger, fear and dissatisfaction they felt antenatally and with their birth experiences. This was at odds with the very positive, verbal birth reports they gave initially (Gillen, 1995). This method has the merit of being felt by the women to be beneficial to their understanding and progress through the life event of birth. Women who are not happy about their maternity care seldom complain. Some who do contact the Association for Improvements in Maternity Services (AIMS), which campaigns on behalf of women (*see* Chapter 18). Midwives can be retrospective while planning ahead and ask multigravid women what they liked about their care and birth and what they would like to do differently in subsequent pregnancies.

Women's Needs and the Organization of Care

Current maternity care is a long way from being woman-centred; mostly it is fragmented and needs drastic reorganization around the woman, her needs and her wants. Women's needs are not being met – comments from women in Redbridge echo many others all over the country:

> *The antenatal staff should make their patients more aware of the choices of giving birth ... I felt there was a lack of involvement. I saw a different person at every visit.*
>
> (Brooks and Black, 1994.)

In one survey, 850 women in North Essex were asked about their birth experiences and expectations; only 14% were offered a choice of where to have their baby and 29% were offered a choice of who to have their antenatal care with (Gready *et al.* 1995). At present, most antenatal care is determined by the professionals alone.

For many the way in which the maternity services operate perpetuates a system in which needs are not being met. However, there are a number of developments in which systems are being changed for the benefit of women. For example, midwifery-led units, day care for at-risk or high-risk women, teams, group practices and caseloads.

Teams

One way of organizing midwifery care is by teams. The first team approach was started to provide the woman with the opportunity to get to know her midwife. The research demonstrated that this was safe and much appreciated by the women and midwives (**Box 5.3**; Flint and Poulengeris, 1987).

A variety of teams have evolved. Some are very successful, others have been discontinued. There are community groups, exclusive hospital-based teams and some that are mixed. The size varies from 2 to 30 midwives and the number of women cared for by the team varies or is unknown. The benefits of teams depends on the group size, their workload and flexibility. The national survey into team midwifery (Wraight *et al.* 1993) identified the characteristics of successful teams. It is very difficult to generalize as to the benefits of reorganization into teams because there is no accepted definition of a 'team'. Change is not easy – it takes time and commitment. The managerial issues, the setting up and the evaluation of the successful Riverside Health Authority community group practices and hospital teams have been well documented by Lewis (1995a–d). Midwives in these groups practices take full responsibility for the care of women throughout their pregnancy. Obstetric consultants are not necessarily named on the notes and are only referred to in the event of a medical complication. Midwives working in this way report increased job satisfaction and enjoy their autonomous role, but Lewis acknowledges that opposition to the changes came from general practitioners (GPs), obstetricians and some midwives. Not all reorganizations have been so well thought out or managed. Some schemes simply pay lip service to the

---

Box 5.3

Women and Midwives Appreciate Team Midwifery – Quotes from Early Research

The women:
• The midwives really want to know about you as a person and do not treat you as a symptom.
• You build up a close friendly relationship over the months and this I feel puts you at ease.

The midwives:
• For the first time I have the support of a closely knit team and am able to confide experiences and discuss difficulties.
• I have appreciated being a 'whole' midwife rather than a 'fragmented' one. I feel that because I know them [the women]; I am better equipped to help them through the difficult stages.

Source: Flint and Poulengers, 1987.

Box 5.4

Key Characteristics of the One-to-One Service, Started in 1993, in Hammersmith Hospitals NHS Trust

Women are cared for by their named midwife, who plans care and provides the majority of care; care is:
• Focused on the needs of individual women and their families.
• Evidence based.
• Community based – midwives provide both community and hospital care, being 'with the woman where and when wanted'.
• Midwives work in partnerships, within group practices of six.
• There is a systematic programme of support and professional development for the midwives, including peer review.

Source: Page et al. 1994.

ideals of improving continuity of carer and Flint acknowledges that:

> *The total effect may be purely cosmetic, no change in working practice, no change in working hours, no greater intimacy between women and midwives.*

(Flint, 1994.)

Some teams may have been set up to fail. There are many difficult issues of power and control between the health professionals involved, as well as problems for individuals.

There are advantages and disadvantages of working within a nonhierarchical team, but this way of working can be difficult to adjust to and the increased on-call commitment may be difficult or impossible for some. An early team scheme, set up in the Rhondda Valley in Wales, involved six midwives who provided care for most of the 300 pregnant women of one GP practice (Russell, 1988). These team midwives were recruited internally and externally, but all were committed to a woman-centred approach, which may be why this scheme continues to work so well. Hall (1996) analyzes the problems and difficulties in providing continuity of care within a team and suggests that team midwifery might be a stepping stone to caseload practice, a better and more effective way of organizing midwifery care.

Caseload Practice

Caseload practice ensures continuity of care and makes it easier for the woman get to know her midwife. A working definition is: 'a midwife with a caseload is the primary provider of midwifery care throughout the pregnancy for a specified number of women' (Hutton, 1995). It is a one-to-one way of organizing midwifery care. **Box 5.4** illustrates the characteristics of one such innovative NHS service. Similar schemes are in existence and evaluations have recently been reported (Henderson and Grant, 1996).

Independent midwifery practice was, until recently, the only example of caseload practice. Generally women have to pay directly for this sort of care; they and the midwives are self-selected and there have been no controlled trials of independent care. An audit, based on the birth registers of independently practising midwives, showed very safe care and many positive outcomes (**Box 5.5**; Weig, 1993). There are less than 100 midwives working independently in this country. Most do so not because they believe in private practice, but because they want to be fully autonomous practitioners who provide continuity of carer and informed choice for women and their families. In many Trusts constricted by policies and attitudes, midwives are finding it difficult to practice autonomously with woman's needs appearing to come second to those of the institution (Hobbs, 1993).

Caseload practice appears to meet women's needs and satisfy midwives' desire for clinical autonomy; they are not necessarily more expensive, as demonstrated by a one-to-one scheme involving 1400 women

---

Box 5.5

Outcomes of Independent Caseload Midwifery

Audit of care for 1285 women by 43 midwives from 1980–91 (there was a high proportion of older and multiparous women):

- 63% 30 years and over; 48.5% were primigravida.
- 75% planned to give birth at home.
- 89% of the women gave birth spontaneously, vaginally.
- 6% were delivered by Caesarean section and 5% had instrumental births.
- 16% had an unplanned transfer to hospital in labour, but only 3% did so because of an obstetric emergency.
- 95% breastfed.
- The perinatal mortality rate was 7.7 per 1000.

Source: Weig, 1993

Box 5.6

Strategies to Prevent Burnout Developed by One Independent Group Practice

The group is self-employed and manage themselves; they:

- Have a high degree of autonomy over how, when and where they work.
- Are self selected, as are the coworkers.
- Are chosen by the group and have a commitment to the same overall philosophy.
- Have their own premises, quite separate from hospital, health centre or GP surgery, which helps with their identity.
- Meet often for debriefing sessions and to arrange time off and holidays.
- Care about each other and want to help in a mutual way.
- See reflection as an integral part of their model.
- Prioritise voicing uncertainty within a safe environment.
- Aim to minimize women's dependence and help them develop their own support networks.

(McCourt and Page, 1996). However, many midwives are anxious about the demands of team and caseload midwifery and it is difficult for them to anticipate the rewards of getting to know women and helping them to fulfil their needs. Midwives expect that being on call so often and for so long will result in burnout. Leap (1996) explored the strategies developed by the South East London Group practice to prevent burnout (**Box 5.6**). This group of independent midwives now contracted in to the NHS. Current evidence demonstrates that caseload care, by enabling midwives to be responsible for their workload, reduces burnout (Sandall, 1996). However, whenever a woman receives care she should have a named midwife and be able to choose who will lead her care.

Who Should Provide Care?

With woman-centred care, it is the woman who will book the midwife, consultant or GP rather than, as is currently the case, the woman being booked by the professional.

(Department of Health, 1993.)

A woman with an uncomplicated pregnancy should, if she wishes, be able to book with a midwife as the lead professional for the entire episode of care including delivery in a general hospital.

(Department of Health, 1993.)

A woman may need or want her maternity care to be mostly provided by her Family Doctor or an obstetrician. She has the right to choose her lead professional and to change for personal or clinical reasons (**Case Study 5.1**).

It is likely that all women will need a midwife; ideally they should be involved in choosing their named midwife. Most women when pregnant for the first time do not know any midwives or obstetricians. They go to their GP first: a recent survey found that only 3% approached a midwife first (Gready *et al.* 1995).

Profiles of the professionals, with an outline of their philosophy of care, should be available to all women (**Box 5.7**).

Antenatal clinics, family planning clinics, GP surgeries and pharmacies could stock the profiles for all the maternity caregivers in their area. Information on how to find out about your nearest midwife could be included in all pregnancy testing kits. For good care, all the maternity caregivers need to be aware of professional boundaries and accepting overlap in their ability to provide some aspects of antenatal care. General education is needed for women to understand the differences in the GPs', obstetricians' and midwives' roles. It is said that GPs see their patients from the cradle to the grave, midwives are the experts in normal childbirth and obstetricians can deal with all high-risk cases. Is this what women want to know?

Box 5.7

Profile of an Independent Midwife, Developed to Inform Women of Personal Beliefs and Professional Expertise

I qualified in 1982, and am married with a daughter, born at home. I believe in informed choice and think that although knowing your midwife is very important, feeling in control is essential for positive birthing. I am fully trained and experienced in normal childbirth, can detect complications and arrange appropriate referral and or treatment. Book with me for continuity, home-based, family-orientated midwifery care (Warren, 1996).

Case study 5.1

Janice

Janice booked with her obstetrician as lead professional, but chose her midwife for postnatal continuity.

Janice contacted her nearest independent midwife at 34 weeks' gestation. She had been seeing her obstetrician throughout her pregnancy, whom she knew from several years of infertility treatment. She wanted to have continuity of care postnatally after her planned Caesarean section.

Three antenatal visits enabled both to get to know each other, and the midwife accompanied Janice to hospital and then gave full postnatal care. This woman planned her care after being fully informed of her options early in her antenatal period.

Selling Midwifery and Midwives

Midwives in many NHS Trusts still wear nurse uniforms and some women are unaware that they have received care from a midwife. Other initiatives may be needed, such as 'Meet the Midwives' coffee mornings or open days at hospitals and health and community clinics. Care and carers must be accessible to the women. The Bradford Bus provides a focus for women to meet the midwives in their area. Originally set up to take antenatal care to those unable or unwilling to travel to clinic, women can now make their initial contact with these visible midwives (Wilkinson, 1995). As a midwife, it is necessary to think yourself into the woman's shoes: 'What would help you choose a carer?' Think of what questions you could ask to find out a carer's view on childbirth. How can women become aware of the different skills, qualities and attitudes of the different professionals? The Association of Radical Midwives (ARM) produced an excellent leaflet, *What is a Midwife*, which describes and clarifies the extent of the role and responsibilities of midwives (ARM, 1989).

Accessing Maternity Services

Information about maternity services should be available in the community to help women make choices about who to see and where to go, as well as decide what type of care she requires.

Confirming the Pregnancy

When her period is late or missed, a woman often chooses to confirm or deny the pregnancy on the basis of a home test kit. These rely on an increased level of chorionic gonadotrophin in the urine, which is most concentrated in the first morning specimen. Reliable home kits mean the woman can choose with whom to share the knowledge of pregnancy without involving health professionals. Traditionally, a woman took a urine sample to the GP's surgery and get the result a few days later. Many still do this as a way of initiating their care. Some women seem to know they are pregnant within a week of conception and many are aware of breast tenderness or fullness, nausea and vomiting long before the second missed period. Many women want to acknowledge their pregnancy as soon as the test is positive, others delay until the growing bulge can no longer be hidden.

Getting Information and Support

If booking is delayed, women need a source of professional information and support – a drop-in centre, a named midwife or a pregnancy hot line. These facilities need to be well known and should be advertised wherever pregnancy tests are sold or available, where preconception counselling takes place and in family planning clinics. Such provision, offering information and support early in pregnancy, is patchy and sparse countrywide, both in and out of the NHS. Independent midwives in Deptford have a shop front base in The Albany, a community centre situated in a shopping precinct. Here, women can have a free pregnancy test and can talk to someone knowledgeable about their options (Demilew, 1994). The Priory St. Centre, York, is a community centre and twice a week there are free pregnancy testing sessions, staffed by women (not NHS employees) who offer support and information about abortion and pregnancy care. The Brierley Midwifery Practice, a NHS team of midwives who care for women wanting home births and for those with mental health problems, holds a weekly drop-in session. These informal sessions, staffed by a team member, offer information or advice to antenatal and postnatal women and their partners or friends (Meyer and Wallace, 1995). For women to plan their maternity care they need to know where to go for help and information early in their pregnancy.

Supporting the Woman who has a Miscarriage or Spontaneous Abortion

The risk of spontaneous miscarriage is substantially less after the first trimester – about 75% of all miscarriages occur before 14 weeks. It was thought that women would suffer more if they had a miscarriage after booking, but it is now known that minimizing the loss is not helpful. It is better to acknowledge the reality of the pregnancy and its subsequent loss than to pretend it never happened. Midwives in some areas are involved in visiting women who have suffered a miscarriage, and they may be better able to provide support if they have already met. Some women may wish to see a midwife at this time and should be offered the option.

Dilemmas of Early Assessment and Diagnosis

With the development of early diagnostic tests, such as chorionic villus sampling performed at around 8–10 weeks, and early risk assessments, such as the Triple test, women need to be aware of what is available to them before 12 weeks. Ideally, with preconception knowledge, women or couples who would benefit from, or want, early diagnostic tests would self-refer at 7–8 weeks to their chosen specialist. One of the reasons for booking early is to arrange tests which detect conditions in the baby that are not treatable, but for which termination of the pregnancy is an option. Such screening tests open up an emotional and ethical minefield and skilled counselling should be available before and after the test. These issues are explored by Rothman, who argues that:

> ... *prenatal diagnosis changes women's experience of pregnancy. That is obviously true for women who receive bad diagnoses, but [is] also true when the results are normal.*
>
> Rothman (1988.)

One woman who decided to have an amniocentesis at 15 weeks to exclude her fears of a spinal cord defect described her experiences as the 'prenatal testing roller coaster, the scariest ride of my life.' During the pre-test ultrasound a sac was seen at the base of the baby's skull and a definite diagnosis was not possible until after the birth. Her baby seems perfectly normal, but the mother's anxiety marred the antenatal period and her doubts continued for months after the birth (Kuba, 1995). There is not a support group aimed at women and their families who receive an ambiguous or unknown ultrasound diagnosis, but there are a number of organizations that offer support and lists of local contacts can be obtained from NHS Trusts and other organizations, such as Community Health Councils (*see* Chapter 18).

Antenatal screening

Antenatal care provision is based on tests and assessments to detect potential problems or deviations soon enough to enable preventative or corrective action. Some health professionals expect that women should take up all screening options and, if an abnormality is found, terminate the pregnancy or have invasive intrauterine surgery. It is a very difficult, highly individual decision – the trauma and stress may linger for years, regardless of the outcome. Openness about the tests and investigations help demystify the technology and prepare women for possible results of the tests.

Research and Information Giving

There is evidence that women are often badly prepared and suffer emotionally as a result of antenatal screening. In 1995 Marteau conducted a review to establish how women can gain the maximum benefits from antenatal testing, and yet suffer the minimum of harm. The review was unable to offer any answers, but concluded that more research is needed before there can be evidence-based provision of antenatal screening. In the past, women were automatically sent for tests such as ultrasound scans and amniocentesis if they were over a certain age. Such routine antenatal tests are being questioned increasingly and good practice expects that a proper explanation should be given when any test is considered. As the importance of choice is being acknowledged and the limitations of tests admitted, some of these procedures are now being offered as a choice. The explanation, in an appropriate form and language, should be given in person wherever possible and backed up with leaflets. It should include:

- The reliability and rate of false-positive and false-negative results.
- An explanation of follow on options.
- An acceptance that the woman can choose not to proceed with further tests, if she wants, at any time.

A woman who wants a ' routine' scan because she treasures the scan picture she has of her first baby may be unaware that the 18 week scan is an anomalies scan. She knows it is a dating scan, but radiologists systematically looks for abnormalities of the organs and limbs. It is unethical to let her proceed in ignorance. Information and choice are linked – choice is not informed if facts are missing or presented in a misleading or biased way. **Box 5.8** shows the results of one survey relating to informed choice and ultrasound scans. Currently NHS clients have to opt out of having an ultrasound scan, but independent clients have to opt in for a routine ultrasound scan.

Women booking with an independent midwife have sometimes rejected the system and are 'anti' routine, others just want continuity. Only 2 of the 32 women (6%) who booked early with the author wanted, and had, an anomalies scan (Warren, 1996). *Changing Childbirth* advises that:

> *Each woman should be approached as an individual and given clear and unbiased information on the options that are available to her, and in this way helped to balance the risks and benefits for herself and her baby.*
>
> (Department of Health, 1993.)

Caregivers need to be sensitive to the individual's capacity and not overload the woman with facts or opinions. It is wrong to make decisions for women except in exceptional cases such as unconsciousness. Paired leaflets, one for women and one for professionals, based on the best available research evidence recognize that pregnancy is a time of choice and decisions (Midwives Information and Research Service and the Centre for Reviews and Dissemination, 1995).

The information leaflets tackle one issue at a time and can be given to a women to help with specific choices; some are useful to all, such as *Ultrasound Scans*, and others, such as *Breech Births*, only to a few. For woman-centred care, the information is needed in a form that is acceptable to the woman before decisions need to be made by her. The caregivers must then support her in her decisions. She must have time to think about and discuss, if appropriate, her options with significant others. Caregivers often underestimate the amount of information wanted by women and fail to give enough (**Box 5.9**).

Armed with unbiased, honest information, the woman can opt in to have the investigations and tests that are right for her (**Case Study 5.2**). History taking can be delayed if that is what the woman wants or if tests are not wanted until 3 or 4 months.

Box 5.8

Information and Ultrasound Scans

• All the women (787) receiving care in one survey were offered an ultrasound scan, only one chose not to have one.
• Retrospectively, 8% could not remember being given a reason for the scan.
• Only 60% of the women remembered being told that the scan was to look for abnormalities or problems.

Source: Gready et al. 1995.

Box 5.9

Women from Three Different Surveys Wanted more Information

• More information was ranked third after kindness and continuity by 1271 National Childbirth Trust (NCT) members who gave birth in 1992 (Newburn, 1993).
• Poor and inconsistent information was what women in Redbridge were given, and they wanted comprehensive and clear information (Brooks and Black, 1994).
• Of the 850 women in Essex asked if they wanted more information without having to ask, 18% said 'Yes, definitely' and 37% 'Yes, to some extent'.

(Gready et al. 1995).

Case study 5.2

Jackie

Jackie, a 34-year-old primigravida, did not wish to involve any health professionals in her early care, but did want to assess her risk for having a baby with Down's syndrome. After reading a newspaper article, she arranged for blood to be taken privately and sent to St James Hospital, Leeds, for a postal Triple Test. She was reassured by the literature and low-risk result. She booked with a midwife at 30 weeks and gave birth at home to a daughter, without the direct involvement of other practitioners. A woman who has had no contact with maternity care providers, but who receives a high-risk Triple Test result by post, may seek support from friends or relatives. With woman-centred care such a woman should also feel that she could, if she wanted, contact a midwife or other maternity carer to talk through her options.

Confidentiality

If a woman is wanting to keep her pregnancy private, a home visit by a uniformed midwife would be inappropriate. Initial visits can be done in the evening or at the weekend by an out-of-uniform midwife. It may not be easy to maintain confidentiality if the midwife is well known. There are many diverse reasons why a woman may wish to minimize the number of people who know of her pregnancy and personal circumstances – she may:

- Live in rented accommodation where children are not allowed.
- Not wish the baby's father to know of her pregnancy.
- Have a lesbian partner.
- Be a celebrity.
- Wish the baby to be adopted.
- Have agreed to be a surrogate mother.

The UKCC gives guidance on confidentiality which states:

> *The client has a right to expect information given in confidence... will not be released to others.*
>
> (UKCC, 1987.)

Some of these women may book late or seek care outside the NHS but should, with woman-centred care, be confidently able to access the system knowing their privacy will be respected.

Antenatal Visits – Where, When and Who does What?

The place for antenatal care affects the time available for the consultation and may affect the quality of the interactions. **Table 5.1** shows some differences in facilities and opportunities provided by the different places for antenatal care.

The British Way of Birth survey of the care of 6000 women in 1981 reported widespread dissatisfaction with antenatal care, with hospital clinics being the most heavily criticized. Comments such as:

- Very overcrowded, you can wait up to two and a half hours just to see a doctor for two minutes.
- It was a waste of time, theirs and mine.
- The clinic was appallingly like a pregnant cattle market.

(Boyd and Sellars, 1982)

Women are now more likely to have shared care with their GP or midwife and one or two visits to the hospital. Community clinics with the GP and/or midwife have always been friendlier, more convenient and preferred by women.

Where

Very little attention has been paid to the effect of the environment on meaningful interaction between woman and carer. This is an area ripe for research. It is important to consider the power implications of 'your place or mine'. Having chosen her lead professional, the woman will follow her or him for antenatal visits. There is limited scope for choice. Obstetric consultants generally hold antenatal clinics at a hospital once or twice a week. Some visit outlying clinics, usually GP group practices, once a month or every 2 weeks. GPs hold weekly antenatal sessions at their surgery on a specific morning or afternoon. It is possible for the woman to arrange antenatal care during normal surgery hours, but this is usually discouraged by the GP. Having a midwife as her lead professional may increase the woman's choices as she/he may hold surgeries at a community clinic, GPs surgery, at the hospital clinic or arrange to visit at home. There are likely to be educational displays and useful posters about parentcraft or recreational facilities for pregnant women at the clinics, but at home the woman may well feel more at ease and more confident in seeking information or questioning routine procedures. Not all clinics have crèches for toddlers or other children and transport or parking can be a problem.

Frequency of Antenatal Visits

The traditional timings of antenatal visits for a woman having a first baby are:

- Monthly during 12–28 weeks.
- An extra visit at 18 weeks for a scan.
- Every fortnight from 28 until 36 weeks,
- Weekly until the baby is born.

This averages out at 13 visits. Many women complain of long waits for short impersonal consultations and duplication of care. Changes in Aberdeen resulted in low-risk primigravidae having an average of 9–10 visits and low-risk multigravid women six antenatal visits (Hall *et al.* 1985). There was no compromise of maternal or child health and the new community-based services were accepted and liked by the women. Maternity services, like the rest of the NHS, are involved in cost-cutting exercises and there is a strong

Table 5.1 A Comparison of the Facilities Available at Different Venues for Antenatal Care					
Where	Hospital antenatal clinic	Community Centre	GP's clinic	Midwife's clinic	Woman's own house
Who Obstetrician GP Midwife	✔ – ✔	± ± ±	occasionally ✔ ±	– ± ✔	– – ✔
Educational Videos Displays Leaflets	✔ ✔ ✔	occasionally – –	– general health general health	– ✔ ✔	– – ✔
Time/Wait	up to 2 hours	up to 1 hours	up to 1 hour	up to 0.5 hour	0.5–1 hour
Consultation	5–10 minutes	10–20 minutes	10–15 minutes	15–30 minutes	30–40 minutes
Opportunity to use others HV	–	✔	✔	occasionally	
SW	✔	occasionally	✔	–	–
Other	✔✔	occasionally	–	–	–
Child care	± crèche, playbox	± crèche, playbox	playbox	playbox	own toys
Easy to socialize with other pregnant woman	no	usually– often women know others in their locality	usually– often women know others in their locality	usually– often women know others in their locality	no
Privacy	should be possible to arrange	should be possible to arrange	should be possible to arrange	should be possible to arrange	Yes

financial incentive to reduce the number of routine antenatal visits. Despite this, little changed until after the publication of *Changing Childbirth* which encouraged review of the pattern of antenatal visits and endorsed the Royal College of Obstetricians and Gynaecologists recommendations of nine visits for primigravidae and six for multigravid women. There is recognition that some women may be anxious at the prospect of fewer antenatal visits – the *Changing Childbirth* report states:

> Time should be taken to explain that a reduction in antenatal visits will not mean any less support during pregnancy but rather that the quality and continuity of care will be improved, and waiting times reduced. The woman should know that she can telephone her midwife if she has any anxieties or worries between check-ups.
> (Department of Health, 1993.)

The benefits from improved continuity, basing care in the community, shorter waiting times and less conflicting advice from fewer carers need to be balanced against any possible disadvantages. Additional services such as 'drop-in' facilities and a 24-hour contact phone number, answered by a person not a message, may be needed to reduce anxieties.

Recent research

More recent work has endorsed the findings of Hall with regard to safety but highlighted some women's concerns. Research in Bedfordshire showed that safety and standards were not compromised by fewer visits, but 46% of the women wanted more antenatal visits. The changes included introducing midwife-led and GP-led care, maximizing community care and women keeping their own notes (Johnson, 1996). .For woman-centred care, safe standards must be maintained and change may need to balance what women want against financial gains. A rigorously conducted randomized controlled trial in Southeast London found no significant differences in clinical variables relating to maternal or perinatal morbidity when women were allocated to a schedule of either traditional care (13 visits) or new style visits (6–7). Women were more likely to be dissatisfied in the new style group and more than half thought some of the gaps were too long. **Box 5.10** shows some of the psychosocial outcomes of this research (Sikorski *et al.* 1996). Of the women invited and eligible to take part in this trial, more than one-quarter declined and of these three-quarters said they did not wish to have

Psychosocial Findings Associated with a Reduced Number of Antenatal Visits

- No difference in feeling encouraged to ask questions or wanting more medical or general advice.
- Less likely to feel listened to and more likely to say they wanted more time to talk.
- Significantly more expressed worries, more so during pregnancy, about whether their baby was thriving.
- More had negative attitudes towards their baby, both before and after the child had been born.
- No difference in confidence about giving birth, satisfaction with the birth or self ratings of coping with the birth.

Source: Sikorski et al. 1996.

fewer antenatal visits. However, when asked about the number of visits in future pregnancies many choose the same schedule of visits as for the first.

Disadvantages of less antenatal care

The above trial was large, involving 2794 women, but the conclusions recommended that further research is needed to investigate the effect of reduced visits on rare clinical problems such as eclampsia. This is a major concern to members of APEC. With fewer visits there is the possibility of missing more cases of pre-eclampsia. Redman and Walker (1992) believe primigravidae are particularly at risk, even with traditional care, because of the current gaps between 20–24 and 24–28 weeks. They suggest that this is the reason for more fetal and maternal deaths during this period. In their book there is a poignant quote from an unnamed woman:

> I can't help thinking that if my antenatal checks had been more frequent, the pregnancy might have lasted long enough for my baby to have had a better chance.
>
> (Redman and Walker, 1992.)

An exciting development, in Bristol, is looking at the affect of allowing women to decide how many visits they want and at what intervals they wish to be seen. This is to be a randomized controlled trial with traditional or a minimum of six visits and the results should be available late in 1998 (Sharp and Jewell, 1996). Some women choose fewer visits, but some, like Jenny, want more antenatal contact (**Case Study 5.3**).

With a reduced schedule, there is also less oppor-tunity for women to get to know the midwives; a multigravid woman cared for by a team of six may only meet each midwife once. There is also less time for one-to-one education in preparation for birth and parenting or for contact with other women, which may be important .

Who Does What during an Antenatal Visit?

There is very little research on the content of the antenatal visit – physical, social or educational. There is evidence of the importance of the psychosocial dimension to antenatal care (Sikorski *et al.* 1996). The physical examination includes testing the urine, particularly for glucose and protein, measuring the blood pressure, looking for oedema, assessing the uterine growth and listening to the baby's heart. In the KYM Scheme (Flint and Poulengeris, 1987) women weighed themselves and tested their urine. Some staff were opposed to this, believing that women would not do the tests. This paternalistic view raises issues of power and control that need to be explored before antenatal care can move forwards. Changes may be made on financial grounds, but may still be beneficial if the result empowers women, increases mutual trust and balances the relationship between the cared for and the carers. Maternity care professionals need to be honest and realistic about what antenatal surveillance can achieve and to ensure there are a range of opportunities for education, information exchange and support.

Social Support during Pregnancy

The ability of a woman to plan her maternity care depends on her knowledge, her circumstances and her resources – financial and social. Although extra social support has not been proved to improve medical outcomes in current pregnancy, there are some long-term benefits and some measurable advantages. These include less suspected child abuse, less nappy rash, a lower incidence of hospitalization for the baby and fewer of the young mothers becoming pregnant during the next 18 months (Enkin, 1994). The Newcastle Community Midwives Care Project involved antenatal education and increased social support by midwives to women at risk because of their poor socioeconomic situation. Food was provided at each session not only to introduce nutritional information in a practical way, but also to provide a social setting. These women felt more confident about childbirth and used less pain relief during labour (Davies, 1991). Longer term benefits were also found 1 year later in another group of women who received extra social support from a midwife during their antenatal period. More had a spontaneous vaginal birth compared with controls and both mothers and babies were judged to be significantly healthier in the first 6 weeks (Oakley, 1992). Such projects are often funded by research money and may stop once the research is finished, despite their apparent success. However, Oakley (1996) was able to follow-up the research commenced in 1986–88. The results of the seven-year follow-up indicates that offering socially disadvantaged women additional support during pregnancy has positive effects on the family and children's health. The *Changing Childbirth* report does not mention social support, but many of the benefits are also found when there is good continuity of care. Purchasers of care need to be persuaded to buy such continuity, but because it is difficult to demonstrate health gain in the short term they can be reluctant to do so.

Opportunities for Receiving and Giving Information

These exist whenever the woman makes contact with her carers, but are not always fully utilized. Friends, relatives, books, magazines and the media are also a source of information on childbirth.

The Antenatal Visit

A women expects her antenatal visit to include more than just an assessment of her health and her baby's well-being. Despite an apparent information explosion, women still want more (**Box 5.9**). Information should be based on evidence and may cause guilt or be rejected if it does not take into consideration the woman's circumstances. Where there is good motivation, interventions can help change behaviour. For example, midwives who want to help pregnant smokers quit can use the strategies in the Health Education Authority training pack for smoking cessation (HEA, 1994). During antenatal visits, open questions should be used to explore possible anxieties and coping strategies, such as:

• What do you think will happen on the day your labour starts?

• How are you feeling about becoming a mother?

There should be time for the woman to explore her hopes and fears, for information to be sought and received and for realistic plans to be made for the birth and the time beyond. It is often claimed that although women who want to birth at home are given full information about the possible dangers of home birth, those choosing to go to hospital are never warned of the dangers of this choice. It is easy to allow one's beliefs to bias the giving of information, by content, omission or emphasis. By virtue of their professional status, maternity caregivers' comments are considered authoritative. It is not always easy to tell someone who wants an elective Caesarean section that she is between 2–4 times more likely to die than if she had a vaginal birth, or that the risks of induction of labour include a higher incidence of fetal distress leading to more forceps and Caesarean deliveries. The *Changing Childbirth* report acknowledges that 'while professionals feel they have an obligation to offer guidance to women who are making choices

---

Case study 5.3

Jenny

Jenny wanted more frequent antenatal visits after her previous experience of pre-eclampsia. Jenny's first baby was born by Caesarean section at 32 weeks because of pre-eclampsia. When pregnant for the second time, she arranged to see her midwife weekly from 28 weeks until she felt safe at 34 weeks. She also tested her urine daily and took her own blood pressure with an automatic sphygmomanometer, loaned by the midwife. Her blood pressure started to rise at 38 weeks and she was admitted and went into spontaneous labour 2 days later and, after a 6 hour labour, gave birth vaginally to a daughter.

about their care, this can sometimes be seen as coercion by the women' (Department of Health, 1993). The challenge is to make such figures meaningful and realistic without being frightening.

Antenatal Education or Preparation for Parenthood

Research into antenatal education has focused on classes and shown a disappointing lack of change in behaviour as a result of class attendance. In general, smoking, alcohol use and diet have not changed and the physical outcomes of birth are unaffected. However, women or couples who go to classes use significantly less pain-relieving medication in labour (Enkin *et al.* 1995). Research is hampered by variation in content, length, size and aims of the classes. Despite the lack of evidence, classes remain very popular, especially evening sessions. The benefits of being part of a group are also difficult to assess, but these are often mentioned by participants as a positive aspect. Preparation for parenthood is changing from lecture presentations to an exploring, enabling, empowering style well covered in the Health Education Authority's resource book, *Approaching Parenthood* (Braun and Schonveld, 1993) . Active birth classes and books encourage women to discover what birth means to them and to encourage active participation in the labour and birth (Robertson, 1993). Classes don't suit everyone. Members of ethnic minorities and socially disadvantaged or very young mothers seldom attend regular classes and alternative approaches are needed to prepare them for birth and parenting. In Salford, renaming pregnancy classes the 'Pregnancy Club' and inviting women individually encouraged young attendees. The sessions are 'feelings' based, using small group discussions and brainstorming techniques (Richardson, 1993). In Bradford, 30% of the births are to Asian women, few of whom attend classes. It was found that they were anxious about the classes, felt their extended family would support and teach them and that domestic chores took priority. A collaborative venture has resulted in highly successful antenatal and birth videos in Urdu and Bengali, with more planned (Walker and Pollard, 1995). Many activity sessions also have discussions about birth and parenting; a woman may wish to try a yoga session or attend her local baths for some aquanatal exercise before choosing a class (**Table 5.2** outlines some of the differences in the classes).

Preparation for parenthood needs further evaluation and should be based on what women say they want or what helps them most to achieve their goals. Local NCT classes are often full and overbooked, but it is not known whether this is because they are better or preferred, or because there are simply far fewer places on these courses than on those run by the NHS. Some question whether it is realistic to try to prepare parents in a class situation. Should women need training and physical preparation for a natural event? Should all women be told about stillbirths or the likelihood of having a baby with a congenital malformation? If women are told that childbirth is painful, does this become a self-fulfilling prophecy? If the word pain is not used in conjunction with labour, but sensations, intensity, rushes or strong tightenings, is this better or dishonest? There are many unknowns. The major difficulty in preparing for birth and parenting is that no two births are the same and as each woman or couple are also unique, it is impossible to make the preparation specific for the individuals. The range of normal is enormous and there are many possible variations from normal, as shown by Anne's and Nadia's stories (**Case Study 5.4**).

The Relevance of Becoming and Being Known

Successful antenatal care provides the opportunity for the relationship between the woman and the professional to develop. It does appear barbaric that a woman should be attended by a stranger at the birth, but how important is it? Nadia from **Case Study 5.4** said of her midwives:

> *They were friends that I'd come to know and trust who supported me through the hardest and most wonderful experience ever.*

It is not known how well the woman needs to know her carer to develop such a trust or what effect the environment of the antenatal contact has. Being empowered by the lead professional antenatally and then being cared for by a midwife or doctor who is kind, sympathetic and has the same philosophy as yours may or may not be important. Many midwives, especially those who work in a labour ward or antenatal clinic have developed techniques to put the woman at ease and get to know her quickly. Most women are more relaxed at home and may find it easier to get to know the midwife when they are the host-

Type or sort	Cost	Venue	Teacher/facilitator	Main content	Other comments	Availability
Table 5.2 Table to Compare and Contrast Different Sorts of Preparation for Birth and Parenthood Classes						
NHS	Free	Hospital Community clinics	Midwife, health visitor and/or physiotherapist	Programme of sessions Try to cover all aspects	Get to know staff and hospital Teaches conformity to hospital norms Sometimes just lectures, not interactive	Widespread Limited evening sessions
NCT	Pay, concessions available	Facilitator's home Village hall Community centre	Trained lay person, already a mother	Aimed at couples Explore emotions and feelings Information for choice	Middle-class, middle-aged whites Time to think about being a parent with like-minded others Questioning system, adverse to NHS	Widespread, may have to travel Evenings and days
Yoga	Pay, concessions available	Mostly home Some centres	Yoga-trained midwives Yoga teachers	Stretching Mental preparation	Gentle pace, focusing on oneself Does not prepare for all eventualities Middle class or hippies	Limited availability Evenings or days
Active birth	Pay, concessions available	Mostly centres	Active Birth teachers Some midwives	Stretching, keeping fit Empowerment – your body, your baby, your birth	Cuts through medical waffle Helps those wanting everything natural Vegetarian and alternative	Limited availability Evenings or days
Aquanatal	Pay, concessions available	Local pool	Midwives Aqua-fit teachers	Physical fitness and stamina	All social classes, young and old Sometimes no childbirth education given Can be too strenuous or too gentle	Limited availability Evenings or days

Anne and Nadia

Anne's and Nadia's stories, told together, can help prepare couples for the range of normal labour and birth. Nadia contracted strongly over 3 days, pausing to have several short sleeps or to eat. Shortly after an assessment found that her cervix was 9 cm dilated, her contractions stopped and she ate lunch. Emily was born, normally, vaginally 2 hours later. Anne woke at 4 a.m., had one contraction every half hour until 6.30 a.m. and then contractions every 5 minutes until Jessica arrived at 7.20 a.m.

Both these women birthed at home and had ruptured membranes before the onset of labour. Neither had any chemical pain relief, Nadia used a warm bath on several occasions, massage with aromatherapy oils and visualization techniques. Both knew their midwife. Getting to know each other, i.e. the mother and midwife, is a two-way process the value of which is not universally accepted.

ess, but it is quite unknown how much time is needed to get to know each other or whether a 1-hour visit equals six 10-minute ones. Home is not always best – the midwife may be ill at ease in a spotless or less than clean house and the woman may be embarrassed and anxious if expecting her drunken or abusive partner to arrive. Women who have had a positive birthing experience may find it impossible to tell if knowing the midwife would have improved the event.

Research shows that knowing the midwife has positive effects, but it is very difficult to quantify or to separate out the effect of continuity of carer. One of the objectives of *Changing Childbirth* is for 75% of women to be cared for in labour by a midwife whom they have come to know during pregnancy. The way this question is addressed has an obvious effect on the response and needs interpreting with caution (**Box 5.11**).

Continuity of Carer – the Evidence

Women who have continuity of carer antenatally are significantly more likely to report that they felt fully involved in the decision making. More women who have previously met the doctor or midwife who was at the birth felt that they had enough information, that they were told enough about the necessary procedures and that their views and wishes were taken notice of (Gready *et al.* 1995). More women in the 'Know your Midwife' Scheme, the first team scheme, felt that their labour had been enjoyable, felt in control and that all their choices had been explained to them. They had fewer episiotomies and epidurals and more breastfed their babies (Flint and Poulengeris, 1987) . The same trends are found for independent midwifery, current teams with meaningful continuity of carer, case load practices and in midwife-led units (Henderson and Grant, 1996; McCourt and Page, 1996). What is not known is why this is? Are the midwives who work in this way different, are they kinder, nicer? Do they communicate better? Or are the women different? Does a 'known' midwife adopt a 'doula' role? A doula is a woman who supports a labouring woman by her continuous presence. She gives reassurance and encouragement, information, advice and physical help such as massage. Research consistently shows significant positive benefits of having a doula that mirror those for continuity of carer (Hodnett, 1995):
• Fewer Caesarean sections.
• Fewer instrumental deliveries.
• Lower use of pharmacological analgesia or epidurals.
• Labour was a more positive experience.

Birth at Home

Very few women choose to give birth at home. Those who do can face difficulties, but many are put off by the attitudes of the midwives and doctors or their partner, friends and families.

Home Births and Professional Support

The advantages of home-based antenatal care and birth at home are many. Flint suggests that every woman should book for a home birth regardless of their intentions and that by doing so the woman will (Flint, 1992):
• Be the focus of her home-based antenatal care.
• Have increased continuity from one or two midwives.
• Labour well at home knowing she can call on a midwife when she wants.
• Have the equipment at hand if labour is quick and the baby 'pops out' at home.
• Will have better care if she does decide to go in, as the staff 'will bend over backwards to ensure that her stay is as pleasant and as comfortable' as if she had stayed at home.

The change in place of birth from home to hospital was influenced by politics and a misplaced belief in the increased safety afforded by the institution and

---

Box 5.11

Measuring Continuity of Carer and Knowing Your Carer

In the Birth Choices survey, whether the woman had met any of her labour carers and whether a midwife or doctor had got to know her and remembered her and her progress from one antenatal visit to the next were used as indicators of knowing and continuity.

• 30% had previously met one of the doctors or midwives present at the birth.
• Of these, 47% would have liked to know them better.
These women said:
• I felt that because I'd met one or two of them before, my baby's birth wasn't just another birth to them.
• The care I had from my community midwife was excellent. I would have rather had her to deliver my baby than the hospital midwives I didn't know.

Source: Gready et al. 1995.

availability of highly trained and qualified staff (**Figure 5.1**). In 1987 a small booklet, *Where to be Born – The Debate and the Evidence*, exploded this piece of well-established medical dogma. The second, expanded edition reached the same conclusions (Campbell and Macfarlane, 1994):

- *There is no evidence to support the claim that the safest policy is for all women to give birth in hospital.*
- *There is some evidence, although not conclusive, that morbidity is higher among mothers and babies cared for in an institutional setting. For some women, it is possible, but not proved, that the iatrogenic risk associated with institutional delivery may be greater than any benefit conferred.*

Despite the availability of such convincing evidence since 1987, maternity caregivers still use scare tactics to put women off the idea of giving birth at home (**Box 5.12**).

It is every woman's right to give birth to her baby at home – no one should make that decision for her. Women are seldom told this and are swayed by professionals, who give information and advice that is seldom evidence based. Advice on rights is given in books (Beech, 1986; Wesson, 1995) and leaflets from organizations such as ARM, the NCT and other support groups. Local home-birth support groups have evolved to support women and parents, give information and ensure that women who make the unusual decision of planning to give birth at home do not feel alone. Home births are rare and the percentage of births that take place outside the hospitals is so small that many midwives and most GPs have not provided care for a woman birthing at home. In 1993 there

were 668,511 births in this country, of which 657,415 were in hospital, 10,569 at home and 527 elsewhere (OPCS, 1995), so home births constituted 1.6% of all the births. It is difficult for professionals to be confident at providing care in unknown (to them) circumstances. This percentage varies from the highest, 2.8% in South East Thames region, to the lowest, 0.7% in the Northern region (OPCS, 1995). The views of midwives, GPs and obstetricians surveyed differ widely – more midwives accept that home birth should not be discouraged on safety grounds than do GPs or obstetricians. In Grampian, few GPs or obstetricians thought that home birth was a viable option and many would try to dissuade women from giving birth at home. More midwives had experience of home birth and were supportive of women's right to choose this option (Bathgate *et al.* 1995). In another small sample, although only two community midwives routinely offered home births, half were strongly positive despite their limited experience (Floyd, 1995). A much bigger study in the Northern Region (with the lowest percentage of home births in the country) looked at the outcomes and the attitudes of the carers for all the requests for home births that reached the supervisors of midwives. During the time of the study there were 139 planned and 93 unplanned births at home. **Box 5.13** gives the outcomes of this study. The midwives were mostly supportive and a surprisingly high number (70%) of the GP's stated that they were in favour of home birth. Having a supportive GP was associated with a higher likelihood of giving birth at home. Women who were put off by their initial encounter with the GP or midwife were not included in the study as there was no way of finding out about this group (Davies and Young, 1995).

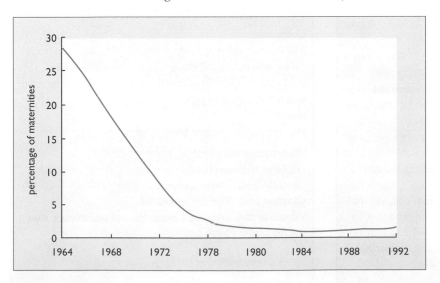

Figure 5.1 Percentage of deliveries at home, England 1964–92 (Campbell and Macfarlane, 1994).

Continuity, Control and Power at Home

It is easier for care to be woman centred when it is provided in the woman's home. Within the NHS, good continuity of carer is often found for women who book for home birth. Most antenatal visits take place at her home or at the GP's surgery, usually with one or two midwives who try hard to be available for the birth. This happens as a routine with caseload practice. Postnatal care usually involves the same midwives. The system does fall down in large teams when the on-call midwife is not the one called to the birth. Many women who book with independent midwives do so to have a home birth with continuity of carer; more than 75% of these have their babies at home (Weig, 1993). An interesting finding from studies of continuity of carer schemes is that the home birth rate increases even when this is not an initial aim. One of the Riverside Teams has a home birth rate of between 11 and 14% (Lewis, 1995b) and the South London independent midwives, who have contracted in to the NHS, have around 60% home births (Leap, 1996). The issues of power and control come to the fore in any debate about home birth. At home the woman feels in control; in hospital she is likely to feel disempowered. Women can only be empowered when the professionals face up to the issues and consider ways of reducing the inequalities in the power equation all through childbirth care. The way language is used reflects power – 'we *let* women deliver in any position'; 'Are women *allowed* to eat and drink in labour?' When a midwife is asked how many deliveries she has done, it reinforces the idea that a woman gives birth to her baby by having the midwife actively do something. In reality, apart from some encouragement, the midwife can sit on her hands and watch the woman deliver or give birth by her own expulsive efforts. Leap (1992) and Shirley and Mander (1996) explore this topic in more depth, and those who want to provide woman-centred care could usefully draw up a list of words not to use or to be used with extreme caution only.

In some places it is easy for a women to choose to give birth at home and to be supported by her midwives and doctors. The GPs support or agreement is not necessary but many women are unhappy at following a course of action that sets them at loggerheads with their family practitioner. A joint statement was issued by the Royal College of Midwives and the Royal College of General Practitioners to clarify responsibilities and to encourage GPs who don't wish to provide home birth care to refer women who want a home birth to another GP or a midwife (RCM and RCGP, 1995). Some caregivers need to change their attitudes and pay more attention to the evidence.

Box 5.12

Home Birth and General Practitioners

- The GP said, 'We don't do those, hospital is much safer'.
- The midwife was not keen but said that if I insisted she would have to come, but only if it was her night to be on call.
- I thought I'd better go in because they said there is no flying squad in our area.
- The community midwife was lovely, she said 'Yes, but don't tell the GPs as they don't like them'.
- The doctor told me that I was risking my baby's life and the last home birth he had attended had nearly ended in disaster with the women having to be rushed in to hospital.
- They told me I would bleed to death as it was my fourth.

Source: Quotes from author's clients.

Box 5.13

Views and Outcomes in the Northern Home Birth Survey

Outcomes:
248 women participated, of whom 11% were dissuaded during pregnancy, 3% changed their minds by choice, 15% booked at hospital for obstetric reasons, 15% transferred in labour and 56% delivered at home.
Views:
Women wanted to give birth at home:

- To feel more in control.
- To be in their own home.
- Because it was more natural
- So their partner could be involved.

Wherever the birth took place, 91% of the women would opt for a home birth again.

Source: Davies and Young, 1995.

Complementary Therapies

'Using alternative therapies offers women more control over their own health' (Jones, 1996). Complementary therapies such as homoeopathy, aromatherapy and acupuncture should work alongside conventional medicine. Midwives and doctors, with dual training, can and should be encouraged to offer both within the NHS. The UKCC acknowledges that midwives who have studied a recognized course in a complementary therapy are competent to advise women and to prescribe if appropriate. All midwives need some understanding of the more common therapies, a willingness to learn more and an awareness of women's rights in this area. The woman must give consent before the midwife can use alternative or complementary therapies in the course of her care. If the midwife is not happy about any substances that the woman wishes to take, she/he has a duty to discuss this with the woman but must: 'respect the right of individuals to self administer substances of their choice ... and be mindful of the need not to override the woman's right' (UKCC, 1994).

There is a high level of scepticism within the medical establishment, so complementary therapies are only slowly gaining acceptance. In the Southampton area, a midwife who has trained in scientific aromatherapy offers an alternative labour preparation service. This is voluntary, in her own time and from her own house. She is attempting to meet the needs of women who wish to avoid using drugs during their labour and birth (Mason, 1996). Women may be more interested in using complementary therapies once they have been accepted by the establishment and are offered within the NHS.

Acupuncture

Skelton (1988) found that women who received acupuncture during labour felt more in control and were generally more satisfied than the control group. Despite this positive finding, most women are reluctant to use acupuncture. In the author's experience, women try acupuncture for specific reasons, such as to stimulate labour when pregnancy is prolonged, but are reluctant to use it in labour. Two midwives in Plymouth offer acupuncture within the maternity unit and at an outpatients clinic. They treat many antenatal conditions (**Box 5.14**), use moxibustion to turn a baby presenting by the breech and try to be available to offer help in labour. They say acupuncture 'allows the woman a greater chance of achieving natural childbirth, helping her stay in control by keeping her as relaxed and comfortable as possible' (Yelland, 1995).

Hypnosis and Multiple Remedies

Women may use more than one sort of alternative therapy (**Case Study 5.5**), such as aromatherapy massage oil, raspberry leaf tea as a herbal uterine stimulant and homoeopathic arnica for bruising. Many self-treat and are attracted to self-hypnosis. Hypnosis, taught by a qualified practitioner, can then be self-induced and has been found to be effective at reducing the need for pain relief in labour. Antenatally, practitioners use hypnosis to treat morning sickness, constipation and insomnia (Brann, 1995).

Aromatherapy

Aromatic plants yield aromatic oils. When distilled, these potent compounds need to be treated with caution. Undiluted, most will at least cause severe skin reactions, but used appropriately they have much therapeutic value. They can be inhaled, used in a compress, in the bath or in a massage oil.

For early pregnancy nausea, the following essential oils can be safely used (Tiran, 1996):

- Ginger.
- Grapefruit.
- Lime.
- Mandarin.
- Petitgrain.
- Sweet orange.
- Tangerine.

Box 5.14

Some of the Antenatal Conditions Treatable by Acupuncture within the NHS at Southampton

Hyperemesis	Abdominal pain	Migraine
Varicose veins	Haemorrhoids	Skin problems
Sciatica	Constipation	Heartburn
Vulval varicosities		

Source: Yelland, 1995.

Tiran and Mack (1995) also recommend that women try acupressure wrist bands. These were initially marketed to combat travel sickness and have been shown in a randomized controlled trial to be effective for some women at alleviating nausea, but not at preventing vomiting during the first trimester (Belluomini *et al.* 1994).

Homoeopathy

Homoeopathy is one of the most accepted of the complementary therapies and, like most of the others, involves a holistic view of health, seeing this as so much more than an absence of disease. This is in keeping with the essence of woman-centred care. The name homoeopathy comes from two Greek words: *homoios* meaning similar and *pathos* meaning suffering. Treatment with remedies, available in differing strengths, is based on the principal of treating like with like. For example, ipececuanha causes vomiting, so its homoeopathic preparation is given for morning sickness.

Homoeopaths treat the whole person, not the disease only, and aim to stimulate the body's natural healing processes. There are a few specific remedies, arnica for bruising and caulophyllum to stimulate contractions, but generally women who want to use homoeopathy have a consultation or several with a registered practitioner and are prescribed individual remedies to suit them. It is acceptable for the woman to self-treat without training, but the guidance for midwives from the UKCC is clear.

Can Planning Antenatal Care Really Help?

Poverty, with the resulting poor nutrition and general illhealth, is a major cause of maternal and perinatal mortality and morbidity. Tew (1990) considers that the greatest reduction in mortality has occurred because of improvements in the general standard of living rather than because of antenatal care or treatments. She suggests that it would be better to spend time and effort on reducing poverty and improving nutrition instead of giving antenatal care.

The cost of antenatal care provision is estimated (or 'guesstimated') by most NHS Trusts and private practitioners charge for antenatal consultations, but it is part of a continuum and so difficult to separate out from total care costs. Continuity of carer antenatally reduces intrapartum costs. The financial cost of new screening tests may be easy to state, but the cost in terms of raised anxiety or expectations is very difficult to assess. If women's self-esteem and self-confidence are lowered by the way childbirth care is delivered, there may be long-term hidden costs in the quality of mothering and parenting in our society. A self-employed woman could have considerable loss of earnings by attending for parenthood preparation and routine antenatal care. To give women what they want, maternity caregivers need to prove that antenatal care is worthwhile – physically, emotionally and socially.

Organizing maternity care so that it gives women what they want makes sense, it works and it is effective. Prevention is not always better than cure and excessive diagnostic effort can indicate pathology that is not there and so cause unnecessary anxiety and intervention. Although antenatal care is preventative

---

Case study 5.5

Alison

Alison used various techniques and therapies to help with her labour. She had been using acupuncture, massage and aromatherapy for her own health care and planned to use them in labour. She had supportive labour companions and midwives at the home birth of her first child. Alison used water to help her relax, she inhaled clary sage and lavender aromatherapy oils when contractions were very strong and found loving touch and massage very helpful. Her acupuncturist gave some treatment when she was despondent over how little she had dilated. She also used Entonox while her perineum was sutured and believes that everything that was used was helpful at times and says of the birth: 'The experience was a challenging, exciting, wonderful, exhilarating, frightening, joyful and momentous one'. This birth took place in Birmingham, with NHS midwives.
Source: Belbin, 1996.

and associated with improved pregnancy outcomes, it is not known how or why it works (Enkin, 1994). Evidence-based knowledge is growing. Continuity of carer, knowing the carer, feeling in control and being able to choose birth options are associated with positive outcomes. What women want is good for them and their babies. Helping a woman to plan her care and providing the range of facilities to meet her needs is vitally important. For effective woman-centred care, midwives and doctors must listen to women and ensure the service they provide is evidence based and responsive to women.

KEY CONCEPTS

- Women need to be fully involved at all times with decisions about their care.

- Professionals must learn to listen to what women say they want and structure their care accordingly.

- Honest, unbiased information is needed by women to plan their care.

- Paternalism is *out* and power-sharing and equality are *in*.

- Expectations are realistic and antenatal care is empowering.

References

Association Radical Midwives: *What is a midwife*. ARM leaflet. 62 Greetby Hill, Ormskirk, Lancs, L39 2DT.

APEC: *Why blood pressure is checked in pregnancy – a woman's guide to screening for pre-eclampsia*. Harrow, (31–33)1996, Action on Pre-eclampsia.

Bathgate W, Ryan M, Hall M: Divided views amoung health professionals on place of birth, *Br J Midwifery* 3(11):583, 1995.

Beech B: *Who's having your baby? A health rights handbook for maternity care*, London, 1991, Bedford Square Press.

Belbin A: Power and choice in birthgiving: a case study, *Br J Midwifery* 4(5):264, 1996.

Belluomini J, Litt R, Lee K, *et al.*: Acupressure for nausea and vomiting of pregnancy a randomised, blinded study. *Obstet Gynaecol* 84(2):245, 1994.

Boyd C, Sellars L: *The British way of birth*. London, 1982, Pan Books.

Brann L: The role of hypnosis in obstetrics, *J Diplom R Coll Obstet Gynaecol* 2(2):95, 1995.

Braun D, Schonveld A: *Approaching parenthood A resource for parent education*, London, 1993, Health Education Authority.

Brooks L, Black M: Local delivery, *Health Serv J* 104(5389):33, 1994.

Campbell R, Macfarlane A: *Where to be born – the debate and the evidence*, 2nd edn, Oxford, 1994 National Perinatal Epidemiology Unit.

Chitty L, Barnes L, Berry C: Continuing with pregnancy after a diagnosis of lethal abnormality: experience of five couples and recommendations for management, *Br Med J* 313(7055):478, 1996.

Davies J: The Newcastle Community Care Project in action. In Robinson S, Thomson A, editors: *Midwives research and childbirth*, London, 1991, Chapman and Hall.

Davies J, Young G: Northern Region home birth survey, *Assoc Community-Based Maternity Care Newslett* 11:6, 1995.

Demilew J: South East London midwifery group practice. *MIDIRS Midwifery Digest* 4(3):270–72, 1994.

Department of Health: *Changing childbirth. The report of the Expert Maternity Group (Cumberlege report)*, London, 1993, HMSO.

Department of Health: *Report on confidential enquiries into maternal deaths in the United Kingdom 1988–1990*, London, 1994, HMSO.

Enkin M: Six myths that can lead us astray, *NZ Coll Midwives J* 11:1321, 1994.

Enkin M, Keirse M, Renfrew M, *et al.*: *A guide to effective care in pregnancy and child birth*, 2nd edn, Oxford, 1996, Oxford University Press.

Flint C: Home births for all, *New Generation* 11(3):16, 1992.

Flint C: *Midwifery teams and caseloads*, Oxford, 1994, Butterworth Heinemann.

Flint C, Poulengeris P: *The KNOW YOUR MIDWIFE report*, 1987 (from 49 Peckarmans Wood, London SE26 6RZ).

Floyd L: Community Midwives' views and experience of home birth, *Midwifery* 11(1):3, 1995.

Gillen J: *Collage work*. MA Thesis, University of Manchester 1995.

Gready M, Newburn M, Dodds R, *et al.*: *Birth choices – women's expectations and experiences*, London, 1995, National Childbirth Trust.

Hall J: The Trouble in Teams. MIDIRS, *Midwifery Digest* 6(1):77, 1996.

Hall M, MacIntyre S, Porter M: *Antenatal care assessed. A case study of an innovation in Aberdeen*. Aberdeen, 1985, Aberdeen University Press.

HEA: *Helping pregnant smokers QUIT: training for health professionals*, London, 1994, Health Education Authority.

Henderson C, Grant J: Team midwifery in Birmingham, update 7, *Newsletter Changing Childbirth Implementation Team*, October, 1996.

Hobbs L: *The independent midwife, a guide to independent midwifery practice*, Rochdale, 1993, Books for Midwives Press.

Hodnett E: Support from caregivers during childbirth. In Enkin

M, Keirse M, Renfrew M, editors: *Pregnancy and childbirth module of the Cochrane Database of Systematic Reviews*. London, 1995, BMJ Publishing Group.

House of Commons Health Committee: *Maternity services chaired by Sir Nicholas Winterton*. London, 1992, HMSO.

Hutton E: *Midwifery caseloads*, NCT Policy Statement, London, 1995, National Childbirth Trust.

Jacoby A, Cartwright A, Garcia J, *et al.*: Finding out about the views and experiences of maternity-service users. In Garcia J, *et al.*, editors: *The politics of maternity care*, Oxford, 1990, Clarendon Paperbacks.

Johnson G: Changes in antenatal care – do they affect standards? *Changing Childbirth Update* 5, 1996.

Jones K: The use of homoeopathy in women and children's health, *Br J Midwifery* 4(4):214, 1996.

Kuba L: The prenatal testing roller coaster: one mother's story, *J Perinat Educ* 4(4):19, 1995.

Leap N: The power of words. *Nurs Times* 88(21):60, 1992.

Leap N: Caseload practice: a recipe for burn out, *Br J Midwifery* 4(6):329, 1996.

Lewis P: Developing a group practice approach to care, *Midwifery Digest* 5(1):104, 1995a.

Lewis P: Refining the model, *Midwifery Digest* 5(2):219, 1995b.

Lewis P: Group practice midwifery and moving the vision on, *Midwifery Digest* 5(3):353, 1995c.

Lewis P: Group practice midwifery – a time for reflection, *Midwifery Digest* 5(4):475, 1995d.

McCourt, Page L: *Report on the evaluation of one-to-one midwifery*, London, 1996, Hammersmith Hospitals Trust/Thames Valley University.

Marteau T: Towards informed decisions about prenatal testing, *Prenat Diagn* 15(13):1215, 1995.

Mason M: Aromatherapy in practice, *Br J Midwifery* 4(6):325, 1996.

Meyer J, Wallace V: Mothers' help, *Nurs Times* 91(50):42, 1995.

MIDIRS and The Centre for Reviews and Dissemination: *Ultrasound screening in the first half of pregnancy: is it useful for everyone?*, Bristol, The Informed Choice Leaflets no 3, 1995, MIDIRS.

Newburn M: Choice, continuity and care, *New Generation* 12(2), 1993.

Oakley A: Social support in pregnancy: Methodology and findings of a one year follow-up study, *J Reprod Infant Psychol* 10(4):219, 1992.

Oakley A, Hickey D, Rajan L: Social support in pregnancy: Does it have long term effects. *J Repro Inf Psycho* 14:7–22, 1996.

Office of Population Censuses and Surveys: Birth statistics: *Review of Registrar General on births and patterns of family building in England and Wales 1993*. London, 1995, HMSO.

Page L, Jones B, Bentley R, *et al.*: One-to-one midwifery practice. *Br J Midwifery* 2(7):444, 1994.

RCM and RCGP: *Working together: Responsibilities in intrapartum care*, Joint Statement, London, 1995, Royal College of Midwives, Royal College of General Practitioners.

Redman C, Walker I: *Pre-eclampsia – The facts*, Oxford, 1992, Oxford Paperbacks.

Richardson A: The pregnancy club, *MIDIRS Midwifery Digest* 3(4):403, 1993.

Robertson A: *Preparing for birth: Background notes for pre-natal classes*, Sevenoaks, 1993, ACE Graphics.

Rothman B: *The tentative pregnancy: Amniocentesis and the sexual politics of motherhood*, London, 1994, Pandora.

Russell C: The Know Your Midwife scheme in Rhondda, *Assoc Radical Midwives Magazine* 36:14, 1988.

Sandall J: Midwives, burnout and continuity of care, *Br J Midwifery*, 5(2):106–11, 1997.

Sharp D, Jewell D. Bristol study of giving women choice over the number and timings of their antenatal care, Study in progress (Details from Department of Social Medicine, University of Bristol, Whiteladies Rd, Bristol BS8 2PR), 1996.

Shirley K, Mander R: The power of language, *Br J Midwifery* 4(6):298,317, 1996.

Sikorski J, Wilson J, Clements S: A randomised controlled trial comparing two schedules of antenatal visits, *Bri Med J* 312(7030):546, 1996.

Skelton I: Acupuncture and labour – a summary of results, *Midwives Chron* 101(1204):132–34, 1988.

Tew M: *Safer childbirth? A critical history of maternity care*, Chapters 7 & 8, London, 1990, Chapman and Hall.

Tiran D: *Aromatherapy in practice*, London, 1996, Bailliere Tindall.

Tiran D, Mack S, editors: *Complementary therapies for pregnancy and childbirth*, London, 1995, Bailliere Tindall.

UKCC: *The midwife's code of practice*, London, 1994, United Kingdom Central Council for Nurses, Midwives and Health Visitors

UKCC: *Confidentiality*, Advisory Paper, London, 1987, United Kingdom Central Council for Nurses, Midwives and Health Visitors

Walker J, Pollard L: Parent education for Asian mothers, *Modern Midwife* 5(9):22, 1995.

Warren C: *Chris Warren profile* (from Eagle Farm House, Cundall, York YO6 2RN), 1995.

Weig M: *Audit of independent midwifery 1980–1991*, London, 1993, Royal College of Midwives.

Wesson N: *Home birth* 2nd edn, London, 1995, Little, Brown and Co.

Whyte A: Fortifying the pregnancy message, *Health Visitor* 69(10);297, 1995.

Wilkinson A: All aboard in Bradford, *MIDIRS Midwifery Digest* 5(3):302, 1995.

Wraight A, Ball J, Seccombe I, *et al.*: *Mapping team midwifery*, Brighton, 1993, Institute Manpower Studies.

Yelland S: Using acupuncture in midwifery care, *Modern Midwife* 5(1):8, 1995.

Yuster EA: Rethinking the role of the risk approach and antenatal care in maternal mortality reduction, *Int J Gynecol Obstet* 50(suppl 2):S59, 1995.

Further Reading

Flint C: *Sensitive midwifery*, London, 1986, Heinemann.
Caroline Flint's liberating book is for all who want to gain confidence in themselves and as midwives.

Page L, editor: *Effective group practice in midwifery Cornwall: Working with women*, Oxford, 1995, Blackwell Science.
This book contains a wealth of detail about the theory and practice to help those wishing to set up effective continuity of care schemes.

Tiran D, Mack S, editors: *Complementary therapies for pregnancy and childbirth*, 1995, Bailliere Tindall.
Useful information on a range of complementary therapies.

6 Assessing Fetal and Maternal Well-Being

LEARNING OUTCOMES

After studying this chapter you should be able to:

- Appreciate the value and limitations of screening techniques.
- Discuss the aims and organization of antenatal care.
- Compare and contrast the value of various screening tests.
- Evaluate the uses of ultrasonography.
- Show an understanding of invasive prenatal screening tests.
- Demonstrate an awareness of the most common fetal abnormalities.
- Evaluate the value of screening during pregnancy.
- Appreciate the importance of providing women with adequate information to enable choices to be made.
- Describe the methods of monitoring well-being and their limitations in practice.

Introduction

The Health of the Nation (1992), a strategy for health in England, highlighted a number of factors that affect health. Although it dealt with many factors that affect the health of individuals, this document did not have a direct bearing upon midwives and the care they offer to pregnant women – it did, however, target issues such as family planning and teenage pregnancies, both of which are within a midwife's remit.

The targeting of health is not a new notion; indeed the Ministry of Health in 1919 foresaw the need to secure the health and welfare of childbearing women and their infants. Ballantyne in 1901 appealed for a proactive approach to antenatal care – his concerns lay with the ignorance of professionals in recognizing such conditions as eclampsia and jaundice (Rhodes, 1995). The care and management of the pregnant woman and her family has come a long way since the 1900s, as has the development of effective screening programmes to facilitate health.

The Aims and Organization of Antenatal Care

Antenatal care has undergone a revolutionary change in the past 20 years. This was essential to tailor the appropriate care to those women who require it. The original concept of antenatal care, when introduced early in the 20th century, was to perform mass screening of the pregnant population, the majority of whom suffered from malnutrition and were in poor general health. In addition, conditions such as rickets, tuberculosis and polio were endemic. The prenatal mortality during this era was high, and maternal mortality was common in most maternity units.

In recent years it has become apparent that the majority of women who attend antenatal clinics are in good health. The 'cattle market' antenatal clinics of the 1970s have thankfully disappeared, with the majority of healthy pregnant women being cared for by general practitioners (GPs) and midwives in the community. However, this does not mean that we should be complacent. Women and babies continue to die as a result of complications that occur in pregnancy and labour. Good antenatal care provides an effective screening programme for women considered to be 'low risk', without the need for multiple hospital visits or excessive intervention. Wald (1994) defines screening as: 'The identification, among apparently healthy individuals, of those who are sufficently at risk of a specific disorder to justify a subsequent diagnostic test or procedure, or in certain circumstances, direct preventative action'. Therefore to screen is to examine for the presence or absence of health to detect or prevent deviations from the norm; it is a major part of the role of midwives. Midwives also have a role in diagnosing (that is, identifying or refuting) conditions with reasonable certainty. In addition, there must be adequate provision for those women who, by nature of their pre-vious obstetric or medical history, might be considered to be at increased risk in pregnancy. To assess risk is to estimate the possibility of occurrence. Antenatal care must be individualized, and may change as the pregnancy progresses. The overall 'package' of antenatal care must take into consideration the wishes of the mother, who will undoubtedly have the best interests of the baby at heart. Preconception care is concerned with risk and sets out to consider the threat that lifestyle and behaviour may have on health.

Preconception and Early Pregnancy Care

'Care' of the mother begins before pregnancy. It is important that women enter pregnancy in good health. Women who smoke may wish to stop (or at least attempt to stop) before conception. In addition, screening for rubella antibodies and immunization should be undertaken by the GP or midwife. If a woman has concerns about toxoplasmosis, her antibody levels should also be checked. There is some evidence that multivitamins and preconception folate may help to prevent the occurrence of neural tube defects, and women planning to conceive should be advised to commence such therapy. A Department of Health campaign in November 1995 recommended that all midwives should advise women to take folic acid. Furthermore, it was stated that responsibility rests with the professionals concerned if such advice is not given (Long, 1996).

The First (Booking) Visit

This may take place in the hospital or in the community.

Establishing the expected date of delivery (EDD)

When the date of the most recent menstrual period is known with certainty, the periods have been regular and the most recent period was 'normal', then the date of delivery may be calculated using Naegele's rule (all gestation calculators are based on this rule). The EDD is calculated by adding 7 days to the date of the most recent menstrual period (LMP), taking away 3 months and adding 12 months:

EDD = [(LMP + 7) – 3] + 12
For example: If a women's last menstural period is: 1: 6: 98.
add 7 days = 8: 6: 98.
minus 3 months = 8: 3: 98.
plus 12 months = 8: 3: 99.

This calculation is only accurate for a 28-day cycle, so days need to be added or taken away for 21-day or 35-day cycles. Confirmation of the dates by an ultrasound scan is undertaken in many, but not all, units. Establishing the dates and the EDD is an important part of the booking visit, as it prevents confusion in later pregnancy should there be a suspicion of poor fetal growth.

Identifying potential problems

There is no doubt that the first hospital or community visit is one of the most important episodes for many pregnant women. The booking visit should ideally be undertaken by an experienced clinician. Many potential pregnancy complications may be missed by an inexperienced observer – it is vital that no obvious clue to a problem in pregnancy is missed. In addition, the booking visit may be a good time to discuss the mode of delivery if an operative delivery has been conducted previously, and to outline the options for prenatal diagnosis. The remainder of the care for the pregnancy may be planned on the basis of the booking visit.

Hospital or community care?

There is a tendency to care for women with no pregnancy complications in the community. This makes a lot of sense, and allows the obstetrician more time for the more complex obstetric problems in the hospital environment. However, there is still some reluctance by hospital consultants to let go of 'their patients', but midwives and GPs in the community are as capable as obstetricians at carrying out a general and abdominal assessment. Problems can just as easily be missed by both junior trainees and senior staff in an overcrowded hospital clinic.

Hospital or home birth?

The choice of the place of delivery should be an informed choice made by the woman. Every woman has a right to have her baby at home (Department of Health, 1993), and there should be facilities in every community for midwifery and medical support. Obviously, not every woman is in a condition or situation suitable for a home confinement. However, if a woman chooses a home confinement and is well informed of the risks, she should be given every support. This can be illustrated by a recent case in Stratford where a woman who had previously had a Caesarean section for breech presentation requested a home confinement. Despite being told of all the complications, the most extreme of which was fetal and possible maternal death in the event of scar rupture, she opted for home delivery, which occurred with no complications! The majority of women continue throughout pregnancy with no complications at all. However, some may require particular screening tests to ensure fetal well-being. It is usual for some tests to be performed on all women for whom pregnancy is confirmed or suspected.

Antenatal Care – The Low-Risk Mother

The majority of pregnant women have no problems in pregnancy, which for them is a normal physiological event. The aim of antenatal care in such women is to screen for problems that may occur in the population of women with no risk markers. The main ones that are detectable include growth retardation, hypertension and pre-eclampsia. These problems may be detected by a midwife or GP, so there is no reason why such women cannot be screened in the community.

How often a women should be seen and examined is debatable, but there is often a tendency to bring low-risk women to clinics for review too often. The fear is often that something will be missed. However, the majority of audits tend to show that antenatal care is often detrimental to the pregnancy in that over-diagnosis of problems leads to unnecessary intervention in many cases.

Monitoring maternal health

Routine clinical examination of the mother includes a general observation of health (anaemia, breathlessness). Weighing has been abandoned in many clinics, although an excessive weight gain may often herald the onset of pre-eclampsia. Blood pressure checks and assessment of urinalysis are the mainstay of screening for pre-eclampsia, however, and remain vitally important. Oedema is important if associated with hypertension, but in itself is not a problem. Assessment of haemoglobin should be carried out to screen for anaemia, and iron supplements prescribed when required. More complex medical problems are managed in hospital clinics and vary according to the condition involved. Diabetics, for example, monitor their own blood glucose levels and have periodic assessments of their glycosylated haemoglobin levels. Epileptics require serological assessments of their anticonvulsant levels during pregnancy, as changes in their plasma volume, glomerular filtration rate, protein binding, liver breakdown and bowel absorption in pregnancy alter the amount of drug in their blood stream. For similar reasons, women on thyroxine also require serial assessments of their thyroid function.

Monitoring fetal health

The simplest screening test for fetal well-being is to ask the mother about her fetal movements. Although not infallible, generally a health fetus moves and kicks vigorously. Any complaint of a deterioration in fetal movements must always be taken seriously. Formal assessments of fetal movement, such as kick charts, are often unhelpful.

The second screening test is, as mentioned above, an assessment of the fetal size by palpation. Abdominal palpation remains the primary method for detecting small-for-dates fetuses. The size of the fetus may be observed and compared to that expected for the given gestational age, but reported detection rates by abdominal palpation during routine antenatal care are poor, ranging between 30% and 50% (Hall *et al.* 1980; Rosenberg *et al.* 1982). In an attempt to improve this the simple tape measure is being increasingly used in antenatal clinics. Measurement of abdominal girth is not helpful in detecting small-for-dates fetuses (Elder *et al.* 1970), but tape measurement of symphyseal fundal height allows detection rates of between 56% (Rosenberg *et al.* 1982) and 86% (Belizan *et al.* 1978). Measurement is best performed from the highest point of the uterus (whether or not in the midline) by minimally indenting the fundus and reversing the marked surface of the tape (to ensure objectivity). Much of the success of tape measurement probably stems from the necessity of the examiner to record a numerical value in the case notes and therefore to consider further when this is at variance with that expected. As with virtually all techniques, an accurate knowledge of gestational age is needed to interpret the clinical findings. In addition to the measurement, an assessment of liquor volume may be made. If the fetus feels small and there is oligohydramnios present, this suggests growth retardation caused by placental insufficiency. The liquor volume is generally a good reflection of fetal health, for reasons that are discussed later. The fetal heart is always auscultated on clinical examination. Whether this is performed using portable Doppler ultrasound equipment or with a Pinard-type stethoscope depends on the preference of the clinician.

Screening Tests and Investigations

The majority of maternity hospitals in the UK perform an ultrasound scan in the first trimester to check the viability of the fetus, confirm or establish the date of delivery, exclude multiple pregnancy and exclude fetal anomaly.

Although all midwives and obstetricians participate in a National Surveillance Screening Programme (NSSP), not all advocate the same screening programmes for all pregnant women. Needless to say, for a woman to be treated as an individual it is the midwives' role to empower her to make informed decisions. A new committee chaired by Sir Kenneth Calman has been formed to ensure that screening programmes are effective (Department of Health, 1996).

Nevertheless, it is reasonable to assume that the NSSP in **Table 6.1** is offered to all pregnant women, with further investigations offered to others (**Table 6.2**). This screening is not necessarily carried out by midwives directly, as they (like all health professionals) operate in a multiprofessional team.

Table 6.1 Probable Routine Surveillance to Assess Maternal and Fetal Well-Being
1. General examination including:
Heart and lungs (first visit)
Weight, oedema, B/P
Urine analysis
2. Abdominal examination
3. Investigations
Full blood count, group
Rhesus factor, syphillis
Rubella status

Table 6.2 Other Possible Screening Investigations
Hepatitis

Haemoglobinopathies
     Sickle-cell disease
     Thalassaemia

Toxoplasmosis
Cystic fibrosis
Cytomegalovirus
Barts/triple/triple plus test /double test   Down syndrome screening
Phenylketonuria
Blood sugars
Alpha-fetoprotein
Human immunodeficiency virus
Fetal anomaly detection

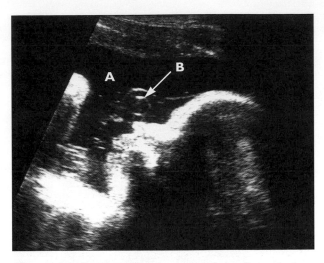

Figure 6.1 Facial profile of a normal fetus. **A**, amniotic fluid; **B**, umbilical cord.

Table 6.3 Capabilities of Ultrasonography
Detect a pregnancy and fetal heart movements from 6 weeks' gestation
Determine the number of fetuses
Determine the fetal position
Placental site localization
Estimate fetal growth and weight
Demonstrate fetal well-being

Ultrasonography

Ultrasonography has made it possible to visualize the fetus *in utero* and either confirm normality (**Figure 6.1**) or detect particular structural abnormalities. This gives women and their partners the opportunity to consider what problems they may encounter during their pregnancy.

Sonography basically means to 'write sound' and derives from the Latin word *sonus* and the Greek *graphein*. It is classified as a non-invasive technique. Almost every pregnant woman in the UK will have a scan. It has become a ritualistic part of antenatal care and is usually performed between 18 and 20 weeks' gestation (Joint Study Group on Fetal Abnormalities, 1989). In a study of 100 maternity units (Proud and Murphy–Black, 1997) it was reported that very few units gave information to enable women to make a choice of whether to have a scan. Occasionally, malformations can be diagnosed within the first trimester of pregnancy as a result of the 'routine' booking scan. Suspicions can arise in the event of finding a smaller fetus which does not comply with most recent menstrual period dates, an empty gestation sac or a fetus which does not possess normal embryonic appearances (**Table 6.3**). In certain circumstances, transvaginal scanning is useful in confirming such suspicions (Rottem *et al.* 1989; Cullen and Hobbins, 1993), because this provides better image resolution when the tissue interfaces are far more intimate to the cervix.

Measurements for gestational age and viability
Crown–rump length
The crown–rump length (CRL) measurement is performed within the first trimester. The fetus at this stage of pregnancy adopts a 'curled' position. It is achieved by placing an ultrasound caliper a the top of the head (crown) and another at the base fo the spine (rump). This scan is usually performed at the antenatal clinic to check viability and provide a baseline measurement for gestational age.

Fetal Nuchal Translucency Screening

This is an area behind the fetal neck where abnormal free fluid is present and can be detected from 10–14 weeks' gestation (**Figure 6.2**). Combined with maternal age, the fetal nuchal translucency can be used to estimate the risk for trisomy, especially Down syndrome (Nicolaides, 1996). Developments with this technique are still relatively new and the preliminary research

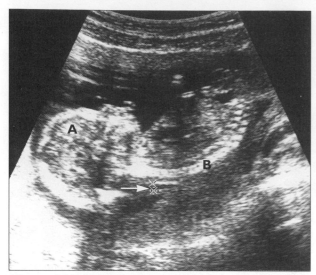

Figure 6.2 Longitudinal section of a fetus with a nuchal translucency. Note the fluid is between the cervical spine and skin (arrow). **A**, head; **B**, fetal spine.

work inconclusive and so in most units this is not used. Well-performed normal population data are required to establish the place of this promising test. However, if a nuchal translucency of more than 3 mm is visualized, other minor markers are often checked.

Biochemical Serum Screening for Down Syndrome and Neural Tube Defects

Down syndrome

Each year in the UK approximately 1000 babies are born with Down syndrome (a rate of 1/600–1/1000 births). Down syndrome is the most common cause of severe learning disability and can be associated with duodental atresia and cardiac malformations. The commonest cause is by non-disjunction, resulting in the triple replication (3 copies) of chromosome 21. Non-disjunction occurs when a cell does not divide equally during meiosis. When this cell combines with the partners's gamete the result is a total of 47 chromosomes (normal count 46). This can happen to a woman of any age and tends to be sporadic. In advanced maternal age (>35 years) the incidence is higher and this is why, until recently, amniocentesis was offered to them. Based on age selection alone, just one-third of Down babies can be detected (**Tables 6.4** and **6.5**). Although the individual risk of Down syndrome is lower in young women, overall, they produce more affected babies by virtue of their large group numbers. A useful comparison of different screening policies for Down syndrome is given in an article by Fletcher *et al.* (1995).

The triple test

Studies involving women carrying Down syndrome fetuses demonstrated that unusual levels of human chorionic gonadotrophin (βhCG) and alpha-fetoprotein (AFP) were present in their blood. In 11 of these women, AFP and unconjugated oestriol (UE3) levels were low in the maternal serum while HCG was high (Bogart *et al.* 1987). In 1988, a screening programme was initiated (Wald *et al.* 1988) to identify women at risk of having a child with either Down syndrome or spina bifida. This test has been available for more than 6 years and has many variations, the most common being the Bart's test or Triple test. To calculate a woman's risk, a logarithmic formula consisting of maternal age and the analysis of three hormones, namely HCG, AFP and UE3, are combined together. This formula determines the likelihood of a particular pregnancy being affected with Down syndrome. The optimal time for taking a sample of maternal blood is at 15–22 weeks' gestation, so it is important to accurately date the pregnancy. This method can detect 60% of Down syndrome fetuses. Oestriol level has been abandoned in some maternity units as, overall, it only enhances the detection rate by a further 7%, and adds to the cost. In an audit of women's views regarding a Down screening programme more explanations and information were identified as essential to decide whether the test was appropriate (Fairgrieve, 1997).

Table 6.4 Maternal age and incidence of Down syndrome		
Maternal age (years)	**Down syndrome risk at amniocentesis at 16 weeks' gestation**	**Risk of Down syndrome at birth**
20	1:1000	1:1000
30	1:600	1:900
35	1:250	1:380
40	1:75	1:100
45	1:20	1:25

Table 6.5 Chromosomal Disorders with Mental Retardation and Physical Disabilities		
Syndrome	**Chromosomes**	**Ultrasound features**
Most common		
Down syndrome (1/600 live births)	Trisomy 21 (47 chromosomes)	Cystic hygroma
		Duodenal atresia
		Heart defects
		Hydrops
		Hydronephrosis
		Short femur length
		Sandal gap toe
		Clinodactyly
		Ectogenic bowel
Edward's syndrome(1/5000 live births)	Trisomy 18 (47 chromosomes)	Growth retardation
		Cleft lip/palate
		Hydrocephalus
		Micrognathia
		Cystic hygroma
		Heart defect
		Exomphalos
		Overlapping fingers
		Rocker-bottom feet
		Choroid plexus cysts
Patau's syndrome (1/5000 live births)	Trisomy 13 (47 chromosomes)	Microcephaly
		Holoprosencephaly
		Cleft lip/palate
		Heart defect
		Polydactyly of the hands/feet
		Rocker-bottom feet
		Renal malformations
		Cyclopia
Other syndromes		
Turner's syndrome (1/5000)	45XO	Small in stature
Note: Survivors of Turner's syndrome have		Cystic hygroma
normal intelligence		Micrognathia
		Lymphoedema
		Ovarian dysgenesis
		Cardiac abnormalities
Triploidy (1/2500)	69 chromosomes	IUGR
Note: Complete extra set of		Cystic abnormal kidneys
chromosomes in a triploidy fetus		Ambiguous genitalia
– the fetus will either miscarry or die		Abnormal heart
a few days into the neonatal period		Omphalocele
		Cleft lip/palate
		Holoprosencephaly
		Hydrocephaly
		'Molar-type' placenta

Invasive Prenatal Diagnosis

Introduction

It is now accepted that prenatal diagnosis has become an integral part of antenatal care, with couples accepting prenatal diagnosis if it helps avoid having a handicapped child. Donnai (1987) stated that:

> It should be ensured that all patients enter a screening programme with full knowledge of the tests and their limitations and having given some thought to their action if a test result suggests that further specific tests are indicated.

To consider embarking upon an invasive test is not easy to do, so professionals should offer as much support as needed to help couples cope with their decision. For a majority of women, positive feelings surrounding their pregnancy are put on hold, because of their private fears and anxieties during the waiting period for results, and for them, this can seem like a lifetime. The purpose of prenatal diagnosis is to provide information to women and couples who may be at risk of having a baby with a genetic or chromosomal abnormality. It permits preparation for bad news and, in essence, helps a woman come to the decision to terminate an abnormal pregnancy. The report by the Royal College of Physicians (1989), *Prenatal Diagnosis and Genetic Screening*, states that:

> The ideal professionals to provide information and counselling would be specially trained health visitors and midwives, who are already the point of first and most frequent contact with mother and child.

This statement is unquestionable, as the UKCC (1994) *Professional Code of Practice* states that a midwife should, 'prescribe or advise on the examinations necessary for the earliest possible diagnosis of pregnancies at risk.' Hence, it is clear that the midwife is regarded as the key person responsible for providing a framework of continuing care for those women who encounter a problem with their pregnancies. **Table 6.6** outlines the risks of invasive prenatal tests.

Chorionic villus sampling (CVS) or placental biopsy

Women with a family history of genetic disease or who have had a baby with a chromosomal abnormality can be offered this early prenatal test, as trophoblastic cells can provide an excellent source of cytogenetic material for DNA, chromosomal and metabolic investigation.

CVS, which came to light in the 1960s and in the mid-70s was primarily used by the Chinese for fetal sexing. It's main advantage is that it can be performed within the first trimester and results can be rapidly available within one week (direct culture) to two weeks (long-term culture). If an abnormality is found then a first trimester termination can be offered (suction and curettage). This is less upsetting for the woman as the procedure is performed under general anaesthetic.

Compared with amniocentesis, CVS has a slightly higher miscarrage risk of 2–3%, in addition to the background risk of spontaneous fetal loss, although the Canadian trial (Canadian Collaborative Trial, 1989) reported that there was no significant difference between the two. Another recent trial evaluating the safety of the procedure, comparing CVS with second trimester amniocentesis highlighted a 4.6% fetal loss rate (MRC Working Party, 1991). It is evident that operator experience can influence the overall loss rate associated with the procedure (Saura *et al.* 1994).

The test can be done either transabdominally (**Figure 6.3**) or transcervically (**Figure 6.4**), the determining factors being placental location. Great controversy arose in 1991, when a 'cluster' of children born in Oxford

Table 6.6 Overall Risks of Invasive Prenatal Tests
Maternal risks
Miscarriage
Premature delivery
Haemorrhage
Haematoma
Infection
Premature rupture of membranes (PROM)
Rhesus isoimmunization
Fetal risks
Premature delivery
Fetal bradycardia
Infection
Haemorrhage – haematoma/vessel in cord
Trauma
PROM
Respiratory difficulties
Limb abnormalities
Death

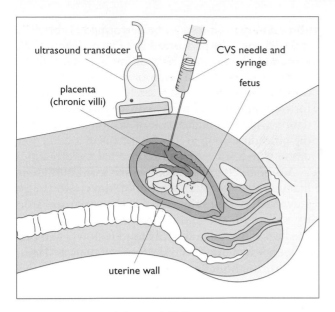

Figure 6.3 Transabdominal CVS.

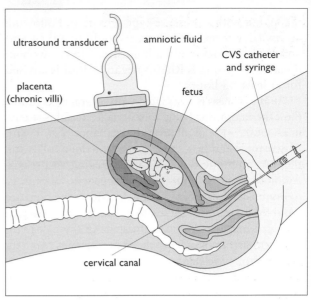

Figure 6.4 Transcervical CVS.

presented with oromandibular limb hypoplasia syndrome. The common associated factor is that their mothers all had CVS performed very early in pregnancy: <10 weeks gestation (Firth *et al.* 1991). Investigations supported the hypothesis that the syndrome was caused by placental vascular disruption, which resulted in hypoperfusion to the fetus. As a result of this, prenatal diagnostic centres perform CVS from ten and a half weeks.

Amniocentesis

Amniocentesis is the most practised invasive procedure and is relatively simple for an operator to do. The test can provide a 99.9% reliable result that can enable women and their partners decide upon the future of their pregnancy. Amniocentesis involves the removal of liquor from the amniotic sac under direct ultrasound guidance from as early as 14 weeks gestation. Liquor is 'straw-coloured' in appearance and contains hundred of fetal cells called amniocytes, which originate from the fetal skin and orifices. The cells are mainly utilized for karyotyping and DNA analysis, but can also be measured for levels of amniotic AFP, acetylcholinesterase for NTDs, as well as bilirubin levels in the prediction of fetal anaemia in a Rhesus-sensitized pregnancy.

Direct ultrasound visualisation helps minimise injury in the fetus, placenta or cord. Initially an ultrasound scan is performed to establish fetal gestational age, viability and a clear pool of liquor. A 21-gauge spinal needle is inserted through the skin of the abdomen, into the uterus and finally into the amniotic sac (**Figure 6.5**). The stylet is removed and at least 20 ml of fluid is aspirated with a syringe. Reassurance is offered to the woman, following removal of the needle by showing her baby to her, with an emphasis placed on the 'beating heart'.

Generally, amniocentesis is slightly uncomfortable – most women say that it is similar to having blood

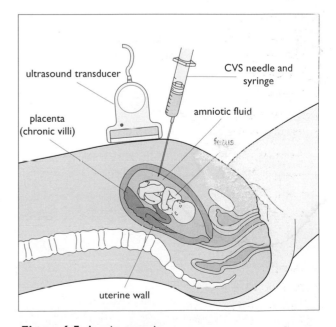

Figure 6.5 Amniocentesis.

taken, but with a pressure-type sensation. Following all invasive tests, a Kleihauer should be taken and anti D immunoglobulin administered to the woman if her blood group is Rhesus negative. Rest is advised for at least 48 hours.

Amniocentesis is associated with several risks (**Table 6.6**), the major one being miscarriage, and this occurs in about 0.5–1% of all procedures (Tabor *et al*. 1986). Miscarriage can be caused by contractions following the test, amniotic fluid leakage, bleeding and sepsis. Amniotic fluid is cultured in a cytogenetic laboratory to establish a karyotype. The cells within the fluid are removed for culture and treated in an incubator so that they can mature. At a certain stage in their growth, about 15 are analysed and the chromosomes counted. Photographs are taken to ensure that each chromosome is paired up with its neighbour. The results can take 2–4 weeks to arrive, and in some instances there will be no result at all because of culture failure – in large centres this can occur in about 1% of cases.

Percutaneous Umbilical Blood Sampling (PUBS)/Cordocentesis

It is sometimes necessary to carry out a percutaneous umbilical blood sample (PUBS/cordocentesis) when information about the fetus is required urgently. If necessary, this can be performed from 17 weeks gestation, with results in 24–48 hours. Fetal blood can allow a variety of tests to be performed (**Table 6.7**).

PUBS has to be performed by an experienced operator and the overall risk of miscarriage largely depends upon the condition of the baby at the time of sampling. Obviously, a severely compromised baby, for example, a fetus with hydrops or growth retardation will be at higher risk of demise as a result of the procedure compared with a fetus in a good condition with a suspected chromosomal abnormality.

A 6-inch, 20-gauge needle is passed transabdominally (**Table 6.8**) with the aid of 'direct ultrasound guidance'. Once in the vessel of the cord (operators try to aim for the umbilical vein), the stylet of the needle is removed and fetal blood is slowly and gently withdrawn using 1 ml syringes for analysis (**Figure 6.6**); throughout the procedure, the fetal heart is monitored.

Table 6.8 Four Sites for Cordocentesis
● Umbilical vein at the placental cord insertion
● Intrahepatic umbilical vein
● Free loop of cord
● Cardiac chambers

Table 6.7 Clinical Investigations from Cordocentesis
Cytogenetic studies
karyotype
DNA analysis
Virology studies
fetal infection
virus [e.g. TORCH – toxoplasmosis, rubella, cytomegalovirus (CMV), herpes]
Fetal biochemistry
Fetal blood gases/acid–base balance
Rhesus status
Blood disorders
alloimmune thrombocytopenia
haemoglobinopathies, e.g. sickle cell, thalassaemia
Inborn errors of metabolism

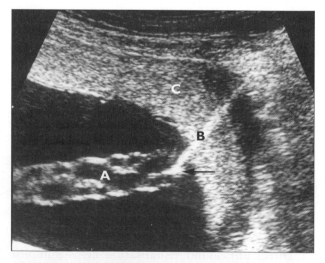

Figure 6.6 Ultrasound image of cordocentesis. Note the needle tip entering at the placental cord insertion (arrow). **A**, umbilical cord; **B**, needle; **C**, placenta.

Fetal Biometry – Ultrasound Assessment of Growth

As already mentioned, ultrasonography can alert the practitioner if things are wrong by enabling observation of the baby *in utero*. Fetal biometry refers to measuring the baby ultrasonically.

Biparietal diameter

The biparietal diameter (BPD) measurement is achieved by obtaining an image in transverse section of the fetal head and measuring the distance between the biparietal eminences (the widest diameter of the fetal skull). This measurement is useful within the second trimester of pregnancy for assessment of gestational age.

Fetal head circumference

Fetal head circumference (HC) measurement proves useful in the late second trimester and third trimester of pregnancy. The HC is the maximum distance around the skull at the level of the biparietal diameter (BPD) and is taken by first measuring the BPD and then introducing a third caliper to trace a line around the fetal skull. The image is frozen and a measurement recorded.

Abdominal circumference

Abdominal circumference (AC) is the preferred measurement to assess fetal growth in the late second and third trimester of pregnancy. It is basically a measurement of the waistline of the baby *in utero*. AC is the largest circumference of the abdomen at the level of the bifurcation of the portal vein and stomach. This measurement, once again, is achieved by using the electronic caliper and freeze frame button.

Femur length

The femur length can be measured from as early as 12 weeks' gestation. Compared with the BPD, it is a more accurate measurement of gestational age in the third trimester. The FL extends from the great trochanter to the lateral femoral condule and elctronic calipers are placed on these parts to obtain a measurement.

Other fetal limbs can be measured this way (tibia, fibula, radius and humerus). In some instances, practioners use these limb measurments to exclude skeletal dysplasia. Such common conditions are osteogenesis imperfecta and achondroplasia (dwarfism).

'Small for Dates' Fetus

Where the fetus is considered to be 'small for dates', then an ultrasound assessment of fetal size should be performed. To interpret the ultrasound data accurately it is essential that the gestational age of the fetus be accurately known. Wrong dates may result in a normal-growth fetus being labelled as growth retarded. Fetal biometry includes the fetal HC or BPD and the AC – because of variations in fetal head shape, the fetal HC is preferable to the BPD. The resultant measurements are plotted on standard growth charts. Two broad categories of 'growth retardation' are recognized.

Symmetrical growth retardation is said to exist where the HC and AC are reduced. The causes of this pattern include placental insufficiency, wrong dates, a small normal fetus, chromosomal abnormalities and even in-utero infection. Racial differences in fetal size and differences due to maternal size are accounted for by using a 'standardized' fetal growth chart. This is a computer-generated individual growth chart that takes into consideration factors such as maternal height, race and parity, but the use of such charts is not widespread.

The other recognized growth pattern is when the fetal HC is within normal limits, but the AC is reduced. This asymmetrical pattern of growth is considered more typical of growth retardation. The reduction of growth in the AC is thought to reflect the use of the fetal liver glycogen stores when the placenta fails to meet the demands of the fetus. The fetal head continues to grow because of the so-called 'brain-sparing' effect, whereby the fetus maintains the circulation to the developing brain at the expense of the blood supply to the viscera.

Both patterns should alert the clinician to a potential problem, although a static measurement is often of little value. The velocity of growth of the fetus is probably a better indicator of the true fetal growth pattern – this must be assessed over a 2-week period. Assessment of growth within a week is not reliable as the increase in fetal size during that period is not sufficient to be detected accurately with ultrasonography.

In addition to fetal biometry, an assessment may be made of the liquor volume, which reflects the renal function of the fetus. Where the fetus is healthy, fetal urine production is normal and thus the liquor volume is normal. Where the fetus is growth retarded, the reduction in the blood supply to the viscera causes a reduction in renal blood flow, and thus in urine production, so the amount of liquor may be reduced. The assessment can be made by looking at maximum pool depth or by using the summation of 'cord-free' pool depths from the four quadrants of the uterus, the amniotic fluid index (AFI). Charts that depict the normal range of AFI for gestational age are available.

The Management of Complications during Pregnancy

Medical Problems

Certain medical conditions may result in abnormalities in the fetus if they are poorly controlled. The best known of these is diabetes. The incidence of miscarriage and fetal anomalies (classically, sacral agenesis is associated with diabetes) is increased when diabetes is poorly controlled around the time of conception. It is vitally important to ensure diabetes is tightly controlled around the time of conception and, indeed, throughout pregnancy.

Epilepsy, too, is a condition that is associated with problems. Sodium valproate is associated with an increased risk of NTDs, and multiple fetal defects have been described with the use of phenytoin. Carbamazepine is one of the safest drugs to use in pregnancy, but is not always appropriate. The aim would be to avoid polypharmacy and attain a safe level of medication. The importance of a medical condition to a woman prior to pregnancy lies in the questions:
• How will the pregnancy affect her medical problem?
• How will her medical problem affect her pregnancy?
As a result of pregnancy, certain conditions may deteriorate to such an extent that there is a risk of maternal death, e.g. congenital cardiac conditions that may lead to cardiac failure, such as Eisenmenger's complex. In such cases, pregnancy should be discouraged. Other conditions may be made worse by pregnancy, such diabetes. In other cases, the disease process itself may have an adverse outcome on pregnancy.

Most of the medical problems that influence the outcome of pregnancy are best managed by a multidisciplinary approach, i.e. obstetric, medical, paediatric, midwifery and often anaesthetic inputs. Management may be conducted through a 'joint clinic', although this may be difficult to organize in smaller units.

The Rhesus Negative Mother

Approximately 17% of women in the UK are Rhesus D negative (Rh –ve) as they do not have protein antigen 'D' on their red blood cells (RBC). This is usually detected from a sample of blood taken at the 'booking' visit. There are five5 major antigens within the maternal blood stream (D, C, c, E and e) but the Rhesus D antigen is the most common one found. Since its discovery, the perinatal mortality rate from haemolytic disease of the newborn (HDN) has decreased from 15 per 10,000 births, in the 1950s, to 0.2 per 10,000 in 1993 (Oxford Regional Health Authority). This can be attributed to early identification of antibodies and the specialised management and treatment of the disease.

Throughout the antepartum and intrapartum period, there is always a potential risk that a Rhesus negative woman in her first pregnancy, may be 'sensitised' (the stimulation of IgG antibodies), if fetal Rhesus D positive (Rh D +ve) blood enters her circulation (feto-maternal haemorrhage, FMH). Anti -D antibodies seek out the fetal Rh D +ve red blood cells (RBC) within the circulation and destroy them (haemolysis). In a subsequent pregnancy, with another Rh D +ve baby, the attack continues, the severity depending on the antibody levels within the woman's blood. If this is not recognised, then hydrops fetalis (abdominal ascites and generalised oedema) or intrauterine death can occur (**Figures 6.7, 6.8** and **Table 6.9**).

There are several ways to prevent fetal hydrops. It is essential that regular samples of maternal blood are taken to ckeck for antibody formation. Most units perform this at booking, 28, 32, or 34 weeks gestation. FMH can happen for various reasons (**Table 6.10**) and for this reason a Kleihauer–Betke test should be perfomed to assess the degree of haemorrhage, so that the appropriate dose of human Anti D immunoglobulin can be given to the woman intramusculary. The National Blood Transfusion Service Immunoglobulin Working Party guidelines, 1991, advises that Anti-D 250 iu is given prior to 20 weeks gestation and 500 iu given after this time.

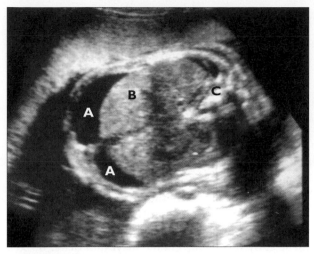

Figure 6.7 Cross-sectional view at thoracic level of fetal hydrop. **A**, hydrops; **B**, fetal lungs; **C**, fetal spine.

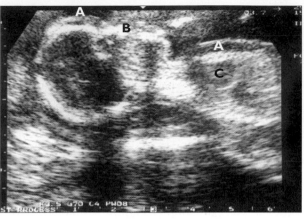

Figure 6.8 Longitudinal view of fetus with hydrops fetalis. Note the 'halo' effect of the oedema around the head and chest. **A**, hydrops; **B**, face; **C**, fetal heart.

In the case of babies who are significantly compromised because of HDN, the treatment is carried out in a specialist centre. Serial amniocentesis for optical density (ΔOD_{450}) starting from 24 weeks gestation, can rapidly provide fetal bilirubin levels which can indicate the severity of the haemolysis. If haemolysis is apparent, then a transabdominal intravascular transfusion (IVT) is performed under direct ultrasound guidance to correct the anaemia. It is also possible for the operator to do this intraperitoneally. Usually, there is a series of transfusions, the last occuring around 32–34 weeks gestation. Following delivery at least one exchange transfusion may be required in the neonatal period.

Table 6.9 Features of Hydrops Fetalis
• With severe hydrops fetalis the fetus has a 'Buddha' type appearance
• Generalized abdominal ascites
• Skin oedema of the body and scalp
• Pericardial effusion
• Pleural effusion of the lungs
• Enlarged liver
• Ascites around the midgut
• An enlarged hydropic placenta
• Polyhydramnios

Table 6.10 When Sensitisation Can Occur and Anti-D Immunoglobulin is Given to a Rhesus Negative Woman
During the following events fetal blood cells cross the placental barrier and mixing occurs – Rhesus sensitization takes place

• Following a miscarriage	• After invasive prenatal testing	• Following delivery
• After termination of pregnancy	amniocentesis	normal vaginal
• Following an antepartum haemorrhage	CVS	caesarean section
• Following an accident, e.g. fall, car-crash	cordocentesis	Instrumental vaginal
	fetal therapy/surgery	• External cephalic version for breech presentation

Hypertension and Pre-eclampsia

Hypertension in pregnancy may predate the pregnancy (essential hypertension) or may arise in pregnancy (pregnancy-induced hypertension). Pregnancy-induced hypertension may be a benign condition (gestational hypertension) in which high blood pressure is the only feature. This tends to have a good prenatal outcome, although occasionally the blood pressure may require treatment. On the other hand, pre-eclampsia is associated with an increased prenatal mortality and is often found in association with proteinuria and oedema. The cause of pre-eclampsia is unknown, but it is thought to originate in the placenta, resulting in the 'maternal syndrome' (a widespread vasculitis that affects every organ in the body and manifests as the typical signs of pre-eclampsia) and the fetal syndrome (growth retardation). Screening for this condition is important because of the associated prenatal mortality, but also because it remains a major cause of maternal mortality. The maternal syndrome is assessed clinically (measurement of blood pressure, assessment of reflexes, testing for oedema) and with laboratory tests. A raised serum urate indicates the condition, and in the latter stages of disease the platelet count falls due to consumption – there may even be a widespread disseminated intravascular coagulation, which becomes evident on testing the clotting system and checking for fibrin degradation products. Liver function test results may be abnormal if the liver is involved, and a syndrome of haemolysis, elevated liver enzymes and low platelet count (HELLP syndrome) may develop. In such cases, the fetus and placenta should always be assessed by Doppler of the umbilical artery, ultrasound biometry and cardiotocography.

The condition of pre-eclampsia is progressive. Although hypertension may be controlled, the underlying disease process continues and may eventually result in eclampsia (a condition in which fits occur and which has a high maternal and fetal mortality). The timing of delivery to prevent this condition requires careful deliberation. Prolongation of the pregnancy is only necessary when there is something to be gained, i.e. to allow the fetus to mature. Where the fetus is beyond 36 weeks' gestation, delivery should be effected where there is concern for either the fetus or the mother.

Growth Retardation

Intrauterine growth retardation (IUGR) is a major cause of prenatal mortality and morbidity. The rate of fetal growth is determined by interaction of the intrinsic drive to grow of the fetus and the extrinsic support it receives during pregnancy to ensure an adequate supply of nutrients, such as glucose, lactate and amino acids, and of oxygen. This necessitates a satisfactory supply of blood to the intervillous space of the placenta and adequate exchange mechanisms. The principal determinant of the intrinsic growth potential of the fetus is probably genetic, although this may be modified by insults in early intrauterine life [e.g. by rubella infection (Naeye and Blanc, 1965).

Owing to the heterogeneity of the small-for-dates group, the degree and nature of prenatal risk to the individual baby varies greatly. At least risk are those that are small merely because of their genetic inheritance; at greatest risk are both those with major malformations and those that are genuinely growth retarded because of uteroplacental insufficiency. The terms 'small for dates' and 'growth retarded' are frequently, but wrongly, used as if synonymous. Small-for-dates is a statistical concept, useful both because it is easily estimated (as long as gestational age and birth weight are known and appropriate criteria agreed to separate normal from abnormal) and because it undoubtedly identifies a group of babies at increased prenatal risk. The major risks are of death (especially intrauterine), intrapartum asphyxia, neonatal hypoglycaemia and, possibly, long-term neurological and intellectual impairment.

To assess the risks of prenatal death and damage, a study in Melbourne of 500 consecutive small-for-dates babies by Dobson *et al.* (1981) is probably the most useful; the prenatal mortality rates for babies with birth weights above the 10th percentile, between the 5th and 10th percentiles and below the 5th percentile were, respectively, 12, 22 and 190 deaths per 1000. Approximately 80% of prenatal deaths of small-for-dates babies occur *in utero* and almost a half occur after 36 weeks (McIlwaine *et al.* 1979); these are certainly potentially avoidable. Also growth retardation is as important a cause of fetal loss during the late second trimester as during the third (Whitfield *et al.* 1986). In addition, the Melbourne study found 13% of small-for-dates babies have low Apgar scores.

There are a number of reasons why intrapartum asphyxia is more common among growth-retarded babies:

- Pre-existing uteroplacental insufficiency is made worse by the effect of myometrial contractions.
- Fetuses have less metabolic reserve to withstand the hypoxic effect of labour because of intrauterine malnutrition.
- Some fetuses are hypoxaemic even before the onset of labour.
- The vessels in the umbilical cord are more vulnerable to compression because of frequent reduction in both amniotic fluid and Wharton's jelly.

Morbidity among small-for-dates neonates may conveniently be divided into three categories (Oh, 1977):

- Fetal problems, e.g. chromosomal abnormalities, congenital infections and other malformations.
- Sequelae of intrapartum asphyxia, e.g. meconium aspiration syndrome, hyperviscosity and postasphyxial encephalopathy,
- Abnormalities of substrate transfer and aberrations of hormonal control, e.g. hypoglycaemia and hypocalcaemia.

Multiple Pregnancy

Multiple pregnancy is, by definition, a high-risk pregnancy. Pregnancy complications such as pre-eclampsia may be more severe in twin pregnancy, and early pregnancy symptoms such as nausea tend to increase. Generally, twin pregnancies that derive from the splitting of a single fertilized egg (monozygotic twin pregnancy) have more complications than those that arise from two or more separately fertilized ova (dizygotic). The background rate of twin pregnancies is around 1:80, although the rate is rising because of the increased number of assisted conceptions (in-vitro fertilization, gamete intrafallopian transfer and intracytoplasmic sperm injection). For triplets the rate is $1:80^2$ and for quads it is $1:80^3$. Antenatal care in multiple pregnancy is largely hospital based, and serial ultrasonography is usually performed to assess fetal growth. In addition to the general obstetric complications that may ensue, women with multiple pregnancies are more prone to develop anaemia, pre-eclampsia and growth retardation. Also, problems may arise that are peculiar to multiple pregnancies, such as the twin-to-twin transfusion syndrome, which results from a placental vascular anomaly, or rare fetal anomalies such as the acardiac acephalic twin maintained as a result of blood supply from its donor twin. Prenatal diagnosis is more complex as serum assessments are not possible. A detailed ultrasound scan may demonstrate markers for chromosomal abnormalities – the nuchal translucency test has potential in these circumstances. When there is the possibility of a trisomic fetus, amniocentesis may be performed, providing there are two separate sacs (i.e., the fetus must be dizygotic).

Breech Presentation

Breech presentation is common before 30 weeks' gestation and has no relevance antenatally until approximately 36 weeks, when the incidence of breech presentation is 3%, the same as that at term. At this point, a decision must be made with regard to the mode of delivery. There is no doubt that a vaginal birth is more risky for the fetus. However, these risks must be balanced against the risks to the mother of caesarean section. The estimated weight of the baby may be calculated from ultrasonic measurements and some clinicians measure the size of the pelvis with radiographic pelvimetry (rarely used today) or computed tomography (CT) scan. This information, together with past obstetric history, is taken into consideration and the final decision made jointly with the patient. Many primigravid women opt for a caesarean section – in some centres all primigravid women with a breech presentation are given a caesarean section (there is no patient choice). The option to turn the baby [external cephalic version (ECV)] may be available, which has been shown to reduce the incidence of breech presentation where routinely practised with minimal complications.

Fetal Surveillance

Cardiotocography

The assessment of fetal heart rate (cardiotocography – the cardiogram displays the fetal heart rate and the tocogram displays the contractions) is the most utilized form of fetal assessment. The essential features of fetal heart rate (**Figure 6.9**) that should be noted are:

- The baseline fetal heart rate. The normal fetal heart rate usually lies between 120–160 beats per minute (b.p.m.). However, a lower rate is often acceptable as long as other features that suggest fetal health are present.

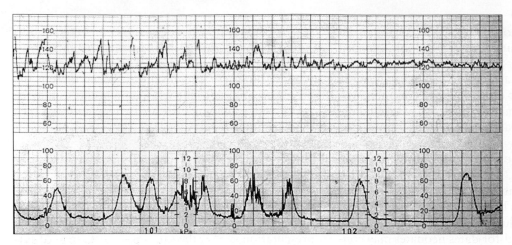

Figure 6.9 The first part of the tracing shows normal reactivity to fetal movements, followed by a period of fetal sleep.

- The variability of the fetal heart rate, i.e. the amount that the fetal heart varies around the baseline. Hammacher *et al.* (1968) describe a variation of less than 5 b.p.m. as abnormal, between 5–10 b.p.m. as the lower limit of normal and between 10–25 b.p.m. as normal. Above 25 b.p.m. is also considered abnormal.

- Reactivity. This is the acceleration of the fetal heart rate in response to fetal movement or uterine activity. An acceleration is defined as a value of 15 b.p.m. above the baseline that exceeds 15 seconds in duration and is associated with fetal movement. Two such episodes would be expected within a 20 minute period.

Episodes of higher variability increase in frequency of occurrence with gestational age until a plateau is reached at 34 weeks, when 55% of the time is spent in a state of high variability. Corresponding to this change, fetal heart rate accelerations (>14 b.p.m. and lasting ≥15 seconds) progressively increase in frequency with gestational age and are associated with clusters of fetal body movements. On average, they occur every 2.5–3.0 minutes from 34 weeks onwards.

The assessment of these features gives a reasonable evaluation of the fetal health at the time of the monitoring. Lavery (1982) reviewed 11 series and calculated a false negative rate for prenatal death of 6.8/1000 following a normal reactive cardiotocograph (CTG). One practical drawback of the test is the relatively high frequency of falsely abnormal test results – about 10–15% in the mature fetus and 20–40% in the early third trimester. The vast majority of abnormal results are due to the fetal sleep cycle, which can

be verified by prolonging the test for up to 120 minutes. In Europe the majority of cardiotocographs are performed without the addition of induced uterine activity, a so-called 'non-stress test'. However, in the US and Canada oxytocin-induced contraction stress tests are occasionally used. There are obvious disadvantages to such tests. It is relatively invasive, it is also time consuming and may precipitate labour or even fetal compromise (Baillie, 1974). The false positive rate for prenatal death using such methods is about 90% (Baskett and Sandy, 1977) and, overall, between 20–50% of positive tests are not followed by signs of fetal distress in labour. However, the false negative rate is low – 0.3/1000 for stillbirth in one large multicentre trial (Freeman *et al.*, 1982).

The recording of a cardiotocograph is of no value if the tracing is misinterpreted. An assessment of a cardiotocograph may vary from one observer to another; indeed, the opinion of one observer may also change when given the same tracing after a period of time. For this reason, objective measures of the fetal heart rate pattern have been developed over the years which include various scoring systems. By far the best to date is the computerized cardiotocograph system (System 8000 – Oxford Medical). Besides being objective and reproducible in its assessments, the computerized system stores data and a review of the trends in serial monitoring may be displayed. However, the computerized system is not a replacement for the clinician, who is responsible for the interpretation of data and the correct management as a result of this information.

The Biophysical Profile

The biophysical profile or score was developed to try and improve detection of the fetus at risk. The CTG has a high predictive value for a good prenatal outcome when the result is normal. However, it has a high false-positive rate (>80%) for poor prenatal outcome (fetal distress in labour, intrauterine growth retardation or low 5-minute Apgar score) and more than 95% for prenatal death (Baskett *et al.*, 1987). Manning *et al.* (1979) found that combining cardiotography with the observation of fetal breathing movements on ultrasound lowered the false positive rate. With this background, Manning *et al.*, 1980) developed a fetal profile by assessing five biophysical variables (**Table 6.11**). Many centres now use variations of these criteria, usually incorporating AFI in the amniotic fluid assessment. Each variable is assigned a score of 2 when normal or 0 when abnormal. Techniques used in the UK and the differences between screening and diagnostic tests are discussed in an article by Green and Statham (1993).

The biophysical profile improves the positive predictive value for abnormal prenatal outcome compared to single biophysical variable testing. The false negative rate is low (0.7/1000) and comparable to that of a contraction 'stress test', but superior to unstressed cardiotocography. In high-risk pregnancies the likelihood of a normal biophysical profile result is higher (>97%) than that with a CTG alone (85–90%). This suggests that the biophysical profile is better able to differentiate altered fetal behavioural states from hypoxia. One drawback in the use of the biophysical profile is that the test itself may be time consuming, as a healthy human fetus may exhibit episodes of absent breathing movements that last for up to 120 minutes. However, the average time taken for a biophysical profile is about 20 minutes (Baskett, 1989).

Doppler Assessment

Doppler assessment may be used to indirectly assess the health of the placenta. The signal obtained as a result of reflected ultrasound waves onto the fetal and placental vessels is actually the velocity of individual particles within the vessel (**Figure 6.10**). The umbilical artery is the vessel most commonly used. The flow velocity initially increases with the contraction of the fetal heart, and then reaches a peak at the end of systole (**Figure 6.10, A**). When the fetal heart stops beating, flow continues during diastole (**Figure 6.10, B**) as the placenta is a low-resistance system. The end of diastole is when the particles accelerate into systole again. When the placenta is diseased, the resistance to flow increases, so flow in diastole is curtailed. When this resistance is high there may be no flow at all in diastole – in severe cases the flow in diastole may even be reversed. The conditions of 'no end diastolic flow' and reversal of flow are pathological and show the placenta to be diseased. Although at this point the placenta is known to be unhealthy, the fetus is not necessarily unhealthy, although it is only a matter of time before its condition becomes compromised.

Although Doppler assessment of the umbilical artery is the most common measurement to be undertaken, by using pulsed colour-flow Doppler vessels within the brain can be analyzed and the degree of circulatory shifts to maintain the cerebral circulation estimated. Whether this measurement is of benefit relative to a sim-

Table 6.11 The Biophysical Profile	
Variable*	**Criteria**
Cardiotocograph	Two or more fetal heart rate accelerations of at least 15 b.p.m. and 15 seconds duration within a 20 minute observation period
Fetal breathing movements	At least one episode of 30 seconds sustained fetal breathing movements within a 30 minute observation period
Fetal movements	At least three separate fetal limb or trunk movements within a 30 minute observation period
Fetal tone	At least one episode of extension with return to flexion of a limb or the trunk within a 30 minute observation period
Amniotic fluid volume	A pocket of amniotic fluid that measures more than 1 cm in two perpendicular planes

*Scoring – Each variable for which the criteria are fulfilled scores 2; if not, it scores 0
*Scores – 8–10, normal; 6, equivocal; 0–4, abnormal

Source: Baskett, 1989

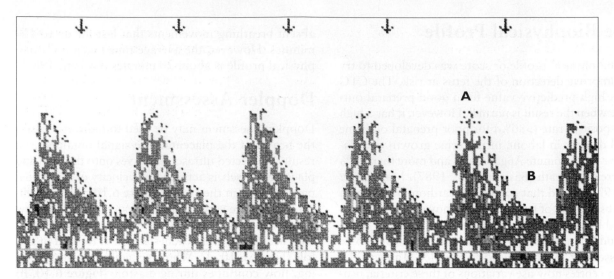

Figure 6.10 Umbilical artery Doppler waveforms where A is the systolic flow, B is the diastolic flow and the resistance index (RI) is given by

RI = (A–B)/A.

ple assessment of the umbilical artery waveform along with other parameters of fetal health is debatable.

Doppler assessment is a useful adjunct to other forms of fetal assessment. For example, a baby that is found to be small for dates warrants a Doppler assessment of the umbilical flow velocity to assess placental health. An abnormal test suggests that the baby is growth retarded due to uteroplacental insufficiency. There is no need to screen low-risk women with regular Doppler assessments, although certain high-risk groups (women with previous growth-retarded babies, systemic lupus erythematosus or antiphospholipid antibody syndrome) may benefit from regular assessment.

Hypoglycaemia may account in part for the very high prevalence of long-term neurological impairment noted during the 1950s in early studies of the postnatal development of small-for-dates infants. The increased incidence of major malformation among the small-for-dates group has already been stressed. Dobson *et al.* (1981) found the rate to be as high as 17% in infants with birth weights less than the 5th percentile. Although data as to the risk of long-term neurological and intellectual handicaps are conflicting, the overall risk is probably increased in small-for-dates babies (Breart and Poisson-Salomon, 1988), especially if growth retardation starts during the second trimester.

The above discussion emphasizes the importance of optimizing antenatal care for the small-for-dates fetus. Clinical management usually follows, to a greater or lesser extent, the sequence:

(1) Detection, by clinical examination, of the fetus as probably small-for-dates.
(2) Confirmation by fetal measurement using diagnostic ultrasound.
(3) Investigation of probable cause, with special attention to fetal abnormality and uteroplacental insufficiency.
(4) Assessment of fetal well-being.
(5) Decision as to the optimal timing and mode of delivery.

Identifying the best time for delivery is based on several pieces of information, including gestational age, the severity of growth retardation, whether or not there is accompanying maternal disease (such as preeclampsia), the results of tests of fetal well-being, past obstetric history, (possibly) the state of fetal lung maturation and the ripeness of the mother's cervix. Individual cases require individual decisions.

It is better to effect planned delivery before severe oligohydramnios occurs, because this may prevent vaginal delivery through severe cord compression during labour. An incompletely resolved question is whether it is better to deliver an apparently healthy small-for-dates baby early because of possible adverse effects on brain development. Ounsted *et al.* (1989) suggest that the prolongation of pregnancy beyond 38 weeks is not associated with an improved long-term developmental prognosis in small-for-dates babies and that this may be positively harmful in some cases (especially when associated with maternal hypertensive conditions). Perhaps Doppler ultrasound studies of cerebral arteries will provide fresh insights and allow greater individualization of management.

The best method of delivery, like timing, depends on a number of factors. The hazards of intrapartum asphyxia have already been discussed. There is evidence that small-for-dates babies tend to tolerate vaginal breech delivery poorly.

Postdates and Postmaturity

'Postdates' and postmaturity are separate entities. The term 'postmaturity syndrome' should be reserved as a description of the affected neonate. Affected neonates occur in only a minority of postdate pregnancies. Although prolonged pregnancy may occur in more than 10% of pregnancies, true postmaturity occurs in about 5%. In true postmaturity there is an increased prenatal mortality, although it is considered safe to allow a pregnancy to progress to 42 weeks' gestation providing there are no other pregnancy complications. At 42 weeks it is acceptable to induce labour, as at this time the risks of induction are less than the risks of leaving the fetus in-utero.

Fetal Anomaly

Women who have had an abnormal baby require extra counselling both after the event and before another pregnancy. The identification of an abnormal fetus in a future pregnancy needs to be discussed at some length, as many of the common fetal anomalies have an increased incidence following an affected pregnancy. In addition, genetic counselling may be appropriate.

Neural Tube Defects (Spina Bifida)

The spinal column begins to develop in early pregnancy from about day 14 to day 25. In most cases this development is successful. However, when the closure of the neural plate fails, then cerebrospinal fluid containing AFP leaks out and quickly crosses over the placenta and into the maternal circulation. The cause of neural tube defects (NTDs) is not yet known, but the abnormality appears to be more predominant in the British Isles, especially Ireland and the northwestern coast of Britain, with a population-based risk of 1/1000. They can have an association with Patau's syndrome (trisomy 13), Edward's syndrome (trisomy 18), triploidy (69 XXX) and others

(**Table 6.5**). Research by the Medical Research Council (1983) suggested that a deprivation of folic acid in the diet may be the cause of the problem. It was suggested that if all women preconception and up to 12 weeks' gestation were given a daily dose of folic acid (400 µg if no risk, 4 mg if history of NTD), then the risk of carrying a baby with spina bifida could be reduced by at least 70%.

Alpha-fetoprotein

Alpha-fetoprotein can be detected at 6 weeks, peaks at 10 weeks, then gradually decreases and levels off at 15 weeks' gestation in the maternal serum. It is initially produced in the embryonic yolk sac in the first trimester; in the second and third trimesters the fetal liver takes over. The optimal time to test the blood is at 16–18 weeks' gestation when levels are stable. Laboratory results are expressed as 'multiples of the median' (MoM). An abnormal result would be greater than 2–3 MoMs, in which case further investigation using a high resolution (level 2) ultrasound scan is required. Hopefully, this would exclude an anomaly and therefore provide the woman with reassurance. However, in some the worst scenario is encountered when the raised AFP is caused by an intrauterine fetal death (IUFD) or spina bifida. In the case of the latter, the architecture of the fetal head may be altered. The cerebellum (normally shaped like a 'dumb-bell' or 'figure of 3') changes and appears 'banana shaped' (**Figure 6.11**). In addition to this, hydrocephaly (**Figure 6.12**) may also be a feature. An accumulation produces a 'lemon-shaped head' (Nicolaides *et al.*). A raised AFP may also be caused by other things (**Table**

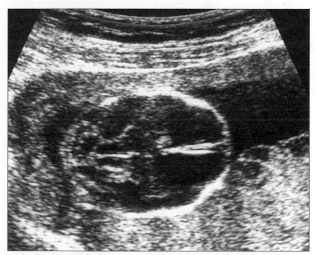

Figure 6.11 Cross-section of fetal skull with a 'banana-shaped' cerebellum.

6.12). If there is insufficient evidence on ultrasonography to confirm or establish why there is an abnormal AFP result that levels of at 15 weeks and there is a strong suspicion of a NTD, then an amniocentesis can be performed to measure acetylcholinesterase (an enzyme produced from fetal neural tissue). The presence of this confirms a defect of the spinal canal, although the resolution of ultrasound equipment in current use should render this unnecessary. Where the AFP level is raised but there is no fetal abnormality, the pregnancy is at higher risk of growth retardation, preterm labour and pre-eclampsia, so therefore careful antenatal surveillance is required. For the important area of informed consent, *see* Smith and Marteau (1995), who discuss serum screening and fetal anomaly scans in connection with informed consent.

Spina bifida occulta

This type of spina bifida occurs in about 10% of fetuses – its presence is caused by failure of the neural arch to fuse. The majority are asymptomatic, will have normal bodily function and do not require surgery. However, in a small minority of cases some infants may have mild urinary or mobility problems. In such cases, there is a dimple, sometimes with hair present on the skin, because of a small defect in the vertebrae which is usually found in the cervical, lumbar or sacral areas of the vertebral column. The spinal cord and nerves are usually normal.

Spina bifida cystica

The cyst-like appearance is due to a herniation of the spinal cord or meninges anywhere along the vertebral column. There are two types, meningocele and myelomeningocele (meningomyelocele).

Myelomeningocele

This is more serious in nature because the spinal cord is damaged, underdeveloped and is present with the nerve roots in the herniated cyst or sac, which also contains the CSF. Depending on the location of the cyst, there s always a degree of neurological damage below the site of the cyst. A cyst present in the lumbar area, for example, results in lower limb paralysis, as well as urinary and bowel incontinence.

Skull and brain malformations

Cranium bifida

This is a serious congenital condition in which there is maldevelopment of the fetal skull and brain (one in every 2000 births). As a result several problems can arise:

- Encephalocele – this is a general term to describe the herniation of brain contents through the fetal skull.
- Meningocele – This is a sac which contains the cerebrospinal fluid (CSF) and meninges. It can be in an open or closed defect.
- Meningoencephalocele – this is a herniation of the meninges and brain through a large portion of the fetal skull.

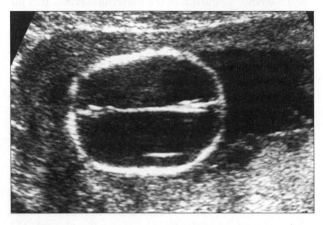

Figure 6.12 Cross-section of fetal skull with hydrocephaly.

Table 6.12 Causes for Raised Alpha-Fetoprotein Levels in Pregnancy
Neural tube defect anencephaly, spina bifida
Abdominal wall defects gastroschisis, exomphalos
Amniotic band disruption
Intra-uterine fetal death miscarriage
Placental problems placenta previa, abruption
Invasive prenatal testing amniocentesis, chorionic villus sampling, cordocentesis
Multiple pregnancy
Miscalculated gestational age
Miscarriage

Anencephaly

Anencephaly is a major intercranial and skull malformation that is not compatible with life. It is four times more common in females than males and has a birth incidence of 1:1000. The cranial vault is absent and the poorly developed fetal brain is exposed. These babies have typical 'gargoyle' features, with bulging eyes and absent forehead. It can be detected on a scan from as early as 12 weeks' gestation and sometimes spina bifida is also be present. If not detected by serum screening, the abnormality is usually found by ultrasonogrpahy. Parents are usually offered termination of pregnancy because of the poor prognosis. If termination is declined, then these babies only survive for a few hours following delivery. Before embarking on another pregnancy, couples should be offered genetic counselling and early ultrasound scans.

Other abnormalities

These are usually discovered in the second trimester, if a women has an anomaly scan.

Head

Choroid plexus cysts

Cerebrospinal fluid (CFS) originates from two glands within the brain, situated in the lateral ventricles. These glands known as the choroid plexus, occasionally contain cysts probably due to the blockage of cellular debris within the cerebrospinal fluid. The cysts can be unilateral, bilateral or multicystic in nature (**Figure 6.13**) and tend to shrink and resolve by 24–26 weeks' gestation. They can have an association with Edward's syndrome. If the cysts are particulary large or other minor markers are identified, then karyotyping can be offered to exlude trisomy; however, this is not the policy in some centres.

Holoprosencephaly

Holoprosencephaly (incidence of 1:5000 live births) is the fusion of the two lateral ventricles, caused by absence of the cavum septum pellucidum. It can be associated with trisomy 13 and other chromosomal abnormalities, can present in different degrees and has a poor prognosis, resulting in either severe mental retardation or fetal death.

Neck

Cystic hygroma

Cystic hygroma (incidence of 1:6000 per live births) presents as a cystic lesion around the fetal neck (**Figure 6.14**), which can extend over the head and chest. It is thought to be due to a defect in the fetal lymphatic system and can be related to Turner's syndrome (karyotype XO). If the lesion occurs very early in the pregnancy then the chances of survival are extremely poor.

Chest

Diaphragmatic hernia

Diaphragmatic hernia (incidence of 1:2000 pregnancies) is caused by a defect or hole in the diaphragm, which then allows the stomach, liver, spleen and intestines to escape into the chest cavity. The fetal lung tissue is denied growth (it can become hypoplastic)

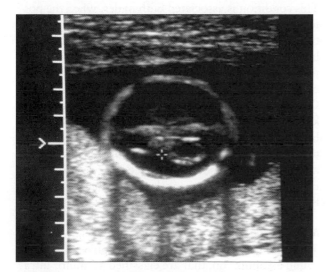

Figure 6.13 A cross-section of the fetal head demonstrating a unilateral choroid plexus cyst within the lateral ventricle of the brain.

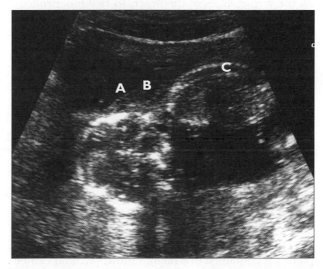

Figure 6.14 Longitudinal section of fetus demonstrating a cystic hygroma at the back of the neck. **A**, skin; **B**, fluid; **C**, spine.

and the heart can be shifted onto the right side of the chest. The prognosis of this condition depends on the severity and size of the hernia.

Heart abnormalities

These can be associated with chromosomal abnormalities, such as Down syndrome and Edward's syndrome, and are usually detected at the 'routine' scan. The chambers, valves and major arteries are examined in a transverse (cross-section) scan to exclude abnormalities. Gaseous exchange occurs within the placenta. However, with a congenital heart defect, transfer of oxygen to the fetal tissues is impaired and can result in heart failure, thus leading to hydrop fetalis.

Hypoplastic left heart

This is a fatal condition in which the left ventricle of the heart is underdeveloped and very small. The baby usually dies a few days after birth.

Fallot's tetralogy

This condition comprises four major defects:
- Ventricular septal defect (hole between the dividing membrane of the heart chambers).
- Narrowing or 'stenosis' of the pulmonary valve.
- Right ventricular hypertrophy.
- Shunting of blood from right to left ventricles.

The abnormal heart causes cyanosis after birth, but corrective surgery is possible.

Transposition of the great vessels

In this condition the pulmonary artery and aorta are on the wrong sides of the heart, so two independent circulations are present. This means that that the baby doesn't receive oxygenated blood to its body because all the blood from the lungs flows to the left side of the heart. After delivery, surgery is performed to correct this.

Abdomen
Exomphalos (omphalocele)

During early fetal development the abdominal gut develops outside the abdomen. In week 10 of embryonic life, the gut contents should return back to the abdominal cavity. When this fails to happen successfully – it becomes an anterior wall defect or exomphalos (1:5000 pregnancies) because herniation of the gut contents occurs within the umbilicus. The exomphalos is contained in a membranous sac, and can be visualized on scan as a mass adjacent to the abdominal wall. Unfortunately it can be associated with other chromosomal defects (e.g. Edward's syndrome),

so karyotyping should be offered. Corrective surgery is performed postdelivery.

Gastroschisis

Gastroschisis (incidence of 1:5000 pregnancies) is similar to exomphalos, except that the abdominal contents are predominantly situated to the right of the umbilical cord and there is no association with chromosomal abnormalities. Because of the exposure of the fetal gut raised levels of AFP may be found in maternal serum. On ultrasonography, loops of bowel are seen floating in the amniotic fluid. The condition is corrected after delivery by surgery – success depends on the size, degree of herniation and condition of the tissue as, occasionally, necrosis of the gut occurs.

Urinary tract abnormalities
Renal agenesis

Oligohydramnios, a reduction in the amount of amniotic fluid, makes ultrasonography diagnosis difficult. A fetus that is curled up and squashed is difficult to examine under these circumstances. If there is difficulty in establishing the cause of the fluid loss, then Hartmann's solution can be infused through a spinal needle into the amniotic cavity to visualize the fetus. If no kidneys or bladder are present then the prognosis is extremely poor. Renal agenesis, or Potter's syndrome (incidence of 1:10,000 births), is caused by failure of the ureteric buds to develop in early embryonic life and is more predominant in male babies.

Posterior urethral valves

This condition is associated with males, when the posterior urethra is obstructed. Urine cannot escape from the bladder, which in turn causes back pressure in the bladder and kidneys. The bladder on ultrasonography is enlarged with a thickened wall and the kidneys can appear hydronephrotic and dysplastic. Oligohydramnios is also present. If there is minimal kidney tissue damage, then the tension of fluid can be relieved by the insertion of a 'pig-tail' catheter into the fetal bladder. This invasive technique, also known as vesicoamniotic 'shunting', is a conservative method until neonatal surgery can be performed to correct the defect.

Minor Markers

There are specific abnormalities, recognised on ultrasound examination, that are classified as 'minor ultrasound markers'. Without chromosomal or genetic association, they do not cause any harm in the fetal or neonatal period. They are simply a variation from the normal, the majority of which turn out to have no relevance. If, however, several are present, then it is likely that there is a problem of a more serious nature. It is then necessary to carry out invasive prenatal testing. If results demonstrate a fetus with a chromosomal abnormality, then the 'marker' is obviously part of that syndrome. Examples of this are choroid plexus cysts, mild renal pelvis dilatation and talipes of the feet. It is important to realize that much stress and anxiety will be present upon diagnosis; this may cause unnecessary worry if the abnormality is found not to be serious.

Concluding Remarks

All health-care professionals and some lay organizations participate in screening programmes for pregnant women and their families. However, the midwife as a member of a National Health surveillance screening team has a major role in screening for the potential health or illhealth of pregnant women and their families.

Their role as supporters, observers, advisors and informers in distinguishing between normality and abnormality is vital. So too is their role in executing and facilitating effective screening programmes in a multiprofessional team.

Although the medical staff mainly deal with diagnosis and prescribing treatment, they also have the responsibilities outlined within the role of the midwife. All have a responsibility to the women in their care and all must be involved in any decisions made with regard to screening – its purpose, acceptability and implications. The choice as to what to do ultimately must rest with the parents, supported by the professionals in whatever they decide.

KEY CONCEPTS

- It is important to remember that although screening tests are available, women may choose to decline them. For women who embark upon prenatal screening, access to information about the test should be made available and easily understood.

- Midwives should ideally possess the ability to impart medical information and perform non-directive counselling to couples, so that they are able to make informed decisions. The cultural, spirital and ethical beliefs of women/families should be taken into consideration

- Effective communication is the key to providing continuity of care for couples trying to make decisions regarding prenatal testing or waiting for test results. Midwives should act as a liaison between prospective parents and medical staff to provide this service. An unhurried and sympathetic manner should help couples come to terms during an emotional and stressful time.

References

Baillie P: Non-hormonal methods of antenatal monitoring, *Clinics in Obstetrics and Gynaecology* 1:103–123, 1974.

Baskett TF, Sandy EA: The oxytocin challenge test and antepartum fetal assessment, *Br J Obstet Gynaecol* 84:39–43, 1977.

Baskett TF, Allen AC, Gray JH, *et al*: Fetal biophysical profile and perinatal death, *Obstetrics and Gynecology* 70:357–60, 1987.

Baskett TF: The biophysical profile. In: *Obstetrics and Gynaecology*, 7:145–59, Edinburgh, 1989, Churchill Livingstone.

Belizan JM, Lillar J J, Nardin JC, *et al*: Diagnosis of IUGR by a simple clinical method: Measurement of fundal height, *Am J Obstet Gynecol* 131:634–64, 1978.

Bogart MH, Pandian MR, Jones OW: Abnormal maternal serum chorionic gonadotrophin levels in pregnancies with fetal chromosome abnormalities. *Prenatal Diagnosis* 7:623–30, 1987.

Breart G, Poisson-Salomon AS: Intrauterine growth retardation and mental handicap epidemiological evidence, *Ballieres Clinical Obstet Gynaecol* 2:91–100, 1988.

Canadian Collaborative CVS –Amniocentesis Clinical Trial Group: Multicentre randomised clinical trial of chorion villus sampling and amniocentesis: First report, *Lancet* i:1–6, 1989.

Cullen MT, Hobbins JC: Transvaginal ultrasound in early prenatal diagnosis. In: Neilson JP, Chambers SE, Obstetric Ultrasound, vol. 1:19–40, Oxford, 1993, Oxford University Press.

Department of Health: *The health of the nation*, London, 1992, HMSO.

Department of Health: *Changing childbirth*, London, 1993, HMSO.

Department of Health press release: *New national screening committee*, 17th July 1996.

Dobson PC, Abell DA, Beischer NA: Mortality and morbidity of fetal growth retardation, *Australian and New Zealand J Obstet Gynaecol* 21:69–72, 1981.

Donai D: The management of the patient having fetal diagnosis, *Balliere's Clinical Obstetric and Gynaecology* 1:737–45, 1987.

Elder MG, Burton ER, Gordon H, *et al*: Maternal weight and girth changes in late pregnancy and the diagnosis of placental insufficiency. *J Obset Gynaecol Brit Commonwealth* 77:481–91, 1970.

Fairgrieve S: Screening for Down's syndrome: What women think. *British Journal Midwifery* 5(3):148–51.

Firth HV, Boyd PA, Chamberlain IZ, *et al*.: Severe limb abnormalities after chorion villus sampling at 56–66 days gestation. *Lancet* 337:762–3, 1991.

Fletcher NR, Hicks JD, Kay JDS, *et al*.: Using decision analysis to compare policy for antenatal screening, *Br Med J* 311:351–56, 1995.

Freeman RK, Anderson G, Dorchester W: A prospective multi-institutional study of antepartum fetal heart rate monitoring. Risk of perinatal mortality and morbidity according to antepartum fetal heart rate test results, *Am J Obstet Gynecol* 143:771–77, 1982.

Green J, Statham H: Testing for fetal abnormality in routine antenatal care, *Midwifery* 9:124, 1993.

Hall M, Chng PK, MacGillivray I: Is routine antenatal care worthwhile?, *Lancet* 2:78–80, 1980.

Hammacker K, Huter KA, Bokelmann J, *et al*: Foetal heart frequency and perinatal condition of the fetus and newborn, *Gynaecologia* 166:349–60, 1968.

Joint Study Group on Fetal Abnormalities: Recognition and management of fetal abnormalities, *Arch Dis Childhood* 64:971–6, 1989.

Lavery JP: Non-stress fetal heart rate testing, *Clinical Obstetrics and Gynecology* 25:689–98, 1982.

Long L: Folic acid campaign by the Health Education Authority, *Br J Midwifery* 4(1), 1996.

Manning FA, Platt LD, Sipos L, *et al*: Fetal breathing movements and the nonstress test in high-risk pregnancies, *Am J Obstet Gynecol* 135:511–15, 1979.

Manning FA, Platt LD, Sipos L: Antepartum fetal evaluation: Development of a fetal biophysical profile, *Am J Obstet Gynecol* 136:787–95, 1980.

Mcllwaint GM, Howart RCL, Dunn F: The Scottish perinatal mortality survey, *BMJ* 11n3–n6, 1979.

Nicolaides KHS, Gabbe G, Campbell S, *et al*.: Ultrasound screening for Spina bifida: Cranial and cerebellar signs, *Lancet* ii:72–4, 1986.

Oh W: Considerations in neonates with intrauterine growth retardation, *Clinical Obstet Gynecol* 20:991–1003, 1977.

Ounsted M: Concepts and criteria of fetal growth. In: *Abnormal Fetal Growth: Biological Bases and Consequences* (Naftolin F, editor), 21–48, Berlin, 1978, Dahlem Konferenzen.

Proud J, Murphy–Black, T: Choice of a scan: How much information do women recieve before ultrasound, *Br J Midwifery* 5(3):144–7, 1997.

Royal College of Physicians report: *Prenatal diagnosis and genetic screening, community and service implications*, p 52, 1989.

Rhodes PA: *A short history of clinical midwifery*, Haigh and Hochland, 1995, Royal College of Midwives.

Rottem S, Bronshtein M, Thaler I, *et al*.: First trimester transvaginal diagnosis of fetal abnormalities, *Lancet* 1:445–6, 1989.

Rosenberg K, Grant JM, Hepburn M: Antenatal detection of growth retardation: Actual practice in a large matenity hospital, *Br J Obstet Gynaecol*, 89:12–15, 1982.

Rosenberg K, Grant JM, Weedie I, *et al*: Measurement of fundal height as a screening test for fetal growth retardation *Br J Obstet Gynaecol* 89:447–50, 1982.

Smith DK, Marteau TM: Detecting a fetal abnormality: serum screening and fetal anomaly scans, *Br J Midwifery* 3(3):133, 1995.

Tabor A, Masden M, Obel EB: Randomised controlled trial of genetic amniocentesis in 4606 low risk women, Lancet ii:1287–93, 1986.

Wald NJ, Cuckle HS, Densem JW, *et al*.: Maternal serum screening for Down's syndrome in early pregnancy. *BMJ* 297–887, 1988.

Wald NJ: *Antenatal and neonatal screening*, Oxford, 1994, Oxford University Press.

Whitfield CR, Smith NC, Cockburn F, *et al*: Perinatally related wastage – a proposed classification of primary obstetric factors, *Br J Obstet Gynaecol* 93:694–703, 1986.

Further Reading

Alexander J, Levy V, Roch S: *Midwifery practice: care topics 1*, 1996, Macmillan.
The focus of this book is on the organization and delivery of antenatal care including preconceptive care and antenatal risk assessment.

Kingston HM: *ABC of clinical genetics*. 2nd edition. London, 1990, British Medical Association.
Helpful, and in-depth understanding of basic clinical genetics which can be used by midwives for counselling.

MIDRIS: Informed choice leaflet 3: Ultrasound scans and 10: Down's syndrome and 4: Spina bifida. Obtainable from MIDRIS, 9 Elmdale Road, Clifton, Bristol BS8 I5.
Based on best available evidence, the leaflets come in pairs, one for women and one for professionals for each topic.

Proud J: *Understanding obstetric ultrasound*, Books for Midwives Press, 1994, Haigh and Hochland.
Clear, concise enjoyable read for midwives who need to know more about ultrasound and prenatal diagnosis.

SAFTA: *Support after termination for fetal abnormality*, 1990, Good News Press.
Informative insight and useful companion about what couples will face when embarking upon a termination for a fetal abnormality. Extremely useful for health care professionals.

Singleton J, McClaren S: *Ethical foundations of health care: responsibilities in decision making*, London, 1995, Mosby.
This book discusses the ethical implications of professional decision making.

7 Women with Special Needs

LEARNING OUTCOMES

After studying this chapter you should be able to:
- Identify the nature and origin of special needs.
- Compare and contrast the range of special needs and discuss the problems faced by pregnant women in these situations.
- Review policy and organizational changes and their relationship to special needs.
- Critically discuss the implications of special needs for midwifery practice.

All continuing, wanted pregnancies are special to the women concerned. Much of social science's contribution to the understanding of reproduction has focused on the experience and needs of women at low risk during pregnancy and birth. It has further emphasized the importance of community rather then hospital sources of care. In this chapter, the needs of women whose circumstances may vary from the familiar patterns of pregnancy and birth are addressed.

First, the changing context of maternity care is considered and the origins of a woman-centred approach to maternity care are reviewed. In so doing, attention is drawn to assumptions about women's circumstances, lives and experiences that underlie this approach.

The nature of special needs are then examined by posing a number of questions:
- What are special needs?
- Who defines special need?
- What issues and challenges do women with special needs present to midwives working within a women-centred approach?
- How can women who require care which is in some way different have their need identified and met?
- Does the organization of maternity care allow for meeting such needs?
- What happens when a midwife encounters needs which are unfamiliar to her?

These questions are designed to encourage the reader to think about the kinds of issues which underlie special needs care.

The experience and context of a broad range of special needs are then explored. Illness pre-dating or arising during pregnancy can present women and their midwives with particular problems. The health and well-being of the fetus or baby may raise other problems. Women vary in their cultural needs. Access to services may be difficult for those who live in a rural area or who live a travelling lifestyle. All women need good communication during pregnancy and birth, so women with hearing or speech difficulties face especial problems, as do those with language differences. Women who live in an institutional setting, such as prison or psychiatric hospital, are particularly constrained in their lives. Multiple pregnancy poses a number of social difficulties in addition to the obstetric implications. Finally, the implications of a history of trauma and of pregnancy or perinatal loss are considered; such experiences require sensitive care not only when they occur, but also in the months and years that follow.

The Changing Context of Maternity Care

The woman-centred approach to midwifery care has developed during a period of change in the maternity services. Dissatisfaction with the maternity services has a long history, as Garcia (1982) pointed out. Much of this was concerned with the place and circumstances of birth rather than what Reid and McIlwaine (1980) described at that time as the 'less fashionable period of pregnancy'. In the 1980s, however, a number of studies concentrated on antenatal care. Consumer opinion of the maternity services was given voice not only in academic surveys, but also through studies undertaken by Community Health Councils and through press and media coverage.

Reid and McIlwaine (1980) drew attention to the shift in emphasis from studies which took the perspective of the providers of services to those which explored the views and experiences of the users or recipients. Early studies from the providers' perspective investigated women's apparent underuse of the services (e.g. Robinson and Carr, 1970) or the circumstances of women who attended too late or infrequently for care (e.g. Mackinlay, 1970, 1972). The shift of emphasis opened up a number of key themes important to the development of a woman-centred approach to midwifery care. Studies which set out to explore women's experiences of care provided a very different picture (e.g. Oakley 1979; Graham and McKee, 1979; Macintyre, 1981). The increasing medicalization of pregnancy and birth, the inconvenient location of care and the impersonal atmosphere of clinics were familiar themes. Other work compared and contrasted user and provider perspectives (e.g. Graham and Oakley, 1981).

A number of innovations in care were introduced and evaluated. Several key themes of these are present either in the current service organization or in the policy changes which herald further reorganization. The innovations largely focused on the location and organization of care, including clarification of the roles of the various practitioners and the aims and efficiency of care. Most schemes involved some change in the location of care, particularly of a move from hospital-based to community-based care. Other schemes explored integration of hospital obstetricians with community midwives and general practitioners (GPs) in community clinics. The basis of the number of visits a woman is required to make during pregnancy was investigated and in some instances rationalized when duplicated or inefficient care was revealed. Women were encouraged to take charge of their own obstetric records during pregnancy.

A central point identified by the research on women's perspectives was that for many women pregnancy and birth are normal processes experienced within the everyday social context of their lives. The innovations in care began to acknowledge some elements of this, particularly in the relocation of care to the community and in the recognition of the role of the midwife in the provision of care. The emphasis on women at low risk during pregnancy overlooked other women's less happy circumstances. Women who suffer illness during pregnancy, or whose social circumstances differ from the norms of the community around them, or who suffer pregnancy or perinatal loss or the extraordinary experience of multiple pregnancy do not necessarily have their needs met by such a system. Although hospital-based care has, of course, continued to be provided, there has been less recognition within the literature of the variety of circumstances of women with special needs.

Identifying Special Needs

Special needs in maternity care can be divided into four groups. First, needs that arise as a result of illhealth or an ongoing condition or disability and that require some form of specialist attention in addition to the familiar regime of care. Second, sets of social and cultural conditions which vary from those of most pregnant women, for example women who are very young or are considered old for pregnancy, and those who are homeless or in prison. Third, some women's actual experience of pregnancy and birth may differ in ways which require additional or different forms of care and support from the carers, for example in pregnancy loss or where there are ambiguous feelings about the pregnancy. Fourth, some women's needs may vary from those of the local population and hence be seen as 'special' by those who provide care, for example when cultural or ethnic needs are different. 'Specialness' may therefore be inherent in the situation and experience of the pregnant woman, be part of the health professionals' perceptions of unfamiliar needs, or be perceived by both the woman and carers.

Special needs imply special care – care which is in some way different from, or additional to, that which is regularly or routinely provided. Specialized care may, of course, be an exciting professional challenge where skills are tested to the full and beyond. But clients and patients who require something different may be seen in a very different light – as making extra work, as a disruption to the routine practice and organization of care. They may be seen as 'difficult' rather than 'special'.

An important aspect of the perception of women with special needs is the attribution of responsibility. Throughout the process of reproduction, women are expected to act responsibly, with planning and forethought. Pregnancies are expected to be planned, regardless of the fallibility of contraceptive methods, the frailty of support from partners or the complexity of making such decisions. During pregnancy, women are given much advice about health behaviour, such as smoking, diet and exercise. Motherhood brings responsibility for care of the baby. Women who have special needs prior to or during pregnancy or birth may be treated as if they were themselves at fault for the situation. Women who, for example, become pregnant at an inadvisable time of life or in disadvantageous circumstances may be regarded as being the problem rather than as having problems.

What are the implications for midwifery practice? In the provision of woman-centred care it might be supposed that all needs are identified and responded to on an individual basis. However, midwives are not free of the norms and values of the social and cultural situations within which they practice, and organization of care implies at least a framework for practice, even if this is delivered in a personal and individual manner. It is important, therefore, that midwives acknowledge the various responses which special needs evoke:

- Why do some conditions elicit sympathy but not others?
- What is the basis of distinctions between 'deserving' and 'less deserving' clients and patients, between the culpable and the innocent?

Categories of Special Needs

The development of a woman-centred approach to maternity care has taken place at the same time as other developments, such as the move away from hospital-based care. There is now an emphasis on pregnancy being a normal, healthy state rather than one bordering on illness. The limitations of the medical model of reproduction have become apparent as the importance of the social context of a woman's experience of pregnancy and birth have been recognized. Much of the midwifery enterprise in recent years has been a claiming back of maternity care as a community-based activity, with the implication that hospital-based care will then be available in less crowded conditions for those women who require specialist obstetric advice throughout pregnancy. Much of the social science literature addresses similar issues; however, there have been very few studies of the experiences of women who have complications of pregnancy or are ill before or during pregnancy.

Illness

The experience of women who either develop an illness or condition during pregnancy or whose illness or condition pre-dates the pregnancy are considered in this section. The implications for care at preconception, antenatal, intrapartum and postpartum stages are discussed.

For women who live with a chronic illness or condition, the process of family planning is additionally complex. For some conditions, for example diabetes, much research and experience of delivery care has contributed to professional knowledge about the effects of the condition on the progress of pregnancy and birth, and the effects of pregnancy on the condition. A set of routines have therefore developed to guide maternity care. The implications of pregnancy, and the need to make alterations to aspects of the diabetic regime before conception, are likely to have been addressed during visits to the diabetic clinic. Thus women report that pregnancy is often raised by their diabetic clinic well before they consider pregnancy for themselves (Thomas, 1997). When diabetic women want to become pregnant further control of the blood sugar level is required. Women report that the experience can be frustrating. They are required to achieve different targets from their usual diabetic regime, and they are also waiting for 'official' permission to become pregnant. Although other couples make decisions based on their circumstances and intentions, women with diabetes have to make professionally sanctioned changes to their bodies before embarking on pregnancy.

Other conditions may raise the issue of whether pregnancy is at all advisable. Women with multiple sclerosis (MS), for example, receive differing advice from their specialists according to the nature and severity of their symptoms and the opinion of their consultant. Women who engage in such complex decision-making may later find a doctor or midwife who questions the wisdom of the decision and assumes that little or no thought has preceded the conception.

Problems which arise during pregnancy present other issues for women and for their carers. At one level this is precisely what antenatal care is intended to achieve – the identification and diagnosis of health problems. There may be a disjuncture between feelings of illness experienced and the perception of the specialists about the risks to mother and baby. The diagnosis of problems when a woman has experienced no symptoms of illhealth is likely to be a shock – for example, for women who develop gestational diabetes. There may be implications for care during pregnancy, including insulin injections if necessary, for delivery of the baby, and for the woman's future. In this situation the pregnant woman has to come to terms with the diagnosis of a possibly recurring chronic illness. In contrast, a woman who experiences hyperemesis (continuous sickness during pregnancy) may feel very ill, but not attract much attention from her carers unless dehydration is severe and she requires hospitalization. In addition, she may not receive much sympathy from family and friends if she is perceived as having the more normal 'morning sickness', which many women experience.

During pregnancy, women may experience a loss of control over conditions that seemed to be well-controlled before pregnancy. In diabetes women may find it difficult to establish a pattern of control over their blood sugar. Women who have controlled epilepsy with drug treatment may experience convulsive attacks during pregnancy. In contrast, many women who usually follow a healthy diet as part of their condition need to make few or no changes during pregnancy.

Women's experiences of labour and delivery in the context of illness or other health problems raise a number of issues. Carers may have particular routines which they follow for certain conditions which may be at odds with the level and exercise of control to which the women and their partners are accustomed. Women with diabetes who are used to testing their own blood and acting accordingly and whose partners have many years of close observation-based experience of the symptoms may find the routines at birth do not run in accordance with their understanding. Where a condition is relatively rare or where its progress is unpredictable, for example in MS, there may be no routines in place.

Postnatal care may not provide enough support for women with an ongoing illness once the main event of the birth is over. Women with diabetes may feel that they are given insufficient help in re-establishing their diabetic control. The exhaustion of birth may compromise the health of women with MS. In contrast, women with hyperemesis often report that the symptoms vanish at the delivery.

Illness during pregnancy has implications for midwives in both the community and the hospital. Where a condition is common a midwife may have gained experience of providing care. Rare conditions require more specialist attention. Good communication between the relevant carers is important, especially where this involves specialists from different departments.

Disability

Women with disabilities face particular problems with pregnancy and childbearing in addition to those they face in their everyday lives (Maternity Alliance, 1996). The concept of disability includes the social consequences of a loss of function in the body, be this caused by disease or loss of a bodily part. It can be argued that the social consequences are the results of a disabling society – a society that is physically and socially designed for the able-bodied discriminates against those who are not able-bodied. For example, sharp edged pavements, bank money dispensers placed too high in the wall and public toilets situated at the top or bottom of flights of stairs all discriminate against people who use wheelchairs.

Mothers with physical or learning disabilities may be subject to the charge of irresponsibility for becoming pregnant. They may be seen as selfish for wanting children: are they able to be fit and proper parents? Many women with disabilities argue that they are as entitled to have children as others, that the effects of their disabilities could be lessened with appropriate help and that apparently able-bodied parents may have other, less identifiable shortcomings.

An essential part of woman-centred midwifery care is good communication. Women need to be able to express their experiences and thoughts about pregnancy and birth, and need clear, appropriate information from their carers. Women with hearing or speech difficulties need services which can circumvent or lessen the effects of these problems.

Women who care for others with disabilities also require particular consideration during pregnancy, birth and the postnatal period. Women who provide the main source of care for a partner or a child with disabilities may find it difficult to attend clinic visits and may require additional help at home if they deliver and stay in hospital.

The maternity alliance has raised these issues in a compilation of the reports from the Disability Working Groups (Maternity Alliance, compiled 1994).

The pack consists of :
• A survey of disabled mother's experiences entitled 'Mother's pride and others prejudice.'
• A charter for disabled parents and parents to be called 'Listen to us for a change.'
• The report of a conference: 'Disabled people, pregnancy and early parenthood.'

Cultural Needs

The processes of pregnancy and birth are deeply social and cultural. All societies mark such transitions in distinct ways. In a multicultural society, maternity services have to identify and meet a variety of social and cultural expectations. Ignorance of cultural needs, shortage of funding and unimaginative organization of existing services can all contribute to difficulties for women who receive care.

Although cultural expectations and practices may differ between groups, midwives (in common with other health-care practitioners) need to develop professional expertise in relating theoretical knowledge to the practical, clinical encounters with women in their care. An individual woman's needs cannot be 'read off' or assumed from the carers' knowledge of cultural differences. This poses a number of problems for the midwife. While she must be alert to possible differences, she must also be sensitive to the life experiences of each individual woman. Not all members of social groups follow the practices of those groups. Assumptions such as 'working-class women think this ...' or 'Punjabi women do that ...' may amount to discriminatory rather than sensitive practice.

Unfamiliar cultural needs provide a professional challenge to the midwife. In a district where a variety of cultural practices exist and where midwifery colleagues have a good working knowledge of these variations a midwife has many opportunities to improve and extend her own knowledge. She will become more experienced by meeting women from different groups and learning what support and advice they find useful and acceptable. She also has the collective experience of her colleagues on which to draw. Where cultural variation is more rare, it is important that a woman's needs are identified and met without this being seen as making additional and unwelcome demands on the midwife's time.

Access to Services

Recent innovations and reorganizations in the maternity services have recognized the importance of providing care in convenient locations. Districts may aim to make services more convenient for more women, but the needs of women for whom the schedule and location of services are not convenient need to be borne in mind. Bus fares and inconvenient transport services may make attendance difficult for women with few resources. Time may also be a factor. Women are entitled to time off work to attend antenatal care, but where a woman is employed in an unofficial capacity, perhaps on short-time work, she may have little redress against her employer.

Rural populations require different arrangements. Where the midwife's caseload is scattered over a wide area the women under her care may face long journeys to attend clinics. Similarly, the midwife may travel considerable distances to meet the women in their own homes. Telephone contact can be very valuable in these circumstances. Use of an air ambulance may be necessary for transport to hospital if complications arise or labour progresses more swiftly than expected. Travelling communities face different problems. Where a family or group are not settled in one place women need a variety of forms of contact with midwifery care. As travellers are often the subject of discrimination and consequently mistrust the services provided for members of (more) settled populations, midwifery care needs to be planned with the needs of this group in mind – for example, domiciliary care may be accepted.

Age of Mother

When pregnancy and motherhood occur at young or mature ages relative to the majority of the population this is often considered to be problematic. Women in these circumstances are often considered to be irresponsible. The obstetric and social implications of pregnancy and giving birth at young or older ages are diametrically opposed. Young mothers find the social disadvantages of their pregnancies emphasized while the obstetric advantages and other health benefits are overlooked. Mature women face the opposite – obstetric and paediatric problems are emphasized, yet the benefits of mature parenthood are not well-addressed.

Teenage pregnancy is usually portrayed in a negative light, but Phoenix (1991) argues that the literature contains some contradictions. Although teenage pregnancy is said to be associated with poor perinatal outcomes, welfare dependence of mothers and poor educational outcomes for mothers and children, other work indicates that there has been on overemphasis on the impact of teenage motherhood. Phoenix argues that teenage mothers are seen in a negative light because attention is focused on age rather than on the socioeconomic circumstances of the mothers. Teenage women become pregnant for a variety of reasons, as do other women. Many do not consider that their chances of employment are high; also, in communities where it is common for members of the peer group to have children in their teens, women may feel old to be having a baby at 18 or 19 years of age.

It is only recently that later motherhood has become unusual. When families were large births sometimes spanned a generation (Berryman, 1991). Later pregnancy may occur in a number of circumstances. For example, a woman may have her final baby when over 40 years old, or may begin motherhood at this age. Where divorce and remarriage occur a second family may be conceived at a later age. More dramatic, but rare, is the issue of postmenopausal

infertility treatment in women of age 50–60 years and beyond. Clearly, there are increased risks to the health of the mother and baby, although these may different for women of different parity, but overemphasis of these does not help the mother.

Institutional Settings

A key feature of woman-centred care is the importance given to understanding a woman's needs within her social context. Community midwives have long established the importance of visiting a woman at home, where she is likely to be more relaxed. Some women spend some or all of their pregnancies within an institutional setting, not in their own home. Such settings include prisons, hospitals and residential care (for example for people with learning disabilities). For some women admission to hospital during the antenatal period is occasioned by a problem with pregnancy itself and time is spent on an antenatal ward. Each of the settings restricts a woman's freedom, to varying extents, of movement within and outside the building, of choice of when to eat and sleep, and of contact and intimacy with family and friends. Visiting hours in maternity and general hospitals are now somewhat relaxed, but access to long-stay psychiatric hospitals is usually more restricted.

Although the overall pattern of antenatal care is now to devolve care from the hospital to the community, a countertrend can be observed in the rising rates of hospital admission during pregnancy (Kirk, 1994). Kirk reported that women were anxious about their partners' and children's welfare. Most were happy about their pregnancies, but some expressed negative feelings about the baby and the need for hospitalization together with feelings of low self-esteem. They did not receive as much information as they required. Many of the women experienced boredom. Women who smoked increased their smoking while in hospital. Lack of privacy when partners and family visited was identified as a particular problem. Kirk (1994) concluded that institutional aspects of hospitalization could be decreased, for example, by encouraging women to wear day clothes, and by providing facilities for making drinks and snacks. However, the rising rates of admission should also be examined critically; attention needs to be paid to whether women could receive the necessary care at home rather than in a hospital setting.

Women prisoners face additional problems – deprivation of liberty is a central and intended feature of the custodial sentence. Remand prisoners, awaiting trial and therefore legally still innocent of the charges laid, may spend lengthy periods in prison. In a review of services for pregnant women prisoners, Wilson (1993) revealed a variety of provision. Antenatal and postnatal care are given, together with antenatal classes; women are usually transferred to the nearest hospital to give birth. As many of the prison population are from disadvantaged backgrounds some women's health improves with regular meals and sleep. However, they face childbirth without the support of family and friends. Some prisons have mother and baby units that provide facilities up to a specified age of the baby (varying between 9 and 18 months). If the length of the sentence goes beyond that age, the date of separation from the child is at the discretion of the prison governor. However, a woman who is deemed unlikely to be able to care for the child after release (for example, if her existing children are all in care or she is physically or mentally ill), is not permitted to keep her child in prison. Enforced separation in such circumstances is unlikely to be helpful when a mother suffers from postnatal depression.

Multiple Pregnancy

The conventional media image of a multiple birth is of a number of healthy babies of the same size, perhaps identical in some cases. The reality is often very different. Multiple pregnancy places a greater physical strain on the mother than does a singleton pregnancy. Complications are more common and women are more likely to be admitted to hospital during the pregnancy. For a large-scale study of triplets and higher order births, included obstetric data and surveys of the views of parents, health professionals and personal social service providers, *see* Botting *et al.* 1990).

Triplets and higher-order births are more likely to be conceived following infertility treatment – 55% of quadruplet and 31% of triplet pregnancies followed some form of infertility investigation compared with 7% of twins and 3% of singletons. Parents of babies from higher order births found themselves accountable for their later difficulties when it was known by relatives and friends that infertility treatment had been obtained. Diagnosis of multiple pregnancy was usually made through ultrasonography – 100% of quadruplets, 97% of triplets and 91% of twin pregnancies were diagnosed in this way. However, the actual number of babies present was not always known until delivery. The importance of good communication at the time of ultrasonography is particularly marked when a multiple pregnancy is detected – this may be the first indication that more than one fetus is present.

Botting *et al.* (1990) point out that multiple birth is not only momentous for the parents, but is also fairly unusual for most hospital staff. There may therefore be many staff present to watch the delivery, in addition to the obstetric and paediatric teams involved in the birth. When women are under general anaesthesia or when the babies are immediately transferred to special care baby unit (SCBU) the provision of photographs may be especially appreciated.

Mothers who experience problems with their own health are not best placed to begin the considerable task of caring for their babies. Not all babies survive the birth and some have congenital or other health problems that are diagnosed at birth. Not all surviving babies are well and fit for discharge from hospital at the same time. Discharge policies vary, but the difficulty faced by parents who care for one small baby or more at home and attempt to visit the other baby or babies in hospital sometimes leads to earlier discharge of the remaining infants than would be usual. Parents of higher order births need additional help at home to care for their babies. Advice and the opportunity to talk through the strategy during the antenatal period is helpful as is the identification of a key professional, such as a health visitor, to coordinate the services required. Multiple births are relatively rare events and social services need to use their resources imaginatively to provide assistance.

Pregnancy and Perinatal Loss

Not all continuing pregnancies result in the birth of a live baby who thrives. Loss is important not only at the time of its occurrence but also in any subsequent pregnancy. Spontaneous loss may occur at any time during pregnancy. The availability of pregnancy testing kits that can confirm early pregnancy has contributed to the experience of loss. Women who might otherwise have experienced a 'late, heavy period' may, if they have had a positive pregnancy test, experience this as an early miscarriage.

It is often assumed that the depth and impact of loss can be predicted from the gestation of the pregnancy – that the early death of a baby born alive would be more upsetting for the parents than a stillbirth or late miscarriage and that early miscarriage is in turn a lesser loss than these. Lovell (1983) termed this the 'hierarchy of sadness' and suggested that the experience of pregnant women and their partners may be different. For example when a baby has lived, if only for a short time, there is a life to be remembered. Where death precedes birth it is more difficult to understand the nature of the 'life'. Early miscarriage may pose greater problems for the woman, who may feel there was little evidence of pregnancy apart, perhaps, for the experience of morning sickness. The attachment that women feel to the fetus may vary greatly at similar gestational ages – a model that incorporates attachment and loss has been proposed (Moulder, 1994).

Termination for fetal abnormality presents women, their partners and the carers with complex and difficult problems. The setting in which care is given may affect the way in which the loss is experienced. For example, where provision is made in a maternity ward the abnormal nature of the loss may be underlined for parents and staff alike.

Loss is likely to have long-term consequences, although there appears to be no straightforward association between psychological status after miscarriage and the experience and outcome of subsequent pregnancy (Garel *et al.* 1994). The experience of live birth following stillbirth requires particularly sensitive care from all staff (Hense, 1994). During the subsequent pregnancy a woman may feel guilt about the previous loss and anxious that it may happen again. She is likely to experience residual grief from the previous loss and may find a fusion between the two pregnancies. Some women may resist attachment to the new pregnancy. There are often feelings of relief when the new baby is born.

There are several implications for midwives in the delivery of care. First it is important that sensitive care should be provided at the time of any loss and that a mother's feelings should be listened to, not assumed. Second, there are important implications for care during subsequent pregnancies during which the previous loss should be acknowledged together with the difficulty and ambiguity that this can raise for the mother in the current pregnancy. Third, midwives need to recognize their own feelings and needs at these traumatic times. The setting within which a midwife is expected to provide care may be far from ideal. It is important to recognize this – midwives can easily feel their professional skills are undermined and hence that they are not providing appropriate support for the women in their care (*see* Chapter 8).

Conclusion

In this chapter the nature and origins of special needs are considered. In the provision of woman-centred care, 'meeting' the needs of individual women is paramount. However, all services need a framework to underpin individual practice. There may therefore still be tensions between routine and personalized care. Being seen as special may bring its own problems. Women who are the subject of research interest may find that the services take a particular interest in the progress and outcome of their pregnancies, which may be of benefit when staff are skilled in communication. Alternatively, women can feel special but depersonalized as the interest centres on the progress and outcomes of the research rather than her experience. Finally, it is important to note that identifying and providing care for women with special needs should be the basis for individual care not for discrimination against groups due to assumptions about the nature and meaning of the differences.

KEY CONCEPTS

- Recent policy changes have emphasized the needs of women at low risk during pregnancy.

- Special needs may arise from illness or disability of the women, the social circumstances of the woman, the woman's experience of pregnancy and birth, and needs or circumstances which are unfamiliar to the midwife.

- Specialness may therefore be inherent in the situation and experience of the pregnant women or be part of the health professionals' perceptions of unfamiliar needs, or be perceived by both women and carers.

- Clients or patients who require different or additional care may be seen as difficult rather than special – as being a problem rather than as having problems.

- Women who have rare conditions may be the focus of research interest, which can result in impersonal care.

- Good communication between all practitioners involved and the women who receive care is especially important for women with special needs.

References

Berryman J: Perspectives on later motherhood. In Phoenix A, Woollett A, Lloyd E, editors: *Motherhood: meanings, practices and ideologies*, London, 1991, Sage.

Botting BJ, Macfarlane AJ, Price FV, editors: *Three, four and more: a study of triplet and higher order births*, London 1990, HMSO.

Garcia J: Women's views of antenatal care. In Enkin M, Chalmers I, editors: *Effectiveness and satisfaction in antenatal care*, London, 1982 Heinemann Medical.

Garel M, Blondel B, Lelong N, Bonefant S, Kaminski M: Long-term consequences of miscarriage: the depressive disorders following pregnancy, *J Reprod Infant Psychol* 12:233, 1994.

Graham H, McKee L: *The first months of motherhood*, London, 1979, Health Education Council.

Graham H, Oakley A: Competing ideologies of reproduction: medical and maternal perspectives on pregnancy. In Roberts H, editor: *Women, health and reproduction*, London, 1981, RKP.

Hense AL: Livebirth following stillbirth. In Field PA, Marck PA: *Uncertain motherhood: negotiating the risks of the childbearing years*, Thousand Oaks, 1994, Sage.

Kirk SA: The needs of women hospitalised in pregnancy. In Robinson S, Thompson AM: *Midwives, research and childbirth*, Vol. 3, London, 1994, Chapman & Hall.

Lovell A: Some questions of identity: late miscarriage, stillbirth and perinatal loss, *Soc Sci Med* 17(11):755, 1983.

Macintyre S: *Expectations and experiences of first pregnancy*, Occasional paper No 5, Aberdeen, 1981, Institute of Medical Sociology, University of Aberdeen.

Mackinlay JB: A brief description of a study on the utilisation of maternity and child welfare services by a lower working class subculture, *Soc Sci Med*. 4:551, 1970.

Mackinlay JB: Some approaches and problems in the use of health services – an overview, *J Health Soc Behav* 13:115, 1972.

Maternity Alliance: *Action on disability and maternity*, London, 1994, Maternity Alliance.

Moulder C: Towards a preliminary framework for understanding pregnancy loss, *J Reprod Infant Psychol* 12:65, 1994.

Oakley A: *Becoming a mother*, Oxford, 1979, Martin Robertson.

Phoenix A: Mothers under twenty: Outsider and insider views. In Phoenix A, Woollett A, Lloyd E, editors: *Motherhood: meanings, practices and ideologies*, London, 1991, Sage.

Reid ME, McIlwaine G: Consumer opinion of a hospital antenatal clinic, *Soc Sci Med* 14A:363, 1980.

Robinson JS, Carr G: Late bookers for antenatal care. In McLachlan G, Sherog R, editors: *In the beginning: Studies of maternity services*, Oxford, 1970, Oxford University Press.

Thomas H: Major illness during pregnancy: women's views, Occasional Paper, Guilford, 1997, Department of Sociology, University of Surrey.

Wilson J: Childbearing within the prison system, *Nurs Standard* 7(18):25, 1993.

Further Reading

Berryman J, Thorpe K, Windridge K: *Older mothers: conception, pregnancy and birth after 35*, London, 1995, Pandora.

A good, comprehensive account of the experiences of women giving birth after the age of 35 years. The book draws on material from Britain, the USA and Australia.

Carty E: Disability, pregnancy and parenting. Chapter 3 in Alexander J, Levy V, Roch S, (eds): *Aspects of midwifery practice*, London, 1995, Macmillan Press.

Deals with rheumatoid arthritis, spinal cord injury, visual impair-

ment and multiple schlerosis. Useful practice check.
Coventry Health Promotion Services, 1996.
*Package developed which contains information on disability and
pregnancy following a project funded by the Changing
Childbirth initiative. Contact: 01203 844092, Sue Kingwell.*
Doyal L: *What makes women sick*, London, 1995, Macmillan.
*This is an excellent overview of the range of women's health prob-
lems.*
Field PA, Marck PA: *Uncertain motherhood: negotiating the risks of
the childbearing years*, Thousand Oaks, 1994, Sage.
*A good collection of articles, based mainly on material from the
USA, addressing a variety of risks associated with
conception, pregnancy, birth and the health of the baby.*

Maternity Alliance Disability Working Group pack, Maternity
Alliance, 15 Britannia Street, London, WC1X 9JP.
*A useful pack including a chapter for disabled parents and
parents to-be. Would be helpful to use points highlighted to
examine and review trust policies and practices.*
Phoenix A, Woollett A, Lloyd E, editors: *Motherhood: meanings,
practices and ideologies*, London, 1991, Sage.
*An excellent collection of articles covering a range of issues in
motherhood.*

8 *Loss during Pregnancy*

LEARNING OUTCOMES

After studying this chapter you should be able to:
- Describe the classification of abortion.
- Identify the factors involved surrounding pregnancy loss.
- Discuss the psychological consequences of pregnancy loss within a framework of loss and grief.
- Consider the ways in which the midwife can provide effective care for parents who are experiencing pregnancy loss.

The role of the midwife is predominantly concerned with caring for women and their families in what is usually a joyous life event. According to government recommendations (House of Commons, 1992; Department of Health, 1993a), the midwife is to become the lead professional involved in care. The role is one of empowerment, advocacy, health promotion and carer. It is this caring role that becomes paramount in the time of loss.

This chapter is divided into two main sections. The first discusses losses in early pregnancy, such as, ectopic pregnancy and abortion, whereas the second section considers loss in later pregnancy. The midwife's role in enabling parents to cope with the loss is examined by exploring theories that relate to grief and grief reactions and by assessing the skills and support needed by midwives to fulfil this role.

Early Pregnancy Loss

Early pregnancy loss includes spontaneous abortion (miscarriage), induced abortion and ectopic pregnancy (**Figure 8.1**). To a lay person the term 'abortion' may have negative connotations in that it could imply that the pregnancy was ended deliberately. In this chapter the term 'miscarriage' is used when spontaneous abortion is discussed.

Spontaneous Abortion (Miscarriage)

Miscarriage is a lay term for spontaneous abortion in which there is premature expulsion of the embryo or fetus from the uterus before 20–24 weeks' gestation (Symonds, 1992; Pernoll and Garmel, 1994). The vast majority (75%) of spontaneous abortions occur before 16 weeks – 62% occur before 12 weeks (Pernoll and Garmel, 1994). Thus early spontaneous abortion (miscarriage) can be defined as the 'loss of a pregnancy up to 16 weeks from the beginning of the last menstrual period' (Houwert-De Jong *et al.* 1990, p. 534).

Incidence of miscarriage

It is difficult to identify precisely how common is miscarriage. This is in part because the majority of miscarriages occur before 12 weeks' gestation, with a significant number before 8 weeks, when the woman may not even be aware that she is pregnant. It has been estimated that the incidence is between 15 and 40% of all conceptions, as compared with fetal and neonatal death at 2% and ectopic pregnancy at 1% (Pernoll and Garmel, 1994), with approximately 700,000 women a year in England and Wales bleeding in early pregnancy (Allan, 1995). The incidence of miscarriage is influenced by the age of the couple and whether they have had previous successful pregnancies. If there is a history of miscarriages then the likelihood of having a further miscarriage increases.

Why miscarriages occur

There appears to be a consensus that approximately one-half of miscarriages are caused by fetal abnormality, with the remainder attributed partly to unknown causes and a variety of other causes (**Box 8.1**; Tindall, 1987; Allan, 1995).

Classification of miscarriage

As **Figure 8.1** suggests, vaginal blood loss in early pregnancy does not inevitably lead to miscarriage. The pregnancy can proceed without further problems. However, many miscarriages occur without vaginal bleeding as the primary symptom.

Threatened miscarriage

Here there is slight vaginal bleeding, the cervix is closed, the uterus is of an appropriate gestational size and there may also be associated mild pelvic pain. Vaginal bleeding in the first trimester can be extremely upsetting, as it inevitably raises the question as to the

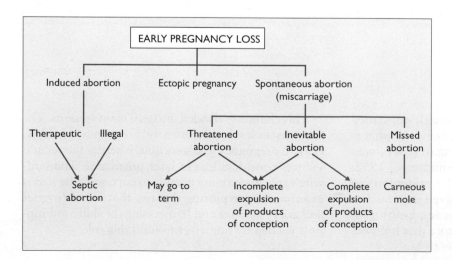

Figure 8.1 Classification of early pregnancy loss.

outcome of the pregnancy. However, approximately one-half of women who bleed in the first trimester go on to have a healthy baby (Symonds, 1992; Allan, 1995). Bleeding in early pregnancy could be attributed to implantation or cervical erosion, or may simply be unexplained. There is little that can be recommended in this situation. Traditionally, the advice has been bed rest, although the only controlled study (Diddle *et al.* 1953) demonstrated that there was no benefit. Avoiding sexual intercourse to reduce local stimulus may also be recommended. Although these measures are unproved, the woman and her partner often feel the need to take some action to try and preserve the pregnancy. In addition, the woman and her partner are likely to need sympathetic care and support throughout this time of uncertainty.

Inevitable miscarriage

When the bleeding and pain increase in severity, abortion is likely to be inevitable. The bleeding is bright red, clots are passed as the cervix is open and the membranes may have ruptured. Some of the products of conception may be passed or retained within the uterus. The pain is severe and cramping in nature, caused by uterine contractions, and it may be accompanied by backache. When miscarriage is inevitable it becomes either complete or incomplete.

Complete miscarriage

In complete miscarriage, all the products of conception are expelled from the uterus. There may be a small amount of a slight reddish discharge, the cervix is closed and the woman may experience little pain. It is important that *all* the products of conception are examined histologically to ensure that there is no evidence of molar gestation. However, before 16 weeks' gestation it is likely that some products of conception may be retained (Allan, 1995), so the woman may require surgical or medical intervention to empty the uterus.

Incomplete miscarriage

In incomplete miscarriage, not all the products of conception are passed, the bleeding continues, the cervix remains open and there is a possible risk of haemorrhage. The woman may need to be admitted to hospital for the retained products of conception to be evacuated, either through suction and curettage or curettage alone – the uterus must be empty of any products of conception. There is the potential risk of haemorrhage (which may necessitate emergency treatment) and infection. Some units offer a medical alternative which allows the woman some choice in how the miscarriage is managed. Pessaries containing misoprostol 800 μg (a prostaglandin analogue) are inserted vaginally and the woman observed in hospital for 6–8 hours. After a vaginal examination, and assuming that the vaginal blood loss is not heavy, the woman can be discharged home – blood loss continues for an average of 10 days.

Missed abortion

Here the fetus has died, but the products of conception have been retained. There may be few external signs of pregnancy, in that the uterus does not continue to enlarge, which indicates that the embryo or fetus has died *in utero*, but the cervix has remained closed. If the uterus fails to expel the products of conception these can be reabsorbed gradually. In some cases there is partial reorganization of the blood clot around the fetus with subsequent development of a carneous (blood) mole. Usually by approximately 21 days (Tindall, 1987) the fetus has miscarried. However, that the fetus has died is often diagnosed on a routine booking scan, which can come as a considerable shock to the woman and her partner. The woman may then be offered the choice of either medical or surgical intervention. Oral medication can be given to induce miscarriage, such as mifepristone 400–600 mg (a prostaglandin analogue; Joshua,

---

Box 8.1

Possible Causes of Miscarriage

1. **Fetal abnormality:**
- Chromosomal.
- Structural.

2. **Known factors:**
- Maternal.
- Infection – *Rubella, Mycoplasma, Chlamydia, Listeria monocytogenes.*
- Immunological.
- Endocrine factors related to the failure of the corpus luteum.
- Systemic diseases, e.g. diabetes, hypertension.
- Anatomical defects, e.g. incompetent cervix, abnormalities of the uterus.
- Trauma, e.g. local injury to the uterus.

3. **Unknown factors.**

1994); if miscarriage is still incomplete after this, then further medication is required. The alternative is the surgical procedure to evacuate the retained products of conception. Whatever choice she makes, the woman needs support and information with an opportunity to discuss all the issues.

Recurrent spontaneous miscarriage

This is commonly defined as when a woman has suffered three consecutive spontaneous abortions before 20–24 weeks' gestation (Pernoll and Garmel, 1994). Although causative factors may be identified (**Box 8.1**), the cause frequently remains unknown. Specialist miscarriage clinics for couples who experience recurrent miscarriages can help to identify specific causes and can provide the necessary psychological support and counselling. Recurrent miscarriage can be very distressing for the parents, but it has been estimated (Pernoll and Garmel, 1994) that even after three pregnancy losses the incidence of a successful pregnancy is 68%.

Isoimmunization

Following any type of pregnancy loss, a woman who is Rhesus negative should be given Rhesus immune globulin within 72 hours to prevent isoimmunization.

Ectopic Pregnancy

This is when a fertilized ovum implants in an area outside the uterine cavity; it occurs in about 1 in 200 pregnancies (Symonds, 1992), although the incidence is increasing (Irvine *et al.* 1994). The most common site is in the Fallopian tubes, although implantation can occur in the ovary, the abdominal cavity or the cervix.

Causes

The main causes relate to factors that either prevent or impede the movement of the fertilized ovum through the Fallopian tubes and into the uterus. Such factors include previous termination of pregnancy and pelvic inflammatory disease (Irvine *et al.* 1994), the presence of an intrauterine contraceptive device (IUCD) and a history of fertility problems.

Recognizing ectopic pregnancy

Recognition is dependent to some extent on the site of the ectopic pregnancy. If it is a tubal pregnancy, the most common form of ectopic ```pregnancy (Pernoll and Garmel, 1994), then the woman has a history of amenorrhoea for 6–8 weeks, develops abdominal pain and then bleeding from the vagina. The pain increases in intensity as the tube ruptures, haemorrhage occurs and the woman may become shocked, which requires hospital admission.

Managing ectopic pregnancy

Again, this is dependent on the site and duration of the pregnancy and the woman's condition. Tubal rupture with haemorrhage means that the woman requires emergency abdominal surgery – attempts are made to preserve the Fallopian tube if possible, but otherwise a salpingectomy may be needed. In some cases laparoscopy is possible rather than a laparotomy. In other cases in which the pregnancy is in a very early stage and the tube is not ruptured, some units administer systemic methotrexate (Pernoll and Garmel, 1994), which facilitates reabsorption of the pregnancy and aids in the preservation of the Fallopian tube.

Induced Abortion

Induced abortion refers to an abortion that is either legal, within the terms of the Abortion Act, or illegal, outside the terms of the Act.

Therapeutic abortion

Legal termination of pregnancy is allowed under the terms of the 1967 Abortion Act as amended by The Human Fertilisation and Embryology Act 1990 section 37. A 24-week time limit is allowed if abortion is performed on the grounds of injury or risk to the woman's physical and mental health, provided the risk is greater than that posed by termination of the pregnancy. It also allows for the termination of pregnancy without time limit if there is the possibility of grave permanent injury to the woman's physical or mental health and if there is a risk of serious fetal abnormality (RCN, 1992). In addition, all legal abortions must be carried out in an institution and by practitioners approved under the terms of the Abortion Act.

It is beyond the scope of this chapter to fully explore the legal and ethical issues of induced abortion as these are complex, with individual practitioners having to decide for themselves on the issues involved. The decision to terminate a pregnancy is often a very difficult one for the woman and the midwife needs to be aware of the physical, psychological, legal and ethical issues of abortion, as they can impact on the woman's next pregnancy. Circumstances such as the termination of a pregnancy for fetal abnormality can be especially challenging for the midwife. Kohn and Moffitt (1994) relate some parent's experiences of feeling that this is a double blow. The parents have to come to terms with the fact that their baby is abnormal and then have to wrestle with the difficult issues of whether or not to terminate the pregnancy.

Illegal abortion

Illegal abortion is an attempt to evacuate the uterus of the products of conception that is not carried out within the terms of the Abortion Act. Illegal abortions are associated with high maternal mortality and morbidity rates, mainly caused by sepsis and haemorrhage.

Septic abortion

Septic abortion may occur following incomplete abortion and induced abortions, particularly illegal abortions, in which bacteria gain access to the genital tract. Pyrexia is evident and there may be a foul-smelling vaginal discharge. The infection may be confined to the products of conception or it may spread more widely – if the bacteria gain access to the blood stream the result can be bacteraemic (endotoxic) shock (Tindall, 1987). Any evidence of infection should be reported and treated promptly with antibiotic therapy.

Methods of Induced Abortion

The method used depends on a number of factors, including the duration of the pregnancy, the physical condition of the woman and the medical facilities and expertise that are available (Burkman, 1994). A common method before 12–14 weeks is by suction and curettage. After 12–14 weeks labour can be induced; for example, by the administration of vaginal prostaglandins. Whatever the circumstances or the method used, the woman needs sympathetic and non-judgemental care.

Effects of Early Pregnancy Loss

This section focuses on the effects on the woman and her partner after early miscarriage or ectopic pregnancy. There are also recognized physical and emotional consequences of induced abortion, but they are not dealt with specifically here.

Physical Effects of Early Pregnancy Loss

For the woman who experiences an early miscarriage, the passage of large amounts of blood and clots and the pain are distressing. She may also have to contend with a hospital admission and the effects of general anaesthesia. For the woman who experiences an ectopic pregnancy there are the physical effects of recovering from emergency surgery, as well as the difficulties of coming to terms with the a lost pregnancy and possibly a damaged or lost fallopian tube, with may impact on her future fertility. The physical consequences alone of early pregnancy loss can be considerable and their impact on the woman can be underestimated.

Emotional Effects of Early Pregnancy Loss

There is now increasing recognition that early pregnancy loss can be an extremely painful emotional experience for parents. Anecdotal accounts from women who have had an early miscarriage, for example, point to it as being a painful experience not just in the physical sense, as this account from Oakley *et al.* (1984) serves to illustrate:

> ... *nothing had prepared me for the despair, the emptiness of grieving for an 'it'. The sheer murderous anger – I didn't know how to behave. The casual attitude of the hospital, the blankness of the GP and the absence of any practical help or information confused me. Was I meant to behave as if nothing had happened?*
>
> (Oakley *et al.* 1984, p. 31)

The feelings expressed here highlight the sense of grief and loss that are commonly felt. Parents often express feelings of shock, numbness, guilt and not knowing how to behave. These are compounded by the perception that early pregnancy loss is somehow an intangible loss that is not publicly acknowledged. In other bereavement situations there are formalized

Table 8.1 Psychological Consequences of Miscarriage			
Authors	**Sample**	**Method**	**Findings**
Friedman and Gath (1989)	67 women 4 weeks after miscarriage	Interviews Depression rating scales Self-rating scales	Depression 32 women considered as psychiatric cases
Turner *et al.* (1991)	300 women 1 month after miscarriage	Not stated	4% had no grief reaction 75% had grief reaction which had resolved 21% had grief reaction which had not resolved
Thaper and Thaper (1992)	Compared 60 women who had a miscarriage with 62 pregnant women who were attending antenatal clinic	Interview General Health Questionnaire Hospital Anxiety and Depression Scale	Women who have a miscarriage experience a significant degree of anxiety
Harker (1993)	115 women 6–7 and 25 weeks after miscarriage	Questionnaire Edinburgh Post Natal Depression Scale (Cox *et al.* 1987) Crown Crisp Experiential Index (Crown and Crisp, 1979)	Depression between 2 and 25 weeks after miscarriage
Prettyman *et al.* (1993)	65 women 1,6 and 12 weeks after early miscarriage	Questionnaire Hospital Anxiety and Depression Scale	First week 41% had anxiety, 22% had depression, declining to 32% with anxiety and 6% with depression by week 12

rites of passage in that there is a funeral and a public recognition that death has taken place. Kuller and Katz (1994) discuss how miscarriage in other cultures is afforded ceremony that allowed a public expression of grief, but this is denied by Western culture.

Psychological Consequences of Early Pregnancy Loss

In recent years there has been a growing recognition of the psychological consequences of miscarriage and a number of studies were carried out to try and identify the psychological consequences using standardized measures – these are summarized in **Table 8.1**.

These findings appear to suggest that for a significant number of women miscarriage is at the very least an unpleasant and upsetting experience; these experiences seem to be unique to the individual with their intensity not appearing to be related to the gestational age of the baby (Stewart *et al.* 1992). For 'an important minority' (Prettyman, 1995) it can provoke severe emotional problems. It is also fair to say that for some women miscarriage may come as a relief and may not be an upsetting experience, as not all view miscarriage as loss (Moulder, 1990). It is also suggested that woman who have an ectopic pregnancy

also experience similar feelings and that their loss is two-fold. First, they have lost their baby and, second, there is the perceived threat to their fertility (Kohn and Moffitt, 1994).

Loss in Late Pregnancy

Loss in late pregnancy may be classified as a stillbirth, in which the baby is born after 24 weeks' gestation and shows no signs of life, or a neonatal death, in which the baby is born alive but dies within the first month. The definition of stillbirth was reduced from 28 to 24 weeks following the Stillbirth (Definition) Act 1992, which gives recognition to the parents' needs after delivery of a viable baby.

When a pregnancy has progressed into the 24th week, it can often be a tremendous shock that the baby dies. Women often anticipate miscarriage up to the 12th week of pregnancy and assume that once this 'critical' period has passed they will progress to term and deliver a live healthy baby.

When birth and death occur simultaneously the effects on the woman and her family can be devastating. Midwives' experiences of childbirth and maternity care are usually associated with joy and happiness. Dealing with unexpected death alongside normal births can prove distressing.

Caring for a woman during delivery can present a special challenge to the midwife, especially when the baby's death is known in advance. The woman's wishes in relation to pain relief should be respected. Staff may offer generous sedation in an attempt to make this extremely painful situation pain free – this may make the staff feel better but is not always helpful to the woman. She may feel a need to be in control and not journey through a fog (Kohner, 1985). It does not help the grieving process if the woman has no recollection of the event.

When stillbirth or neonatal death occurs during a vaginal delivery, there is a great deal of activity in the delivery room. There may be obstetricians, paediatricians and midwives actively attempting resuscitation while the parents are helpless onlookers. It is important that they are supported through this trauma. Eventually, on reflection, the parents may derive some comfort from knowing that attempts were made to save the baby.

Loss and Grief

Loss and grief are intrinsically linked within the context of bereavement. It is essential that midwives have a knowledge of these concepts to facilitate the grieving process.

Loss

The experience of losing a baby at any stage of the pregnancy can be devastating for the parents, with potentially adverse psychological consequences. An understanding of loss and grief can help midwives to provide the appropriate individualized care. This particular loss is complex in that it involves the loss of expectations. From the time that the woman and her partner know that she is pregnant they may begin the process of attachment and acquanticeship with the baby (Sandelowski and Black, 1994), which can include making plans for the future and thinking of names. Thus, the complex process of adjusting to changes in their roles and the perception of themselves begins. The loss of a wanted pregnancy may be particularly acute for individuals who have had fertility problems. The experience of loss is unique to the individual as each may have particular expectations of the future – midwives need to be aware of this.

Grief

The grief following pregnancy loss can be similar to that experienced following other types of bereavement. There are parallels between the stages of grief as described by Parkes (1986) and Ramsey and DeGroot (1984) in their work on bereavement, as presented in **Table 8.2**.

Many of these components can manifest at the same time, for example guilt anxiety and anger can accompany depression (Jones and Jones, 1990); in addition these components can also manifest as behaviours, cognitions, physical symptoms or affects. It is also worth noting that grief as a concept is poorly understood (Jacob, 1993) and that it is a constantly changing process. People are not locked in one stage of grief, but may move backwards and forwards through various stages. Littlewood (1992) argues that it may be unrealistic to pin the stages down to portions of time, with the expectation that an individual will recover at a certain point. It may well be that full recovery from grief is not always possible and that,

Table 8.2 Theoretical Approaches to Grief	
Parkes (1986)	**Ramsey and DeGroot (1984)**
Shock, numbness and the pain of grieving	Shock
Manifestations of fear, guilt, resentment	Disorganization
Disengagement, apathy and aimlessness	Guilt
Gradual hope and a move in a new direction	Anger Aggression Resolution Acceptance and integration

in a sense, the parents may always grieve for the loss of the baby. However, such theoretical frameworks have some use in increasing understanding and awareness of what parents may experience.

Stages of Grieving

In the accounts of parents' experiences of pregnancy loss, it is possible to find similar themes. They describe the shock and numbness when they first realized that the pregnancy had ended, with the feeling that no one really understood what they were going through. Friends and family may try to help by playing down the significance of the loss – by saying, in the case of miscarriage for example, that it was not a real baby and that they can always try for another one. By all accounts such comments are not helpful, because what the parents have lost is that particular baby who was special and unique to them.

Fear, Anger and Guilt

Any one or a combination of these emotions may be found in the experience of pregnancy loss. The parents may worry, if this was their first loss, that this may happen again, so raising all kinds of doubts and concerns that they may never have more children. There is a strong expectation in British culture that at some point couples will have children, so pregnancy loss may threaten this expectation and view of themselves as parents. This may be the case particularly with parents who have had more than one miscarriage, as the likelihood of having a successful pregnancy diminishes with each successive miscarriage (Allan, 1995).

Anger is a common emotion following pregnancy loss. It may be directed at the parents themselves or at the people around them. This includes the health professionals who may become a focus for this anger and resentment because it was perceived that they could do nothing to prevent the loss. The way that the parents are treated by health professionals is also influential as the health professionals' actions may be interpreted as meaning that they do not care. The woman who has a miscarriage, for example, may feel a mere number in a fast-moving impersonal system. Guilt may also be an emotion. If no cause can be identified for the loss, then the parents may blame themselves or each other.

Disengagement, Apathy and Aimlessness

Parents can often feel isolated from family and friends. Pregnancy loss is not usually a topic of everyday conversation, as it incorporates the taboo subjects of sex, reproduction and death. This may make it difficult for friends and family to discuss it or to know what to say. The couple themselves may become so immersed in their own feelings of grief that they can find it difficult to support each other. Social encounters are frequently painful and require emotional energy – indeed, it may be extremely difficult even to take a walk, as some women report that pregnant women, babies and children appear to be everywhere and only serve as a reminder of what they have lost. Such social disengagement may lead to feelings of depression (Friedman and Gath, 1989) and a sense of loss of purpose.

Moving in a New Direction

This is a final stage in which eventually the grief begins to resolve and the person can move forwards. Even when parents feel able to grieve openly, they may feel pressure to move forwards and 'get over' the loss before they are ready. Although the pain subsides, the loss is something that may never be forgotten.

Men and Pregnancy Loss

Until recent years very little attention was paid to how men may feel following pregnancy loss. However, there is now an awareness and recognition that in miscarriage, for example, men may experience feelings of grief similar to those of women (Kohn and Moffitt, 1994; Murphy, 1996). Men also report feeling shocked and numbed when they learn that the baby has died, and some may feel angry and frustrated that there was nothing that they or the medical profession could do. They may cope by focusing on distractions, such as work, or by trying to be positive and thinking of the future. The experience may also be made worse because they have their partners' obvious grief to contend with. Some men may feel that it is their role to be strong and supportive when their partner is openly distressed about the pregnancy loss.

Kohn and Moffitt (1994) consider that the feelings of loss are attributable to the disruption of plans for the future and, indeed, that some men can become very quickly attached to the baby and so feel the loss keenly. There is an assumption that the loss is the woman's and not the man's, so there may be little provision for male grieving.

It may be important to acknowledge that the impact of both early and late pregnancy loss can have adverse effects on both partners and that the man's feelings should also be considered.

The Midwife's Role

Following the death of a baby, the midwife is often the key person to deal with the family in the initial grieving process. She needs to acknowledge her own beliefs and values and recognize the individual needs of the family for whom she is caring. Grieving is unique to each person and the midwife, through her knowledge of grief theory and the deployment of appropriate counselling skills, should be able to facilitate mourning.

Factors that influence grief reactions are age, gender, culture, religion and how others in the immediate social circle respond to their loss. Individuals within a family may react differently to the loss and the midwife should be sensitive to their feelings.

Each Loss as Unique

The anecdotal accounts of the experience of miscarriage in particular indicate that people react very differently and with varying degrees of intensity. SANDS (1995)

suggest that health professionals should treat each parent individually and sensitively and understand '... what the loss means to the parents.' Kohner (1985) also advises midwives to recognize the importance of the loss to the parents. She suggests that professionals: '... work openly and flexibly, to communicate honestly with parents, to avoid assumptions and judgements, and sometimes to risk making mistakes.'

Stillbirth and neonatal death can be described almost as a 'non-event' (Bourne, 1968) in which there is guilt and shame with no tangible person to mourn. It is important that steps are taken to help remember the loss and to mark the death. The taking of photographs, videos, footprints and locks of hair are all reminders for the parents that their baby existed. It may not be appropriate for the parents to have these mementos in the early days of the loss, but they can be kept in the maternity unit along with an entry in the remembrance book until the parents feel ready. The parents could also be offered, if appropriate, the opportunity to see and hold their baby. If the parents have not named their baby, this should be encouraged as it will help create memories where few exist (**Case Study 8.1**) (Raphael-Leff, 1991).

The Need for Information

Whether preceding an anticipated death or immediately afterwards, parents need to be given clear, concise and factual information. The unreality of the situation makes it difficult for them to absorb

---

Case study 8.1

Margaret

Margaret, a 20-year-old traveller, delivered a stillborn baby girl at term, having presented at the labour ward with a history of no fetal movements for 24 hours. No explanation could be found. She left the hospital after 12 hours, stating that she did not want to see the baby and that the hospital should take care of the funeral arrangements.

On visiting the home the following day, the community midwife noted that in accordance with custom all the possessions of the baby had been disposed of.

During conversation, Margaret produced a photograph of the baby from under a cushion. She commented that the baby did not look dead. The midwife explained that the baby was

dead and that the dark red colouring of the lips is not present in a live baby. She then encouraged Margaret to see her baby in an attempt to realize that her baby was dead. When the midwife returned to the hospital to arrange this, the baby had been buried that morning, robbing Margaret of the opportunity to see her baby.

Her family had believed that all possessions relating to the baby had been destroyed. Hiding the photograph was the only means that Margaret had of actualizing the death. This case study illustrates the importance of giving mothers and of fathers time to make decisions relating to their babies.

complex information (Palmer and Noble, 1986), so information must be given with skill and sensitivity. Kirk (1984) describes the difficulty in breaking bad news gently while ensuring that the message remains clear. It may be necessary to repeat information as

parents only retain a small amount when shocked and upset. This is a time when their hopes and dreams have been shattered and their 'dream child' exists no more. If stillbirth occurred and the labour has resulted in a Caesarean section, the woman may be anaesthetized and her partner may be alone to deal with the news of the baby's death. He will need support to cope with this news and with breaking it to his partner.

Parents also need practical information about procedures such as registration and funeral requirements, particularly in the case of stillbirth and neonatal death (see **Box 8.2** for legal requirements relating to stillbirth and neonatal death). It is also important that staff are aware of the religious and cultural beliefs when giving this information (**Box 8.3**). The SANDS (1995) document provides excellent guidelines for carers and recommends the use of protocols for guidance when dealing with bereaved parents. Providing the addresses of support groups, such as the Stillbirth and Neonatal Society (SANDS), Support After Termination for Abnormalities (SAFTA) and the Miscarriage Association, may also be very helpful to parents.

Postmortem examinations are usually requested following the loss of a baby. It is essential that this request is made with sensitivity for the parents' feelings – the parents will need support and time to make the decision. The information upon which they base their decision must be clear and concise; postmortem examinations should not be carried out without the written consent of the parents.

In addition to such procedural information, certain practical information must also be given. Women who

---

Box 8.2

Legal Requirements Relating to Stillbirth and Neonatal Death

Stillbirth

A certificate of stillbirth is given to the parents by the midwife or doctor who examined the baby at delivery. This must be taken to the Registrar of Births and Deaths within 42 days for the stillbirth to be registered. Registration must take place before the baby can be buried.

Neonatal death

All deaths must be registered within 5 days. The birth and the death must be registered – they can be done simultaneously.

Box 8.3

Time for Decision Making

You pay a routine antenatal visit to Sarah, who is expecting her second child. According to your records she is 12 weeks' pregnant with no major problems identified. She answers the door; however,. when she sees you she seems very hostile, but lets you in. You ask how she is and she angrily tells you that she had a miscarriage a week ago – why didn't you know and what is the point of your visit. You try to explain that there must have been a breakdown in communication, offer your apologies and try to talk with her. Unfortunately, she still appears angry and despite your best efforts to talk to her it seems appropriate to leave, but she agrees to let you visit again.

When you leave it seems obvious that this breakdown in communication has damaged your relationship with her, which now needs to be painstakingly built up again, and you feel angry and upset at this.

What explanation could there be for her reaction?

What could you do to help her?

Box 8.4

Physical Manifestations of Grief

- Hollowness in the stomach.
- Tightness in the chest.
- Tightness in the throat.
- Oversensitivity to noise.
- A sense of depersonalization.
- Breathlessness.
- Weakness in the muscles.
- Lack of energy.
- Dry mouth.

Source: Worden, 1991.

Support for Carers

have lost a baby need to know when the vaginal blood loss will cease and how to cope with lactation. Mander (1994) suggests that not all women view lactation after pregnancy loss as negative and may feel comforted by the knowledge that their baby would have been well nourished.

Parents need information about grief and mourning, as this may be the first major loss in their lives. They need to be aware of the psychological and physical manifestations of grief, as many of the physical symptoms, as described by Worden (1991), may be misinterpreted as part of normal childbirth (**Box 8.4**). Protocols are often used in hospitals to assist midwives to advise parents of the practical issues that surrounding the birth of a baby. Again, the SANDS (1995) document *Guidelines for Professionals* provides clear, constructive advice to avoid errors being made. In addition, the woman who has had an ectopic pregnancy or a Caesarean section will need help and advice towards recovering from major surgery.

Counselling Bereaved Parents

Counselling skills are essential for midwives to enable them to deal with families in distress. However, each midwife should recognize that the use of counselling skills and counselling itself are quite different (Thomas, 1994). It is essential that midwives recognize the different expressions of grief and the situations in which professional counsellors are required. Such counsellors may be employed within the maternity unit or by general practitioners (GPs) in the community.

Klaus and Kennell (1982) suggest ways to intervene to facilitate mourning through a series of meetings between the parents and appropriate health professionals. The first two are to explain what has happened, give support, warn about the grief reactions and, where appropriate, encourage the parents to see the baby. Sharing and expression of feelings are encouraged. Later, a third meeting is arranged to discuss any problems.

The provision across the country of such counselling and follow-up after pregnancy loss appears to be patchy, so it is perhaps an appropriate area for midwives to develop. Not all parents require professional counselling – sometimes a person with good listening skills is all that is necessary. The parents may also prefer support through group networks, such as SANDS and SAFTA, so those who have suffered a pregnancy loss could be given information about such support groups. It should be recognized that each person's need for support is unique.

Providing care and support for bereaved families is emotionally and physically demanding, with a great deal of time and energy spent in dealing with the distress of families. There may be distress experienced by the midwife caring for the parents and she may in some way feel a responsibility for what has occurred. Support for carers, therefore, should always be considered an integral component of the provision and delivery of care to parents who have lost a baby (Kohner, 1985; Jones and Jones, 1990; Raphael-Leff, 1991; Mander, 1994). Midwives need education and training to enable them to care for families in crisis. Indeed, Raphael-Leff (1991) advises '... personal exploration of what death in the face of birth means to people who have chosen as their life work a profession which helps life come into being.'

Experienced midwives can provide support and guidance to junior staff by acting as role models to help them acknowledge the situation (Lugton, 1989). Carers may feel that they have failed the family, which can produce feelings of guilt, resentment, helplessness and defeat (Stack, 1982). Although the acquisition of counselling skills is an essential part of the midwife's role, Thomas (1994) advocates training and support for carers. The House of Commons (1992) Select Committee on Health recognized the importance of skilled care for bereaved parents in recommending that all units ensure that carers receive appropriate training. There needs, therefore, to be some kind of mechanism which provides support and training for the carer to cope with the demands of caring for parents after pregnancy loss. SANDS (1995) recommends that: '... the need for training should be recognized in policies for the management of pregnancy loss and the death of a baby and should be specified in contracts with purchasers.'

Staff have the right to work in a supportive atmosphere. This can be in the form of informal staff support groups or provided in a more structured way. Staff need time to reflect after a traumatic situation and managers should be aware of their needs. The use of clinical supervision is an identified method of supporting staff, as reinforced in the document *A Vision for the Future* (Department of Health, 1993b). Clinical supervision of midwifery practice can be defined as '... professional support, counsel and advice to practising midwives' (UKCC, 1995). Midwives who are supported by their managers, peers and supervisors of midwives are more likely to provide effective support to the families in their time of loss.

Conclusion

In this chapter, some of the issues surrounding loss in pregnancy and childbirth have been explored. It is hoped that readers will use the text as a basis from which to extend their knowledge and skills. A further reading list is provided for those who want a more extensive coverage of the subject than is possible in one chapter.

Bereavement during childbirth can be one of the most challenging aspects for midwives, in a role which is predominantly concerned with creativity and new life. However, the profound nature of loss in childbirth can provide those concerned with opportunities for personal and professional development by being with women at a time of great need.

KEY CONCEPTS

- Pregnancy loss can be considered as a bereavement situation that evokes a grief reaction.
- The reaction to pregnancy loss is unique for each individual.
- It is important that midwives acknowledge the impact of the loss and provide appropriate support and follow-up.
- Support and training is an essential component to enable midwives to help families through bereavement.

References

Allan A: Types and causes of miscarriage, *Modern Midwife* 5(3):27, 1995.

Bourne S: The psychological effects of stillbirth on women and their doctors, *J R Coll Gen Pract* 16:113, 1968.

Burkman RT: Contraception and family planning. In DeCherney AH, Pernoll ML, editors: *Current obstetric and gynecologic diagnosis and treatment*, 8th edn, London, 1994, Prentice Hall.

Cox JL, Holden JM, Sagovsky R: Detection of post natal depression: development of the 10 item Edinburgh post natal depression scale. *Br J Psychiatry* 150:782, 1987.

Crown S, Crisp AH. *Manual of the Crown Crisp experiential index*, London, 1979, Hodder and Stoughton.

Department of Health: *Changing childbirth*, Report of the Expert Maternity Group, London, 1993a, HMSO.

Department of Health: *A vision for the future*, London, 1993, HMSO.

Diddle J, Diddle AW, O'Connor KA *et al*: Evaluation of bed rest in threatened abortion, *Obstet Gynaecol* 2:63, 1953.

Friedman T, Gath D: The psychiatric consequences of spontaneous abortion, *Br J Psychiatry* 155:210, 1989.

Harker L: Emotional wellbeing following miscarriage, *J Obstet Gynaecol* 13:262, 1993.

House of Commons: *Health Committee Second Report. Maternity services*, London, 1992, HMSO.

Houwert-De Jong MH, Bruinse HW, Eskes TKAB et al: Early recurrent miscarriage: histology of conception products, *Br J Obstet Gynaecol* 97(June):533, 1990.

Irvine LM, Hicks JL, Blair–Bell C *et al*: The incidence of ectopic pregnancy in the City and Hackney Health District of London 1990–1991, *J Obstet Gynaecol* 14:29, 1994.

Jacob S: An analysis of the concept of grief, *J Adv Nurs* 18:1787, 1993.

Jones A, Jones K: Support for parents after a child's death, *Nurs Stand* 4(46):32, 1990.

Joshua A, editor: *Guy's Hospital 1995–96 nursing drug reference*, 3rd edn, London, 1995, Mosby.

Kirk E: Psychological effects and management of perinatal loss. *Am J Obstet Gynaecol*, 149:45, 1984.

Klaus M, Kennell J: *Parent–infant bonding*, 2nd edn, St Louis, 1982, CV Mosby.

Kohn I, Moffitt PL: *Pregnancy loss — a silent sorrow*, London, 1994, Hodder and Stoughton.

Kohner N: *Midwives & stillbirth*, London, 1985, Royal College of Midwives/Health Education Council.

Kuller JA, Katz VL: Miscarriage: a historical perspective, *Birth* 21(4):227, 1994.

Laurent C: Marking the loss, *Nurs Times* 87(January):26, 1991.

Littlewood J: *Aspects of grief. Bereavement in adult life*, London, 1992, Routledge.

Lovell H: Mothers reaction to perinatal death, *Nurs Times* 82(46):40, 1986.

Lugton J: *Communicating with dying people and their relatives*, London, 1989, Lisa Sainsbury Foundation/Austin Cornish.

Mander R: *Loss and bereavement on childbearing*, London, 1994, Blackwell Scientific Publications.

Moulder C: *Miscarriage: women's experience and need*, London 1990, Pandora.

Murphy F: *The experience of early miscarriage from a male perspective*, unpublished MSc Thesis, Swansea, 1996, University of Wales.

Oakley A, McPherson A, Roberts H: *Miscarriage*, Glasgow, 1984, Fontana.

Palmer CE, Noble, DN: Premature death: dilemmas of infant mortality, *J Contemp Soc Work* 16:332, 1968.

Parkes CM: *Bereavement. Studies of grief in adult life*, 2nd edn, Harmondsworth, 1986, Penguin.

Pernoll ML, Garmel SH: Early pregnancy risks. In DeCherney AH, Pernoll ML, editors: *Current obstetric and gynecologic diagnosis and treatment*, 8th edn, London, 1994, Prentice Hall.

Prettyman R: The psychological sequelae of miscarriage, *Matern Child Health* 20(6):207, 1995.

Prettyman RJ, Cordle CI, Cook GD: A three month follow-up of psychological morbidity after early miscarriage, *Br J Med Psychol* 66:363, 1993.

Ramsey R, DeGroot W: A further look at bereavement. Cited in: Abnormal grief and its therapy, *Psychiatry Pract* 4:114, 1984.

Raphael-Leff J: *Psychological processes of childbearing*, London, 1991, Blackwell Scientific Publications.

RCN: Abortion: the nurse's responsibilities, *Nurs Stand* 7(3):35, 1992.

Sandelowski M, Black BP: The epistemology of expectant parenthood, *West J Nurs Res* 16(60):601, 1994.

SANDS: *Pregnancy loss and the death of a baby. Guidelines for professionals*, London, 1995, Stillbirth & Neonatal Death Society.

Stack J: *Reproductive casualties*, New York, 1982, Perinatal Press.

Stewart A, Harker L, Ford J: An unfinished story. Helping people to come to terms with miscarriage, *Prof Nurse* 7(30):656, 1992.

Symonds EM: *Essential obstetrics and gynaecology*, 2nd edn, Edinburgh, 1992, Churchill Livingstone.

Thaper AK, Thaper A: Psychological sequelae of miscarriage: a controlled study using the General Health Questionnaire and the Hospital Anxiety and Depression Scale, *Br J Gen Pract* 42:94, 1992.

Thomas J: Maternity bereavement counselling: How it has changed, *Br J Midwifery* 12(10):509, 1994.

Tindall VR: *Jeffcoate's principles of gynaecology*, 5th edn, London, 1987, Butterworth.

Turner MJ, Flannelly GM, Wingfield M *et al*: The miscarriage clinic: an audit of the first year, *Br J Obstet Gynaecol* 98:306, 1991.

UKCC: *Consultation on proposed amendments and additions of the midwives rules*, London, 1995, UKCC.

Worden W. *Grief counselling and grief therapy*, 2nd edn, London, 1991, Routledge.

Further Reading

Pipes M: *Understanding abortion*, London, 1986, Women's Press.

This book addresses a sensitive and difficult area. The prime aim is to support women through a difficult situation.

Mander R: *Loss and bereavement in child bearing*, Oxford, 1994, Blackwell Scientific Publications.

A research-based text covering all aspects of loss, it also addresses grief in staff carers.

Oakley A, McPherson A, Roberts H: *Miscarriage*, London, 1990, Penguin Books.

An extremely readable text, written from a sociological and psychological perspective, useful for professionals, women and their partners.

Raphael B: *The anatomy of bereavement*: *A handbook for the caring professions*, 1984.

This book is a presentation of case studies and research findings. It is informative and direct in its approach.

Dickenson D, Johnson M: *Death, dying and bereavement*, London, 1993, Sage Publications.

This book uses an interdisciplinary approach using literature, theology, sociology and psychology. There is a wide range of contributors with sensitively written chapters.

SANDS: *Pregnancy loss and the death of a baby. Guidelines for professionals*, London, 1995, Stillbirth & Neonatal Death Society.

unit 2

From Birth to Health after Birth

9 The Physiology and Clinical Management of Labour

After studying this chapter you should be able to:

- Demonstrate an understanding of the physiological processes underpining the process of labour.
- Discuss the advantages and disadvantages of interventions in labour.
- Demonstrate an appreciation of the value of individualized care.
- Identify the factors which may contribute to a positive labour experience.
- Assess the progress of labour and utilize professional judgement in assisting the labour process.
- Recognize problems which may occur during labour and birth and demonstrate an understanding of the appropriate actions.
- Evaluate the limitations of current methods of intrapartum fetal surveillance.
- Consider the influence of research findings on current midwifery practice and on future developments.

Physiology, Biochemistry and Pharmacology of Parturition (Labour)

It is paradoxical but not uncommon to find a lack of knowledge about events that occur frequently – parturition is no exception. In particular, the initiation of labour and ripening and effacement of the cervix remain areas of uncertainty.

Anatomy and Physiology of the Uterus Regarding Labour

The uterus consists of two main functional components – the myometrium and the cervix (Gee and Olah, 1993). During pregnancy the myometrium must grow and remain relaxed. At the same time, the cervix must be strong enough to obstruct delivery. Labour denotes a dramatic change. The muscle has to contract to produce tension in the wall of the uterus, to dilate the cervix. It is becoming clear that nature has orchestrated a complex series of biochemical and physical changes to achieve this (Granston *et al.* 1989; Osmers *et al.* 1993). Even more amazingly, the processes have to be reversible and repeatable. There is no evidence to suggest that repeated delivery results in loss of cervical function, as might be evident by pre-term deliveries or miscarriage with increasing number of pregnancies the woman may carry.

The Myometrium

The myometrium consists of smooth muscle (Danforth, 1954), which contracts slowly compared to skeletal and cardiac muscle. Each muscle cell contracts spontaneously or can be activated by the action of adjacent cells. Throughout the pregnancy contractions occur, but these are characterized by the recruitment of few muscle fibres. Therefore the activity is not propagated throughout the myometrium. It is said to be *decremental*.

Oestrogens, produced by the pregnancy itself in the placenta, increase muscle mass and increase the electrical activity. Hence the contractile activity of the myometrium increases as pregnancy proceeds. By term, the mother notices the activity as 'Braxton Hicks' contractions. These contractions typically remain below the 'pain threshold'. It must be pointed out that the origin of pain associated with contractions is poorly understood. It may be due to tension in the cervix or to ischaemia in the myometrium due to interference with blood supply by the contraction.

Labour is characterized by a marked escalation in myometrial activity so that contractions become regular and painful. The muscle activity is now coordinated because of the formation of specialized cell-to-cell junctions called *nexuses*, which permit the rapid transmission of electrical activity throughout the myometrium. This activity is now termed *propagated*. Nexus formation is promoted by oestrogens and prostaglandins. Prostaglandins are manufactured within the uterus itself from the large stores of arachidonic acid, the precursor of prostaglandins, which is to be found in the cells of the decidua (the decidua is formed from what was the endometrium).

The Cervix

The cervix is a tubular structure consisting predominantly of collagen fibres (Danforth, 1954). These fibres are inelastic and wound tightly around the canal of the cervix, which means that they readily resist dilatation. No energy is expended to maintain this competence. The problem lies with delivering the conceptus. Forceful dilatation can damage the collagen structure, resulting in permanent weakness and predispostion to midtrimester miscarriage or premature delivery in future.

The collagen fibres are held together by a 'gel' composed of glycoproteins (Osmers *et al.* 1993). In the solid state the glycoproteins bind together the collagen fibres, which are strong and inelastic, like concrete binds steel reinforcing to produce a stable structure. In preparation for labour, there is a change in composition due to removal of structural glycoproteins, which bind the collagen fibres, and their replacement with glycoproteins which merely fill the space between the fibres.

In addition, glycoproteins can change their properties rapidly depending on the amount of water associated with them. The most familiar glycoprotein to us is gelatine. As with gelatine, cervical glycoproteins can be changed from solid to liquid by adding water, which can produce increases in cervical compliance of the order of 20-fold.

In the body the exact mechanisms that produce the changes in cervical state are not yet known. However, the process can be recognized clinically in what is known as *ripening* and can be documented by using semi-objective means, e.g. the Bishop score (cervical consistency, dilatation, length, position within the pelvis and station of the presenting part). It is known that oestrogens and prostaglandins promote ripening.

Effacement is shortening of the cervix to the point where it sometimes has barely any thickness. The redistribution of tissue from the cervix to the lower part of the uterus, just above the cervix, is recognized clinically as *formation of the lower segment*. The process of ripening facilitates this redistribution by permitting the tissues to become more 'fluid' and thus to 'flow'.

Formation of the lower segment permits the head to begin its descent down the birth canal. This is recognized clinically as engagement of the presenting part.

Dilatation can take place once the cervix has become compliant and once effacement has taken place. For women in their first labour, the processes, generally speaking, follow the sequence ripening, effacement and dilatation. In second and subsequent labours, dilatation will often be taking place while the other processes are occurring. Why this should be so is unclear, but the process of the first labour is unlike those that follow and there are marked differences between the behaviour of nulliparas and multiparas.

Labour Onset and Progress

The Onset

It is highly likely that the agents which determine the onset of labour are manufactured within the uterus and act over relatively short distances – this is known as the *paracrine* effect. This makes investigation difficult because both access to specimens is problematic and the agents involved in labour are short-lived because of rapid degradation.

The trigger is unknown. In the mother, levels of oestrogens rise as pregnancy progresses giving them dominance over progesterone, the hormone that maintains pregnancy. This increases myometrial activity and 'ripens' the cervix (**Figure 9.1**). Prostaglandin production and storage in the decidua between the membranes and the wall of the uterus is also promoted by oestrogens. Prostaglandins promote both uterine activity and cervical ripening. They 'potentiate' the effects of oxytocin, i.e. in small amounts prostaglandins amplify the effect of oxytocin. Oxytocin levels reach a plateau in early pregnancy. There is no peak at the time of labour, but the release of prostaglandins at the onset of labour permits oxytocin to have its effect.

The fetus may play a part. The fetal adrenals, in conjunction with the placenta, synthesize oestrogens (particularly oestriol) and the fetal pituitary is known to release oxytocin. How much influence the fetus has is unknown.

Thus, by the end of pregnancy the scene is set for the uterus to contract and the cervix to undergo ripening ready to efface and dilate. Proper integration of these processes is the key to efficient labour.

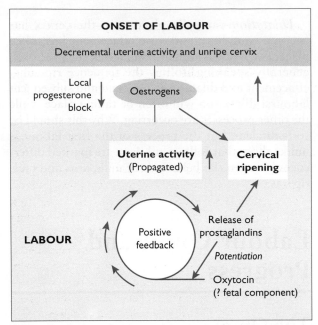

Figure 9.1 Proposed schema for the transition from pregnancy to labour.

There is some evidence to show that contractions release prostaglandins, perhaps by simple disruption of the decidua. These prostaglandins further potentiate the effect of oxytocin, creating more frequent and stronger contractions. *This is a positive feedback system.* Nature usually works with negative feedbacks, which are safe; i.e. the stimulus is cut off as the action increases. Positive feedback, however, drives itself until there is a break in the process. For labour this is delivery. If labour is obstructed, the process may continue until the uterus ruptures! This is certainly the case for multiparas, but for some unknown reason not in nulliparas whose uteruses tend to become inert. Stimulation of the uterus with either oxytocin or prostaglandins has to be done with care otherwise the lack of a natural safety valve can easily result in overstimulation.

Interaction of Cervix and Myometrium

When the myometrium contracts it generates tension within the wall of the uterus (Gee *et al.* 1988). This tension is transmitted to the cervix which, if compliant, will deform. Initially, this results in effacement and subsequently dilatation. When the cervical tissue has been redistributed and dilated to the point where there is continuity between the uterus and the vagina,

i.e. no cervix can be detected by clinical examination, the term 'full dilatation' is used; at this point the first stage ends and the second begins.

There is an important paradox which is evident in everyday practice. Multiparous women dilate their cervixes more rapidly than nulliparous women (Beazley and Kurjak, 1972), which could be attributed to more uterine activity but in fact they do it with less (Al-Shawaf *et al.* 1987). The cervix and its ability to ripen more efficiently must be the key. The ripe, compliant cervix not only dilates more readily, but also dissipates some of the wall tension created by the myometrium, thereby producing an apparent reduction in uterine activity.

Effects of Labour on Placental Circulation

Placental perfusion is impaired during each contraction (Borell *et al.* 1964; Janbu and Neshein, 1987). Some studies have related this to intrauterine pressure (Borell *et al.* 1964), suggesting that blood flow is markedly reduced or even ceases when intrauterine pressure rises above the blood pressure in the uterine arteries that lead to the placenta – at about 35 mmHg. This does not necessarily mean that the fetus is compromised. The fetus has several minutes of oxygen within its own circulation. Providing relaxation of the contraction occurs on time and there is adequate time between contractions for recovery of oxygen saturation, the fetus has no problems. It is merely like us holding our breath. However, if we overstimulate the uterus so that the fetus cannot recover between contractions, or if the fetus is already compromised, a cumulative asphyxia may result.

Fetal tolerance places a limit on the forces which can be employed and the duration over which it can be applied (Gee and Olah, 1993).

Progress of Labour

Efficient progress in labour depends upon the interaction of the following three variables:
- Powers.
- Passages.
- Passenger.

The *passenger* has changed little (Gee, 1994). The geometry of the head is complex. Its degree of flexion or deflexion affects the presenting dimensions. Flexion and rotation are encouraged by the relative geometries of head and pelvis and by effective powers. Since we have no control over the former, it has become customary to concentrate on manipulating the powers when the mechanism of labour gives rise to delay.

The *passages* are usually equated with the bony pelvis. In times gone, by pelvic pathology due to poor nutrition in childhood and adolescence gave rise to deformation of the pelvis, resulting in marked reductions in pelvic dimensions. Cephalo-pelvic disproportion (CPD) was the result. Frank cephalo-pelvic disproportion (CPD) is rare in the UK today (Gee, 1994), yet an undue emphasis is placed upon the pelvis. Two-thirds of women who require Caesarean delivery for 'failure to progress' in their first labours deliver successfully in their second, despite the same pelvis and the probability of a larger baby. The absence of pelvic pathology is almost certainly why pelvimetry is rarely used now because it carries little prognostic value.

The *soft tissues* have been relegated to the second division. In the first stage, the cervix offers resistance and in the second, the pelvic floor. Episiotomy is a surgical cure for obstruction from the latter and Caesarean section for the former. It is a pity that the pharmacological means of manipulating the cervical state has not been persued with the same vigour that has been seen with the myometrium. That the cervix can obstruct labour is conjectural by there are a lot of clues to this effect and abnormal biochemistry in the cervical connective tissues has been associated with delay (Ganstrom *et al.* 1991).

The *powers* have received most attention. The physiology of smooth muscle was well researched during the 1960s and the availability of oxytocin added a further stimulus. Of the 3 P's, the powers is the only one over which we have developed any influence short of resorting to surgery and the increased morbidity and mortality which is incurred.

in the latent phase and dilating properly in the active phase. The latent phase begins at the onset of labour and finishes at about 3 cm dilatation, by which time the cervix has usually effaced. The active phase lies between 3 cm and full dilatation (**Figure 9.2**; Friedman, 1967).

There are two fundamental problems with the management of labour – knowing when labour has begun and deciding whether labour is in the latent or active phases. Labour can be assumed to be present when there are regular, strong contractions that result in cervical change; the active phase is not entered unless 3 cm dilatation has been reached. Some define labour only when there are signs of active cervical dilatation; with such a definition, the latent phase does not exist. Delay in the latent phase does not respond well to oxytocin (Cardozo *et al.* 1982; Chelmow *et al.* 1993).

Friedman determined that cervical dilatation in the active phase should ideally achieve a minimum of 1 cm/hour. He rarely found straightforward deliveries with rates less than this but this limit has not been statistically determined for a given population.

There is no upper limit for progress above which labour should be slowed down even if we had the means. Terms like precipitate labour and precipitate delivery in relation to spontaneous labour had validity until it was recognised that the morbidity and mortality associated with them were the result of delivery in inappropriate settings rather than the speed of the process *per se*.

Monitoring Progress

Cervicography is the graphical recording of cervical dilatation with time in labour. Cervicograms are an aid to the management of labour (Beazley and Kurjak, 1972; Philpott and Castle, 1972; Studd, 1973). They are not, in themselves, a diagnosis. Poor progress may be due to a number of factors: poor contractions, malposition, malpresentation, CPD or obstruction from the soft tissues. Clinical assessment may establish a cause but often this is not the case, demonstrating how far short we are from an ideal understanding of the processes.

Cervimetrically, the first stage of labour, may be divided into two portions – the latent and active phases. For practical purposes the cervix is effacing

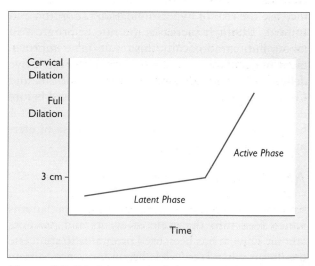

Figure 9.2 Friedman cervimetric pattern.

Patho-Physiology of Management Interventions

Oxytocin

Oxytocin is a peptide released from the posterior part of the pituitary, and is usually given intravenously in labour. It increases the firing rate of quiescent smooth muscle cells and slows the conduction of electrical activity, thereby encouraging recruitment of more muscle fibres per contraction and hence increasing the strength of weak contractions (Caldeyro-Barcia *et al.* 1957). The sensitivity of the uterus varies greatly from one labour to the next, even for the same woman. Therefore, dosage is titrated against activity, the optimal contraction rate being three contractions every 10 minutes.

The increase in uterine activity is initially proportional to dosage. As contraction frequency increases beyond this, the amplitude of contractions declines and the basal tone rises (Caldeyro-Barcia *et al.* 1957). This is serious because placental blood flow is restricted, as noted earlier, and there is decreasing intervals between contractions for recovery. Therefore, fetal distress is the usual result of over-stimulation. Luckily, oxytocin is rapidly degraded. Stopping the infusion when hyperstimulation occurs results in loss of effect within 2–3 minutes. Uterine relaxants such as the β-adrenogenic agent ventolin can also be used.

In clinical trials, oxytocin has been shown to increase the amount of pain the mother perceives and increase the risk of hyperstimulation (Thornton and Lilford, 1994). It increases the rate of progress in labour but, paradoxically, this results in no improvement in outcome in terms of decrease in operative deliveries nor in neonatal well-being (Thornton and Lilford, 1994). When oxytocin has been used before delivery it is customary to maintain it for at least 1 hour afterwards, as otherwise there is a risk of uterine atony and postpartum haemorrhage.

Amniotomy

Amniotomy releases endogenous prostaglandins which feed into the cycle of events and promote labour. Thus, it has been used profitably to stimulate the uterus when labour has begun but is not 'getting into gear' so to speak. However, it does commit us to delivery within a relatively short period of time, say 24 hours, because the procedure almost invariably introduces infections. Arguments for its ability to improve the forces between the head and cervix have not been substantiated.

Clinical trials on its routine use in labour show that it results in slightly faster labour (by about half an hour), but this confers no benefit in terms of operative delivery rates or neonatal well-being (UK Amniotomy Group, 1994). It may reduce the incidence of hyperstimulation when used with oxytocin. Therefore most practitioners combine the two if intervention is to be made.

Summary and Conclusion

The onset of labour demands integration of events in both the myometrium and the cervix. Prolonged labour is associated with increased morbidity and mortality of mother and child. The major part of labour management is directed towards detecting delay. Unfortunately, interventions like amniotomy and oxytocin which augment the powers and accelerate the rate of progress have not produced the expected improvements in clinical outcome (Frigoletto *et al.* 1995; Cammu *et al.* 1996). This should stimulate us to ask why. Perhaps events outside the myometrium should be considered. It may be that subtle changes elsewhere may be fruitfully considered; e.g. in the cervix and/or general make up and well-being of the mother.

Clinical Management of Labour: A Midwifery Perspective

Every childbearing woman in the UK has the right to midwifery care in labour in whatever environment she chooses to have her baby. Her experience of labour may remain etched in her memory for many years, if not for ever, and will be revisited and retold on many occasions. This fact is evident to any midwife who has cared for a woman in labour in the presence of a female companion who has herself given birth. The readiness of women to discuss their own labour experience and the detail recalled gives some idea of the importance of this life event and the emotions that it arouses, even many years later.

Role of the Midwife

The midwife is in the privileged position of providing care and support during a vulnerable time in a woman's life. Her responsibility is to monitor the condition of the mother and the fetus *in utero*, to recognize any abnormality that may require referral to a doctor and to act appropriately. The aim of midwifery care is to deliver a healthy baby to a healthy, satisfied mother. Supporting and encouraging the mother helps to reduce anxiety. A meta-analysis of controlled trials compared the effects of continuous intrapartum support by a trained support person (who may or may not have had obstetric training and was not necessarily known to the mother previously) with usual hospital care. The results consistently showed clear benefits (Hodnett, 1994). 'Support' included continuous presence during the period of active labour, if not for the whole of labour – in 8 out of 11 trials comforting touch and words of praise and encouragement were the minimum. The result was a reduction in the need for pain-relieving medication and operative vaginal birth, and an Apgar score of more than 7 at 5 minutes. No known risks were demonstrated and some trials showed a more positive evaluation of the labour experience. This reflects the effect of support and encouragement generally seen as part of the role of the midwife.

Social and psychological support must also take into account cultural differences. Midwives need to be aware of different cultural backgrounds to meet the specific needs of the various ethnic groups. Stereotyping of women from ethnic groups may lead to a lower standard of care and a feeling of resentment (Alibhai, 1988). Asian women who did not say please and thank you caused some offence to midwives who did not realize that these words were rarely used in Urdu (Bowler, 1993). The important principle is to treat everyone as an individual regardless of background and to tailor midwifery care to each individual's specific needs. Need can only be assessed where there is adequate communication and a willingness to listen.

The mother has a need for information on her progress in labour in order to be able to make choices and she needs to be reassured if labour is progressing normally. We are advised that words have a very strong influence, both positive and negative; indeed, in the case of pregnancy and childbirth words are remembered in detail and often quoted 10–15 years later (Flint, 1986). When a group of women were interviewed 15–20 years after their first birth their recollections were extremely clear and so emotionally charged that 9 out of 20 wept as they relived the experience (Simkin, 1991).

This partnership between the mother and the midwife develops if there is communication and trust. An observational study of information-giving in labour revealed that the communication skills required to satisfy the mother's need for information are not always evident within the midwifery profession (Kirkham, 1989). Midwives were seen effectively to block conversation by failing to answer questions or by changing the subject, although when questioned all stated the importance of satisfying the mother's need for information. The *Changing Childbirth* report (Department of Health, 1993) echoed the recommendations of the Winterton report (House of Commons, 1992), advocating choice, continuity and control for childbearing women and recommending 'woman-centred' care. To provide effectively the information necessary for the mother to be in a position to make an informed choice midwives must constantly update their practice. The standard of practice expected from the midwife '... shall be that which is acceptable in the context of current knowledge and clinical developments' (UKCC, 1994). Maternal satisfaction is as important an outcome measure as morbidity, particularly with regard to interventions in labour (Walkinshaw, 1994). Care in labour is therefore a balancing act between the priorities of the midwife to provide a safe standard of care and the needs of the mother to enjoy the benefits of a positive experience of labour (Drayton, 1990). Imagine, then, the significant contribution of supportive, professional care to the whole process of labour, when given by a well-informed midwife who is able to empower the mother.

Midwifery care in labour requires a sympathetic, well-informed midwife capable of:

- Providing emotional support and encouragement.
- Observing and recording fetal and maternal conditions throughout labour.
- Recognizing any deviation from normal and taking appropriate action.

The First Stage of Labour

The early stage of labour often takes place in the woman's own home, even if a hospital birth is planned, with the preference being to remain there until such time as the contractions become regular and strong. If a home birth is planned, preparations for this can be finalized and the family can settle in for the birth. The woman and her partner are best prepared if they have an understanding of the process of labour and have had prior opportunity to discuss the options available. The midwife at this stage needs to reassure the couple that all is well and to agree on the plan of care. Some mothers are keen to document their preferences for labour, whereas others are content to await events and deal with them as they arise. The advantages of the 'known' midwife are in evidence at this stage of the pregnancy, as both mother and midwife know the preferences expressed and the discussions which have taken place and so ideally are working from a mutually agreed knowledge base. It is important that the initial assessment and record of progress are documented in the mother's notes, along with an agreed plan of care. This may be invaluable if another opinion is sought, if there is any need to question any decisions or actions or if care is handed to another person.

The first stage of labour is generally recognized as being from the onset of regular uterine contractions to full dilatation of the cervix. As a woman may experience several 'false starts' this is usually modified to 'pains plus progress', and as such is often a retrospective diagnosis. Care must be taken in confirming a diagnosis of labour, as the decision may initiate intervention for failure to progress in a labour which was not properly established in the first place. Care in a supportive environment with adequate fluid intake and such foods as the mother may wish to eat help maintain her physical and mental well-being. The freedom to remain mobile and active during contractions not only helps alleviate the discomfort of labour, but also allows the mother to retain an element of control. The inclusion of the partner and any support people in the discussion helps to foster a good relationship and enhance the confidence of the mother, while respecting her choice.

Latent Phase of Labour

The stage of labour from 0 to 3 cm is known as the latent phase, which, if acknowledged, is recognized as being from the onset of regular uterine contractions to the beginning of the active phase. The recommended maximum duration of this phase varies; it has been stated as 20 hours in primiparous women and 16 hours in multiparous women (Friedman, 1978). A working party set up by the World Health Organization (WHO)

recommended in 1988 that this phase of labour should not last longer than 8 hours, but it is important that care be tailored to the individual rather than blanket policies be applied (Walsh, 1994). This can be an extremely demoralizing time, as the contractions may be sufficiently painful to prevent adequate rest and the apparent lack of progress may be seen as a sign that labour is not proceeding 'normally'. It is important to understand that descent of the presenting part and effacement of the cervix are the indicators of progress at this stage. Coping mechanisms, such as relaxation, hydrotherapy and transcutaneous nerve stimulation or any distraction techniques, along with explanation, reassurance and patience should help to instil confidence. Home is probably the ideal place for many mothers at this stage of labour, but for when it occurs in the hospital environment an appropriate area needs to be provided where care can be given without detriment to other client groups and without undue haste to 'augment' the labour process. Reports that prolonged latent phases result in an increased Caesarean section rate can be criticized for including women who may not actually have been in labour (Walsh, 1994).

The decision to enter the hospital environment is usually made by the mother herself when she feels it is appropriate. Admission to hospital may increase the mother's anxiety levels, which can have a diminishing effect on the strength and frequency of contractions; this is usually transitory, but it may reduce the mother's self-confidence. Adrenaline is known to reduce uterine muscle contractions and an increased concentration of plasma adrenaline has been associated with anxiety and prolonged duration of labour (Zuspan *et al.* 1962; Lederman *et al.* 1978). When two systems of care were compared, that which delayed admission to hospital had a beneficial effect by reducing interventions and improving labour outcomes; this suggests that a longer hospital stay rather than a longer labour is a detrimental factor (Klein *et al.* 1983).

Active Phase of Labour

The active phase of labour is generally recognized as being from 3 cm onwards in the presence of regular uterine activity. Contractions become progressively stronger and closer together until approximately 3–4 contractions occur every 10 minutes. Induced or augmented labours may result in hyperstimulation of the uterus, in which as many as 5 contractions occur in 10 minutes. This allows very little respite for the mother and baby and does not mimic the normal labour process.

The midwife is the monitor of labour. Electronic equipment is often used to provide a continuous recording of fetal heart rate and uterine activity, and may facilitate the monitoring process. Injudicious use of such equipment may give rise to a false sense of security in the belief that a printed record demonstrates a good standard of care. In the absence of a good reason to use electronic fetal monitoring and without a professional suitably trained to interpret the information it may hinder the monitoring process.

Careful monitoring of the progress of labour is required to detect deviations from normal and initiate the appropriate intervention to maximize the chances of a low-risk outcome. However, the normal rate of progress for one woman may not be normal for another so account has to be made for variations when guidelines and protocols are drawn up. The partograph is a composite record of a woman's general condition, well-being of the fetus and also a graphic record of the progress of labour and descent of the fetus (cervicograph). The record itself does not display how the woman is feeling; therefore it is important for the midwife to actively communicate with the woman throughout. The partograph and how the woman feels are both important. The partograph has been in use since 1970 to provide a graphic record of labour (WHO, 1988). This not only provides a rapid means of recording large amounts of data, but when used properly aids the diagnosis of normal or abnormal progress in labour. WHO (1988) advocated the use of an alert line and an action line on the cervicograph (**Figure 9.3**) to facilitate the recognition of prolonged labour and allow arrangements to be made for transfer to an appropriate setting, if required. This is particularly important in areas of the developing world where cephalopelvic disproportion may result in obstructed labour, maternal dehydration and exhaustion, uterine rupture and vesicovaginal fistula. Prolonged labour also predisposes to maternal sepsis, postpartum haemorrhage (PPH) and neonatal infection. However, well-planned alert and action lines may also reduce the risk of unnecessarily aggressive management in countries where intervention in the normal labour process is common.

It is important to involve the partner or other support persons actively in the care of the mother. Although midwives are aware that pain may be considered a normal aspect of labour, the distress at witnessing such discomfort in a loved one may require frequent reassurance and explanation.

The midwife monitors:
- **The condition of the mother,** which involves observation and recording of pulse, blood pressure and temperature (at appropriate intervals), urinalysis (to detect the presence of protein or ketones) and assessment of psychological well-being. Positive efforts may be required to encourage frequent micturition to aid the progress of labour and

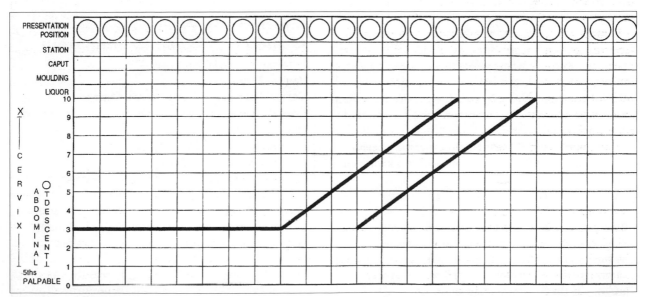

Figure 9.3 Cervicograph (part of the partograph indicating progress) showing alert line (top) and action line (bottom). (Courtesy of Liverpool Women's Hospital.)

maintain comfort. Assessment of psychological well-being is equally important – observation of how the mother is coping with contractions and ensuring that she is kept informed of progress facilitate choice regarding position and method of pain relief (*see* Chapter 10). The frequency of recording vital signs depends on the history and progress in labour, but generally for temperature is every 4 hours and for pulse rate at least every 2 hours in established labour.

- **The condition of the fetus,** which involves regular observation and recording of the fetal heart rate and rhythm, and interpretation of the cardiotocograph recording (if used) and of the colour of the amniotic fluid (if known). Fetal heart rate is usually recorded at least half hourly and often quarter-hourly in the light of information regarding intermittent fetal heart-rate monitoring as recommended by Spencer and Ward (1993).

- **The progress of labour** – cervical dilatation is the prime parameter of progress in the first stage. The frequency, strength and duration of contractions need to be assessed and documented. Dilatation, continuing painful contractions and descent of the presenting part are all indicators of progress.

In cephalic presentations the assessment of how much of the head is palpable above the pelvic brim (usually measured in fifths) is a skill that can be learned. It provides evidence of descent of the fetal head. Vaginal examination to assess cervical effacement and dilatation provides evidence of progress and more information about the descent, position and attitude of the fetus (flexion or extension of the head). Vaginal examination should always be preceded by abdominal palpation (**Box 9.1**).

Vaginal examination in many units is performed at regular intervals, often approximately every 4 hours, but logically should be performed when any information gained is likely to be both meaningful and provide a basis on which to either initiate change or reassure that all is well (**Box 9.2**). It is helpful if examinations are performed by the same person, since assessment of dilatation, caput succedaneum and moulding are subjective, any progressive changes are more likely to be noted. Vaginal examinations can be

---

Box 9.1

Information Which May Be Gained by Abdominal Palpation

Fundal height. Small or large for gestational age may influence management, particularly with regard to monitoring a growth retarded fetus.

Number of fetuses. Undiagnosed twins are now rare with the frequent use of ultrasound scanning, but not every woman has a scan.

Lie of fetus. Oblique or transverse lie causes obstructed labour. Should be longitudinal.

Presentation. Breech presentation is frequently undetected in pregnancy. Normally cephalic.

Position. Knowing where the fetal back is assists with auscultation of the heart beat.

Descent. Engaged or not engaged; fifths palpable above the pelvic brim demonstrate progressive descent of the head over a period of time.

Attitude. Flexion or extension of the head in a cephalic presentation may be determined, provided it is known on which side the fetal back is.

Uterine activity. Frequency, duration and strength of contractions.

Bladder. A full bladder is usually easily palpated in labour as the organ becomes displaced up into the abdomen. A full bladder is not only uncomfortable, but can also hinder descent of the presenting part and may predispose to problems in the third stage of labour.

Box 9.2

Information Which May Be Gained by Vaginal Examination

External genitalia. Normality.

Vagina. Normality.

Cervix. Position, consistency, length, dilatation.

Presentation. Cephalic, breech, face, brow, compound, cord presentation.
- Attitude of flexion and/or extension.
- Well or poorly applied to cervix.
- Caput succedaneum, cephal haematoma and/or moulding.

Position. Identifying landmarks, e.g. fontanelles, buttocks.

Station. Above or below ischial spines.

Membranes. Intact or ruptured.

Liquor. Colour and amount.

Note: Any history of bleeding before means that vaginal examination should not be performed.

performed in whatever position the woman feels most comfortable. As the orientation will be different, the midwife may find it useful to draw a diagram of her findings to interpret the position (Flint, 1986).

Midwives and obstetricians need to be sensitive to the woman's feelings when performing vaginal examinations. The procedure may be extremely uncomfortable – simply reassuring the woman that the examiner will stop if the woman so requests, and complying with this, can make all the difference. Also, some women may have suffered sexual abuse, so vaginal examination may reawaken traumatic feelings. The feeling of powerlessness felt by survivors of childhood sexual abuse during such examinations has been described (Menage, 1993; Cassin, 1996), and flashbacks may be experienced during childbirth because of the intensity of the experience (Kitzinger, 1990); since as many as 25% of midwifery clients may have experienced sexual abuse (Tidy, 1996) midwives need to be aware of and sensitive to behavioural clues. Also, there is a difference between consent to vaginal examination and acquiescence (Clement, 1994).

Nutrition in Labour

It is a widely held belief that food and drink should be withheld once labour has begun. The risk of regurgitation and aspiration of acidic gastric contents during obstetric anaesthesia was first described by Mendelson (1946). This is a serious complication and was the cause of two maternal deaths between 1988 and 1990 (Department of Health, 1994). However, prohibiting food and fluid intake for all women in labour on the assumption that they may require an anaesthetic at some stage is too restrictive, especially as there is no guarantee that withholding food and drink ensures that the stomach is empty. A more serious outcome of restricting food is the development of ketosis, which impairs myometrial activity. Small meals of low-fat, low-residue food at frequent intervals, if required, have been advocated, particularly when no problems are envisaged (Crawford, 1978). Hunger is an unpleasant experience and, although many women have no desire to eat in labour, the denial of food to someone who is using a great deal of energy and who wishes to eat is unreasonable. Adequate fluids should be provided to prevent dehydration – hot drinks may be comforting and may bring a semblance of normality. Delayed gastric emptying has been demonstrated in labouring women who received opiate analgesia (Nimmo *et al.* 1975) so a limited oral intake may be beneficial, but fluids

should still be available. Policies aimed at preventing gastric aspiration, such as food and fluid restriction and routine administration of antacids in labour, are partly effective but offer no guarantees; the recommendation is for good anaesthesia technique if a general anaesthetic should be required (Johnson *et al.* 1989). The belief that women in early labour should be encouraged to load up on carbohydrate and fluids to prepare for the work of active labour (Hazle, 1986) appears to be a sensible suggestion and could be done in the form of small frequent snacks.

Position and Mobility

'The important factor when a woman is in labour is not where she finally delivers but the ability to move around restlessly during labour' (Flint, 1986). In medieval Europe women were expected to continue household duties until the second stage of labour. By adopting an upright posture for labour many women find it easier to cope with pain and are able to rock or rotate the pelvis at will and to use the effect of gravity to aid descent of the fetus. This mobility can also help the mother to feel in control. It is said that Louis XIV promoted the dorsal position for birth to allow him to observe his mistress during the birth process (Gupta and Lilford, 1987). The custom of women taking to their beds in labour is believed to have gained favour as men became more involved in midwifery and obstetrics about 300 years ago (Milner, 1986). The dorsal position risks causing compression of the maternal venae cavae with resultant fetal hypoxia (Humphrey *et al.* 1974). The ability to freely change posture and position can be used to widen the pelvic diameters and affect the progress of labour. Walking up and down stairs has been used to aid descent of a high head, as it is believed that movement of the lumbar spine enables the head to enter the pelvis (Stevenson, 1994). Crawling on all fours is thought to aid rotation from an occipitoposterior position to an anterior position – it may be performed before labour begins or may be comfortable in labour (Flint, 1986). Women need to be able to adopt positions to suit during labour; those that increase the pelvic outlet, usually upright or squatting (as adopted by primitive peoples), can aid the progress of labour (Russell, 1982). A review of the literature on upright versus recumbent posture in labour shows that there is less need for analgesia or augmentation of labour when upright postures are used (Nikodem, 1994). As no adverse effects on maternal, fetal or neonatal conditions were demonstrated, the benefits of mobilization and upright positions need to be communicated to women in labour and the choice left to them. The fetal heart can be monitored by using hand-held Doppler equipment, which does not interfere with mobility.

Interventions

Any interference with the natural process of labour needs to be carefully considered on an individual basis. The effects of one intervention may actually necessitate another, so initiating a 'cascade of interventions' where each one may reduce the chance of a favourable outcome (Inch, 1989).

Artificial rupture of the membranes

Artificial rupture of the membranes (ARM) may have been practised as long ago as 100 AD by Soranus of Greece; since the middle of the 18th century it has been used in the management of labour. By the end of the 1970s ARM was an almost routine procedure in labour, as it was believed to shorten the duration of labour and so be beneficial. One survey based on 3000 self-completed questionnaires showed that ARM was most commonly performed at a dilatation of 3–5 cm, was less common in home deliveries, resulted in an increase in the rate and strength of contractions and a greater need for pain relief (Newburn and Borton, 1989). A multicentre, randomized, controlled trial was conducted on 1463 nulliparous women in spontaneous labour at term with a singleton, cephalic fetus. One group had ARM early in labour and the control group was left as long as possible. It was shown that routine early ARM resulted in only a modest shortening of labour with no affect on Caesarean section rate, operative vaginal birth, use of analgesia, blood transfusion or neonatal intubation and so could not be recommended (UK Amniotomy Group, 1994).

ARM in early labour has been shown to result in more cardiotocograph abnormalities, particularly in the last hour of labour, and in an increased use of epidural analgesia (Barrett *et al.* 1992). The overall consensus is that the membranes should be left intact when labour is progressing normally. However, there are those who believe in the Active Management of labour.

Active Management of Labour

The Active Management of labour is an empirical approach to the management of labour first documented in 1969 by Professor O'Driscoll and colleagues (O'Driscoll *et al.* 1969; Duignan, 1985) from the National Maternity Hospital, Dublin. 'Empirical' here means a form of care put in place which is thought to be beneficial but may have no sound scientific basis. It should have been tested by clinical trial, but this has happened only recently.

No purpose was seen in defining poor uterine activity or malrotation of the head because, at the end of the day, the only influence available was via the powers, using oxytocin.

The study was confined to nulliparous women and was prospective but uncontrolled. Oxytocin stimulation in nulliparas was deemed safe. Care was taken to define labour, amniotomy was performed early to check for meconium, parenteral narcotics were used for analgesia and progress was determined by regular cervical assessment. Progress was considered aberrant if the rate of cervical dilatation fell below 1 cm/h, in which case oxytocin was administered.

As 55% of the women required oxytocin, this became the 'norm'. The Caesarean section rate was only 5%. Unfortunately, because there were no controls, it is impossible to say whether these data (which took 25 years to produce) represent improvement over prior practice.

Meta-analysis (the statistical lumping together of research data to produce enough for further analysis) has failed to show any major benefits from the individual components of Active Management (Thornton and Lilford, 1994). In fact, Active Management was originally devised to solve a problem with the throughput of patients in a delivery suite. The fact that no woman had prolonged labour – they were either delivered vaginally or by Caesarean section – meant the each woman was allocated a midwife to provide support for the duration of the labour. It is this component which appears to have a beneficial effect.

Two studies from the USA examined the whole package of 'Active Management' (Lopez-Zeno *et al.* 1992; Frigoletto *et al.* 1995). One claimed to show a marked reduction in Caesarean section due to Active Management, but this was only achieved by removing certain categories of patient. The other showed no change in operative delivery rates. A third study also showed no benefit (Cammu and van Eeckhout, 1995). Two of these randomized studies show how an intervention, in these cases the performance of research into labour, produced apparent reductions in operative delivery. The original claims for Active Management may have been caused by this effect rather than the measures being researched, an effect known as the Hawthorne effect. Its presence is the reason for conducting randomized controlled trials whenever possible to test the benefits of clinical interventions.

Thus, Active Management, although clear, simple and thus attractive, was not rigorously tested until recently. In most peoples' hands it has not lived up to expectations. Failure to progress in labour is still the major indication for Caesarean section (Kiwanuka and Moore, 1987).

Induction of labour

Providing that pregnancy is progressing normally, most women wait for the spontaneous onset of labour. Induction of labour is most likely for post-term pregnancy which, by definition, is 42 weeks or more (WHO, 1977). Post-term pregnancy appears to be more common in primigavidae and women with previous post-term births (Alfirevic and Walkinshaw, 1994). There is evidence that pregnancies of more than 42 weeks' duration have a higher perinatal mortality rate (Bakketig and Bergsjo, 1989). Although not all post-term pregnancies are pathological, there is no agreement so far as to what constitutes a safe method of assessing pregnancies which go beyond 42 weeks (Alfirevic and Walkinshaw, 1994). Sweeping of the membranes, involving detachment of the membranes from the lower uterine segment during digital vaginal examination, successfully induces labour in prolonged pregnancy (Grant, 1993). This procedure may be uncomfortable, but may be considered preferable to an oxytocic infusion or vaginal prostaglandin.

Women need to be adequately prepared for induction of labour, so appropriate explanation must be given before an individual consents to this procedure. Some women may see induction as an easy way out of an uncomfortable pregnancy but may not be aware of any associated risks. If the midwife has a good relationship with the woman she can 'prescribe' natural methods of inducing labour, such as sexual intercourse [prostaglandin, which is present in large amounts in seminal fluid, is effective in bringing about cervical 'ripening' (Gaskin, 1991)]. Care must be taken when labour is induced with prostaglandin or oxytocin to avoid uterine hyperstimulation. Induced labours are generally longer and associated with more instrumental deliveries, an increased risk of PPH and a higher incidence of low Apgar scores than are spon-

taneous labours. Consideration needs to be given to individual risk factors when induction is contemplated (Cardozo, 1993).

These data must be interpreted against the background of the indication. Induction of labour would not normally be within the province of the midwife's role; i.e. she would not normally be the decision maker regarding management.

Fetal heart rate monitoring

Assessment of fetal well-being during labour involves regular auscultation of the fetal heart rate to detect changes that may be significant. Pinard is credited with the introduction of the fetal stethoscope in 1876, although apparently his was not the first version (Gibb and Arulkumaran, 1992). Electronic fetal heart rate monitoring (EFM) became popular in the 1970s, after the association between fetal acidosis and changes in the fetal heart rate was found (Beard *et al.* 1971); it was introduced without prior evaluation or research into its benefits in general for women in labour. It was assumed that continuous monitoring would detect those fetuses likely to suffer damage caused by intrapartum asphyxia, thus ensuring delivery before permanent neurological damage could occur.

Although there was a fall in the stillbirth and perinatal mortality rate after the introduction of continuous EFM, it could not be attributed directly to this intervention. There was no demonstrable fall in incidence of cerebral palsy in normal birthweight infants, which was generally believed to be due to intrapartum asphyxia (Pharoah *et al.* 1990). The immobility imposed by continuous monitoring on women in labour was not always welcome and predisposed to other interventions, such as an increased need for analgesia and a slower progress in labour [requiring oxytocin therapy (Inch, 1989)]. The use of continuous EFM increases the operative delivery rate, although this increase is less when EFM is used in conjunction with fetal blood sampling (MacDonald *et al.* 1985; Neilson, 1994).

Several trials have since explored the effects of continuous EFM versus intermittent auscultation. One particular study of 12,964 women looked at intermittent auscultation that involved, in the first stage of labour, every 15 minutes listening to the fetal heart for 60 s after a contraction and, in the second stage, listening for 60 s after every contraction (MacDonald *et al.* 1985). Fetal blood sampling was used in both continuous and intermittent groups when required. Although there were more neonatal seizures in the intermittent monitoring group, equal numbers in each group were found to have severe disabilities at 1 year of age. The results suggest that continuous EFM confers no benefit over intermittent monitoring in medium-risk and low-risk women, other than in relatively long labours. The findings that continuous monitoring in low risk women predisposes to increased intervention with no benefit to mother or baby were reflected in a report by the 26th RCOG Study Group on Fetal Surveillance (Spencer and Ward, 1993) whose recommendations include:

- 'Fetal monitoring is an integrated part of, not a substitute for, care and support during labour and should be conducted in a manner suited to the needs and wishes of the woman.'
- 'There should be written guidelines for the practice of fetal surveillance within each provider unit, be it a consultant unit, general practitioner unit, community hospital or a midwifery practice.'
- 'Auscultation is the method of choice for women at the normal end of the continuum of fetal risk.' A Doppler device is recommended if the mother is mobile.
- 'The standard of intermittent auscultation evaluated by randomized controlled trial is as follows: auscultation for one complete minute beginning immediately after the end of a contraction, repeated every 15 minutes during the first stage

and while not pushing in the second stage, and after every maternal effort while pushing. All values should be recorded.'
- 'EFM should be used whenever there is an increased risk of fetal hypoxaemia and/or acidaemia developing during labour.'
- 'Difficulty in obtaining or interpreting a continuous fetal heart record, or difficulty in obtaining a fetal blood sample, are circumstances that require the involvement of senior medical staff.'
- 'EFM should not be used without the facility for fetal blood pH measurements.'

It should be remembered that a cardiotograph (CTG) is simply a screening test designed to detect those fetuses *at risk* of damage caused by hypoxia in labour (**Boxes 9.3** and **9.4**). This is true of all measures of fetal surveillance currently used, such as fetal pH, liquor volume and the presence of meconium. These tests are limited in their ability to reliably detect fetal hypoxia and must be recognized as such. It is recommended that the term 'fetal distress' should not be used (Spencer and Ward, 1993).

As there is now a wealth of evidence that continuous EFM of low-risk women is not only of no demonstrable benefit but is also potentially harmful, in that it risks unnecessary intervention, it is necessary to reduce the practice. This has not proved easy, as one review of 1000 consecutive postnatal transfers showed (Beckwith, 1995). Although the unit in question boasted a predominantly midwifery-led approach and 65% of their clientele was expected to be low risk, the survey showed that 64% of women received continuous EFM. It appeared that EFM was being used whenever there was any deviation from the normal so the notion of 'high risk' was explored.

Box 9.3

Factors Identifiable before Labour Which Suggest the Need for Continuous EFM

- Suspected intrauterine growth retardation.
- Antepartum haemorrhage.
- Hypertensive disorders.
- Medical disorders, e.g. diabetes, thyroid, renal and connective tissue.
- Previous caesarean section.
- Previous intrauterine death and/or bad obstetric history.
- Maternal substance abuse.
- Multiple pregnancy.
- Gestation greater than 42 weeks.
- Preterm.
- Abnormal antepartum fetal monitoring.
- Malpresentation.
- Liquor volume reduced or absent.

Box 9.4

Factors Identifiable during Labour Which Suggest the Need for Continuous EFM

- Maternal tachycardia and/or pyrexia.
- Maternal request.
- Prolonged, augmented or induced labour.
- Abnormal fetal heart rate on initial CTG or on auscultation.
- Presence of fresh meconium.

Attempts were made to establish strict criteria for EFM and to identify those women for whom it need not be used, such as those with epidural analgesia. Once instituted, the change of policy reduced the incidence of EFM from 64% to 24% with no adverse outcomes. One midwife's comment that CTG monitoring acted as a sort of talisman without which some midwives felt there was an increased risk of being accused of negligence (Symon, 1994), is probably an accurate reflection of midwives' fears of litigation.

EFM also allows a midwife to monitor simultaneously several women in labour, but this does not allow time to provide the individual support and encouragement which has proved to be beneficial. The introduction of central monitoring stations, which allow the CTGs of several women to be viewed from a central point, has the potential to further reduce the individual supervision and may be used inappropriately where there are staffing constraints (Spencer, 1994). There is some evidence to recommend a short CTG on admission of low-risk cases to identify the 'at risk' fetus not previously identified (Ingemarsson *et al.* 1986). There is not a consensus as to which women benefit from continuous monitoring. Some data suggest the use of EFM for those with previous Caesarean section, because fetal heart rate changes may indicate scar rupture, but this is not generally agreed (Scott, 1991). The restriction of mobility imposed by EFM may hinder the progress of labour and increase the chances of a Caesarean section being needed.

There is, however, no value in imposing continuous EFM on a woman when the pregnancy is believed to be at risk if the appropriate actions are not initiated in response to an abnormal trace. It is now believed that most cases of cerebral palsy result from events that occur in the antenatal period rather than from intrapartum events, although this may present as an abnormal CTG in labour (Freeman, 1990). A review of singleton, term, normally-formed babies who either died or developed cerebral palsy also concluded that birth events are contributing factors in only a few cases of cerebral palsy; however, this study also showed a failure to respond to signs of severe fetal distress in this group, particularly in those babies who died (Gaffney *et al.* 1994). CTGs were missing in a third of the cases where the baby died.

Cardiotograph Interpretation

When describing or discussing cardiotocographs it is important that the same language and classification be used by all the professionals involved, which can only be achieved by regular meetings to review clinical situations (Neilson, 1993). It is vital that the attendant has the knowledge to interpret the trace and knows the action to take if an abnormality arises. Interpretation of CTGs can be broken down into its basic components – baseline rate, variability, accelerations, and decelerations.

Baseline Rate

The normal baseline rate was accepted as being 120–160 beats per minute (b.p.m.) for many years, based on data gained by auscultation using Pinard's stethoscope. However, since the introduction of continuous EFM, a wealth of information has been recorded and the recommendation now is that a baseline rate of 110–150 b.p.m. should be regarded as normal for a term fetus (FIGO, 1987). The rate is modulated by baroreceptors, chemoreceptors and the autonomic nervous system (composed of the sympathetic and parasympathetic nervous systems). Sympathetic impulses increase the heart rate and parasympathetic impulses have the opposite effect. The sympathetic nervous system dominates in early pregnancy, which results in a higher baseline rate.

Baseline bradycardia

This is a baseline rate of less than 110 b.p.m. according to FIGO (1987) recommendations for more than 10 minutes. Less than 100 b.p.m. is usually considered a pathological pattern and a rate of less than 80 b.p.m. almost certainly results in fetal asphyxia unless action is taken. It is important to examine other factors of the trace, such as variability, and to consider earlier patterns.

Tachycardia

Tachycardia is a baseline rate of more than 150 b.p.m. at term (FIGO, 1987) for more than 10 minutes. The cause may be fetal hypoxia, maternal or fetal infection, drug treatment (e.g. β-adrenergic agents), extreme prematurity or fetal tachyarrhythmias.

Variability

Variability is generated by the constant interaction between the sympathetic and parasympathetic nervous systems. It has been described as the 'band width' of the baseline heart rate and measures the oscillatory amplitude (Gibb and Arulkumaran, 1992), which should be assessed during a period when there are no accelerations or decelerations. The normal is thought to be 11–25 b.p.m., although some accept 5–15 b.p.m. as being normal. Normal fetal heart rate variability is a very important indicator of fetal well-being. It may be reduced or absent as a result of cerebral or myocardial asphyxia, but it can also be reduced by drugs such as opiate analgesics and diazepam, the rest phase of fetal rest–activity cycles and, rarely, by cardiac conduction defects such as heart block (Wood and Dobbie, 1989).

Accelerations

An acceleration is a rise above the baseline of more than 15 beats for more than 15 seconds. Accelerations are considered to be a good prognostic sign and the presence of at least two in a 20-minute CTG is regarded as a reactive trace. The absence of accelerations may be the first indicator of a problem that affects the fetus.

Decelerations

A deceleration is a fall in the heart rate below the baseline of more than 15 beats for more than 15 seconds. Decelerations can be categorized according to their shape and their relationship to the time of contractions.

Early decelerations

Early decelerations (**Figure 9.4**) are synchronous with contractions and are associated with head compression of the fetus, usually during late first stage and the second stage of labour as the head descends further into the pelvis. The decelerations mirror the contractions. Early decelerations are not thought to be harmful.

Late decelerations

Late decelerations (**Figure 9.5**), as the name suggests, are late in relation to the timing of contraction. They are believed to be caused by poor blood flow to the uteroplacental space and indicate fetal hypoxia. The pattern occurs particularly in growth-retarded fetuses. The speed of recovery of the heart rate and the variability may indicate the degree of fetal compromise (Gibb and Arulkumaran, 1992). Sometimes the decelerations may be shallow and appear insignificant, but it is the *timing* that denotes the seriousness of these

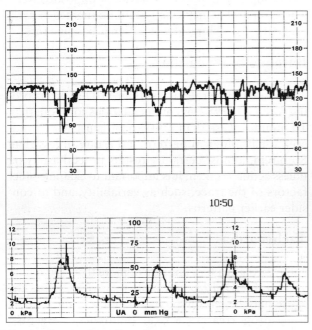

Figure 9.4 Early decelerations: top, fetal heart rate (FHR); bottom, uterine activity (UA).

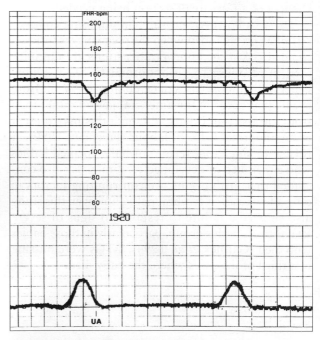

Figure 9.5 Late decelerations: top, fetal heart rate (FHR); bottom, uterine activity (UA).

decelerations. If the baseline variability is already reduced or absent then a deceleration does not have to reach 15 beats below the baseline to be significant. Reduced or absent variability with late decelerations is an ominous sign.

Variable decelerations

Variable decelerations (**Figure 9.6**) are the most common fetal heart rate pattern seen during labour. They are variable in timing and shape and often look dramatic, so give cause for concern. They are believed to be caused by a physiological response to cord compression. Early decelerations that fall to 40 beats or more below the baseline are usually classed as variable. During a contraction the cord becomes compressed, which results in an interruption of blood flow to the fetus. The soft-walled vein is affected first, restricting the oxygenated blood flow to the fetus and causing a fall in blood pressure. The healthy fetus responds by increasing its heart rate, seen as a small acceleration. As the pressure on the cord increases the stiffer walled arteries become compressed, leading to increased systemic pressure, so baroreceptors are stimulated and there is a rapid fall in heart rate. The lowest point of the deceleration is when both arteries and vein are occluded. As the cord compression is released the blood flow through the arteries is restored first and the process reverses.

The accelerations before and after the deceleration are called 'shouldering' and are typical of cord compression decelerations. Provided that the interval between contractions is sufficient to restore normal oxygenation a healthy fetus probably tolerates cord compression for a considerable time. A change in maternal position often relieves the compression and resolves the deceleration trace. These decelerations do not indicate fetal hypoxia if the trace shows good variability and accelerations. The important feature is how the trace changes over a period of time, particularly with regard to the baseline rate and baseline variability. A progressively developing hypoxia is usually indicated by reduced variability and a change in baseline rate (Gibb and Arulkumaran, 1992).

Other Factors

The deceleration is an expression of the insult, whereas the variability is an expression of fetal reserve (Gibb and Arulkumaran, 1992). A healthy, normally grown, term infant has good reserve and usually tolerates the stress of labour well. However, a CTG cannot be assessed in isolation – the clinical situation must be viewed as a whole. A CTG can only be classed as normal, suspicious or pathological and must be supported by fetal blood sampling to achieve a diagnosis.

Factors which affect the interpretation of CTGs and the actions taken are:
- Maturity of the fetus – earlier intervention may be required in preterm labour.
- Uterine activity – hyperstimulation of the uterus can be corrected.
- Stage of labour – changes in the CTG may be acceptable if birth is imminent.
- Drugs – narcotics and sedatives slow the fetal heart rate while caffeine increases it.
- Pre-existing maternal conditions – medical disorders, antepartum haemorrhage.
- Pre-existing fetal conditions – intrauterine growth retardation (IUGR).

Fetal Heart Rate Abnormalities

If auscultation reveals an abnormal fetal heart rate then it is reasonable to investigate further by continuously monitoring the heart rate and analyzing the recording. If the abnormal finding is discovered immediately before birth in an otherwise uncomplicated

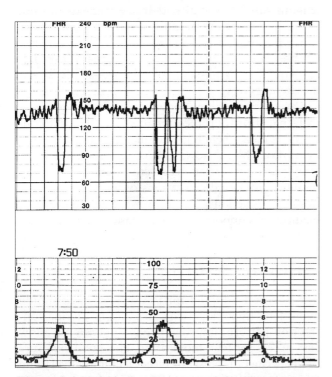

Figure 9.6 Variable decelerations: top, fetal heart rate (FHR); bottom, uterine activity (UA).

labour, then it is reasonable to progress to birth, as an uncompromised fetus is expected to have good reserve. The problem arises when an abnormal CTG persists for any length of time, as this requires a full assessment of the likely effects on the fetus. An understanding of the significance of the various fetal heart rate patterns is essential so that appropriate measures can be taken to restore fetal oxygenation.

If the CTG is suggestive of hypoxia then corrective measures, such as turning the woman on her side (to avoid aortocaval compression and maximize venous return) and reducing the stimulus to the uterus by decreasing oxytocic infusion (if one is used), will increase placental perfusion. The value of administering oxygen to the mother is unclear, as it is known that fetal haemoglobin has a high affinity for oxygen so, providing the mother is not hypoxic, the fetal requirements ought to be met. Maternal oxygen therapy is recommended by Wood and Dobbie (1989) as a rise in maternal P_{O_2} gradient potentially increases the maternofetal oxygen transfer. Recent tests using near infrared spectroscopy in term fetuses with uncomplicated labour showed that administering oxygen to the mother for 15 minutes resulted in a significant increase in fetal cerebral oxygenation (Aldrich *et al*. 1994).

Suggested therapeutic measures are (Wood and Dobbie, 1989):
• Change maternal posture.
• Check blood pressure; correct any hypotension.
• Improve maternal oxygenation.
• Assess uterine activity; discontinue oxytocin infusion.
• Vaginal examination to exclude cord prolapse and assess progress in labour.
• Consider fetal blood sampling or operative birth.
It is vital that the written records document the recognition of an abnormal CTG, the interpretation of this and the actions taken. If the decision is made to continue observation for a longer period or to inform medical personnel, then this also must be documented.

Second Stage of Labour

The stages of labour as they are defined today were first described at the beginning of the nineteenth century (Denman, 1824). The second stage is recognized as being from full dilatation of the cervix to the complete birth of the baby. The diagnosis is made when a vaginal examination reveals that no cervix can be felt.

The head may be visible at the introitus without full dilatation. The urge to bear down is not always present at the start of the second stage (especially if an epidural analgesia has been given) but many women complain of a change in the nature of the contractions. Much has been written in recent years about how long the second stage should last and how it should be conducted. Sometimes the urge to bear down may be irresistible, but to push would be inappropriate because the cervix is not fully dilated. This can occur with a breech presentation or an occipitoposterior position. Every encouragement may be needed to assist a mother not to push in these circumstances, which may involve utilizing alternative positions to relieve the pressure on the cervix and to provide the best degree of comfort.

The transition into the expulsive phase of labour is sometimes heralded by a change in the mother's behaviour, by expression, words or actions. A great deal of reassurance may be needed at this stage as the feelings are often overwhelming and the mother may be at her lowest ebb. Once she is able to push, it is often easier to cope because of the active participation and the realization that the end is near. Until the urge to push is present in the second stage of labour, then it is merely an extension of the first stage with little or no added stress to the fetus. It has been demonstrated that fetal acid–base parameters do not change in the second stage of labour when there is no active pushing (Piquard *et al*. 1989). The frequency of observations can be maintained as that for the latter part of the first stage of labour, usually at 15-minute intervals.

Once active pushing commences then the effects of maternal effort plus the pressure exerted by the contractions mean there is greater likelihood of decreased intervillous blood flow, so it is wise to monitor the fetal heart rate after every contraction for 1 full minute. Any late decelerations or variable decelerations that take longer to recover are detected by this method. It is important that all observations are documented at this stage.

Position for Birth

The position adopted for the second stage should avoid fetal hypoxia, create an efficient uterine contraction pattern, improve pelvic dimensions, allow easy access for fetal monitoring, give good exposure of the perineum, present a clear field for delivery and be comfortable (Stewart, 1984). Comfort is of paramount importance as far as the woman is concerned, but as it is not easy to guarantee comfort at this stage the position which minimizes discomfort and enhances maternal effort is welcome. The dorsal position for birth is not recommended because, apart from the fact that pushing is 'uphill', compression of the maternal venae cavae is likely to result in fetal hypoxia (Humphrey *et al.* 1974). This hypoxic effect is likely to worsen as the time spent in second stage increases (Johnstone *et al.* 1987). A semirecumbent position is often used, although there is a tendency to slip down the bed unless well supported.

Squatting position

In primitive cultures the squatting position has been used for birth throughout history – birth stools have been described in the *Bible* and in ancient illustrations. In recent years birth chairs and birth cushions have gained favour to provide support in this position. The squatting position enables women to feel more in control and produces a more effective bearing-down reflex (Gupta and Lilford, 1987) (**Figure 9.7**). Although the birthing chair uses the principle of the upright position to aid descent of the fetus and prevent maternal caval compression, it does have disadvantages.

An increased rate in PPH and perineal lacerations has been demonstrated (Turner *et al.* 1986), although it is acknowledged that more blood may have been

collected for measurement than would be the case if the birth had been conducted on a bed. The squatting position using a birth cushion has been linked with more labial lacerations, but also with a more intact perineum; it was readily accepted by the women using it (Gardosi *et al.* 1989). The squatting position has been shown radiologically to increase the diameters of the pelvic outlet by approximately 20–30% (Russell, 1969).

Encouraging the mother to try different positions for birth helps to find the one most comfortable and most suitable for her individual needs. Standing to give birth suits some mothers; kneeling (**Figure 9.8**) and the all-fours position may direct the pressure of the advancing head anteriorly rather than towards the perineum. For the midwife, assisting at deliveries in which different positions are used makes for a more stimulating role and an invaluable learning experience (Flint, 1986).

Duration of Second Stage

For many years a strict time limit was applied to the second stage of labour, as reflected in older midwifery textbooks which recommend one hour in a primigravid labour and half an hour in a multigravid labour (Sweet, 1988). Some advocated the abandonment of 'stages of labour' in favour of a 'labour and birth process', which looked at progress rather than duration (Crawford, 1983) provided that the mother and baby were well. Until pushing commences the second stage is merely an extension of the first stage with no additional attendant risks. If the mother is

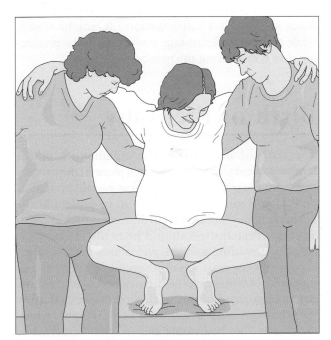

Figure 9.7 Supported squatting position.

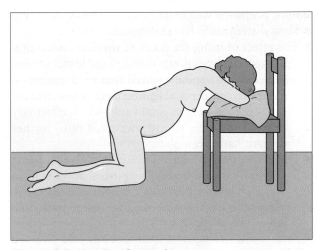

Figure 9.8 Kneeling forwards.

encouraged to adopt a posture that prevents aorto-caval compression, then once pushing begins the risks of fetal acidosis are minimized. A decision to intervene with an assisted birth should only be made when there is no progress, or if the fetal or maternal condition warrants it, rather than when a specified time has elapsed (Sleep *et al*. 1989).

Pushing Technique

Many midwives were taught that women should be instructed to push in the second stage of labour. As soon as a contraction commenced, midwives would diligently encourage the mother to take a deep breath, hold it, then push as long and hard as she could, and then let the breath out and repeat the process. This would ensure that none of the contraction was 'wasted'. The delivery room has been said to resemble a rugby scrum with everyone peering at the woman's vulva and urging her to exert greater effort (Thomson, 1988). Beynon, an obstetrician, observed in 1957 that in two cases where the women were asked to stop pushing the head advanced slowly and steadily, without exertion, and the babies were born with no perineal trauma, even though the baby was the first in both cases. This prompted Beynon to conduct a trial on normal primigravidae with vertex presentations in which no suggestion to push was given to one group of 100 women as compared with a control group of 393 women who delivered over the same period. The results showed that 83 of the 100 delivered entirely spontaneously, with the average duration of second stage being 63 minutes. There were six forceps deliveries (despite ultimate encouragement to push), half the number in the control group, and the suture rate was 39% compared with 63%. The explanation proposed was that:

• Slow distension is less traumatic.
• The effect of using the force of uterine contraction to push the fetus down through the lower uterine segment and vagina ensured that no dragging on the transverse cervical ligaments or connective tissue supporting the vaginal vault, which effectively gripped the baby's head, occurred until further descent had taken place
• The earlier part of each contraction pulls the vagina taut preventing it from being pushed down in front of the presenting part and it is undesirable to push before this has taken place. The urge to push does not usually coincide with the start of a contraction.

Other studies compared spontaneous and directed pushing. One controlled study found that the mean duration of the second stage in the experimental group was twice as long as that in the control group, but this group also had longer first stages and greater use of pethidine; the perineal trauma rate was similar in both groups (Thomson, 1993).

Another factor to be considered is the length of time that each push should last. This was explored by Caldeyro-Barcia (1979), who investigated the effects of strong, prolonged bearing-down efforts, combined with breath-holding, on the fetus. Spontaneous bearing-down efforts lasted 5–6 seconds whereas, when requested to make a prolonged effort, the push lasted about 9 seconds. He demonstrated that longer, stronger bearing-down efforts combined with breath-holding resulted in an increased intrathoracic pressure, a drop in venous return, a subsequent drop in cardiac output and a drop in maternal arterial pressure. The longer the bearing-down effort, the more marked was the fall in arterial pressure, which in turn caused a drop in placental perfusion, resulting in fetal hypoxia and seen as decelerations in the fetal heart rate. Pushing efforts lasting 18 seconds, during which the intrauterine pressure did not returned to normal, greatly reduced blood flow to the placenta, resulting in late decelerations and fetal hypoxia. It is recognized that the second stage of labour conveys most risk to the fetus, but it is likely that it is the conduct of the second stage that really matters. It appears that instruction to the mother as to how and when to push should be reserved for those few who need it and should only be based on known physiology. If there is an urge to push and the presenting part is not visible, for a better outcome it may be worthwhile actively to discourage pushing until the presenting part is distending the pelvic floor.

Birth of the Baby

The birth of her baby is the culmination of the mother's efforts. Ideally this takes place in the privacy of a calm environment with as few people present as necessary. If additional staff are to be present at the birth, then they should be introduced to the couple in advance. Preparation should be made for the new baby by providing a warm, welcoming environment. Equipment for resuscitation should be checked and prepared, if this should be deemed necessary, and the parents informed of this likelihood. More maternity units now provide 'home from home' rooms, which look more like bedrooms and in which emergency equipment is not obviously visible.

Some women like to be constantly reassured of their progress and others feel that talk is a distraction in the latter part of labour and at birth. It may be necessary to speak very closely to the mother's ear or to gain eye contact to communicate, as many women retreat into a world of their own in the presence of such overwhelming sensations. The mother may have expressed a preference to cradle the baby close to her as soon as it is born or may prefer the baby to be cleaned before being handed to her. She may wish to take her time to explore the baby herself, including discovering its sex. It is important to be aware of such preferences and to make every effort to cooperate, to help make it a day to remember with pleasure. Once the birth is completed the mother should be made comfortable and the couple given time to adjust to their new role as parents. If the baby is to be breast-fed then this should be encouraged at this time. Where possible there should be no rush to remove the baby for weighing or examination, which should be done in the presence of the parents and where they can see and touch their baby.

Water Birth

Water has been associated with a feeling of well-being for many centuries – spa towns and public baths have flourished in the past. The interest in water for labour and childbirth is more recent, but has grown in popularity over the past decades (Odent, 1983; Balaskas and Gordon, 1990). Some women choose to use the pool for first-stage immersion only and some choose to give birth in the water. Labour and birth in water results in shorter labours and avoids the use of intra-muscular or epidural drugs, but has been associated with a slight increase in perineal tears, an increase in intact perinea and no significant increase in PPH (Garland and Jones, 1994). Some tragedies have been reported in connection with the use of a birth pool, although not all of the babies who died were actually delivered in water and no deaths were thought to be directly related to birth in water (Alerdice *et al.* 1995).

Women have commented on how much more relaxed they feel while in the water and how much more difficult it was to cope with contractions if they have to leave the water for any reason (Robinson, 1996). No labour is totally risk-free. The *Changing Childbirth* recommendations support client choice (Department of Health, 1993) – the option of labour in water is in response to client demand. Guidelines for midwives who attend water birth have been issued by the Royal College of Midwives; most maternity units have formulated their own guidelines (which incorporate inclusion and exclusion criteria) and also their own training programme (Harmsworth, 1994). It is vital that a midwife only undertakes care in situations for which she has been fully prepared (UKCC, 1993, 1994). On-going audit is recommended on the use of pools for labour and delivery; at present it is generally offered only to low-risk mothers.

Multiple Birth and Breech Birth

The care in labour of a woman with twins and/or breech presentation follows the same principles as care in labour for all women, but with 'added extras'. Twin deliveries and breech presentation both have increased risk of perinatal morbidity and mortality. The obstetrician is almost certainly involved in a breech or twin birth, although if twins are both cephalic the midwife usually conducts the delivery with other appropriate professionals available. In order for the midwife to keep the woman fully informed of progress and likely events, she must herself have a good knowledge of the processes involved. She must also understand the role and responsibility that is hers and the significance of other members of the team, i.e. obstetrician, anaesthetist and paediatrician.

If more than two babies are present, then birth is usually by elective Caesarean section. It is particularly important to prevent an overfull bladder in labour to facilitate descent of the presenting part, and careful monitoring of the fetus and/or fetuses is required. In breech presentations it is vital that the cervix is fully dilated and the breech low in the pelvis before any active pushing commences. It is important that all midwives understand and are familiar with the principles of breech delivery, even though they may not have the opportunity to become competent in practice. A significant number of breech presentations are not detected until labour, but undiagnosed breeches are more likely to be born vaginally and with no added morbidity or mortality (Nwosu *et al.* 1993). The mechanism is taught as part of the midwifery education programme and therefore all midwives should be able to conduct a breech birth if required. Intense support is required for the woman and her partner, so at the time of delivery it is usual to have extra midwifery staff present to assist with the preparation for birth. This allows the midwife responsible for care to concentrate on the mother. The need for infant resuscitation should be anticipated and preparations made for this.

The Infant

The baby should be delivered into the appropriate environment. Routine use of nasopharyngeal mucus extractors is no longer justified – usually the baby responds to the change of environment and the initiation of respiration takes place. It is important to keep the baby warm and this is best achieved by placing the baby next to the mother's skin and gently drying the baby. The Apgar score is used to assess the baby's condition and relies on assessment of colour, heart rate, respiratory effort, muscle tone and reflex response at 1 and 5 minutes of age. It has been suggested for some time that the Apgar score is outmoded and particularly irrelevant in assessment of the preterm neonate (Crawford *et al.* 1973). There is concern that a low Apgar score may be erroneously interpreted as being synonymous with asphyxia, which is a particular cause for concern in medicolegal work (Marlow, 1992). However, the Apgar score has value as a means of assessing the condition of the baby at birth and should be measured as accurately as possible.

Umbilical cord pH provides another assessment of the neonate's condition and can be obtained by double clamping the cord and taking a specimen in a heparinized syringe for analysis. The base deficit of cord blood measures the metabolic component of fetal acidosis and is a better indicator of intrapartum hypoxia; it also correlates with long-term outcome (Sharif *et al.* 1993). Ideally this sample should be obtained as soon as possible after birth, although it need not be analyzed immediately; however, this may involve cord clamping earlier than the mother or midwife may wish.

Infant resuscitation

All midwives should be skilled in infant resuscitation; it is part of the preparation for birth that any resuscitation equipment be checked and that the midwife be familiar with its use. A minute may seem like a long time if the baby is not responding to the normal stimuli of touch and cold that initiate respiration. Regular updates in infant and maternal resuscitation should be incorporated into the in-service training programme of all maternity units. The principles of resuscitation can be broken down into an ABC format:

- A = Airway. Is it clear? Gentle suction may be required.
- B = Breathing. Is the baby breathing? Is it regular or gasping respirations? Administration of oxygen via a mask held over the baby's face may be all that is needed.
- C = Circulation. Is there a good heart rate that is able to pump oxygenated blood around the body and turn the baby a healthy pink colour? If not, positive pressure oxygen may be indicated. In extreme cases external cardiac massage may be required.
- D = Drugs. Administration of an opiate antagonist may be required to neutralize the sedative effect of maternal analgesic drugs once the baby's need for oxygen has been met. If the baby is not responding this indicates the need for more expert resuscitation efforts, possibly with intubation and the administration of cardiac stimulants or sodium bicarbonate to counteract acidosis.

Perineal Care

The prevention of perineal trauma is very much at the forefront of midwifery care – it gives many midwives a sense of pride to complete a birth with no perineal trauma. However, this should not be at the expense of trauma to the vaginal mucosa. Birth technique was focused on reducing the diameter of the presenting part by flexing the head to minimize distension of the perineal tissues and controlling the rate of birth to prevent trauma. In 1967 the Central Midwives Board ruled that midwives could perform episiotomies in emergency situations. Between 1967 and 1978 the episiotomy rate for all deliveries in England and Wales rose from 25% to 53%, with a 70% rate in primiparae (MacFarlane and Mugford, 1984).

The reason for episiotomy was usually to prevent more widespread trauma (rigid perineum) or to expedite birth for fetal or maternal reasons. A randomized controlled trial compared a group of women allocated to a policy of liberal episiotomy to prevent a tear to those with a policy that allowed episiotomy for fetal indications only (Sleep *et al.* 1984). The result was episiotomy rates of 51% and 10%, respectively. There was more perineal trauma in the restricted group, but also more intact perinea. No other significant differences were demonstrated. The evidence is that a policy of routine episiotomy cannot be supported.

Attempts have been made to prepare the perineum for the stretching that occurs during childbirth. Perineal massage to stretch the perineum during the last 6 weeks of pregnancy has been recommended (Avery and Van Arsdale, 1987; Tritten, 1987). However, this practice was opposed by almost one-third of women allocated to the technique and it has not been shown to significantly reduce trauma (Kaufman, 1994).

Episiotomy and perineal trauma rates vary considerably between midwives, indicating that clinical expertise plays a part. It would appear that more research needs to be conducted into the various techniques employed by midwives during childbirth (Floud, 1994a). The general consensus is that a slow, unhurried delivery with minimum expulsive effort on the part of the mother contributes to a better perineal outcome, but whether a 'hands on' or a 'hands off' approach should be used is debatable (Floud, 1994b).

Third degree tear

A tear is classed as third degree if the anal sphincter is torn. There is a growing tendency to adopt the American system where 3° involves the anal sphincter and a 4° tear where there is mucosal involvement. However, any tear to this degree has serious implications for a woman's social and childbearing future, as most result in some degree of residual sphincter defect and approximately one-half of the women experience anal incontinence (Sultan *et al.* 1994). It occurs in less than 1% of vaginal deliveries and a retrospective study by Sultan *et al.* (1994) showed that factors associated with third-degree tears are:
- Forceps delivery.
- Primiparous delivery.
- Birth weight >4000 g.
- Occipitoposterior position at delivery.

However, it must be remembered that the tear may also be caused by the posterior shoulder, not the head; therefore judging the perineum at delivery of the head may not indicate the degree of trauma involved.

Because the effects of third-degree tear can be socially disabling, attention needs to be directed towards both prevention and improvement of repair technique.

Third Stage of Labour

The third stage of labour is the most accurately timed in that it is from the birth of the baby to the delivery of the placenta and membranes. It is said that interference with the natural delivery of the placenta came about when women took to their beds to deliver, so it became necessary to tie off the cord to prevent soiling of bed linen with blood.

Ultrasound imaging of the mechanism of the third stage following the administration of an oxytocic showed that the area of the uterus not covered by the placenta became thickened immediately after birth (>2 cm), whereas the site of placental attachment remained thin (<1 cm). This stage lasted a median of 3 minutes and was followed by a contraction phase when the placenta-site wall gradually thickened to more than 2 cm, during which time the placenta separated. The detached placenta then slid down towards the cervix and was expelled. There was no evidence of retroplacental haematoma formation (Herman *et al.* 1993). If cord traction was applied before the placenta-site wall had thickened, the procedure was not effective – in five women with a prolonged third stage the placenta-site wall remained thin for 50–120 minutes, indicating that contraction and thickening had to occur before separation.

Active Management of the Third Stage

In the 1930s ergometrine was identified as the active oxytocic component of ergot and its use became widespread in the prevention and control of PPH. Synthetic oxytocin became available in the 1950s and in 1963 Embrey *et al.* recommended a combination of ergometrine and oxytocin to combine the benefits of the slower acting but sustained effect of ergometrine with the quicker but shorter lasting effect of oxytocin. Cord clamping and controlled cord traction were also employed. PPH was a common cause of maternal mortality – the use of oxytocics in the treatment of haemorrhage has indisputably reduced the mortality rate.

An analysis of nine published controlled trials over the period 1950–90 showed that routine use of oxytocic drugs reduced the risk of PPH by about 40% (Prendiville *et al.* 1988). Some unpleasant side effects were associated with the use of ergometrine, such as headache, nausea, vomiting, hypertension and vasoconstriction, particularly when given by the intravenous route. Active management was shown to have no effect on Apgar score, neonatal respiratory problems or rate of breastfeeding at discharge (Elbourne, 1994). An Australian study compared active management using intramuscular oxytocin 10 units to a policy using intramuscular syntometrine. The results showed a similar rate of PPH in both groups, but syntometrine was associated with nausea, vomiting and hypertension (McDonald *et al.* 1993). This suggests that with a different choice of oxytocic the protective effect of reducing blood loss need not include the unpleasant side effects. Syntocinon is not licensed for intramuscular use in the UK at present. In recent years there has been a trend to reject routine interventions – the prophylactic use of syntometrine has been one of these. Physiological management of the third stage has become more popular because more women are being involved in the decision-making about their care and are aware that there are choices to be made.

Physiological Management

Physiological management of the third stage involves no administration of oxytocic drugs and leaving the cord unclamped until pulsation ceases. Natural methods to stimulate the production of oxytocin, such as breastfeeding, are encouraged. Once signs of placental separation are observed, such as a gush of blood or an urge to push, the woman is encouraged to adopt an upright position and push the placenta out, a process that can take 20–60 minutes. Note that:

• Women at risk of PPH are not good candidates for physiological management.
• A physiological third stage must follow a normal physiological first and second stages of labour.
• Midwives who practise physiological management must be competent to do so.
• If physiological management is attempted, but active intervention is needed then management must proceed actively.

Perineal Repair

Repair of perineal trauma is usually performed by the midwife who cares for the woman in labour. This promotes continuity of care and avoids any unnecessary delay. Perineal suturing is a technique taught to midwives in training, but the opportunities to acquire this skill in practice vary considerably. Perineal pain following birth can mar what should be a happy time for the mother, and considering that up to 1000 women per day in England and Wales are likely to require repair of perineal trauma following birth, the extent of this becomes evident (Sleep *et al.* 1984). An overview of controlled trials that compared suture materials and techniques employed in perineal repair showed that derivatives of polyglycolic acid (Dexon and Vicryl) were superior for all layers (Grant, 1989). Polyglycolic acid sutures are absorbed by hydrolysis, which does not set up an inflammatory tissue reaction. A continuous subcuticular suture for skin closure is also more comfortable than interrupted sutures (Grant, 1989).

Isager-Sally *et al.* (1986) recommend that the subcuticular technique for skin repair be taught to those professionals learning to perform perineal repair as it should not be more difficult to learn than the interrupted method. A continuous technique has been described that is said to be quick to perform and have excellent cosmetic results (Olah, 1994). One maternity unit set up an intensive training programme to ensure that all the midwives were skilled in perineal repair using polyglycolic acid sutures and subcuticular skin closure (Brownlee, 1994). All new staff are taught this method and are competent by the end of their allocation to delivery suite. A tissue adhesive has also been shown to be effective in providing skin closure with a greater degree of comfort postnatally (Adoni and Anteby, 1991). One small retrospective study appeared to show a satisfactory outcome for those women with perineal tears which were left unsutured (Head, 1993).

Problems during Labour

The midwife is acknowledged as being the expert in normal labour. Rule 40 of the Midwives Rules (UKCC, 1993) requires that:

> *In any case where there is an emergency or where she detects in the health of a mother and baby a deviation from the norm, a practising midwife shall call to her assistance a registered medical practitioner.*

However, once complications develop the midwife still retains responsibility for the care of the mother and is expected to cooperate with medical colleagues who participate in the care of mothers and babies in an atmosphere of mutual recognition of each other's roles (UKCC, 1994). It can take a great deal of midwifery skill and tact to support and encourage a woman through a complicated labour so that she retains some control and derives satisfaction and fulfilment. By acting as the woman's advocate and making sure that her voice is heard the midwife can truly be 'with woman', as the term 'midwife' suggests.

Failure to Progress in Labour

There are no hard and fast rules as to when to intervene in a labour which is not progressing. Some units have a very active policy (*see* Active Management of Labour). Many units have their own locally drawn-up policies for management of such situations, but it must be remembered that the woman needs to be presented with the facts so that she is involved in making the choice. Midwives should also be involved in local policymaking. Written clinical guidelines and protocols show that attempts have been made to be proactive and provide evidence of a standard of care, but they are no substitute for professional judgement (Tingle, 1995).

Operative and Instrumental Deliveries

If the decision is made to deliver the baby by forceps, ventouse or Caesarean section then the midwife is in an ideal position to ensure that the mother is aware of what the procedure entails and approximately how long events will take. 'Soon' or 'not long' are not very informative answers when a woman is asking how long it will be before her baby is born, particularly if she is distressed (Kirkham, 1989). She would have no idea if this meant minutes or hours, particularly if this is her first labour. Sometimes, when an emergency situation arises, it is not possible to give a full explanation before action must be taken; in such circumstances it is beneficial to speak to the woman and her partner as soon as possible after the event to answer questions and to put events into perspective. It is the unanswered questions that often return to haunt the mother and may affect how she feels about this baby or a future pregnancy.

Caesarean section

If labour progresses to a Caesarean section or if a Caesarean birth is planned the midwife has a vital role to play in continuing to care for and support the mother. She would usually 'receive' the baby at delivery and provide its initial care complying with any requests that the mother may have expressed. The Caesarean section rate in the UK between 1985 and 1990 was 11.8% (Department of Health, 1994). There has been a steady rise in the caesarean section rate – fear of litigation has been quoted as being a significant reason for this (Francome, 1989). Emergency Caesarean performed under general anaesthetic appears to be particularly traumatic and has a longer recovery period, both physically and psychologically. The initial feelings of relief and gratitude may soon be replaced by feelings of disappointment and guilt (Steele, 1990). It is important that an explanation is given as to why the operation was necessary and that this is understood. If there is insufficient time to do this adequately before the birth, then the opportunity should be found as soon as possible afterwards. The midwife is often the best person for this 'debriefing'.

Following one Caesarean section what are the implications for subsequent births? This obviously depends on the individual factors involved. A 'trial of scar' is usually the term given to an attempt at vaginal birth in a subsequent pregnancy: 60–70% will deliver vaginally. It is normally considered to be a high-risk event and is recommended to take place in a consultant unit. Management of the labour and birth process may be fairly rigid, involving close fetal and maternal monitoring (Walsmley and Hobbs, 1994). Interventions that reduce mobility and the application of a time scale to labour reduce the chance of a normal birth, as already discussed.

Forceps and/or ventouse birth

Women who have an instrumental delivery are more likely to be primiparous, to have a longer second stage and to have epidural analgesia than are those who have a normal birth (Johanson *et al.* 1993). Maternal trauma is significantly less when the vacuum extractor rather than forceps is used (Vacca and Keirse, 1989), although it carries a higher failure rate. The chignon or artificial caput succedaneum that results disappears within a few days and any scalp abrasions are usually superficial. There is no increased incidence of jaundice requiring phototherapy following birth by vacuum extraction as compared with forceps delivery (Rajkhowa *et al.* 1994). The available evidence indicates that ventouse extraction is preferable for non-rotational deliveries to forceps when assistance is required to give birth, but every effort should be made to ensure that factors are as favourable as possible to achieve an unassisted birth.

Shoulder Dystocia

Shoulder dystocia is an infrequent obstetric emergency with a reported incidence of 0.1–0.38% (Resnick, 1980) rising to 0.9% (Omu *et al.* 1995) and 1.4% (Nocon *et al.* 1993) of all vaginal deliveries. It is associated with a high perinatal mortality and morbidity rate; further, because it is not predictable, it is also not preventable. The term shoulder dystocia refers to deliveries where the anterior shoulder becomes impacted against the symphysis pubis, thus preventing the shoulders from descending into the pelvis and following the normal rotation and birth. Fetal complications include asphyxia, brachial plexus palsies and fractures of the humerus or clavicles. It can also result in fetal or neonatal death. The situation first becomes evident when the head is delivered slowly and with difficulty, but the neck does not appear and the chin retracts against the perineum. Restitution may occur but no further descent takes place. The baby's face becomes increasingly congested as attempts to deliver it by traction are unsuccessful. This is a frightening situation, so it is important that the midwife has a plan of action if it arises as time is of the utmost importance if the baby is to be delivered unharmed (*see below*).

Certain risk factors have been associated with shoulder dystocia, but they have not proved reliable predictors – the condition has occurred when no risk factors were evident. The most consistent risk factors are increasing parity, fetal weight, particularly >4500 g, and a previous large infant. The identification of an extremely large fetus clinically is very unreliable (Rydhstrom and Ingemarsson, 1989). Various manoeuvres have been proposed for the management of shoulder dystocia.

McRobert's manoeuvre

McRobert's manoeuvre (**Figure 9.9**) involves exaggerated flexion of the mother's legs against her abdomen to cause an upward rotation of the symphysis pubis. Although the pelvic diameters do not change, the angle of inclination is reduced from 26° to 10°, which may free the anterior shoulder (Gonik *et al*. 1983). Experiments using a computerized laboratory model consistently demonstrate a reduction in the force needed to deliver the shoulders using McRobert's position compared with the lithotomy position (Gonik *et al*. 1989).

All-fours position

The all-fours position, with the weight resting evenly on all four limbs, maximizes the pelvic diameters. Simply moving the mother into this position sometimes results in an easy birth which could not be accomplished by other means. The advice is to deliver the posterior shoulder when attempts to deliver the anterior shoulder have failed. It is reported that in births managed thus there is enough room to insert the hand up to the wrist along the curve of the sacrum to free the posterior shoulder (Gaskin, 1988; McLean, 1989). This position may be difficult to adopt if the woman has a regional anaesthetic, is obese or is attached to monitoring equipment.

The midwife is often the practitioner faced with the problem of shoulder dystocia, so it is essential that there is a structured plan of action like a 'fire drill' (**Box 9.5**; Dignam, 1976). Shoulder dystocia is a bony dystocia, not a soft tissue dystocia. In the past it was recommended that a large episiotomy be performed to allow room to manoeuvre, but there is no empirical evidence to suggest that episiotomy affects the outcome (Nocon *et al*. 1993). It is difficult to know how severe the degree of shoulder dystocia will be so it is important to try those measures that are likely to be

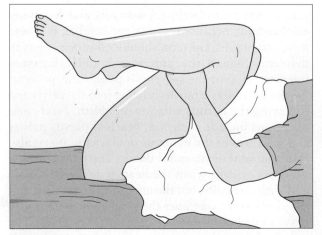

Figure 9.9 McRobert's manoeuvre.

Box 9.5

Plan of Action in Cases of Shoulder Dystocia – 'Fire Drill'

• **Note time** of delivery of the head.
• **Call medical aid** once shoulder dystocia is evident. This should include an obstetrician, a paediatrician and an anaesthetist.
• **Ensure that the shoulders** are in the anteroposterior diameter of the pelvis and attempt McRobert's manoeuvre with gentle to moderate traction, particularly if the mother is in the dorsal or semi recumbent position.
• **If this is unsuccessful,** immediately try the all-fours position and attempt to deliver the posterior shoulder with maternal effort or by inserting the first two fingers under the curve of the sacrum and applying pressure across the armpit to pull the baby down. It may be possible to reach in and locate the posterior arm and sweep this out.
If these measures do not succeed, a general anaesthetic may be required to achieve delivery.

successful first to minimize delay. Prompt recognition and the speedy implementation of a plan of action is vital. Accurate, contemporaneous record keeping is particularly important. Gross *et al.* (1987) stated that if shoulder dystocia occurs and is managed by the standard technique then, even if damage results, this should not constitute medical malpractice.

Retained Placenta

The placenta is generally thought to be retained if it has not been delivered 1 hour after the birth of the baby (Begley, 1990), although some may state a shorter time limit where the third stage has been managed actively. Management of this situation requires close observation of the mother's condition and careful estimation of any blood loss. After ensuring that the bladder is empty, a further attempt is usually made to deliver the placenta using controlled cord traction – an oxytocic drug may be given if it has not already been administered. If this is unsuccessful manual removal under general or regional anaesthesia is indicated and blood should be taken for cross-match purposes. Manual removal of the placenta carries a risk of infection and a course of antibiotics is usually prescribed. The risk of repetition of retained placenta in a subsequent pregnancy has been shown to be 2.4 times the risk for those without a previous history of retained placenta (Hall *et al.* 1985).

Postpartum Haemorrhage

Blood loss of more than 500 ml is said to constitute PPH. Estimates of blood loss at delivery are notoriously inaccurate. In the triennium 1988–91, 11 deaths were directly attributable to PPH. Only one of these followed a spontaneous delivery, but other complicating factors were present (Department of Health, 1994). It seems that fit, healthy women can withstand blood loss of up to 1000 ml at delivery without detriment (Gyte, 1992), but as true blood loss may be double the estimated amount (Brant, 1967) it is reasonable to retain the existing definition. A steady blood loss that continues over a period of time can easily be underestimated and in such circumstances it may be useful to weigh soiled pads and linen to assess the amount accurately. Careful ongoing assessment of the mother's condition is required – a fall in systolic pressure to less than 100 mmHg and a pulse rate of more than 100 b.p.m. are considered indicators of failure to compensate. Warning signs, such as facial pallor, minor changes in pulse rate and coldness of fingers, ears and nose, need to be observed, documented and reported to appropriate personnel (Brant, 1967).

New Developments

Developments in midwifery and obstetric practice may require the acquisition of new skills and may or may not become an integral part of the midwife's role (UKCC, 1994). It is in the interests of the midwife, and women to be aware of new developments, their implications and risks.

Intrapartum Fetal Assessment

Interpretation of fetal heart rate patterns is recognized as being imperfect in the assessment of fetal wellbeing. Measurement of amniotic fluid volume has been proposed as a valuable addition to the admission test to identify those fetuses at risk of hypoxia in labour (Teoh *et al.* 1992). It has also been suggested that changes in the fetal electrocardiogram reflect hypoxia and the fetal response may be a sensitive indicator of fetal well-being (Cockburn, 1996). Increasing myocardial hypoxia results in a build-up of lactic acid, which correlates with a rise in the T/QRS ratio and can be monitored throughout labour.

Another means of assessment under evaluation is near infrared spectroscopy, which is said to allow continuous qualitative measurements of changes in fetal brain oxygenation. Biological tissue is relatively transparent to light in the near infrared part of the spectrum, which means that cerebral concentrations of oxyhaemoglobin can be measured in a substantial part of the fetal brain (Aldrich *et al.* 1994).

However, all of these techniques require further evaluation and any new recommendations regarding intrapartum fetal surveillance should be based, where possible, on randomized controlled studies that include follow-up for a minimum of 2 years (Spencer and Ward, 1993).

Scope of Midwifery Practice

Once trained and assessed as competent in a particular skill the midwife is fully responsible and accountable for her actions. Provided that the midwife works within her sphere of responsibility and within Health Authority or Trust guidelines, and is a member of a trade union then she is usually protected by her indemnity insurance (Cavanagh and Williams, 1992).

Fear of litigation is voiced by many midwives, but hospital policies and guidelines can protect the midwife's practice. Providing she can show that her decisions were in accordance with hospital policy, or that she can justify her actions if they were not, then any claims against her can be defended. Cultivating a good standard of record keeping is of enormous benefit in organizing individual care planning and recording the reasons for any actions taken.

Midwives are becoming more specialized and their field of practice is becoming increasingly extended. Adequate training and assessment must be provided for any new skills (UKCC, 1992). A questionnaire was sent out to consultants, senior registrars, labour ward managers and senior midwives in hospitals in the West Midlands region to gauge opinion on whether midwives should perform ventouse deliveries. The majority felt that it would be safe for lift-out procedures and the suggestion was that there should be training of selected midwives (Rajkhowa *et al.* 1995). Midwives are already performing ventouse deliveries (Benns, 1995; Mulholland, 1997). It has also been suggested that midwives, given appropriate training, could perform the physical examination of the newborn, term baby (Rose, 1994).

The more skilled a midwife is, the better the quality of care she can deliver. The more knowledgeable a midwife is, the better able she is to facilitate informed choice. The skill of enabling women to make an informed choice does not necessarily come naturally, but needs to be learned and practised like any other (Rosser, 1996). It is acknowledged that midwifery practice must be evidence-based, but it must also be flexible enough to take account of individual circumstances in order to give truly individualized care of the standard deserved and expected today.

KEY CONCEPTS

- The uterus has two component parts, the cervix and corpus. For efficient delivery there must be an integration of the cervix and myometrium of the corpus.
- The trigger for labour is unknown.
- Fundamental problems with the management of labour are knowing when labour has begun and deciding whether labour is in the latent or active phase.
- First labour is unlike those that follow and there are marked differences between the behaviour of nulliparas and multiparas.
- Progress in labour depends on the Passenger, which has changed little; the Passages, i.e. the bony pelvis and soft tissues, which have been relegated to the second division; the Powers, which can be manipulated, but cannot solve all problems.
- The potentiation of oxytocin by prostaglandins produces a positive feedback in labour. Positive feedback is risky.
- The midwife is the principal caregiver in normal labour and delivery and continues to give care with the obstetrician in complicated labour and delivery.
- In order to facilitate informed choice the midwife must have sufficient knowledge of the options available. Giving unbiased information on which choices are to be made is a skill that needs cultivating.
- The 'simple' aspects of midwifery, such as giving support in labour and a policy of non-intervention, have been shown to be the most effective in improving birth outcomes in low-risk pregnancy.
- Support during labour makes all the difference to the outcome and experience of the woman and is of fundamental importance.

References

Adoni A, Anteby E: The use of histoacryl for episiotomy repair, *Br J Obstet Gynaecol* 98:476, 1991.

Alderdice F, Renfrew M, Marchant S, *et al*: Labour and birth in England and Wales: Survey report, *B J Midwifery* 3(7):375, 1995.

Aldrich CJ, Wyatt JS, Spencer JAD, Reynolds EOR: The effect of maternal oxygen administration on human fetal cerebral oxygenation measured during labour by near infrared spectroscopy, *Br J Obstet Gynaecol* 101(6):509, 1994.

Alfirevic Z, Walkinshaw SA: Management of post-term pregnancy: to induce or not? *Br J Hosp Med* 52(5):218, 1994.

Alibhai Y: Maternity care: black women speak out, *New Society* 1st April:2, 1988.

Al-Shawaf T, Al-Mogharaby S, Akiez A: Normal levels of uterine activity in primigravidae and mothers of high parity in spontaneous labour, *J Obstet Gynecol* 8:18, 1987.

Avery MD, Van Arsdale L: Perineal massage. Effect on the incidence of episiotomy and laceration in a nulliparous population, *J Nurse-Midwifery* 32(3):181, 1987.

Bakketig LS, Bergsjo P: Post-term pregnancy: magnitude of the problem. In: Chalmers I, Enkin M, Keirse MJNC, editors: *Effective care in pregnancy and childbirth* Vol. 1, p. 765, Oxford, 1989, Oxford University Press.

Balaskas J, Gordon Y: *Water birth*, London, 1990, Unwin.

Barrett JFR, Savage J, Phillips K, Lilford RJ: Randomized trial of amniotomy in labour versus the intention to leave membranes intact until the second stage, *Br J Obstet Gynaecol* 99(1):5, 1992.

Beard RW, Filshie GM, Knight CA, Roberts GM: The significance of the changes in the continuous fetal heart rate in the first stage of labour, *J Obstet Gynaecol Br Common* 78:865, 1971.

Beazley, JM and Kurjak, A. Influence of a partogram on the active management of labour, *Lancet* ii:348, 1972.

Beckwith J: Lock up your monitors, *MIDIRS Midwifery Digest* 5(4):441, 1995.

Begley CM: A comparison of 'active' and 'physiological' management of the third stage of labour, *Midwifery* 6(1):3, 1990.

Benns N: Ventouse deliveries conducted? (Letter), *Br J Midwifery* 3(10):565, 1995.

Beynon CL: The normal second stage of labour, a plea for reform of its conduct, *J Obstet Gynaecol* 64:815, 1957.

Bowler I: Midwives' attitudes to clients of Asian descent, *Nurs Times* 89(23):58, 1993.

Brant HA: Precise estimation of postpartum haemorrhage: difficulties and importance, *Br Med J* i:398, 1967.

Brownlee ME: Synchronised suturing, *MIDIRS Midwifery Digest* 4(1).51, 1994.

Borell U, Fernstrom I, Ohlson L, Wiqvist N: The influence of uterine contractions on the utero-placental blood flow at term. *Am J Obstet Gynecol* 93:44, 1964.

Caldeyro-Barcia R: The influence of maternal bearing-down efforts during second stage on fetal well-being, *Birth Fam J* 6(1):17, 1979.

Caldeyro-Barcia R, Sica-Blanco Y, Poseiro JJ, Gonzalez-Panizza U, Mendez Bauer C, Alvarez H, Pose SV, Hendricks CH. A quantitative study of the action of synthetic oxytocin on the pregnant human uterus, *J Pharm Exp Ther* 121:18, 1957.

Cammu H, van Eeckhout E: A randomised controlled trial of early versus delayed use of amniotomy and oxytocin infusion in nulliparous labour, *Br J Obstet Gynaecol* 103:313, 1996.

Cardozo L: Is routine induction of labour at term ever justified? *Br Med J* 306(6881):840, 1993.

Cardozo L, Gibb DMF, Studd JWW, Vasant RV, Cooper DJ: Predictive value of cervimetric patterns in primigravidae, *Br J Obstet Gynaecol* 89:33, 1982.

Cassin A: Sexual abuse and motherhood, *Nurs Times* 92(15):38, 1996.

Cavanagh S, Williams E: A case of prolonged labour? The acceptance of the ventouse, *MIDIRS Midwifery Digest* 2(4):431, 1992.

Chelmow D, Kilpatrick SJ, Laros RK: Maternal and neonatal outcomes after prolonged latent phase, *Obstet Gynecol* 81:486, 1993.

Clement S: Unwanted vaginal examinations, *Br J Midwifery* 2(8):368, 1994.

Cockburn J: The fetal electrocardiogram in the monitoring of fetal wellbeing, *Maternal Child Health* 21(1):14, 1996.

Crawford JS: *Principles and practice of obstetric anaesthesia* 4th edn, Oxford, 1978, Blackwell Scientific Publications.

Crawford JS: The stages and phases of labour: an outworn nomenclature that invites hazard, *Lancet*, July 30th (ii):271, 1983.

Crawford JS, Davies P, Pearson JF: Significance of the individual components of the Apgar score, *Br J Anaesth* 45:148, 1973.

Danforth DN: The distribution and functional activity of the cervical musculature, *Am J Obstet Gynaecol* 68:1261, 1954.

Denman T: *An introduction to the practice of midwifery* 6th edn, London, 1824, E Cox & Son.

Department of Health: *Changing childbirth, Part 1: Report of the expert maternity group*, London, 1993, HMSO.

Department of Health: *Report on confidential enquiries into maternal deaths in the United Kingdom 1988–1990*, London, 1994, HMSO.

Dignam WJ: Difficulties in delivery, including shoulder dystocia and malpresentation of the fetus, *Clin Obstet Gynaecol* 19:577, 1976.

Drayton S: Midwifery care in the first stage of labour. In Alexander J, Levy V, Roch S, editors: *Intrapartum care: a research-based approach*, London, 1990, Macmillan Education Ltd.

Duignan N: Active management of labour. In Studd J, editor: *The management of labour*, p. 99, Oxford, 1985, Blackwell Scientific Publications.

Elbourne DR: Active versus conservative third stage management. In Enkin MW, Keirse MJNC, Renfrew MJ, Neilson JP, editors: *Pregnancy and childbirth module*, Cochrane Database of Systematic Reviews, 05352, Cochrane Updates on Disk, Oxford, 1994(1), Update Software.

Embrey MP, Barber TC, Scudamore JM: Use of Syntometrine in prevention of postpartum haemorrhage, *Br Med J* i:1387, 1963.

FIGO: Guidelines for the use of fetal monitoring, *Int J Gynaecol Obstet* 25:1159, 1987.

Flint C: *Sensitive midwifery*, London, 1986, Heinemann.

Floud E: Protecting the perineum in childbirth 2: risk of laceration, *Br J Midwifery* 2(7):306, 1994a.

Floud E: Protecting the perineum in childbirth 3: perineal care today, *Br J Midwifery* 2(8):356, 1994b.

Francome C: *Changing childbirth: interventions in labour in England and Wales*, London, 1989, Maternity Alliance.

Freeman R: Intrapartum fetal monitoring – a disappointing story, *New Engl J Med* 322(9):624, 1990.

Friedman EA: *Labor. Clinical Evaluation and Management*, , New York, 1967, Meredith.

Friedman EA: *Labor: Clinical evaluation and management* 2nd edn, New York, 1978, Appleton- Century-Crofts.

Frigoletto FD Jr, Lieberman E, Lang JM, *et al.*: A clinical trial of active management of labor, *N Engl J Med* 333:745, 1995;.

Gaffney G, Sellers S, Flavell V, Squier M, Johnson A: Case-control study of intrapartum care, cerebral palsy, and perinatal death, *Br Med J* 308:743, 1994.

Gardosi J, Hutson N, Lynch CB: Randomised, controlled trial of squatting in the second stage of labour, *Lancet* ii:74, 1989.

Garland D, Jones K: Water birth, 'first stage' immersion or non-immersion? *Br J Midwifery* 2(3):113, 1994.

Gaskin IM: Shoulder dystocia: controversies in management, *Birth Gazette* 5(1):14, 1988.

Gaskin IM: Prostaglandins: a time honoured method of labour induction, *Birth Gazette* 7(2):24, 1991.

Gee H: Trials of labour. *Contemp Rev Obstet Gynaecol* 6:31, 1994.

Gee H, Olah KS: Failure to progress in labour. In Studd J, editor: *Progress in obstetrics and gynaecology* Vol. 10, p. 159, London, 1993, Churchill Livingstone.

Gee H, Taylor EW, Hancox R: A model for the generation of intra-uterine pressure in the human parturient uterus which demonstrates the critical role of the cervix. *J Theor Biol* 133:281, 1988.

Gibb D, Arulkumaran S: *Fetal monitoring in practice*, Oxford, 1992, Butterworth– Heinemann.

Gonik B, Stringer CA, Held B: An alternative manoeuvre for management of shoulder dystocia, *Am J Obstet Gynecol* 145(7):882, 1983.

Gonik B, Allen R, Sorab J: Objective evaluation of the shoulder dystocia phenomenon; effect of maternal pelvic orientation on force reduction, *Obstet Gynaecol* 74(1):44, 1989.

Granstrom L, Ekman G, Ulmsten U, Malmstrom A. Changes in the connective tissue of corpus and cervix uteri during ripening and labour in term pregnancy. Br J Obstet Gynaecol 1989; 96:1198-1202.

Granstrom L, Ekman G, Malmstrom A: Insufficient remodelling of the uterine connective tissue in women with protracted labour, *Br J Obstet Gynaecol* 98:1212, 1991.

Grant A: The choice of suture materials and techniques for repair of perineal trauma: an overview of the evidence from controlled trials, *Br J Obstet Gynaecol* 96:1281, 1989.

Grant JM: Sweeping of the membranes in prolonged pregnancy, *Br J Obstet Gynaecol* 100(10):889, 1993.

Gross TL, Sokol RJ, Williams T, Thompson K: Shoulder dystocia: a fetal–physician risk, *Am J Obstet Gynecol* 156:1409, 1987.

Gupta JK, Lilford RJ: Birth positions, *Midwifery* 3(2):92, 1987.

Gyte G: The significance of blood loss at delivery, *MIDIRS Midwifery Digest* 2(1):88, 1992.

Hall MH, Halliwell R, Carr-Hill R: Concomitant and repeated happenings of complications of the third stage of labour, *BJ Obstet Gynaecol* 92:732, 1985.

Harmsworth G: Safety first, *Nurs Times* 90(11):30, 1994.

Hazle NR: Hydration in labour. Is routine intravenous hydration necessary? *J Nurse-Midwifery* 31(4):171, 1986.

Head M: Dropping stitches, *Nurs Times* 89(33):64, 1993.

Herman A, Weinraub Z, Bukovsky I, Arieli S, Zabow P, Caspi E, Ron-El R: Dynamic ultrasonographic imaging of the third stage of labour: new perspectives into third stage mechanisms, *Am J Obstet Gynecol* 168(5):1496, 1993.

Hodnett ED: Support from caregivers during childbirth. In Enkin MW, Keirse MJNC, Renfrew MJ, Neilson JP, editors: *Pregnancy and childbirth module*, Cochrane Database of Systematic Reviews, 03871, Cochrane Updates on Disc, Oxford, October 1994, Update Software.

House of Commons Health Committee: *Maternity services* 2nd report, London, 1992, HMSO.

Humphrey MD, Chang A, Wood EC, Morgan S, Hounslow D: A decrease in fetal pH during the second stage of labour when conducted in the dorsal position, *J Obstet Gynaecol Br Common* 81:600, 1974.

Inch S: *Birthright. A parents guide to modern childbirth*, 2nd edn, Appendix 5, London, 1989, Green Print.

Ingemarsson I, Arulkumaran S, Ingemarsson E, Tambyraja RL, Ratnam SS: Admission test: a screening test for fetal distress in labour, *Obstet Gynaecol* 68(6):800, 1986.

Isager-Sally L, Legarth J, Jacobsen B, Bostofte E: Episiotomy repair – immediate and long term sequelae. A prospective randomised study of three different methods of repair, *Br J Obstet Gynaecol* 93(5):420, 1986.

Janbu T, Neshein B: Uterine artery blood velocities during contractions in pregnancy and labour related to intra-uterine pressure, *Br J Obstet Gynaecol* 94:1150, 1987.

Johanson R, Wilkinson P, Bastible A, *et al.*: Health after childbirth, *Midwifery* 9(3):161, 1993.

Johnson C, Keirse MJNC, Enkin M, Chalmers I: Nutrition and hydration in labour. In Chalmers I, Enkin M, Keirse MJNC, editors: *Effective care in pregnancy and childbirth* Vol. 2, Oxford, 1989, Oxford University Press.

Johnstone FD, Aboelmagd MS, Harouny AK: Maternal posture in second stage and fetal acid–base status, *Br J Obstet Gynaecol* 90:623, 1987.

Kaufman K: Method of teaching perineal massage and effects on perineal trauma. In Enkin MW, Keirse MJNC, Renfrew MJ, Neilson JP, editors: *Pregnancy and childbirth module*, Cochrane Database of Systematic Reviews, 07526, Cochrane Update on Disk, Oxford, 1994(1), Update Software.

Kirkham M: Midwives and information-giving during labour. In Robinson S, Thomson AM, editors: *Midwives, research and childbirth* Vol. 1, London, 1989, Chapman and Hall.

Kitzinger J: Recalling the pain, *Nurs Times* 86(3):38, 1990.

Kiwanuka AI, Moore WMO: The changing incidence of caesarean section in the Health District of Central Manchester, *Br J Obstet Gynaecol* 94:440, 1987.

Klein M, Lloyd I, Redman C, Bull M, Turnbull AC: A comparison of low risk women booked for delivery in two systems of care: shared care (consultant) and integrated general practice unit, *Br J Obstet Gynaecol* 90:118, 1983.

Lederman RP, Lederman E, Work BA, McCann DS: The relationship of maternal anxiety, plasma catecholamines, and plasma cortisol to progress in labour, *Am J Obstet Gynecol* 132:495, 1978.

Lopez-Zeno JA, Peaceman AM, Adashek JA, Socol ML: A controlled trial of a program for the active management of labor, *N Engl J Med* 326:4501992.

MacDonald D, Grant A, Sheridan-Periera M, Boylan P, Chalmers I: The Dublin randomized controlled trial of intrapartum fetal heart rate monitoring, *Am J Obstet Gynecol* 152:524, 1985.

MacFarlane A, Mugford M: *Birth counts: statistics of pregnancy and childbirth*, London, 1984, HMSO.

Marlow N: Do we need an Apgar score? *Arch Dis Child* 67(7):765, 1992.

McDonald SJ, Prendiville WJ, Blair E: Randomised controlled trial of oxytocin alone versus oxytocin and ergometrine in active management of third stage of labour, *BMJ* 307:1167, 1993.

McLean MT: Managing shoulder dystocia, *Midwifery Today* 12:24,46, 1989.

Menage J: Women's perception of obstetric and gynaecological examinations (correspondence), *Br Med J* 306:1127, 1993.

Mendelson CL: The aspiration of stomach contents into the lungs during obstetric anaesthesia, *Am J Obstet Gynecol* 52:191, 1946.

Milner I: Choosing a natural or an active childbirth, *Nursing* 3(2):39,43, 1986.

Mulholland L: Midwife ventouse practitioners, *BJ Midwifery* 5(5):255, 1997.

Neilson JP: Cardiotography during labour, *Br Med J* 306(6874):347, 1993.

Neilson JP: Fetal blood sampling as adjunct to heart rate monitoring. In Enkin MW, Keirse MJNC, Renfrew MJ, Neilson JP, editors: *Pregnancy and childbirth module*, Cochrane Database of Systematic Reviews, 07018, Cochrane Update on Disk, Oxford, 1994(1), Update Software.

Newburn M, Borton H: Rupture of the membranes in labour, *New Generation* 8(3):9, 1989.

Nikodem VC: Upright vs recumbent position during first stage of labour. In Enkin MW, Keirse MJNC, Renfrew MJ, Neilson JP, editors: *Pregnancy and childbirth module*, Cochrane Database of Systematic Reviews, 03334, Cochrane Update on Disk, Oxford, 1994(1), Update Software.

Nimmo WS, Wilson J, Prescott LF: Narcotic analgesics and delayed gastric emptying during labour, *Lancet* i:890, 1975.

Nocon JJ, McKenzie DK, Thomas LJ, Hansell RS: Shoulder dystocia: An analysis of risks and obstetric manoeuvres, *Am J Obstet Gynecol* 168(6):1732, 1993.

Nwosu EC, Walkinshaw S, Chia P, *et al.*: Undiagnosed breech, *Br J Obstet Gynaecol* 100(6):531, 1993.

Odent M: Birth under water, *Lancet* ii:1476, 1983.

O'Driscoll K, Meagher D: *Active management of labour*, London, 1993, Mosby.

O'Driscoll K, Jackson JA, Gallagher JT: The prevention of pro-longed labour, *Br Med J* ii:477, 1969.

Olah KS: Subcuticular perineal repair using a new, continuous technique, *Br J Midwifery* 2(2):67, 1994.

Omu AE, Al-Quattan F, Al-Ashkanane L: Shoulder dystocia: a continuing obstetric challenge, *J Obstet Gynaecol* 15:373, 1995.

Osmers R, Rath W, Pflanz MA, Kuhn W, Stuhlsatz H, Szeverenyi M: Glycosaminoglycans in cervical connective tissue during pregnancy and parturition, *Obstet Gynecol* 81:88, 1993.

Pharoah PD, Cooke T, Cooke RWI, Rosenblum L: Birth-weight specific trends in cerebral palsy, *Arch Dis Child* 65(6):602, 1990.

Philpott RH, Castle WM: Cervicographs in the management of labour in primigravidae. I The alert line for detecting abnormal labour. *J Obstet Gynaecol Br Common* 79:592, 1972.

Piquard F, Schaefer A, Hsiung R, *et al.*: Are there two biological parts in the second stage of labour? *Acta Obstet Gynecol Scand* 68(8):713, 1989.

Prendiville W, Elbourne D, Chalmers I: The effects of routine oxytocic administration in the management of the third stage of labour: an overview of the evidence from controlled trials, *Br J Obstet Gynaecol* 95:3, 1988.

Rajkhowa M, Johanson R, O'Brien PMS: Forceps or ventouse? *Maternal Child Health* 19(8):248,252, 1994.

Rajkhowa M, Abukhalil I, Chapman G, O'Brien PMS: Should midwives conduct ventouse deliveries? *Br J Midwifery* 3(2):88, 1995.

Resnick R: Management of shoulder girdle dystocia, *Clin Obstet Gynaecol* 23(2):559, 1980.

Robinson J: Safer out of the water? The politics of pool use, *Br J Midwifery* 4(2):100, 1996.

Rose SJ: Physical examination of the full term neonate, *Br J Midwifery* 2(5):209, 1994.

Rosser J: How would you like us to monitor your baby? *Br J Midwifery* 4(1):45, 1996.

Russell JGB: Moulding of the pelvic outlet, *J Obstet Gynaecol Br Common* 76:817, 1969.

Russell JGB: The rationale of primitive delivery positions, *Br J Obstet Gynaecol* 89:712, 1982.

Rydhstrom H, Ingemarsson I: The extremely large fetus – Antenatal identification, risks and proposed management, *Acta Obstet Gynaecol Scand* 68:59, 1989.

Scott J: Mandatory trial of labour after caesarean delivery: an alternative viewpoint, *Obstet Gynaecol* 77(6):811, 1991.

Sharif K, Olah K, Gee H: Umbilical cord blood pH and base deficit: time dependent change at room temperature, *J Obstet Gynaecol* 13(2):107, 1993.

Simkin P: Just another day in a woman's life? Women's long term perceptions of their first birth experience, *Birth* 1(4):203, 1991.

Sleep J, Grant A, Garcia J, Elbourne D, Spencer J, Chalmers I: West Berkshire perineal management trial, *Br Med J* 289:587,1984.

Sleep J, Roberts J, Chalmers I: Care during the second stage of labour. In Chalmers I, Enkin M, Keirse MJNC, editors: *Effective care in pregnancy and childbirth* Vol. 2, p. 1129, Oxford, 1989, Oxford University Press.

Spencer JAD: Electronic fetal monitoring in the United Kingdom, *Birth* 21(2):106, 1994.

Spencer JAD, Ward RHT: *Recommendations arising from the 26th RCOG study group: Intrapartum fetal surveillance*, London, 1993, RCOG Press.

Steele K: Caesarean section: what it feels like for the mother, *MIDIRS Midwifery Digest* No 13 (April), 1990.

Stevenson J: Managing first stage problems, *Midwifery Today* 31:33, 1994.

Stewart KS: The second stage. In Studd J, editor: *Progress in obstetrics and gynaecology* Vol. 4, Edinburgh, 1984, Churchill Livingstone.

Studd, J. Partograms and nomograms of cervical dilatation in management of primigravid labour, *Br Med J* 4:451, 1973.

Sultan AH, Kamm MA, Hudson CM, Bartram CI: Third degree obstetric anal sphincter tears: Risk factors and outcomes of primary repair, *BMJ* 308:887, 1994.

Sweet BR: *Mayes Midwifery* 11th edn, London, 1988, Baillière Tindall.

Symon A: Midwives and litigation 2: a small-scale survey of attitudes, *Br J Midwifery* 2(4):176, 1994.

Teoh TG, Gleeson MD, Darling MRN: Measurement of amniotic fluid volume in early labour is useful admission test, *Br J Obstet Gynaecol* 99(10):859, 1992.

Thomson AM: Management of the woman in normal second stage of labour: a review, *Midwifery* 4:77, 1988.

Thomson AM: Pushing techniques in the second stage of labour, *J Adv Nurs* 18(2):171, 1993.

Thornton JG, Lilford RJ: Active management of labour: current knowledge and research issues, *Br Med J* 309:366, 1994.

Tidy H: Care for survivors of childhood sexual abuse, *Modern Midwife* 6(7):17, 1996.

Tingle J: Clinical protocols and the law, *Nurs Times* 91(29):27, 1995.

Tritten J: Preventing tears, *Midwifery Today* 1(2):16,44, 1987.

Turner MJ, Romney ML, Webb JB, Gordon H: The birthing chair: an obstetric hazard? *J Obstet Gynaecol*, 6:232, 1986.

UK Amniotomy Group: A multicentre randomised trial of amniotomy in spontaneous first labour at term, *Br J Obstet Gynaecol* 101(4):307, 1994.

UKCC: *Scope of professional practice*, London, 1992, United Kingdom Central Council for Nursing, Midwifery and Health Visiting.

UKCC: *Midwives rules*, London, 1993, United Kingdom Central Council for Nursing, Midwifery and Health Visiting.

UKCC: *The midwife's code of practice*, London, 1994, United Kingdom Central Council for Nursing, Midwifery and Health Visiting.

Vacca A, Keirse MJNC: Instrumental vaginal delivery. In Chalmers I, Enkin M, Keirse MJNC, editors: *Effective care in pregnancy and childbirth* p. 1216, Oxford, 1989, Oxford University Press.

Walkinshaw SA: Is routine active medical intervention in spontaneous labour beneficial? *Contemp Rev Obstet Gynaecol* 6(Jan):13, 1994.

Walmsley K, Hobbs L: Vaginal birth after lower segment caesarean section, *Modern Midwife* 4(4):20, 1994.

Walsh D: Management of progress in the first stage of labour. *Midwives Chron* 107(1274):84, 1994.

Wood PL, Dobbie HG: *Electronic fetal heart rate monitoring*, London, 1989, Macmillan Press.

World Health Organization: *Manual of the international statistical classification of diseases, injuries and causes of death*, vol 1:733, Geneva, 1977, WHO.

World Health Organization. The partograph: A managerial tool for the prevention of prolonged labour, Geneva, 1988, World Health Organization.

Zuspan FP, Cibels LA, Pose SV: Myometrial and cardiovascular response for alterations in plasma epinephrine and norepinephrine, *Am J Obstet Gynecol* 84:841, 1962.

Further Reading

Enkin M, Keirse MJNC, Renfrew M, Neilson J: *A guide to effective care in pregnancy and childbirth* 2nd edn, Oxford, 1995, Oxford University Press.

This reference book is a condensed version of the large two-volume edition and provides up-to-date evidence-based information on practice issues. Contains useful lists of various forms of care and their effectiveness.

Gauge S, Henderson C: *CTG made easy*, Edinburgh, 1992, Churchill Livingstone.

A collection of case studies illustrating all types of CTG in labour. It allows readers to interpret and decide upon action and provides an analysis, actual management and outcome.

Gibb D, Arulkumaran S: *Fetal monitoring in practice*, Oxford, 1992, Butterworth–Heinemann.

This comprehensive book details the principles of CTG interpretation in a simplified way and provides examples of normal and abnormal CTGs with an explanation of their physiology and significance. Explains the terminology used and gives a wide coverage of aspects of intrapartum fetal monitoring.

Mason D, Edwards P: *Litigation. A risk management guide for midwives*, London, 1993, Royal College of Midwives.

This easy-to-read booklet, written by lawyers, describes aspects of practice likely to involve litigation and explains how to avoid this. It emphasizes the value of good record keeping and an acceptable standard of practice

10 *The Control of Labour Pain*

LEARNING OUTCOMES

After studying this chapter you should be able to:

- List the main groups of pain control methods available in labour.
- Describe the side-effects of each method.
- Discuss who is the decision maker in relation to each method.
- Outline the main research issues relating to each method.

Despite being experienced by a large majority of women, the pain of labour is unique and isolating; it may have also have certain common or shared characteristics. Our understanding of and response to pain has been shown to be influenced by a range of factors such as culture (Zborowski, 1952), prior experience (Beecher, 1956) and expectation of pain (Johnson and Rice, 1974). Control, in the sense of locus of control as a personality characteristic, has also been shown to influence tolerance of pain and the resultant behaviour (Johnson *et al.* 1971).

Throughout childbearing the feeling of being in control is known to matter more to the mother than any interventions which may be recommended (Green *et al.* 1990; Chard and Richards, 1992). In the context of pain remedies in labour, there are two significant aspects of control. First is the person who controls the remedy – this may be whoever makes the decisions about the remedy or it may be the person who administers it. Rajan (1993) emphasizes the benefits to the mother of being able to choose and be involved in decision-making concerned with pain control. Following her research, Rajan (1993) recommended that the mother be supported in her choice of a method, over which she may exert direct control, such as transcutaneous electrical nerve stimulation (TENS) and inhalational analgesia.

The second way in which control operates is whether the remedy actually does control the pain. The effectiveness of pain remedies had been assumed and was thought to be a major desire of mothers, until Morgan *et al.* (1982) demonstrated that mothers are not more satisfied by a birth experience which is pain free.

Morgan et al.'s (1982) study has necessitated a differentiation between the traditional goal of pain relief in labour from the control of pain (Mander, 1992). This relief of pain implies eradication of pain, as in the dictionary definition 'the removal of a burden' (Macdonald, 1981). This term is inappropriate for four reasons:

- Relief implies a passivity in the mother which is unacceptable in a system of care that focuses on the mother making choices to determine her care.
- Perceptions of passivity are aggravated by limited information given to the mother about the costs of pain relief, including the medicalization of her birth experience and the potential for long-term pathology (Mander, 1996). Thus, she is limited in her contribution to decision making about her care – as a result the likelihood of informed consent recedes.
- Despite pharmacological and anaesthetic advances, it is still not possible to guarantee that any method, except perhaps general anaesthesia (GA), will eradicate pain (Simkin, 1989).
- As mentioned already, Morgan *et al.* (1982) showed that total removal of pain may not be the mother's major concern.

Although pain relief may not be desired, desirable or realistic, pain control is a more woman-centred concept because:

- It allows the mother to decide the pain level she is prepared or is able to experience.
- The mother becomes an active participant not only in the decision, but also in implementing the method.

Apparent Control of Pain Control

As mentioned above, the control of pain may be related to the decision to implement and/or the administration. Increasingly, the mother is presented with choices about pain control for labour. The ultimate choice emerges during labour, which may not be an ideal time for the mother to practise logical, assertive decision making.

It is likely that the mother obtained information about methods of pain control during her pregnancy, and she will base her decisions in labour on this. For a minority of UK mothers, the source of this information is from childbirth education (Perkins, 1980); for others the sources are friends, relatives and the media.

The mother's decision may be implemented by her, by her midwife or by her medical attendants. In this section who controls labour pain remedies is examined in terms of who administers them. The list is not exhaustive, but demonstrates some issues which deserve consideration.

Methods Administered by the Mother

The mother carries immediate or direct responsibility for the selection, timing and administration of certain pain control methods.

Inhalational analgesia

A major principle in the use of premixed nitrous oxide and oxygen (50% N_2O and 50% O_2 delivered by the Entonox apparatus, supervised by a midwife in the UK) is its self-administration. The mother is unable to overdose on this analgesic gas, because an inappropriately high intake causes sleepiness and the mask or mouthpiece falls away. The mother is taught, ideally during pregnancy with reinforcement during labour, the principles of self-administration to achieve maximum pain control.

Transcutaneous electrical nerve stimulation

The mother appears to be in control when using TENS, both in its application and also in physiological terms. The mother, or more likely her partner, applies the electrodes to the precise lumbar area after having been taught where during pregnancy. The mother's hand-held pulse generator–amplifier provides a below-pain-threshold barrage of impulses. These electrical impulses physiologically exploit 'the patient's own in-built neurobiological [pain] control mechanisms' (Woolf and Thompson, 1994).

Relaxation

Childbirth education teaches the mother a range of relaxation techniques that enable the mother to assume control by minimizing sympathetic activity within the autonomic nervous system (Sherwood, 1995). She learns to simultaneously increase the activity of the more vegetative parasympathetic component. These techniques enable the mother to diminish her sensation of pain and to control the intensity of her reaction to that pain (Edgar and Smith-Hanrahan, 1992).

Hydrotherapy

Although sometimes used sequentially, it is necessary to differentiate water used to control labour pain, or hydrotherapy, from its use as a birth medium, or water birth. The instrumental role of mothers in increasing the availability of pools for labour and birth has been identified (Alderdice *et al.* 1995). Additionally, a mother's increased control in labour when water is used has been demonstrated by Swedish researchers (Waldenström and Nilsson, 1992), who found that mothers who bathed during labour were less likely to have labour augmented with oxytocin; the difference becoming significant in the second stage. The mother's need to utilize analgesic medication was also reduced. The difference was significant relative to pethidine and inhalational analgesia.

Methods Administered by the Midwife

Certain pain control methods are applied or administered directly by the midwife.

Massage

Massage in labour is known alternatively as 'counterpressure' (Simkin, 1989) or 'back rubbing'. This rather primitive response to pain, i.e. holding, rubbing or squeezing the affected part, may be self-administered. Although psychological benefits associated with human touch may endure (Malkin, 1994), the pain-controlling effects last only as long as the massage (Simkin, 1989). This relatively short-term effect serves to increase the mother's control in that if she decides to discontinue massage, both the action and effects cease immediately.

Opioid drugs

The mother, with her midwife, is able to control through her decision making whether systemic analgesics, such as diamorphine or pethidine, are appropriate (UKCC, 1989). Because there is a risk that these drugs may cause neonatal respiratory depression, the decision to use them is influenced by the mother's progress in labour.

Methods Administered by a Medical Practitioner

There are certain interventions which provide pain control, and which require a medical practitioner to administer them.

Epidural analgesia

Increasingly in the UK, the mother may choose whether to take advantage of the 24-hour on-demand epidural services that are widely available (Morgan, 1993a). The mother's control may be further enhanced if the epidural medication is delivered by a patient-controlled analgesia (PCA) system (Park and Fulton, 1991).

General anaesthesia

As there is a risk of acid aspiration pneumonitis (Mendelson's syndrome), general anaesthesia in maternity care has been largely superseded by other methods. This is mainly caused by the serious contribution of anaesthesia to maternal mortality (Morgan, 1987). Thus, only 0.79% of midwives reported its use in an authoritative survey (Steer, 1993). Although the mother controls whether to permit a general anaesthetic or not, her control ceases totally once the anaesthetic is in progress.

Methods of Pain Control

Because the mother's control over pain remedies in labour appears considerable, it is necessary to examine in detail the significant methods used. Again, this list is not exhaustive, because of constantly developing knowledge and the mother's opportunities to employ less well known methods. Here the focus is on the methods used to control pain, their mode of action and relevant research, especially that which informs maternal control. Because of their apparently greater potential for maternal control which has emerged (above) the nonpharmacological methods will be considered first.

Nonpharmacological Methods

Pain-control methods that avoid using medication or drugs have become more desirable because of our increasing realization of the vulnerability of the fetus to environmental threats, particularly 'unnatural' or artificial substances. In spite of, or perhaps because of, the widespread assumption that naturally-occurring phenomena are safe, we should examine this assumption and the methods to which it is applied with caution.

The nonpharmacological methods involve varying degrees of intervention or invasiveness. Here, these methods are considered in ascending order of involvement of nonmaternal factors, on the assumption that the smaller the nonmaternal input the greater the mother's control.

Relaxation and Psychoprophylaxis

Relaxation and psychoprophylaxis have the least non-maternal input, as they require no specialized equipment or personnel. These methods are predominantly psychological in their implementation. The nonmaternal contribution comprises the childbirth educator who teaches the methods in groups during pregnancy and the labour companion who reinforces that teaching during labour.

According to Steer (1993), relaxation is the non-pharmacological method of pain control most frequently used in UK. He reports that 34% of mothers used relaxation, a frequency lagging some way behind N_2O and O_2 (60%), but not far behind the second most frequently used method, pethidine (36.9%).

'Relaxation' and 'psychoprophylaxis' are used synonymously in UK, but the history of these approaches illuminates certain differences. Together with education and breathing exercises, relaxation has been one of the cornerstones of prepared childbirth since Dick-Read introduced this concept (1933). Lamaze (1970) followed Dick-Read by applying Pavlovian concepts to relaxation in childbirth and introduced the term 'psychoprophylaxis', aiming to prevent pain through using psychological methods. In North America the name 'Lamaze' replaced the term that he introduced (Sloane, 1993).

Although differing on questionably important aspects, both approaches to childbirth education focused on similar crucial areas (Sloane, 1993;

Melzack and Wall, 1991). The only difference in the recommended practices is found in Lamaze's advocacy of the use of coping strategies to distract from the pain, including counting backwards, singing or reciting. Such techniques would have been inappropriate in Dick-Read's regime due to his questioning of the reality of labour pain. For the mother espousing Dick-Read's approach, learning the nature of labour became fundamental, thus avoiding learning the existence of labour pain.

As mentioned above, all pain-control techniques that include relaxation teach the mother to minimize sympathetic activity in the autonomic nervous system (Sherwood, 1995). The less widely used relaxation techniques include biofeedback, therapeutic touch, acupressure, hypnotherapy, guided imagery and music therapy (Nichols and Humenick, 1988). By suppressing sympathetic activity the mother is able to break the tension–anxiety–pain cycle first identified by Dick-Read and subsequently supported authoritatively by McCaffery and Beebe (1989). Relaxation techniques vary in their approaches, but share this feature in common (Jacobsen 1938; Benson *et al.* 1977).

A mother attending childbirth education is encouraged to practise relaxation, not only at group sessions, but also at other times. Her labour companion should be involved, so that that person is able to provide support and reinforcement when the practice becomes the reality of childbirth (Schrock, 1988).

As relaxation techniques constitute but one component of a package of childbirth education, it is difficult for researchers to isolate them in order to evaluate their effectiveness. Authoritative research in this area has involved various inputs, described as 'prenatal classes of a standard format' (Timm, 1989) or 'psychoprophylactic preparation classes' (Enkin *et al.* 1972).

In spite of the limitations of research into relaxation during childbirth, relaxation has been researched in a range of chronic pathological conditions, such as a study that involved headache sufferers (Philips, 1988). Relaxation significantly reduces the sensory component of pain, but (particularly importantly if this work is applicable to labour pain) Philips (1988) found that the emotional component of pain was equally lowered. Thus, the aggravating effect of anxiety on pain was reduced by relaxation. However in general, the relevance of research on relaxation in pathological conditions to the pain of childbirth must be questioned.

An issue not infrequently raised about the mother's intention to assume control of her birth experience, relating to intervention or nonintervention (such as pain control), is the risk of failure of her chosen method (Drife, 1995). This is thought sufficiently disconcerting to lead not only to 'personal disappointment but also [to feeling] that she has let the side down'. This oft-repeated assertion is contradicted by authoritative research (Green *et al.* 1990), which found that mothers with high expectations of assuming control were more likely to be able to achieve control and a more satisfying birth experience.

Thus, although evidence about the effectiveness of relaxation in labour is lacking, there is a strong suggestion that attempts to use it, if unsuccessful, may not in themselves be as harmful as has been assumed.

Hypnotherapy

The extent of nonmaternal involvement in hypnotherapy in labour is marginally greater than that required by more conventional forms of relaxation. This is associated with the more intensive training necessary to prepare the mother to practise self-hypnosis during childbirth. The training regime comprises weekly sessions during the first and third trimesters with three-weekly sessions in the middle trimester (Crasilneck and Hall, 1985). This considerable time investment decreases the likelihood of hypnotherapy being widely used (Baram, 1995), as reflected in Steer's data (1993) in which only four mothers out of a sample of 6459 employed hypnotherapy (0.07%).

Hypnotherapy has been defined as 'the use of hypnotic techniques to induce a compliant and suggestible trance-like state in the treatment of conditions with a large psychological component' (Booth, 1993a).

It is unclear how hypnotherapy works. It has been compared with the 'mesmerizing' effects of tedious activities such as motorway driving (Booth, 1993), sometimes known as 'highway hypnosis' (Puskar and Mumford, 1990). To explain its mode of action, Hilgard (1973) suggested that an individual's consciousness comprises several levels of awareness. This differentiation permits the subject to function at a level other than the one at which pain is perceived, resulting in the nonrecognition of pain. At the same time, a 'hidden observer' maintains awareness of all activities and permits total recall as well as pain perception when the hypnotized state ends.

An alternative explanation, involving the 'gate theory' of pain control, is that hypnotherapy may operate by closing the 'gates' comprising the inhibitory interneurones in the substantia gelatinosa of the dorsal horns of the spinal cord (Melzack and Wall, 1965). According to this explanation, hypnotherapy

permits the mother to reinterpret the painful stimuli of uterine contractions as benign sensations. In this way the gates in the substantia gelatinosa are prevented, by descending impulses, from opening and allowing the perception of pain. As with more conventional relaxation (*see above*) the autonomic stress response is reduced (Simkin, 1989).

Whether a mother is suitable to use hypnotherapy is influenced by her 'hypnotizability'. This uncertainty has given rise to some concern and much research about the value of hypnotherapy in childbirth (Spanos *et al.*, 1994). Only 15% of the general population are 'highly suggestible and easy to hypnotize'; an equal proportion are 'difficult to hypnotize' and the remainder are variably able to enter a hypnotic state (Baram, 1995).

Research has tended to equivocate about the effectiveness of hypnotherapy in the control of labour pain (Spanos *et al.* 1994). However, a randomized controlled trial (RCT) involving 82 mothers, which was not considered by Spanos, demonstrated clear benefits (Freeman *et al.* 1986). These researchers were unable to demonstrate any significant reduction in the mothers' use of pharmacological analgesia, but the number of assisted births was lower, though not significantly. More importantly, however, and achieving statistical significance ($p = 0.08$), was that 52% of the hypnotherapy group were 'very satisfied' with their labour, whereas this applied to only 23% of the controls. The possibility of the Hawthorne effect cannot be discounted, leading to further questions about the mode of action and effectiveness of hypnotherapy.

The 'bad press' to which hypnosis is vulnerable may discourage the mother from using hypnotherapy. Not unrelated to the media impression of hypnosis, the inclusion of 'compliant and suggestible' in the definition of hypnotherapy (above) may cause concern about the mother's ability to assume control while practising hypnotherapy.

Massage

Everyday forms of massage that we all utilize to treat minor trauma such as bumps are obviously self-administered. In such situations the individual has complete control over this remedy. The massage that springs more easily to mind, however, and attracts publicity is usually applied by another. Thus, when used in labour, the mother's control over massage is marginally reduced.

In the study reported by Steer (1993) almost one-fifth (1178 or 19.3%) of mothers reported receiving massage to relieve pain during childbirth; but the midwives reported using it far less frequently (515 or 5%) for individual mother's labours. It may be that this discrepancy is associated with confusing terminology (above) or with the different significance attached to massage by those involved.

As there is a difficulty with terminology it may be helpful to define massage:

The application of hand pressure to soft tissues, usually muscles tendons or ligaments, without causing movement or change in position of a joint to decrease pain, produce relaxation, and/or improve circulation.

(Haldeman, 1994; Mobily *et al.* 1994).

The basic movements include: effleurage, pétrissage, tapotement, hacking, kneading and cupping (Malkin, 1994). Each movement features different pressure, direction, speed, hand position and motion to achieve specific desired effects on the tissues beneath.

The main mode of action of massage is thought to be that of 'closing the gate' to prevent the passage of pain stimuli being perceived in the higher centres of the central nervous system (CNS). The tactile stimulation and positive feelings that result when a caring and empathetic form of touch is applied serve to enhance the pain-controlling effects of massage (Ferrell-Torry and Glick, 1993). The benefits of massage are further reinforced by the relaxation response that the experience engenders.

It is recommended that massage during labour should be intermittent (Simkin, 1989). This is because of the likelihood of pain increasing when massage ceases, due to the nervous system becoming accustomed or adapting to the stimuli and the sense organs ceasing to respond to them. This endorses the midwife's use of back rubbing which is ordinarily applied during contractions.

In spite of massage being so frequently used, research into its effectiveness is lacking (Steer, 1993). This may be associated with the limited significance attached by health-care providers to this remedy, as demonstrated above. Alternatively, it may be because of the many methodological weaknesses to which such research is prone, as observed by Haldeman (1994), who regrets the shortage of 'serious' RCTs. This lack leads to the question of whether midwives should apply an intervention, albeit as basic as back rubbing, whose effects are inadequately evaluated. The mother's seeking and appreciation of this intervention may justify its use, but the implications for the midwife, her practice and her litigation risk also merit consideration (Chalmers, 1993).

Hydrotherapy

Hydrotherapy is the first of the nonpharmacological methods considered here that involves the use of a nonhuman agent – the bath or pool and the water that it contains. Water in various forms has long been used for healing and comfort, but using water during labour to increase comfort, as hydrotherapy is defined here, is relatively novel (Brown, 1982). The rapid increase in the use of hydrotherapy becomes apparent when comparing the data reported by Steer (1993), relating to the 1990 data collection, with those reported by Alderdice *et al.* (1995), collected in 1992–1993. In Steer's sample of 6459 mothers, none reported using water to increase comfort. Two years later, however, Alderdice *et al.* (1995) found that only 5 out of 219 provider units (2.3%) had no experience of using water for labour.

The benefits of hydrotherapy, which have led to this meteoric increase in use, are attributable to either one or both of two phenomena (Garland and Jones, 1994). First, the 'hydrothermic' effect results from water being a conductor of heat, releasing muscle spasm and, hence, relieving pain. Second, the 'hydrokinetic' effect eradicates the effect of gravity and associated discomforts, such as pelvic pressure. These two effects facilitate relaxation and so reduce anxiety and fatigue.

Bathing has been assumed to encourage vaginal and intrauterine contamination and lead to maternal and/or neonatal infection, so Waldenström and Nilsson (1992) investigated retrospectively the likelihood of infection after bathing. Their sample comprised 89 mothers who bathed following spontaneous rupture of the membranes (SRM); the control group comprised 89 mothers who did not bathe after SRM and whose SRM–delivery interval was comparable. There was no difference in infection rates between the two groups. In terms of their use of medication, though, the researchers found marked differences, such as:

- The 'bathing' mothers required less augmentation of labour.
- The mothers' pain experience was similarly positively affected by bathing.
- The use of analgesic medication was consistently lower in the bathing mothers.
- Their use of pethidine and Entonox was significantly reduced.

Although research relating to the benefits and safety of hydrotherapy has been inconclusive (McCandlish and Renfrew, 1993), a recently completed RCT raises important issues (Cammu *et al.*, 1994). This study involved 120 low-risk, first-time mothers who spent 1 hour of labour in a bath. Assessment of the mothers' pain after 25 minutes of immersion showed the bathing group's pain had increased less markedly than that of the control group who stayed in bed. After 1 hour, that is on completion of the bathing mothers' immersion, there was no difference. Thus, the authors conclude that bathing has a 'pain stabilizing', rather than a 'pain-relieving' effect. The mothers are reported as having appreciated bathing's soothing and relaxing effects.

The aggressively active approach to the management of labour for these 'low-risk' mothers merits comment, even concern, in relation to their ability to assume control of labour. All 120 mothers experienced elective artificial rupture of the membranes and application of a fetal scalp electrode before the cervix was 5 cm dilated. Like Robinson (1994), we must question each mother's control over her labour. Her experience does not seem to accord with the Swedish findings mentioned above or with Beech's observation:

> *A woman in a pool is very much more in control of her labour, and it is a great deal more difficult for the staff to intervene. Therein lies the rub.*
> Beech (1995)

Transcutaneous Electrical Nerve Stimulation

Unlike other remedies considered here, TENS was developed recently and specifically to control pain (Wall and Sweet, 1967). Its development followed the introduction of gate control theory. However, Steer (1993) observes that the use of TENS does not correlate with its 'high profile in the media', as only 335 mothers (5.5%) used it.

The mode of action of TENS comprises closing the gate to the passage of pain impulses, which has been shown to result from a below-pain-threshold barrage of electrical impulses (Sjölund *et al.* 1990). The barrage, felt as gentle electric shocks, is produced by a hand-held current generator that the mother controls. The other crucial action of TENS is to stimulate the release of endorphins, which are one of a group of opiate-like peptides produced physiologically. Endorphins modulate the transmission of pain perceptions and, thereby, raise the mother's pain threshold to produce relaxation and feelings of well-being (Hawkins, 1994).

In labour, the mother sets the current generator or TENS unit at just below her pain threshold and maintains it there between contractions. The mother increases the intensity of the electrical stimulation during each contraction to compete with the pain (Simkin, 1989).

Research into the effectiveness of TENS, like other 'complementary' methods, is fraught with methodological pitfalls. Thus, considerable uncertainty exists about the benefits of TENS in childbirth. An exception to this uncertain picture is the study by Harrison *et al.* (1987), comprising a double blind RCT in which 150 mothers participated. This showed that mothers using TENS were less likely to use any other form of analgesia, indicating beneficial effects and considerable satisfaction with it.

Some of the problems faced during research into less orthodox methods of pain control are illustrated by the work of Hardy (1991) on TENS. Her RCT remains incomplete, but data on the 80 TENS mothers and 67 controls show that (disregarding Entonox use) more TENS mothers used no additional analgesia. This result, however, did not reach the level of significance. The midwives tended to assess the TENS mothers' pain as more severe than the mothers' and more severe than the controls'. Thus Hardy (1991) questions whether the midwives were uncomfortable in providing care for the TENS mothers. She continues by asking whether midwives find it easier to care for narcotized mothers over whom they are able to exert greater control. This line of thought suggests clearly that using TENS permits the mother to assume more control over her situation.

Acupuncture

The nonmaternal contributions necessary for the mother who chooses acupuncture include the assistance of an acupuncturist to both insert the needles and teach her how to manipulate or otherwise stimulate them. Additionally, the mother must make use of a nonhuman agent in the form of the needles themselves. As well as these fundamental nonmaternal inputs to acupuncture, which may be regarded as alien, the mother must also accept a rationale about health that is unconventional and may also be regarded as alien. It is impossible to say which of these extraneous factors is most significant, but they probably contribute to the limited use of acupuncture (Steer, 1993); only one mother in a sample of 6459 (0.02%) used it. Acupuncture's theoretical framework draws on traditional Chinese medicine (Bond, 1979), which teaches that health requires a balance between opposing energy forces; imbalance causes illhealth or disease (Arthurs, 1994). The energy takes two forms: the negative female passive 'yin', and a positive male active 'yang' (Bond, 1979). Collectively this 'energy' is known as 'Chi'. Each individual's vital energy flows through 12 paired interconnected body channels or meridians (Chapman and Gunn, 1990), to which the 365 acupuncture points relate.

The mode of action of acupuncture has been hypothesized as taking one or more of four forms (Simkin, 1989):

- First, psychological effects are associated with the cultural components and the need for preparation for acupuncture, comparable to childbirth education (Chapman, 1984).
- Second, conviction that acupuncture works causes the higher centres to 'close the gate' to the passage of pain impulses (Melzack, 1975).
- Third, the needles activate pain-inhibiting mechanisms in the CNS (Bond, 1979). It may be that endogenous opioid production in the brain stem is enhanced by acupuncture. Arthurs (1994) supports this by his observation of the sedation which occurs 1 hour after acupuncture.
- Fourth, the closure of the gate to pain impulses may be by the presynaptic inhibition of sensory fibres at the level of the dorsal horn due to the stimulation of large diameter sensory fibres.

Acupuncture's psychological benefits are borne out by laboratory research (Yang *et al.* 1984), which showed that the analgesic effects of acupuncture lasted only for as long as stimulation was maintained. This is reminiscent of the relatively short-term benefits of massage (above). However, unlike massage, the emotional response, i.e. not being upset by the pain, was shown to be longer lasting.

The effectiveness of acupuncture was demonstrated in people who suffered from chronic pain by Chapman and Gunn (1990), who found that 50–80% of the sample benefited. This figure may be compared with those who received sham acupuncture, which was 50% effective, and placebo controls in whom 30% found some relief.

In the introduction to this section, it is suggested that for some mothers acupuncture may be unacceptable. However, if the mother is able to take advantage of this form of pain control it may facilitate her control as, according to Skelton and Flowerdew (1988), acupuncture made each mother in their sample 'more in control of the labour and delivery'.

Other Nonpharmacological Methods

Other approaches to pain control in labour are infrequently used and/or under-researched. Positioning and mobilizing exemplify strategies which attract inter-est, often because of issues associated with the mother's control, but have been inadequately researched (Roberts, 1989). Similarly under-researched and having attracted little interest in child-bearing is homoeopathy (Castro, 1992). The effects of the mother's environment on her labour pain, including both the place of birth and the labour companions, is beginning to receive the interest it deserves. Unfortunately, much of the research has been undertaken in settings less than relevant to the UK (O'Driscoll and Meagher, 1980; Sosa *et al.* 1980; Kennell *et al.* 1988).

As mentioned above, it is not possible here to compile an exhaustive list of the nonpharmacological techniques that the mother could consider employing in labour. The development of knowledge is so rapid that, were such a list to be prepared, it would be out of date before publication. Thus, the focus here is on remedies which are frequently used and which inform important issues relating to control.

Pharmacological Methods

As with other interventions pharmacological methods of pain control vary hugely in their effects, their duration and degree of control which the various contributors assume.

Inhalational Analgesia

Currently only N_2O (50%) and O_2 (50%), Entonox, is permitted to be used by a labouring mother under the supervision of a midwife in UK. Higher concentrations are not permitted for midwives' use because of the risk of anaesthesia, i.e. rendering the mother unconscious (Melzack and Wall, 1991). Entonox is the most widely used agent for controlling labour pain in UK (Steer, 1993), with 60% of mothers having used it.

Bonica and McDonald (1990) state that the attraction of Entonox lies in it being 'moderately effective without causing significant maternal or neonatal depression'. Its effectiveness depends on the mother being appropriately instructed in its use.

Having a low lipid solubility, N_2O rapidly reaches analgesic levels in the mother's circulation (Dickersin, 1989) and the cessation of analgesia is equally rapid when inhalation ceases. The mother should begin her self-administration of Entonox 'some 10–15 seconds before the painful period of each contraction' (Bonica and McDonald, 1990). These authors quote research showing that good pain relief is achieved in 60% of mothers and that a further 30% achieve partial pain relief.

Being self-administered, Entonox allows the mother a high level of control over the administration. Effectiveness, though, is less controllable as it depends upon the instruction given to her and her ability to follow it. Entonox is unlikely to affect the mother's control over her birth experience.

The blue cylinders with white quartered tops are becoming less familiar as more clinical areas ensure a continuous supply of Entonox by piped delivery from a central depot. Entonox is administered via a two-stage valve system – the first reduces the pressure of the gas and the second comprises an on-demand valve which opens in response to the negative pressure of the mother's inspiration.

Although relatively safe for the mother and baby, concerns have emerged relating to the potential of Entonox to harm staff. Teratogenic and other pathological effects have been reported among those who frequently administer N_2O, such as dentists (Newton, 1992). A study of 14 midwives showed that their exposure levels to N_2O greatly exceeded those stipulated in countries where upper limits have been imposed. Newton (1992) concludes that midwives must take 'personal responsibility' for their safety when Entonox is administered and should seek institutional safety precautions.

Opioid Drugs

Although the terms may be used interchangeably (Melzack and Wall, 1991), narcotics and opiates are subtly different. Opiates are derived, naturally or synthetically, from the opium poppy, but narcotics are those which cause sleepiness or ultimately narcosis, i.e. insensibility. The opioids that are used in labour are also narcotics.

Their powerful action makes the opioids appropriate during labour. Steer (1993) reports that of 6459 mothers, 2247 (36.9%) had received pethidine, 128 (2.1%) had received diamorphine and 107 (1.8%) had received meptazinol.

There are two sites in the CNS where the opioids are active. First, in the midbrain a system of periaqueductal grey matter indirectly inhibits the spinal cord's ability to transmit pain impulses. Second, in the substantia gelatinosa of the dorsal horn of the spinal cord, high concentrations of enkephalins and opiate

receptors are present. The opioids are, thus, able to limit the transmission of pain impulses, especially to the higher centres (Melzack and Wall, 1991). Opiates also have other less specific effects, including their mood elevating effect through the limbic system.

As well as achieving analgesia, the depressant effects of opiates produce sedation and, crucially important perinatally, respiratory depression. The latter is more problematical because of the easy transplacental transfer of these drugs, although Cawthra (1986) questioned whether this applied to pethidine. Although sedation may be welcomed by the mother, the reports of 'dizziness, dysphoria and drowsiness' that accompany it are not (Moore and Ball, 1974). Kitzinger (1987) links these unwelcome side-effects with the mother's reduced control: 'They ... also cause confusion and can make a woman feel powerless to cope actively with labour.' The excitatory effects of the opiates on the gastrointestinal tract result in the all too familiar nausea and vomiting, as well as the more ominous delay in gastric emptying, associated with Mendelson's syndrome (Park and Fulton, 1991).

Recent research gives rise to concern about the effect of opiates on more general and longer term neonatal behaviour (Mander, 1992). Crowell *et al.* (1994) showed the unhelpful effects of opiates on new mothers' breastfeeding. They recommend that better support in labour and postnatally prevents the need for opiates and the ensuing neonatal problems and encourages the mother to persevere with breastfeeding.

The main features of the opiates used most frequently in labour are now considered.

Diamorphine

The chemical structure of diamorphine results in greater lipid solubility than that of morphine, which allows faster penetration into cerebral tissue. This rapid diffusion permits an equally rapid conversion into morphine, the active agent (Park and Fulton, 1991). Diamorphine is less likely to cause gastrointestinal upsets than morphine and there are greater positive psychological effects. Intramuscular administration of diamorphine results in the drug taking effect within 5–10 minutes, and lasting for 3 hours.

The long-term effects of diamorphine cause concern (Robinson, 1995). Swedish research suggests that diamorphine given during labour is associated with a greater risk of drug addiction when the baby reaches adulthood. Thus, it is not only the mother's control that is jeopardized when diamorphine is used.

Pethidine hydrochloride

Pethidine is a synthetic analgesic, which is metabolized in the liver; this is significant because the neonatal liver is immature, thus prolonging pethidine's neonatal effects. Administered intramuscularly, pethidine's analgesic effect begins within 15 minutes and continues for 2 hours.

A pilot study on the second stage of labour produced the surprise finding that both the first and second stage of labour were longer if pethidine had been administered (Thomson and Hillier, 1994). A literature review found no research to contradict this finding, but rather that the effects of this most frequently used drug have 'not been adequately assessed'. This is an example of the nonavailability of information that the mother requires if she is to assume control of her birth experience.

Meptazinol

Meptazinol may be preferable to pethidine because neonatal respiratory depression is less marked (Park and Fulton, 1991). The analgesic action begins within 15 minutes and continues for at least 4 hours (Knights, 1986).

General anaesthesia

General anaesthesia (GA) is not a conventional form of pain control, but it raises important issues. Used to facilitate either the birth of the baby or placenta in emergency situations, GA is appropriate when there is insufficient time or expertise for regional anaesthesia.

General anaesthesia is used infrequently in maternity care. Steer's data show that 238 mothers out of 6459 (3.9%) were anaesthetized during labour. This small number is probably because of the increasing availability of regional anaesthesia and the serious risks associated with GA. Morgan (1987) recounts the abysmal record of the contribution of obstetric GA to maternal mortality. Although the total number of maternal deathscaused by or associated with GA peaked between 1964 and 1969 (during which time there were 100 such deaths), of greater significance may be the *proportion* of maternal deaths caused by or associated with GA. Despite the rising birth rate at that time, the number of maternal deaths caused by other factors was falling markedly. The proportion of direct maternal deaths caused by GA, however, rose from a stable level of 2.5% to 3.5% between 1952 and 1963 to 13.0% between 1982 and 1984 (Cloake, 1991). A majority of maternal deaths caused by or associated with GA were caused by the aspiration of acid stomach contents into the mother's lungs during the induction of GA in labour (Mendelson's syndrome) (Morgan, 1987). Vanner (1993) suggests that the current maternal mortality figures caused by Mendelson's syndrome are only slightly better than they were in the 1950s, in spite of the widespread use of cricoid pressure.

Unsurprisingly, the possibility of maternal death does not feature in the information given to the mother about to undergo a GA, but the risk of the mother being aware during GA has attracted publicity (Beech, 1995). This 'awareness' results from a light GA being administered to minimize transplacental transfer of the anaesthetic agents that cause neonatal depression. This clearly benefits the baby, but may mean that the mother is insufficiently anaesthetized and remains conscious but incapable of communicating. The extent of the problem emerges in Beech's quote of Crawford's estimate of 1% of mothers being aware during GA; she converts this into 400 women every year. This constitutes the ultimate lack of control by the mother.

Epidural analgesia

A surgical technique similar to lumbar puncture permits injection of slow-acting local anaesthetics, such as bupivicaine, into the lumbar epidural space. The cannula, through which the local anaesthetic is delivered, is sited and the initial injection administered by an obstetric anaesthetist. The administration may be on an intermittent or 'top-up' basis by a suitably trained midwife, or through a 'patient-controlled analgesia' delivery system. Alternatively, a shorter-acting local anaesthetic, such as lignocaine, is injected as a test dose or epidural opioids may be administered epidurally. This blocks pain impulses through the afferent sensory spinal nerves that traverse the epidural space and transmit pain impulses from organs such as the uterus to the CNS. The efficient binding properties of bupivicaine with maternal plasma proteins allow a small proportion, about 20%, to cross the placenta to the fetus.

An effective epidural eradicates the pain of uterine contractions (Howell and Chalmers, 1992) or, as Morgan *et al.* (1982), on the basis of their authoritative 1000 woman study, modestly claimed, 'an epidural is strikingly more effective ... than any other analgesic method.' The proportion of epidural blocks that are effective, though, is difficult to estimate as data are not readily available. Simkin (1989), however, maintains that the success rate of lumbar epidural analgesia is 67–90%. This is supported by one of the few studies to even mention the possibility of epidural failure, which reports a failure rate of 15% (Kitzinger, 1987).

Unfortunately, as well as pain impulses, nonpain motor impulses also tend to be blocked (Pursey, 1994), causing immobility and the mother to become bedfast for at least as long as the epidural block is effective. Additionally, sympathetic nerve fibres are blocked, which results in vasodilatation in the lower body. Vasodilatation may cause sudden, severe and potentially life-threatening maternal hypotension. To avoid the dire effects of this eventuality, an intravenous infusion is established before siting the epidural.

The tendency of continuous epidural analgesia to prolong labour, particularly the second stage, is well recognized (Williams *et al.* 1985). Such delay may be associated with malrotation of the presenting part (Howell and Chalmers, 1992). Chestnut *et al.* (1987) showed that an epidural 'topped up' after cervical dilatation reached 8 cm was associated with a prolonged second stage and instrumental assistance, i.e. forceps, for the birth. A study involving 85 mothers of whom 38 chose epidural analgesia (Williams *et al.* 1985) demonstrated the increased incidence of a series of obstetric procedures, recognized as the 'cascade of intervention' (Jouppila *et al.* 1980). This has been identified by some observers in obstetric practice and may have been aggravated by the introduction of an effective pain-control method (Varney Burst, 1983). The cascade may be associated with neurological changes mentioned above that cause relaxation of the pelvic floor and encourage malposition of the fetal head, incomplete rotation and delay in, especially, the second stage. Oxytocic drugs are used to correct the delay, but these are associated with fetal hypoxia (Yudkin, 1979; Keirse and Chalmers, 1989; Evans, 1992). Thus, interventions to expedite the birth, for example forceps or Caesarean section, may become necessary (Howell and Chalmers, 1992). The lack of authoritative data on the neonatal effects as well as on the long-term maternal effects, such as headache, backache and bladder malfunction, has been highlighted (Howell and Chalmers, 1992).

The proportion of maternity units with the facilities, in the form of suitably trained anaesthetists and midwives, to provide a 24-hour on-demand epidural service correlates inversely with the number of small maternity units in a region (Morgan, 1993a). The proportion varies between 100% in the Oxford region and 28% in Wales.

In the UK, epidural block is used to control pain in more than 19% of labours (Steer, 1993). This seemingly low and benign figure conceals wide variations. The epidural rate may be as low as the 14% quoted for Northern Ireland (Morgan, 1993a). On the other hand, epidural rates as high as 87% have been reported (Mander, 1995), but published rates do not yet exceed 67% (Morgan, 1993b). These not inconsiderable variations may serve to reflect mothers' limited control when in labour and are discussed below.

Reality of Pain Control

Having considered the apparent control of pain and the methods of pain control, the reality of the control of pain is now examined to evaluate where control may actually be situated. To draw together the strands which have emerged already, the input of the three main contributors to pain control and the associated decision making are reviewed here. These participants comprise the mother, midwife and medical practitioner (**Figure 10.1**) and are considered in that order.

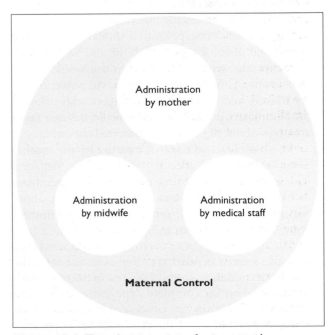

Figure 10.1 The administration of pain control.

Mother

Although the ultimate decision regarding pain control supposedly rests with the mother, her input into this decision may be limited by her lack of information or by her difficulty in understanding the inevitable jargon. Equally likely, though, as has recurred in our examination of the methods, is the lack of research-based information, particularly studies that address the mother's unique concerns.

The reality of the mother's control in the context of hydrotherapy is obvious; as shown by mothers successfully increasing the availability of pools for labour and birth. Data show the large proportion of provider units in which it has been necessary, in the past, for the mother to provide her own pool to enable her to labour and/or give birth in water (Alderice *et al.* 1995). More recently these researchers show the proportion of units (105 out of 219 or 48%) which have been able to provide this facility, resulting in the women not being required to provide their own pools. Thus, the instrumental role of the mother in controlling policy and bringing about change becomes evident.

Compared with the mother's obvious control in relation to hydrotherapy, the midwife's control is lacking (Anderson, 1994). This manifested itself in the case known as the 'East Herts Midwives'. Two midwives were suspended from practice in January 1994 following a home birth in a pool. As required by their employers the midwives asked the mother to leave the pool for the birth, but she could not comply. The midwives were disciplined for nonadherence to trust policy, despite not being permitted to leave a mother in the second or third stage of labour and being unable to remove the woman from pool as this would constitute assault. This case demonstrated the power of policy makers and nonmidwife managers who enforced the disciplinary procedure. Additionally, this case raises concerns about the reality of maternal choice.

The high level of control exerted by the mother using hydrotherapy (Beech, 1995) and by managers has been perceived by some of our medical colleagues as threatening. This has resulted in jibes about 'aquatic fanatics' and, more seriously, in mothers being discouraged from using hydrotherapy.

The mother's support network has attracted considerable interest in relation to the success of her childbearing experience. In the UK, research on support has focused on her complete experience, rather than her labour or pain. In other countries, however, research has addressed the effects of her supporters on her pain experience, but the non-UK settings make this research less than relevant to the present discussion (O'Driscoll and Meagher, 1980; Sosa *et al.* 1980; Kennell *et al.* 1988) – an omission that deserves to be corrected.

Midwife

Maternal control of the use of inhalational analgesia in the form of Entonox is both apparent and real. What has emerged, however, is the limited control that the midwife exerts when Entonox is used, with particular reference to her own health.

The lack of research-based information emerged in relation to an intervention frequently applied by the midwife, i.e. massage. Criticism of the limited availability of research may also be levelled at other forms of pain control, but the midwife's reluctance or inability to utilize existing research should also be taken into account. For example, research on the effects of opioid drugs on breastfeeding (Richards and Bernal, 1972; Rajan, 1993) is underused.

As identified already, the decision regarding pain control is made by the mother, with research-based information being provided by her carers, such as the midwife. Attempts have been made to alter the information-giving role of the midwife in the context of TENS. This follows a suggestion by nurses' and midwives' statutory bodies (Ralph, 1991), who state that the midwife may 'encourage, advise on and use TENS equipment to relieve labour pain'. Even disregarding the inconclusive research evidence on TENS, such 'encouragement' is clearly beyond the midwife's role. Thus, the mother's control of her decision making is being threatened by those who seek to control midwives.

Medical Practitioner

Certain issues relating to the medical control of pain remedies are raised by epidural analgesia. The location of the decision to utilize epidural analgesia has been shown in only a minority of labours to be lodged with the mother (Morgan, 1993a). The mothers in whose labours epidural analgesia was used stated that they made the decision in 47% of cases (1101 mothers). The decision was made by medical staff for 360 mothers (15.8%) and by the midwife for 281 mothers (12%). This evidence seriously questions maternal autonomy.

Not inconsiderable variations in epidural rates in UK have been highlighted (above). What are the implications of these variations for the mother's control? One explanation for the wide variations in epidural rates relates to the enthusiasm of obstetric anaesthetists to share the benefits of this pain control method. Anaesthetists have consistently applied staunch pressure to increase the availability of the services which they provide. An example is: 'A higher priority should be accorded by health boards to obstetric anaesthesia ...' (SHHD, 1985). Such pressure may benefit mothers, but may not be entirely altruistic, as it has been labelled 'empire building' (Reynolds, 1989) and 'professionalization' (Mander, 1993).

While the pressure by anaesthetists at the policy-making level is explicit, pressure at the clinical level is more circumspect. An example of this pressure may be found in a booklet for mothers 'to explain' events during labour (Stewart and West, undated). This booklet devotes almost four times more text on epidural than on all other pain control methods. The effect of such pressure on the mother's ability to control her birth experience may only be surmised as being prejudicial.

The limited availability of research-based information to facilitate a mother's decision making about epidural analgesia causes serious concern (Mander, 1994; Howell and Chalmers, 1992). Research has focused largely on techniques and drugs to be injected (Mander, 1992). The limited research into the mother's anxieties has been dismissed as methodologically unsound (Kitzinger, 1987). The more methodologically respectable research into the woman-oriented long-term effects has been similarly questioned because of its retrospective nature (MacArthur, 1991). Until authoritative research is undertaken that focuses on the mother's concerns, she will face difficulty in decision making and giving informed consent to this intervention (Howell and Chalmers, 1992).

An advantage of epidural analgesia suggested by the Maternity Alliance (1986) is that it permits the mother to retain her self-control. While recognizing the significance of such control, the mother should be in a position to balance this increased form of control against the other aspects of control, which are reduced by epidural analgesia.

The widespread availability of a '24-hour on-demand' epidural service (above) may reflect the success of obstetric anaesthetists' proselytizing. Unfortunately, the services which are available do not invariably meet the demand that has been created, as Rajan (1993) observed:

too often, extraneous factors may ... interfere with the arrival of pain relief. For instance, in this study a great deal of unnecessary suffering was caused when [responses to] requests for epidural analgesia were delayed because of the nonavailability of an anaesthetist

Many midwives have found themselves using their full range of interpersonal and midwifery skills to support a mother whose expectations of her epidural analgesia have not been fulfilled. If the mother is encouraged, as demonstrated above, to take advantage of an epidural service, those who provide it should ensure that both the service and the technique functions effectively. Rajan (1993) drew attention to the gulf between the perceptions of the mother and those of her carers in evaluating the effectiveness of pain control. Disconcertingly, the staff were found to be significantly more likely to agree with each other's perceptions than with the mother's. Rajan (1993) is pessimistic about the likelihood of the mother being able to exert control, or even choice, over her pain control. This pessimism is reflected in her view of the likely effectiveness of the mother's pain control when she states 'it is the professionals' opinions and judgements that are likely to prevail when more effective methods are requested, or needed, by the women.'

Although the concept of the mother's choice has become central to the care provided by midwives, the reality of this choice and the mother's control of her pain remedies is questioned. As Winterton observed relating to maternal choice, the decision-making by the mother about the control of her pain may be 'more illusory than real' (House of Commons, 1992).

KEY CONCEPTS

- The mother's control over her birth experience has been shown to benefit that experience.
- Control over pain control is said to reside with the mother, but this may not be the case.
- Research-based knowledge about many nonpharmacological pain control methods is lacking.
- Research-based knowledge which does exist is not always well utilized.
- Certain pain control methods, including mainly nonpharmacological methods, permit the mother more control over birth experience than do other methods.

References

Alderdice F, Renfrew M, Marchant S *et al.*: Labour and birth in water in England and Wales: survey report, *Br J Midwifery* 3(7):375, 1995.

Anderson T: Trust betrayed: the disciplining of the East Herts midwives, *MIDIRS* 4(2):132, 1994.

Arthurs G: Hypnosis and acupuncture in pregnancy, *Br J Midwifery* 2(10):495, 1994.

Baram DA: Hypnosis in reproductive health care: a review and case reports, *Birth* 22(1):37, 1995.

Beech BL: Conscious during a general anaesthetic caesarean operation, *AIMS J* 7(3):8, 1995.

Beecher HK: Relationship of significance of wound pain to pain experienced, *J Am Med Assoc* 161(7):1609, 1956.

Benson H, Kotch JB, Crassweiler KD *et al.*: Historical and clinical considerations of the relaxation response, *Am Sci* 65(4):441, 1977.

Bond MR: *Pain: its nature, analysis and treatment*, Edinburgh, 1979, Churchill Livingstone.

Bonica JJ, McDonald JS, : The pain of childbirth. In Bonica JJ, Loeser JD, Chapman CR *et al.*, editors: *The management of pain*, 2nd edn, Philadelphia, 1990, Lea & Febinger.

Booth B: Hypnotherapy, *Nurs Times* 89(40):42, 1993.

Brown C: Therapeutic effects of bathing during labour, *J Nurse-Midwifery* 27(1):165, 1982.

Cammu H, van Clasen K, Wettere L *et al* 'To bathe or not to bathe' during the first stage, *Acta Obstet Gynaecol Scand* 73(6):468, 1994.

Castro M: *Homoeopathy for the mother and baby: a guide to pregnancy, birth and the postnatal year*, London, 1992, Macmillan.

Cawthra AM: The use of pethidine in labour, *Midwives Chron* 99(1183):178, 1986.

Chalmers I: Effective care in midwifery: research the professions and the public, *Midwives Chron* 106(1260):3, 1993.

Chamberlain G, Wraight A, Steer P: *Pain and its relief in childbirth*, Edinburgh, 1993, Churchill Livingstone.

Chapman CR: New directions in the understanding and management of pain, *Soc Sci Med* 19(12):1261, 1984.

Chapman CR, Gunn CC: Acupuncture. In Bonica JJ, Loeser JD, Chapman CR *et al.*, editors: *The management of pain*, 2nd edn, Philadelphia, 1990, Lea & Febinger.

Chard T, Richards MPM: Introduction. In Richards MPM, Chard T, editors: *Obstetrics in the 1990s: current controversies*, Oxford, 1992, McKeith Press.

Chestnut DH, Vandewalker GE, Owen OL *et al.*: The influence of continuous epidural bupivicaine analgesia on the second stage of labour and method of delivery on the nulliparous woman, *Anesthesiology* 66(6):774, 1987.

Cloake M: Report on confidential enquiries into maternal deaths in the UK 1985–7: a summary of the main points, *Health Trends* 23(1):4, 1991.

Crasilneck HB, Hall JA: *Clinical hypnosis: principles and applications*, 2nd edn, Orlando, 1985, Grune & Stratton.

Crowell MK, Hill PD, Humenick SS: Relationship between obstetric analgesia and time of effective breast feeding, *J Nurs Midwifery* 39(3):150–6, 1994.

Dickersin K: Pharmacological control of pain during labour. In Chalmers I, Enkin M, Kierse MJNC, editors: *Effective care in pregnancy and childbirth*, Vol. 2, Oxford, 1989, Oxford University Press.

Dick-Read G: *Natural childbirth*, London, 1933, W Heinemann.

Drife J: On political correctness in the delivery room, *Observer* 29 October:70, 1995.

Edgar L, Smith-Hanrahan CM: Nonpharmacological pain management. In Watt-Watson J, Donovan MI, editors: *Pain management: nursing perspective*, St. Louis, 1992, Mosby.

Enkin M *et al.*: An adequately controlled study of the effectiveness of PPM training. In Morris N: *Psychosomatic medicine in obstetrics and gynaecology*, Basal, 1972, Kargar.

Evans S: The value of cardiotocograph monitoring in midwifery, *Midwives Chron* 105(1248):4, 1992.

Ferrell-Torry A, Glick OJ: The use of therapeutic massage as a nursing intervention to modify anxiety and the perception of cancer pain, *Cancer Nurs* 16(2):93, 1993.

Garland D, Jones K: Waterbirth, 'first stage' immersion or non-immersion? *Br J Midwifery* 2(3):113, 1994.

Green JM, Coupland VA, Kitzinger JV: Expectations, experiences and psychological outcomes of childbirth: a prospective study of 825 women, *Birth* 17(1):15, 1990.

Haldeman S: Manipulation and massage for the relief of backpain. p.1251–62, In Wall PD, Melzack R, editors: *Textbook of pain*, 3rd edition, Edinburgh, 1994, Churchill Livingstone.

Hardy J: *A randomised controlled trial into the use of TENS in labour research and the Midwife Conference proceedings 1990*, Manchester, 1991, University of Manchester.

Harrison RF *et al.*: Pain relief in labour using transcutaneous electrical nerve stimulation (TENS): a TENS/TENS placebo controlled study in two parity groups, *Br J Obstet Gynaecol* 93(7):739, 1986.

Hawkins J: Use of TENS for pain relief in labour, *Br J Midwifery* 2(10):487, 1994.

Hilgard ER: A neodissociation theory of pain reduction in hypnosis, *Psychol Rev* 80(5):396, 1973.

House of Commons: *Health Committee second report: maternity services*, London, 1992, HMSO.

Howell CJ, Chalmers I: A review of prospectively controlled comparisons of epidural with non-epidural forms of pain relief during labour, *Int J Obstet Anesth* 1:93, 1992.

Jacobsen EJ: *Progressive relaxation*, Illinois, 1938, University of Chicago.

Johnson JE, Rice VH: Sensory and distress components of pain, *Nurs Res* 23(3):203, 1974.

Johnson JE *et al.*: Contribution of emotional and instrumental response processes, *J Pers Soc Psychol* 20(1):55, 1971.

Jouppila R *et al.*: The effect of segmental epidural analgesia on maternal prolactin during labour, *Br J Obstet Gynaecol* 31(3):1, 1980.

Kierse MJNC, Chalmers I: Methods for inducing labour. In Chalmers I, Enkin M, Kierse MJNC, editors: *Effective care in pregnancy and childbirth*, Vol. 2, Oxford, 1989, Oxford University Press.

Kennell JH *et al.*: Medical intervention: the effect of social support, *Paediatr Res* 23:211A, 1988.

Kitzinger S: *Some women's experiences of epidurals – a descriptive study*, London, 1987, National Childbirth Trust.

Knights J: Use of meptazinol in routine obstetric practice in a district general hospital, *Midwives Chron* 99(1183):182, 1986.

Lamaze F: *Painless childbirth: psychoprophylactic method*, Chicago, 1970, Regnery.

MacDonald AM: *Chambers twentieth century dictionary*, Edinburgh, 1981, Chambers.

Malkin K: Use of massage in clinical practice, *Br J Nurs* 1(6):292, 1994.

Mander R: The control of pain in labour, *J Clin Nurs* 1:219, 1992.

Mander R: 'Who chooses the choices?' *Modern Midwife* 3(1):23, 1993.

Mander R: Epidural analgesia: 2 Research basis, *B J Midwifery* 2(1):12–16, 1994.

Mander R: Forum on maternity and the newborn: pain in labour, *Midwives* 108(1289):180, 1995.

Mander R: Failure to deliver: ethical issues relating to epidural analgesia in uncomplicated labour. In Frith L, editor: *Midwifery ethics*, 3:51–71 Oxford, 1996 , Butterworth-Heinemann.

MacArthur C: *Health after childbirth*, London, 1991, HMSO.

McCaffery M, Beebe A: *Pain: clinical manual for nursing practice*, St. Louis, 1989, Mosby.

McCandlish R, Redfrew M: Immersion in water during labour and birth: the need for evaluation, *Birth* 20(2):79, 1993.

Maternity Alliance: Editorial: benefits and risks of pain relief, *Maternity Action* 25(5):3, 1986.

Melzack R: How acupuncture can block pain. In Weisenberg M, editor: *Pain clinical and experimental perspectives*, St Loius, 251–7:1975, Mosby.

Melzack R, Wall PD: Pain mechanism: a new theory, *Science* 150(971), 1965.

Mobily PR, Herr KA, Nicholson AC: Validation of cutaneous stimulation interventions for pain management, *Int J Nurs Stud* 31(6):533, 1994.

Moore J, Ball HG: A sequential study of intravenous analgesic treatment during labour, *Br J Anaesth* 46(May):365, 1974.

Morgan BM: Mortality and analgesia. In Morgan BM, editor: *Foundations of obstetric anaesthesia*, London, 1987, Ferrand Press.

Morgan BM: Obstetrical anaesthesia. In Chamberlain G, Wraight A, Steer P, editors: *Pain and its relief in childbirth*, Edinburgh, 1993a, Churchill Livingstone.

Morgan BM: Mobile epidurals: combined spinal epidural analgesia in labour, *MIDIRS Midwif Digest* 3(3):312, 1993b.

Morgan BM, Bulpitt CJ, Clifton P *et al.*: Analgesia and satisfaction in childbirth, *Lancet* ii:808, 1982.

Newton C: Hazards of N_2O exposure, *Nurs Times* 88(39):54, 1992.

Nichols FH, Humenick SS: *Childbirth education: research practice and theory*, Philadelphia, 1988, WB Saunders.

O'Driscoll K, Meagher D: *Active management of labour: the Dublin experience*, 2nd edn, London, 1986, Baillière Tindall.

Park G, Fulton B: *The management of acute pain*, Oxford, 1991, Oxford Medical Publications.

Perkins ER: *Education for childbirth and parenthood*, London, 1980, Croom Helm.

Philips HC: Changing chronic pain experience, *Pain* 32:165–72, 1988.

Pursey M: Mobile epidural — the only epidural without anaesthesia, *Paediatr Post* (3):3, 1994.

Puskar K, Mumford K: The healing power, *Nurs Times* 86(33):50, 1990.

Rajan L: Perceptions of pain and pain relief in labour: the gulf between experience and observation, *Midwifery* 9(3):136, 1993.

Ralph C: *Transcutaneous nerve stimulation: Registrar's letter*, London, 1991, UKCC.

Reynolds F: *Epidural analgesia in obstetrics*, London, 1989, Baillière Tindall.

Richards MPM, Bernal JF: Effects of obstetric medication on mother–infant interaction and infant development. In Morris N, editor: *Psychosomatic medicine in obstetrics and gynaecology*, 3rd International Congress, London, 1972, Karger Basel.

Roberts J: Maternal position during the first stage of labour, 55:883–92, 1989. In: Chalmers I, Enkin M, Kierse MJNC: *Effective care: Pregnancy and childbirth*, Vol 2, Oxford University Press.

Robinson J: Use of heroin in labour — AIMS' concern, *AIMS J* 7(2):9–10, 1995.

Schrock P: The basis of relaxation. In Nichols FH, Humenick SS: *Childbirth education: practice research and theory*, Philadelphia, 1988, WB Saunders.

Sherwood L: *Fundamentals of physiology: a human perspective*, Minneapolis, 1995, West Publishing.

SHHD: *Obstetric anaesthesia and analgesia in Scotland*, Edinburgh, 1985, National Medical Consultative Committee, Scottish Home and Health Department.

Simkin P: Non-pharmacological methods of pain relief during labour. In Chalmers I, Enkin M, Kierse MJNC, editors: *Effective care in pregnancy and childbirth*, Vol. 2, Oxford, 1989, Oxford University Press.

Sjölund BH, Eriksson M, Loeser JD: Transcutaneous and electrical stimulation of peripheral nerves. In Bonica JJ, Oesler JD, Chapman CR *et al.*, editors: *The management of pain*, 2nd edn, Philadelphia, 1990, Lea & Febinger.

Skelton IF, Flowerdew MW: Acupuncture and labour: a summary of results, *Midwives Chron* 101(1204):134, 1988.

Sloane E: *The biology of women*, 3rd edn, New York, 1993, Delmar.

Sosa R, Kennell JH, Klabes M *et al.*: The effect of a supportive companion on perinatal problems, length of labour and mother–infant interaction, *New Engl J Med* 303(11):597, 1980.

Spanos NP, Carmanico SJ, Ellis JA: Hypnotic analgesia. In Wall PD, Melzack R, editors: *Textbook of pain*, 3rd edn, Edinburgh, 1994, Churchill Livingstone.

Steer P: The methods of pain relief used. In Chamberlain G, Wraight A, Steer P: *Pain and its relief in childbirth*, Edinburgh, 1993, Churchill Livingstone.

Stewart M, West C: *The birth of your baby at the Simpson Royal Infirmary*, Edinburgh, undated, Royal Infirmary of Edinburgh.

Thomson AM, Hillier VF: A re-evaluation of the effect of pethidine on the length of labour, *J Adv Nurs* 19(3):448, 1994.

Timm MM: Prenatal education evaluation, *Nurs Res* 28(6):338, 1989.

UKCC: *A Midwive's Code of Practice*, London, 1989, United Kingdom Central Council.

Vanner RG: Mechanisms of regurgitation and its prevention with cricoid pressure, *Int J Obstet Anaesth* 2(4):207, 1993.

Varney Burst H: The influence of consumers in the birthing movement, *Topics Clin Nurs* 5(1):42, 1983.

Waldenström U, Nilsson C: A warm tub bath after spontaneous rupture of the membranes, *Birth* 19(2):57, 1992.

Wall PD, Sweet WH: Temporary abolition of pain, *Science* 155:108–9, 1967.

Williams S, Hepburn M, McIlwaine G: Consumer view of epidural anaesthesia, *Midwifery* 1(1):32, 1985.

Woolf CJ, Thompson JW: Stimulation-induced analgesia: transcutaneous electrical nerve stimulation (TENS) and vibration. In Wall PD, Melzack R, editors: *Textbook of pain*, 3rd edn, Edinburgh, 1994, Churchill Livingstone.

Yang Z, Cai T, Wu J: Psychological aspects of components of pain, *J Psychol* 118(2):135, 1984.

Yudkin P, Frumar AM, Anderson ABM *et al.*: A retrospective study of induction of labour, *Br J Obstet Gynaecol* 86(4):257, 1979.

Zborowski M: Cultural components in responses to pain, *J Soc Issues* 8(1):16, 1952.

11 *Psychosocial Support during Labour*

LEARNING OUTCOMES

After studying this chapter you should be able to:

- Discuss the emotional outcomes of labour.
- Identify some factors that influence the birth experience.
- Recognise the effect of the physical and psychosocial environment on the birth experience.
- Consider the influence of support from caregivers in facilitating a positive experience of labour.

Introduction

The Health Committee Second Report (House of Commons, 1992) for maternity services (the Winterton Report) identified that:

> *the way women respond to and express satisfaction with their experience of using the maternity services is largely dependent on the extent to which they consider their needs are met sufficiently during the process.*

For the first time in the recent history of the provision of maternity care, the opinion of women themselves was sought to establish a responsive and appropriate maternity service (House of Commons, 1992, p. xii). It was this evidence which established the principles of continuity of care, choice of care and place of delivery, and that women should have control over their own bodies throughout pregnancy and childbirth. These factors have subsequently become major elements in a common theme representing what women want from maternity services.

Since the Winterton Report and its subsequent policy document, *Changing Childbirth* (Department of Health, 1993), the provision of maternity care has focused more on some of the specific psychosocial needs of women. There is no question that pregnancy and impending childbirth create anxiety for many women (Combes and Schonveld, 1992). Neither is there any doubt that women want the safe arrival of a healthy infant after a healthy, low-risk pregnancy and birth. However, current evidence suggests that care in labour should not be at the expense of a satisfying birth experience. To reduce anxiety and prepare women realistically midwives must be aware of the psychosocial factors associated with birth. Given the right environment and conditions, both physical and emotional, women can adopt coping mechanisms which allay anxieties (*see* Chapter 4). Some of the psychosocial factors that influence the psychological outcome of labour are therefore explored in this chapter.

The Birth Experience

Emotional Outcome of Labour

Giving birth is unquestionably one of the most significant and memorable events in any womans life. Every woman has her own story to tell about her birth experience. Memories of childbirth, the events and the people involved may be positive or negative, and ultimately may have short term and long-term emotional and psychological repercussions (Green *et al.* 1990; Oakley *et al.* 1996). Womens long-term memories surrounding birth have been shown to be accurate and vivid (Simkin, 1991). Simkin's study explored the long-term impact of a woman's first birth and the factors associated with long-term satisfaction and dissatisfaction. The main factors that led to greater feelings of satisfaction, as recalled by the women in this study 15–20 years after giving birth, included feelings of personal accomplishment or accomplishment as a couple, feeling in control, belief that the experience of birth increased their self-esteem or self-confidence and positive memories of the professionals involved in the birth. Similar findings to these have more recently been reported by Ogden *et al.* (1997). This was a small study involving 25 women 3–5 years after their homebirths. Simkin (1991) also identified that some of the women who experienced a less satisfying birth seemed to accept a negative self-image, whereas others continued to feel anger and consequently became more assertive afterwards.

Assessing satisfaction associated with birth is currently becoming integral to the provision of maternity care as satisfaction surveys are implemented in many clinical audits. Shearer (1990), however, cautions researchers who attempt to measure women's satisfaction with the birth. She emphasizes that satisfaction is an odd, simplistic word to use to describe the jumble of partly formed confused emotions at a time when women experience the upheaval in their lives that a baby brings. Bramadat and Dreidger

(1993) also highlighted the potential difficulty in measuring satisfaction. As they identified, women may be satisfied with one aspect of the birth experience and yet dissatisfied with another. Asking women whether they are satisfied with their experience of birth generally is likely to be misleading. As Shearer (1990) ,suggests, it is more advantageous to identify womens responses to specific aspects of care. Aspects of care that have been shown to influence feelings about labour and satisfaction with the birth experience include communication and information giving (Kirkham, 1989), management of pain (Niven, 1994), place of birth (Campbell and MacFarlane, 1994), social support and support from partner (Niven 1985) and support from caregivers (Hodnett, 1995).

Intervention in labour that is either routine or unnecessary has also, in recent years, been increasingly recognized as one of the main areas of dissatisfaction for many women. These include medical interventions, such as artificial rupture of the membranes (ARM), intravenous oxytocic infusion, instrumental delivery, episiotomy and Caesarean birth. It must be remembered that intervention may also include aspects of care which disrupt the spontaneous process of birth and therefore incorporates:

- Policies such as imposition of time constraints on the first, second and third stages of labour.
- Restriction of the position of a woman for labour and birth.
- Routine electronic fetal monitoring.
- Active encouragement of maternal effort in the second stage of labour.

Some of these practices were introduced in the belief that they improved fetal and maternal outcome, but unfortunately such beliefs were not always founded on research. Sheila Kitzinger, in her evidence to the Health Committee, suggested that intervention can also be subtle:

Having to put on a gown, being put to bed as if you were ill, not being able to eat and drink when you want to, the constant checking of labour against the clock, being surrounded by strangers who talk over you and about you, rather than to you ...

(House of Commons, 1992, p. xxiii.)

In fact, it has for some time been recognized that there are certain interventions regarded as routine that are likely to be of little benefit, ineffective or even harmful (Enkin *et al.* 1995). These include, among many others, routine directed pushing during the second stage of labour, pushing by sustained bearing down, routine withholding of food and drink in labour, lying flat on the back for the second stage and the liberal use of episiotomy.

In recent years, some policies which suggest that labour must be actively managed and that the physical care of mother and baby is the only consideration have been challenged. The importance of improving the birth experience for women has become increasingly recognized. It is, however, important to remember that physical and psychological consequences of labour must be considered simultaneously, particularly as physical problems are likely to cause emotional distress or psychological illhealth. Recent research, for example, highlights that the extent of maternal morbidity following childbirth has not been adequately recognized (MacArthur et al. 1991). Backache, stress incontinence, fatigue, perineal pain and dyspareunia were some of the problems most frequently identified by the women in this study. An increased awareness by midwives of the factors that cause or contribute to morbidity helps in recognition and treatment. It is evident that currently such problems are rarely identified and adequate postnatal support and advice in the postpartum period is not readily available (Bick and MacArthur, 1994), see Chapter 14.

There is some suggestion that the long-term effects of some forms of intervention, such as instrumental delivery, may also increase the incidence of postnatal depression, reduce a womans confidence in her mothering ability or interfere with natural attachment processes (Raphael-Leff, 1991). There is also increasing evidence that events surrounding birth can leave women feeling out of control of both these and their bodies, resulting in an experience so distressing that it may lead to psychological problems such as posttraumatic stress disorder (PTSD). It has been suggested that childbirth itself can be a primary trigger for PTSD or it can retraumatize survivors of previous stress (Crompton, 1996). Crompton reminds us that when there is trust, respect and the locus of control is with the woman she may in fact be protected from psychological disorders such as PTSD.

Andrea Robertson (1994) suggests that women who use their innate behaviours, born of instinct and hormonal physiology (p. 7) to manage labour use less drugs, which overall may promote physical and emotional well-being in both mothers and their babies. Robertson is a promoter of active birth, which she defines as one in which the woman is empowered to give birth using her own resources and abilities. Such philosophies have created a major rethink of many aspects of traditional midwifery practice. Empowering the woman and offering her choice throughout pregnancy and birth are elements intrinsic to *Changing Childbirth* (Department of Health, 1993). Midwives as practitioners and educators must therefore continue to reflect and evaluate their practice, acknowledging the well-being of the woman, her baby and her family both physically and emotionally.

Birth is normally a time of great happiness for a woman and her family. The contribution of midwives and doctors should enhance this by providing low-key support when all is going well, complemented by more sophisticated care when complications occur.

(Department of Health, 1993, p.31.)

Aspects of Pain Control in Labour

As suggested previously, control and management of pain in labour is one facet of care which may influence a womans perception of the birth and her feelings of satisfaction. It has been demonstrated that even when women have effective pain relief in labour, some later perceive the overall experience as dissatisfying (Morgan *et al.* 1982). Morgan's study demonstrated that a number of women who had no pain relief in labour reported high pain scores and yet, when asked postnatally, expressed a sense of satisfaction with the birth experience. Conversely, women who had total pain relief with epidural anaesthesia expressed lower levels of satisfaction. Comments made by some women in this group illustrate their feelings of having the birth taken away from them, or having no sense of achievement, and therefore reflect feelings of not being in control of events. Simkin's study (1991) also suggested that women were less satisfied with their birth when they used more pain medication.

The way pain is perceived is dependent on many psychosocial factors. The degree of pain and the quality of pain felt is determined by previous experience and how well such experiences are remembered. Perception of pain is also dependent on understanding what causes the pain and an ability to grasp its consequences, which altogether encompasses even the culture in which people mature (Melzack and Wall, 1988).

Pain, particularly labour pain, is not simply a consequence of trauma or disease. Relating labour pain to most other pathological acute and chronic pain conditions has led to an overall perception that labour pain can best be treated with modern pharmacological methods. Until recently, psychological methods of pain control were often perceived as ineffective (Moir, 1986). However, the increasing demand of complementary methods of pain control for labour suggests that women do not necessarily see drugs as ideal. The use of water in labour as a method of pain control, for example, has the added dimension of providing an environment in which the woman is able to literally immerse herself, in surroundings over which she has some control and which limits intervention by professionals in attendance. Women therefore seem to have unique expectations of how they want to control the pain of labour. A study undertaken to investigate some of the psychological factors that influence pain perception in labour explored womens views of labour pain (Moore, 1995, University of Wolverhampton). The women in this small study were asked if they saw labour pain as different from other forms of pain. Some of their responses suggest that women do see it differently:

'Different because you gain something special at the end of labour.' (Subject 5, primiparous.)

'It is different because its a pain that can be completely controlled and at the end you have something that makes you feel proud and totally fulfilled. Any other pain is just irritating.' (Subject 2, multiparous.)

'It will be different I think because after all the sweat and anguish I will have a baby and the pain will be gone.' (Subject 9, primiparous.)

'Worth the discomfort, not pain associated with illness but natural event.' (Subject 4, primiparous.)

The differences between women's perceptions of pain and professionals perceptions of womens pain was demonstrated by Rajan (1993) in a secondary analysis of the findings of a survey undertaken by the National Birthday Trust (NBT) of pain relief in labour (Chamberlain *et al.* 1993). The NBT study surveyed the perceptions of pain and pain relief of over 1000 women and the professionals who cared for them, including midwives, obstetricians and anaesthetists. Rajan (1993) identified, for example, that although 23% of the women themselves considered breathing and relaxation to be their first method of pain relief used, obstetricians and anaesthetists gave epidural anaesthesia as the first method of pain relief used. Overall, the professionals perception of pain relief was restricted to the use of drugs in labour. Pethidine was seen as an adequate form of pain relief by the doctors, whereas women believed it to be ineffective. Rajan (1993, p. 144) concluded that:

On the whole the level of agreement between women and professionals about the effectiveness of the different methods of pain relief in labour is quite low ... particular effort should be made to avoid stereotyping of the labour experience.

Stereotypical views may encompass many misperceptions. Pain is a subjective experience every woman's pain is what she alone feels, and is as tolerable or as bad as she says it is. Methods of pain relief must therefore be made available that meet the needs of each individual. For some women this will be a conscious decision to be totally pain free and to have an epidural as soon as possible. For others it will be important to use the minimal amount of drugs possible. It is, however, paramount that the woman is given an informed choice. This involves her having a knowledge of what methods are available and being supported in her choice by having appropriate information made available as to the effectiveness of each method and the possible effect on her and her baby (see Chapter 10).

Labour is a physiological process thatembraces certain patterns of pain behaviour. An understanding of pain behaviour in normal labour helps a midwife to be supportive at the same time as empowering the woman. Patterns of birthing behaviour are described by Robertson (1994) and can be a valuable guide to both the woman and her midwife in assessing progress in labour. In early labour, a woman is often restless and nervous. She usually wants to talk, needs company, is unable to sleep, walks around and makes eye contact. In established labour, she rests between contractions, avoids conversation and eye contact, needs unobtrusive company and finds her own positions and breathing patterns. Midwives should perhaps consider that it is unusual for most women to place themselves in a position that increases pain or causes greater discomfort. It is therefore not appropriate to ask her to change her position to adopt one which may look more comfortable to the midwife.

The period of transition may appear disconcerting as women often express feelings of being unable to cope any longer. At this time, the reassurance and encouragement of a midwife will help most women overcome their distress. The woman often makes a last-minute request for drugs and may become irrational. This is followed by a more calm period as the second stage of labour begins, a sense of purpose returns and expulsive effort naturally takes over to bring the baby into the world.

The Labour Environment

The birth environment can be defined as the surroundings in which birth takes place. However, an environment consists of more than bricks and mortar, or the furniture and decor environment is emotional as well as physical. The environment is therefore established not only by the setting, but by the people who support the woman in labour, by their attitudes and beliefs, by policies and practices and by the degree of empathy and understanding which exists. Medicalization of childbirth has come to signify institutionalization, i.e. birth in a hospital environment, within a clinical setting, surrounded by the paraphernalia of increasing technology and the inherent rules and routines of hospital practice.

It has been suggested that the hospital environment is often the cause of high intervention rates during labour in industrialized countries (Keirse *et al.* 1983). Hospitals perpetuate a sick model that, naturally, does not reflect a philosophy of pregnancy and childbirth as a normal healthy event. Women who are hospitalized during pregnancy or childbirth, for example, are permitted by staff to receive visitors, usually family or other members of the social network. Such visiting is restricted or monitored by hospital personnel, thus often isolating her from the very people who may provide a valuable support network. Although such policies have become less rigid over recent years, they may still disempower the childbearing woman. In her own home she is normally able to open her own door and invite in or deny access to whom she chooses. In hospital this is virtually impossible, even in the intimacy of the labour ward environment. It is still not uncommon for midwives or medical personnel to enter a woman's labour environment without requesting her permission. It is, unfortunately, difficult for staff to maintain privacy at all times as well as maintain security. Visiting restrictions and rules are again becoming more necessary as security measures are increased to protect women and their babies from the possibility of abduction and other criminal activity. The hospital environment is therefore likely to create insecurity, and increase stress and anxiety.

A link between the physiological aspects of labour and environmental influences was originally demonstrated using animal studies. Newton (1987) reminds us of experimental research that showed that birth was delayed in mice when they were continually disturbed. In the same experiment Newton and colleagues demonstrated that, after the initial delay, labour speeded up when the disturbances continued. The concept became known as the fetus ejection reflex, which Newton hypothesized is physiologically similar to the milk ejection reflex, because it is triggered by the release of oxytocin as the genital tract is stimulated at term, thus causing uterine contraction. Provoked stress and the adrenaline response are therefore factors which may both inhibit and precipitate labour. Odent (1987) recognized this phenomena as a response sometimes apparent in human labour, identifying instances in which women have given birth rapidly because of threatening circumstances. Most midwives are also aware of instances in which a womans labour has been unexpectedly inhibited or conversely progressed extremely rapidly in stressful or threatening situations. Odent emphasized the importance of the human environment in which birth attendants are aware of the involuntary process of birth and the significance of this process not being disturbed.

The Expert Maternity Group (Department of Health, 1993), referring to the results of a MORI survey, highlighted the limited choice women currently have in choosing the place of birth. Although 98% of women now give birth in hospital, 72% would have liked a choice in the system of care and place of delivery, 22% would have liked a home birth and 44% would have liked a midwife-led domino-style delivery (p. 23). There is as yet little evidence that compares the effect of hospital and home births in the UK. Home is a familiar environment in which a woman can feel safe and relaxed throughout labour, where she can maintain privacy and be surrounded by the people of her choice who will give her support and reassurance. However, women may also be reassured by feeling that they are in a place where technology and specialist services are readily available. A balance can be provided by making maternity units less institutionalized with systems of care which enable women and their families to receive the type and standard of care that will meet their physical, emotional, social and psychological needs.

In fact, the Health Committee (House of Commons, 1992, p. xcviii) recommended that a hospital delivery unit should:

> ... *afford privacy; look like a normal room rather than an operating theatre; enable refreshments for the woman and her partner or companions; ensure the feasibility of the woman being in control of her labour ... [and] enable the woman to have with her a midwife she has been able to form a relationship with during her pregnancy.*

This has, in turn, been reflected by the Report of the Expert Maternity Group in *Changing Childbirth*:

> *The environment in which birth takes place is important to a woman and her partner, and it should be as supportive and comfortable as possible ... she should be free to move around and adopt new positions as labour progresses ... it is essential that the privacy of the woman and her partner are respected and that they are not subjected to unnecessary interruptions.*
>
> (Department of Health, 1993)

A feature of the human environment which has been the subject of recent study is midwifery culture. Culture is described as a shared set of norms, values, assumptions and perceptions (both explicit and implicit), and social conventions that enable members of a group, community or nation to function cohesively (Schott and Henley, 1996). An element of midwifery culture was examined within one locality in the UK through a very informative, thought-provoking and challenging ethnographic study (Hunt and Symonds, 1995). The authors present a detailed description of the labour ward culture, thus providing an insight into aspects of midwifery practice and organization of the work in a fairly typical labour environment. This sociological perspective of some of the rituals and routines of the labour ward, the terminology and jargon used by midwives and the processes of communication specific to the labour ward enable midwives to reflect on the cultural influences. The use of specific labour ward terminology such as the labourers (women in established labour) and the nigglers (women in early labour usually seen as not doing much) illustrates how midwives in the study distinguished between what they perceived as the real work of the labour ward and the presence of women in early labour who were more likely to be seen as a nuisance factor, intruding on the real work. As the study suggested, the criteria for admission to the labour ward seemed to relate more to dilatation of the cervix than assessment of the individual or emotional needs of the woman. Overall, the study serves to remind us that childbirth is the work of women, both the women who give birth and those who provide midwifery care, and that this work takes place within the constraints of a medicalized organization.

Support by Caregivers in Labour

There can be little doubt that one of the most significant influences of care in labour is the type and quality of support received by women. Research demonstrates that support which brings about a positive outcome is both physical and emotional (Keirse *et al.* 1983), and includes aspects of care such as rubbing the womans back or holding her hand, maintaining eye contact, the presence of a friendly companion, the provision of explanations and encouragement, and the promise that a labouring woman will not be left alone. Current research continues to identify many of these aspects of care in providing effective support for women in labour.

A review of all the controlled trials conducted in several countries worldwide was undertaken to assess the effect of continuous support in labour compared with the more usual forms of hospital care (Hodnett, 1995). This review included studies in which the support was provided by various people, including midwives, student midwives, nurses and lay women (trained or untrained). The results of these studies indicate that the continued presence of a trained support person reduced the duration of labour, reduced the likelihood of drugs for pain relief and reduced the incidence of operative vaginal delivery, regardless of whether or not the support person was the woman's chosen birth partner. It was also shown that 5-minute neonatal Apgar scores were greater than 7-minute scores when continuous support was provided by a trained person. The presence of a trained support person also reduced the likelihood of a Caesarean birth. The main interventions specified in the trials included the continuous presence of the support person, comforting touch and words of praise and encouragement. The power of such skills used by an appropriately trained person can hardly be more apparent. Hodnett (1995, p.5) suggests that the findings of this review present some implications for practice:

> *Given the clear benefits and no known risks associated with intrapartum support, every*

effort should be made to ensure all labouring women receive support, not only from those close to them but also from specially trained caregivers ... This support should include continuous presence, the provision of hands-on comfort and encouragement.

Depending upon the circumstances, ensuring the provision of continuous support may require the following:

alterations in the current work activities of midwives such that they are able to spend less time on ineffective activities;

continuing education programmes which teach the art and science of labour support;

changes to more flexible methods of staffing labour wards which will permit the staff census to match more closely the patient census.

Other studies, more qualitative in nature, also reflect many of the elements of support identified in the controlled trials. A Swedish study which explored women's experience of the encounter with the midwife during childbirth reinforced the value of what is termed presence (Berg *et al.* 1996). The findings of this phenomenological study demonstrated three main themes to the encounter between a woman and her carer for a woman in labour to be seen as an individual, to have a trusting relationship and to be supported and guided on her own terms. The presence of the midwife was identified as the overall theme and was seen as the key feature in facilitating a positive birth experience for this particular group of women. A similar phenomenological study conducted in England demonstrated the need for positive interaction between a woman and her midwife as paramount to the type of care which women perceived as beneficial, enabling them to feel safe, strong and feeling in control of events (Choucri, 1997).

The ability to provide emotional support for woman in labour is something every midwife acquires in the early days of her career. The provision of emotional support encompasses communication and information giving skills and can be further enhanced by the skills of counselling as identified in Chapter 20. Taylor (1991) proposes that there may be certain constraints in the acquisition of such skills. She suggests that the hierarchical institution, as well as midwives own personal defences, can inhibit emotional contact. To change deep-rooted beliefs that labour is pathological, Taylor (1991) goes on to suggest that midwives should work to develop relationships with the medical profession to achieve greater respect and a higher profile, to provide continuity of care for women in labour to reduce some of the defences that obstruct emotional involvement and finally to increase self-awareness to recognize the anxieties that inhibit the development of relationships.

Many schemes are now being established to provide care throughout pregnancy and childbirth, and to facilitate continuity of carer and choice of care, as well as to empower women. However, the effectiveness of many of these programmes currently being set up in maternity services has not yet been thoroughly evaluated. One scheme that has been evaluated, however, was established in Glasgow. The scheme, set up in a busy consultant unit, provided care for healthy women throughout pregnancy. Each woman was supported by a named midwife, or an associate midwife if the named midwife was not available. A randomized controlled trial, involving 1299 women, compared the midwife-managed care with traditional shared-care, and demonstrated that women were significantly more satisfied with the maternity care undertaken by midwives during the antenatal, intrapartum and postnatal periods (Turnbull *et al.* 1996).

The authors of this study concluded that midwife-managed care enhances womens satisfaction with maternity care. A further study examined changes in midwives attitudes to their role following the implementation of the programme (Turnbull *et al.* 1995). Midwives working in the midwife-managed unit became more positive in their attitudes, at the same time demonstrating no increased stress. It is therefore proposed that patterns of care throughout childbirth can have a positive influence on women and midwives. The type of support given by midwives and others at the time of labour has a lasting affect on women's lives. Midwives have it in their power to ensure that women have adequate support in a supportive environment.

KEY CONCEPTS

- Satisfaction with the birth experience is a complex concept and therefore difficult to assess and measure.
- The long-term effects of labour may influence a woman's experience of motherhood and therefore her potential well-being and that of her family.
- Psychological methods of pain relief are most often acknowledged by women as important and yet may be undervalued by professionals.
- The effect of the labour environment may influence labour physiologically and psychologically.
- The midwife's skills in supporting and facilitating a positive birth experience are paramount.

References

Berg M, Lundgren I, Hermansson E, Wahlberg V: Womens experience of the encounter with the midwife during childbirth, *Midwifery* 12:11, 1996.

Bick D, MacArthur C: Identifying morbidity in postpartum women, *Modern Midwife* 4(12):10, 1994.

Campbell R, MacFarlane A: *Where to be born? The debate and the evidence*, 2nd edn, Oxford, 1994, National Perinatal Epidemiology Unit.

Chamberlain G, Wraight A, Steer P: *Pain and its relief in childbirth: The results of a national survey conducted by the National Birthday Trust*, Edinburgh, 1993, Churchill Livingstone.

Choucri L: *Care by midwives: Womens experiences*. in Moore S, editor: *Understanding pain and its relief in labour*, Edinburgh, 1997, Churchill Livingstone.

Combes G, Schonveld A: *Life will never be the same again: learning to be a first time parent*, London, 1992, Health Education Authority.

Crompton J: Post-traumatic stress disorder and childbirth, *Br J Midwifery* 4(6):290, 1996.

Department of Health: *Changing childbirth: Report of the Expert Maternity Group*, London, 1993, HMSO.

Enkin M, Keirse MJNC, Renfrew M, Neilson J: *A guide to effective care in pregnancy and childbirth*, 2nd edn, Oxford, 1995, Oxford University Press.

Green JM, Coupland VA, Kitzinger JV: Expectations, experiences and psychological outcomes of childbirth: a prospective study of 825 women, *Birth* 17(1):15, 1990.

Hodnett ED: Support during childbirth in support from caregivers during childbirth, *The Cochrane Pregnancy and Childbirth Database*, Issue 1, 1995, CD Rom database.

House of Commons, *Health Committee second report, maternity services*, London, 1992, HMSO.

Keirse MJNC, Enkin M, Lumley J: Social and professional support during childbirth. In Chalmers I, Enkin M, Keirse MJNC, editors: *Effective care in pregnancy and childbirth*, Vol. 2, p. 805, Oxford, 1983, Oxford University Press.

Kirkham M: Midwives and information giving during labour. In Robinson S, Thomson A, editors: *Midwives, research and childbirth*, Vol. 1, p. 117, London, 1989, Chapman and Hall.

MacArthur C, Lewis M, Bick D: *Health after childbirth*, London, 1991, HMSO.

Melzack R, Wall P: *The challenge of pain*, London, 1988, Penguin Books.

Moir D: *Pain relief in labour*, Edinburgh, 1986, Churchill Livingstone.

Morgan B, Bulpit CJ, Clifton P, Lewis PJ: Effectiveness of pain relief in labour: survey of 1000 mothers, *Br Med J* 282(11):689, 1982,.

Newton N: The fetus ejection reflex revisited, *Birth* 14(2):104, 1987.

Niven C: How helpful is the presence of the husband at childbirth? *J Reprod Infant Psychol* 3:45, 1985.

Niven C: Labour pain: Long term recall and consequences, *J Reprod Infant Psychol* 6:83, 1988.

Oakley A, Hickey D, Rajan L: Social support in pregnancy: does it have long-term effects? *J Reprod Infant Psychol* 14:7, 1996.

Odent M: The fetus ejection reflex, *Birth* 14(2):104, 1987.

Rajan L: Perceptions of pain and pain relief in labour: the gulf between experience and observation, *Midwifery* 9:136, 1993.

Raphael-Leff J: *Psychological processes of childbearing*, London, 1991, Chapman and Hall.

Robertson A: *Empowering women: Teaching active birth in the 90s*, Sevenoaks, 1994, Ace Graphics.

Schott J, Henley A: *Culture, religion and childbearing in a multiracial society*, Oxford, 1996, ButterworthHeinemann.

Shearer MH: Commentary: Pondering the study of womens psychological outcomes, *Birth* 17(1):24, 1990.

Simkin P: Just another day in a womans life? Womens long-term perception of their first birth experience. Part 1, *Birth* 18(4):203, 1991.

Taylor M: Providing emotional support, *Nurs Times* 87(22):66, 1991.

Turnbull D, Reid M, McGinley M, Sheilds NR: Changes in midwives attitudes to their professional role following the implementation of the midwifery development unit, *Midwifery* 11:110, 1995.

Turnbull D, Homes A, Sheilds N, *et al.*, Randomised, controlled trial of efficacy of midwife-managed care, *The Lancet* 348(9022):213, 1996.

Further Reading

Hunt S, Symonds A: *The social meaning of midwifery*, Basingstoke, 1995, Macmillan.

This book is based on an ethnographic study of the labour ward. The labour ward culture is explored, including many aspects of practice such as work routines, patterns of care and aspects of communication which cannot fail to lead every midwife who is working with women in labour to reflect on practice.

Moore S: *Understanding pain and its relief in labour*, Edinburgh, 1997, Churchill Livingstone.

A comprehensive text presenting the psychological and social aspects of pain and pain in labour, as well as physiology and methods of pain control, both pharmacological and nonpharmacological.

Robertson A: *Empowering women: Teaching active birth in the 90s*, 1994, Ace Graphics.

A must for every midwife and student midwife who wants to know anything about the empowerment of women in childbirth and how this may be incorporated into educational programmes.

House of Commons, *Health Committee second report, maternity services*, London, 1992, HMSO.

The Winterton Report makes very interesting reading. Chapter 2, What women want, outlines some of the evidence presented to the Committee, including psychological and social aspects. The section on the wider context (p. xxvi) should be of particular interest (maternity benefits and maternity leave). It is essential reading in conjunction with Changing Childbirth (Department of Health, 1993) to analyse and evaluate progress.

12 Management of the Newborn Baby: Midwifery and Paediatric Perspectives

ADAPTATION: FETUS TO INFANT AND NEONATAL RESUSCITATION

Embryogenesis, fetal development and transition from fetal to extrauterine life is a wonder that becomes more marvellous as it is studied in greater detail. The process is as normal as it is essential and is achieved with remarkable ease in the healthy term fetus during an uncomplicated delivery.

Unfortunately, the process is not always straightforward. The effects of fetal hypoxia, perinatal asphyxia or failure of cardiovascular adaptation to extrauterine life can be disastrous, with devastating effects that the child may have to live with for the rest of its life. Those of us involved in perinatal care have the responsibility to make every effort to prevent or avoid such problems, to detect signs that things are going wrong and to intervene when necessary. This is a dilemma: consider, as you read this chapter, the balance between our wish for relaxed natural delivery and our duty to intervene at a certain threshold.

In this section, the physiological processes that underlie adaptation to extrauterine life are reviewed, our ability to detect problems during parturition considered briefly and an outline of neonatal resuscitation given.

Adaptation: Fetus to Infant

The fetus leads a very protected existence during intrauterine life, so at birth body systems have to adapt if he/she is to survive the independent existence of extrauterine life. The rates at which body systems physiologically adjust to extrauterine life varies considerably.

The Rate of Change

The respiratory and cardiovascular transition from placental oxygenation to gas transfer through the lungs occurs in phases. The first phase is completed within minutes of birth, and is discussed in detail below. Further changes in cardiorespiratory function continue until a mature pattern of circulation is achieved around day 10.

Hepatorenal function changes almost as quickly. The fetus, at term, swallows around 800–1000 ml of liquor each day and passes large quantities of dilute urine. After birth, water intake diminishes, fluid loss through respiration and other insensible losses increases and urine production falls rapidly to avoid dehydration. Waste products that have been dialysed through the placenta into the maternal circulation must be dealt with by the infant's kidney and liver, yet clinical symptoms caused by accumulation of waste metabolites are rare. The most common, 'physiological neonatal jaundice', only exceptionally causes clinical problems.

Other organ systems must function in an integrated fashion after delivery to provide homeostasis. Blood glucose, for example, is maintained by continuous supply from the placenta, but after birth intermittent bolus feeds must be swallowed, digested and absorbed, while hepatic, pancreatic and endocrine functions work to keep the blood sugar in the narrow target range: 2.5–7 mmol/l.

Cardiorespiratory Changes

An understanding of the cardiorespiratory changes (**Figure 12.1**) that occur during the transition from fetus to infant is of prime importance to the midwife, because appropriate action at delivery can have life-saving consequences for the infant.

Fetal pattern of circulation

In-utero pulmonary vascular resistance (PVR) is high because the vessels in the lungs are constricted and resistant to flow. Only 10% of the fetal cardiac output goes through the lungs, whereas the entire cardiac output will do so after birth. In the fetus, the high PVR is maintained while the O_2 tension in the pulmonary blood vessels is kept low, and the pattern of fetal circulation ensures this (**Figure 12.1**). Blood returns to the right atrium from two sources: oxygenated blood from the placenta is streamed through the foramen ovale into the left heart, then pumped into the fetal aorta to provide oxygenated blood for the brain and coronary arteries; in contrast, most of the deoxygenated blood from the fetal tissues is directed through the ductus arteriosus into the aorta, to return to the placenta.

Changes at delivery

Events during normal labour and delivery are usually beneficial, and prepare the fetus for rapid cardiovascular change (**Figure 12.1**). The stress of labour induces high levels of catecholamines, adrenaline and noradrenaline, which promote beneficial cardiovascular changes and, in association with steroid production,

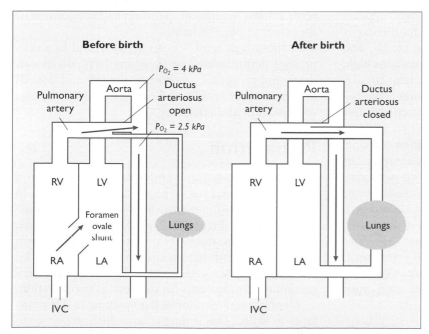

Figure 12.1 The cardiovascular changes from fetal to newborn pattern of circulation: RV, right ventricle; LV, left ventricle; RA, right atrium; LA, left atrium; IVC, inferior vena cava. (Reproduced with permission from Dear and Newell, 1996.)

induce surfactant secretion. Catecholamines also reverse fluid movement in the lung, so that the lung 'dries out'. Squeezing of the thorax during vaginal delivery further empties the lungs of fluid. Clamping the cord increases resistance to flow down the aorta, which increases left atrial pressure and reduces flow through the foramen ovale. External stimuli and cord clamping induce the newborn infant to breathe. As the lungs are drawn open by the first breath, the pulmonary vessels are stretched and exposed to an increased amount of O_2. Pulmonary blood vessels relax and PVR falls. Release of large amounts of prostacyclin and NO augments pulmonary vasodilatation.

Once PVR falls, right heart pressure falls below the pressure in the left heart (**Figure 12.1**). The foramen ovale, in the atrial wall, has a valve-like structure and closes. Oxygenated blood flows through the ductus arteriosus, and it constricts.

Most of these changes occur more quickly than one can read about it! The PVR continues to fall during the following hours or days, the foramen ovale becomes structurally closed, the ductus closes off completely and a mature pattern of circulation is established within 2 weeks of birth.

Failure of cardiovascular adaptation

At birth, PVR falls because of ventilation and oxygenation, so if the fetus is hypoxic at delivery these events may not occur. If the infant becomes hypoxic in the period after delivery, the process may be reversed. Commonly, a newborn infant who appears pink and vigorous may become momentarily cyanosed, but responds immediately to O_2 and improved ventilation. If, however, PVR remains high, the clinical picture known as persistent fetal circulation (or persistent pulmonary hypertension) results – this is a severe neonatal illness that often requires intensive care.

The process of cardiovascular adaptation is crucial to the health of a newborn infant. There are three circumstances that most commonly lead to persistent fetal circulation, each of which has avoidable elements. The most common of these are fetal hypoxia and perinatal asphyxia. Meconium aspiration is also often associated with persistent fetal circulation. The third most common cause is severe congenital pneumonia.

At this point, it may be useful for you to write a list of body systems and the changes each must undergo in the first week of life.

Conclusion

The transition from fetus to infant is complex and involves every body system. The single most important event is the rapid drop in PVR and the ensuing cardiovascular changes. This is ensured by the avoidance of fetal hypoxia and by adequate oxygenation and ventilation immediately after delivery. This is the rationale behind the resuscitation strategy which is now discussed.

Resuscitation of the Newborn

Their body appearing so senseless and their face so blue ... let the midwife take a little wine in her mouth and spout it into its mouth, repeating it often, if there be occasion.

(Aristotle, 384–322 BC.)

Perinatal hypoxia can have disastrous consequences; indeed, if we take into account the anguish of parents whose infant has suffered birth asphyxia, irrespective of the eventual outcome, then the avoidance of perinatal hypoxia must be one of the most important responsibilities charged to the midwife, obstetrician and paediatrician. Prevention of fetal hypoxia is the ideal, but cannot be achieved every time, so neonatal resuscitation is a basic skill of midwifery. Effective resuscitation requires preparation and recognition of the infant in need of help.

In the infant who is born apnoeic and hypoxic, prompt action aimed at reversing hypoxia avoids death and gives the expectation of a full and normal life. In no other area of medicine are simple measures so important and effective.

Preparation

Care of the mother and child includes preparation for resuscitation, even if the need is not expected. In hospitals, the equipment usually comprises a resuscitation station (**Figure 12.2**; platform, radiant heater, supply of O_2 and mechanical suction), equipped with bag and mask, intubation equipment and drugs. O_2, suction apparatus and a bag and mask are the very minimum requirements for delivery in any situation.

All of us require training and updating in our resuscitation skills. This is particularly difficult, yet critically important, for the carer who delivers infants away from paediatric support, when there is little opportunity for the frequent practice of resuscitation. This is a challenge that must be confronted in small, geographically isolated units. Also, as more mothers opt for home delivery it may be that senior midwives, trained by paediatric consultant staff, should provide continuing in-service training for their colleagues.

Finally, whether delivery is in hospital or the shopping centre, the practising midwife should know how to summon help. The commendably high levels of training given to the ambulance paramedics means that they are our best allies out of the hospital.

Prevention and Prediction

Prevention of fetal and perinatal hypoxia is integral to the practice of effective midwifery. Assessment begins at the booking clinic and includes information obtained during pregnancy and observations made during labour. Increasingly, research-based evidence provides the rationale for midwives' practice. We are now more aware of the risk of hypoxia in the antenatally compromised fetus in a pregnancy complicated, for example, by intrauterine growth retardation, placental insufficiency or toxaemia. One salutary and practically important point is that it is not possible to predict with certainty that an infant will be born in good condition. A recent study (Arya *et al.* 1996) in a large district general hospital reviewed the outcomes of 1312 very low risk deliveries selected from over 32,000 deliveries: 3% of these babies required advanced resuscitation.

Recognition

Prompt recognition of the need for resuscitation is paramount. Virginia Apgar's scoring system provides a record of the infant's cardiorespiratory status and vigour (**Table 12.1**). Points are given for each variable, the sum being the Apgar score which is traditionally calculated after 1, 5 and 10 minutes. The Apgar score has been used as a predictor of the likelihood of hypoxic–ischaemic brain damage, but it was not intended for this and is not reliable. Nevertheless, carefully recorded Apgar scores can be most useful to discussion in this area.

Three clinical pictures can be deduced from the Apgar scoring system:

- The infant with a very low Apgar score is pale, floppy, make no respiratory effort, does not respond to oral suction and pulse is slow. This infant needs urgent advanced resuscitation with assisted ventilation.
- The infant with an Apgar score of 4–7 has a pulse below 100 beats per minute (b.p.m.), breathes irregularly and is blue. There is some response to suction and some muscle tone. This infant may well respond to stimulation, but often needs facial O$_2$ or bag and mask ventilatory support.
- The infant with an Apgar score >7 has a normal heart rate, breathes and responds to stimuli. This infant, fortunately representing the majority of infants, needs no resuscitation and so can be dried, wrapped in warm towels and given to the mother.

It is not necessary to calculate the Apgar to determine need for resuscitation. Most important is the heart rate and respiratory effort. An infant with a slow heart rate is hypoxic. When hypoxia is corrected, the heart rate returns to above 100 (b.p.m.), the first response to successful resuscitation.

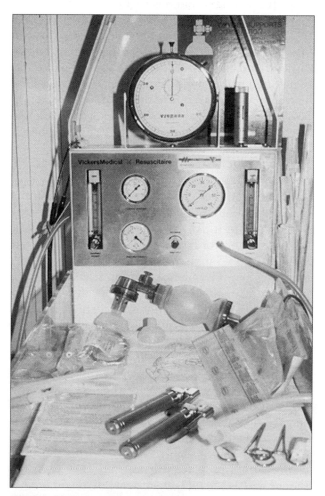

Figure 12.2 Resuscitation station.

Table 12.1 Apgar Score Chart			
Score	**0**	**1**	**2**
Heart rate	Absent	<100 b.p.m.	>100 b.p.m.
Respiratory effort	Absent	Irregular, slow	Regular, cry
Muscle tone	Limp	Some flexion in limbs	Well-flexed limbs
Reflex irritability	Nil	Grimace	Cough/cry
Colour	White	Blue	Pink

Resuscitation

Resuscitation involves a series of steps and the resuscitator should be guided in these by frequent assessment of pulse, respiratory effort and colour. This concept is nicely captured in the inverted triangle of **Figure 12.3**.

The steps of neonatal resuscitation are clearly shown and the shape of the triangle reminds us that although many infants require suction and stimulation, few require drugs.

Step 1 – position, dry, warm, stimulate

This is the first step. Place the baby on its back with the head tilted backwards, gently extending the neck. It is very easy to overextend the neck, which does not help achieve an airway.

Keeping an infant dry and warm is essential. Hypothermia is dangerous, preventable (**Figure 12.4**) and more rapid in the low-birthweight infant. A warm, draft-free room with warm towels and an overhead heater is ideal.

Clear the anterior oropharynx with a mucus aspirator – of a design which prevents direct exposure of the user to secretions or low-pressure mechanical suction. Avoid suction behind the tongue, which may lead to vocal cord spasm and make resuscitation difficult.

Tactile stimulation is often used – some still like to smack a baby's bottom. Do not blow cold gases at a naked infant. Holding a baby upside down by the feet should be a criminal offence. Those fortunate to work in the NHS know that a towel that has been through a hospital laundry is stimulation enough when rubbed up and down an infant's trunk!

Step 2 – oxygen

Facial O_2 is best given by blowing O_2 through a funnel onto the infant's face.

Step 3 – bag and mask ventilation

In skilled hands, bag and mask ventilation with O_2 is very effective. The infant is positioned as described above, the soft mask placed over the baby's mouth and nose, and the baby's jaw is *lifted into* the face mask (**Figure 12.5**). Care must be taken to lift the mandible and not the soft tissue under the jaw, which may lift the tongue and obstruct the airway.

Ventilate at 40–60 breaths per minute using 100% O_2. Squeezing the bag should move the infant's chest visibly and symmetrically – listening for air entry is difficult and can be misleading. Bag and masks are often fitted with a pop-off valve, set at 30 cmH$_2$O. If a higher pressure is required the valve is occluded. The best indicator of a good airway and adequate ventilation is improvement in the baby's pulse and colour.

Step 4 – tracheal intubation and ventilation

Intubation requires the correct equipment and training. In the absence of either, it is almost always best not to attempt it. Any of the newborn endotracheal tubes is suitable for resuscitation. Tube size for a term infant is 3.0–3.5 mm; for preterm, 2.5 mm. Whether midwives should undertake endotracheal resuscitation is an issue that be determined locally.

Tracheal intubation requires no force. A neonatal laryngoscope, with a bright light, is passed over the tongue to look down into the oesophagus. Drawing back, the epiglottis appears and the tip of the laryngoscope is advanced, above the epiglottis, into the vallecula. With slight extension of the neck and gentle lift with the laryngoscope, the cords are visualized and the tube passed under direct vision. Ventilation is provided either by a bag and mask attached to the endotracheal tube or by an O_2 supply from the resuscitaire with a pressure valve. Inspiratory pressures should be 20–25 cmH$_2$O, at a rate of 40–60 breaths per minute, using 100% O_2.

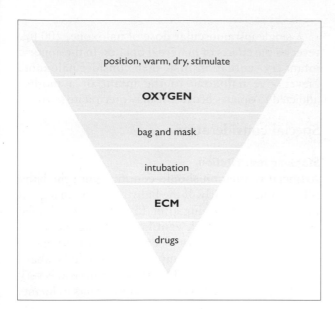

Figure 12.3 Neonatal resuscitation: the inverted triangle. (Adapted from Chameides Hazinski, 1994, with permission from American Heart Association, Dallas.)

Most babies who need resuscitation recover quickly once satisfactory ventilation with O_2 is obtained. This fact is central to understanding resuscitation of the newborn. Unlike adult resuscitation, primary cardiac problems are rare – bradycardia means hypoxia. The correct treatment is oxygenation and ventilation, which will be followed by recovery.

Rarely, an infant does not respond. When this occurs, first think of simple explanations:
- An airway has not been achieved.
- The bag and mask are not applied correctly.
- The soft tissues under the jaw are compressed.
- The endotracheal tube is in the oesophagus or too far into the trachea.
- The airway or endotracheal tube is blocked.
- The oxygen supply is not connected.
- Inadequate inspiratory pressure is being used.

Even more rarely, failure to recover during resuscitation can be caused by other problems, notably persisting severe metabolic acidosis, pneumothorax, massive blood loss, congenital diaphragmatic hernia, severe pulmonary hypoplasia, hydrops fetalis, pleural effusions, marked abdominal distension or congenital laryngeal problems.

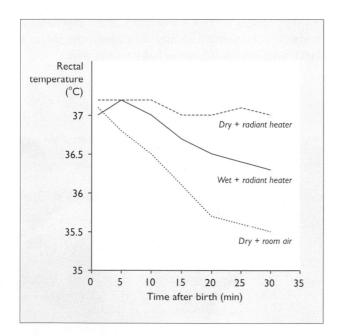

Figure 12.4 Prevention of hypothermia – core temperature may fall very rapidly if the infant is not dried and wrapped. (Reproduced with permission from Dear and Newell, 1996.)

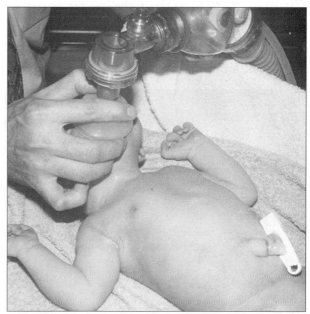

Figure 12.5 The finger is applied to the mandible and the infant's face lifted into the mask.

Step 5 – external cardiac massage

Institute cardiac massage when the pulse remains below 60 b.p.m. or falls to less than 30 b.p.m. The aim of massage is to compress the heart between the sternum and vertebral column, for which there are two techniques:

- Place the fingers of one hand so that the index finger is between the nipples and the other fingers below it on the sternum. The top finger is then lifted and the next two fingers mark the point for compression (**Figure 12.6**). This is higher than the position in the adult to avoid damage to abdominal organs.
- The resuscitator's hands are placed around the infant's lower thorax with the thumbs over the sternum, one thumb upon the other (**Figure 12.7**).

External cardiac massage (ECM) is performed at 120 per minute, pausing after each 3–5 compressions to inflate the chest. Help should be sought urgently.

Step 6 – drugs

The most important drug for resuscitation is O_2. Other drugs are rarely required (**Table 12.2**), and most midwives are not licensed to give them. In the infant in asystole or severe bradycardia, adrenaline is used. Emergency intravenous access is achieved by passing a catheter 5–10 cm into the umbilical vein, until blood can be withdrawn. If the first intravenous dose of adrenaline produces no effect, the endotracheal dose may be given intravenously. Bicarbonate is given after prolonged hypoxia for correction of the acidosis.

A single intramuscular dose of naloxone, 200 μg, reverses the effects of maternal opiates. In the apnoeic infant try ventilation first, then consider naloxone. Never give naloxone to the infant of a mother addicted to opiates because it may precipitate seizures.

Special considerations

Stopping resuscitation

Artificial ventilation should continue until the baby is breathing regularly. If the baby is pink with a good pulse but not breathing after 15–20 minutes, he/she should be transferred, ventilated, to the Neonatal Unit. If an infant is born recently dead, full intensive resuscitation may be attempted, but should be abandoned after 10 minutes of asystole, as survival is very unlikely and brain damage invariably occurs in infants who survive in these circumstances.

Post-resuscitation care

After resuscitation, most infants need not be separated from their parents. After prolonged resuscitation, temperature and blood sugar should be checked. After an acidotic cord gas or prolonged hypoxia, blood gas analysis is indicated.

A close eye should be kept on the infant for a number of hours after resuscitation. Even the infant who is going to suffer severe hypoxic ischaemic encephalopathy may appear well for a few hours. If the experienced midwife is concerned in any way about the infant's behaviour, admission to the baby unit is wise.

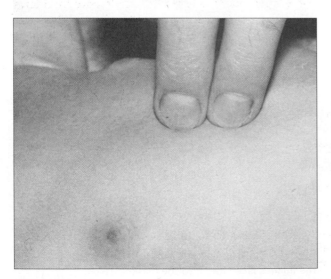

Figure 12.6 External cardiac massage using one hand.

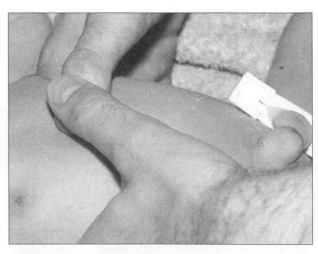

Figure 12.7 External cardiac massage – the bimanual technique.

Meconium aspiration syndrome

The presence of thick, fresh meconium in the liquor indicates that a carer who is skilled in tracheal intubation before delivery should be present, to prevent aspiration of the meconium.

When the head is delivered, wipe the infant's face and clear meconium from the mouth. At delivery if the infant is not breathing regularly, direct laryngoscopy should be performed. Meconium should be aspirated with a wide-bore catheter or endotracheal tube, under direct vision, before the first breath. Once the airway is cleared of meconium, then resuscitation proceeds as described above. If the infant cries lustily no immediate action is necessary. Consider emptying the stomach when resuscitation is complete.

Parents

The tension and anxiety in the parents of a newborn infant who requires resuscitation is hard to imagine. A few kind words of reassurance during resuscitation will earn much appreciation and help reduce anxiety.

CARE OF THE NEWBORN

Care of the newborn begins at birth when a full examination of the infant is conducted. This is the first of the many screening tests after delivery used to determine any underlying abnormality at the earliest opportunity. Early detection of abnormalities is essential to ensure the best possible future for the infant. Abnormalities may be determined through specific screening tests, but careful observation of the infant by both the midwife and the mother during the delivery of routine care may also lead to the early detection of problems that require further investigation.

Examination of the Baby at Birth

Just about the first question asked by every parent, after they know the baby's sex, is 'Is he/she all right?' Behind this question are the queries 'Is the baby breathing?', 'Is he/she normal?', 'Are any parts missing?'. A quick glance at the baby usually enables the midwife to reassure the parents, but a more systematic examination should be carried out before the baby leaves the delivery room to ensure that any problems present at birth are identified at once.

The midwife should examine the baby in view of the parents, should explain to them what she is doing and answer their questions as they arise. As the baby can rapidly lose heat when undressed the examination should be carried out as quickly as possible, having ensured beforehand that the room is warm. The midwife should wash her hands before touching the baby to minimize risks of cross-infection.

The weight of the baby is needed to satisfy the queries of friends and relatives and also to plot on a centile chart – babies whose weights are either above the 90th or below the 10th centiles for their gestation are at risk of becoming hypoglycaemic, so this information should be noted and blood glucose estimations considered. The head circumference is measured around the widest part of the head, and the baby's length measured. This is quite difficult to obtain accurately, but the baby should be laid flat in the cot, one leg gently extended and a tape-measure held against the baby to measure from the crown of the head to the heel of the extended leg. Average measurements of weight, length and head circumference for a term, Caucasian baby are 3.5 kg (7 lb 12 oz), 50 cm and 35 cm, respectively (Gairdner and Pearson, 1971). It

Table 12.2 Drugs used in the resuscitation of the newborn – DRUGS ARE RARELY NEEDED			
Drug	**Route**	**Preparation**	**Volume**
Adrenaline	IV (intravenous)	1:10 000	0.1 ml/kg
	ET (endotracheal)	1:1 000	0.1 ml/kg
Sodium bicarbonate	IV (intravenous)	4.2% (or 8.4% diluted 1:1 with water)	2–4 ml/kg (over 2–5 min)
Volume expansion/blood	IV (Intravenous)	Human albumin solution (4.5%) Normal saline (0.9%) O-negative blood	15 ml/kg
Naloxone	IM (intramuscular)	400 g/ml	0.5 ml

is a good idea to develop a personal system for examining babies – working from head to toe and then front to back is one way.

General Appearance

Blue extremities are common in the first few hours after birth while the peripheral circulation stabilizes and so are not significant. Lips and mucous membranes should be pink. Congestion of the face may be evident if the cord was around the baby's neck, but should not be confused with cyanosis, which could indicate a heart or respiratory abnormality; cyanosis is usually also evident on the trunk. A baby who seems to be pale may be anaemic and one who is very red (plethoric) may have an excess of red blood cells.

The term baby has plenty of subcutaneous fat and the skin folds usually contain vernix caseosa, a lard-like substance present *in utero* to protect the skin from the effects of the fluid in which the baby lies. Post-term babies may have dry, peeling skin. Any bruises or other blemishes should be noted.

The baby should be breathing easily at a rate of 40–60 breaths per minute, with no grunting or sternal recession. He/she should have good muscle tone, which keeps the limbs flexed, and should respond to handling by waking and moving. The cry should not be high-pitched or irritable, which could indicate brain damage.

Head

Moulding of the head, where skull bones over-ride at the sutures, and oedema of the scalp (caput succedaneum) are common after birth because of the pressure exerted on the head by the birth canal. The fontanelles should not be tense, but their size can vary considerably even when there is no abnormality. The eyes are checked for normality – the lens should be clear and there should be no discharge. Subconjunctival haemorrhages (crescent-shaped lesions of the conjunctiva), caused by a sudden increase in thoracic pressure as the chest is compressed by the birth canal, are not uncommon and disappear within a week or two (Swanwick, 1989). The ears are examined for normal shape and position, the top of the ear should be roughly level with the eyes. Low-set ears are associated with a number of abnormalities, Potters, Aperts and Edwards syndromes (Levene and Tudehope, 1993). Skin tags may be present on the face in front of the ear.

The baby's mouth should be opened gently and the inside inspected. Occasionally a congenital tooth may be present, which should be removed (Gandy, 1992). The midwife should feel the palate with her (clean) little finger to check for a cleft. The sucking reflex may be noted.

Minor skin blemishes may be present on the face at birth and can cause the parents great concern. It is important for the midwife to be able to identify these so that appropriate reassurance can be given. Tiny white spots on the nose, known as milia, are present in about 40% of babies and are hypertrophic sebaceous glands. A small capillary haemangioma is often seen on the upper part of the face, particularly the bridge of the nose or the eyelids – this is often called a 'stork mark' and, like milia, disappears during the first months of life (Walker and Champion, 1992). A more extensive capillary haemangioma, known as a 'port wine stain', is permanent and can be quite disfiguring, but laser or cryotherapy may be offered later to fade it (Swanwick, 1989). The baby's neck should be examined for swellings and the head flexed and rotated to ensure free movement.

Chest and Abdomen

The shape of the chest and abdomen is noted – the rib cage should move symmetrically with respiration and the abdomen should be rounded. The position of the nipples is observed and the apex beat palpated just below the left nipple. The number of vessels in the cord can be counted, if this has not already been done, but with care so as not to introduce infection; the base of the cord should be inspected for protrusions, in case a small exomphalos (bowel herniating through the umbilicus) is present.

External Genitalia

The position of the urinary meatus on the penis is located in male infants and the presence of both testes in the scrotum confirmed. In baby girls, the labia are separated to check the urethral and vaginal orifices. If there is any doubt about the sex of the baby a paediatrician should see the baby and the parents to decide urgently how the situation is to be handled.

The baby's rectal temperature may be taken to confirm the patency of the anus and to check for chilling or pyrexia. The presence of meconium on the thermometer and any urine passed should be noted.

Limbs

These are inspected for equal length and normal movement. The hands should be opened and the fingers counted. Toes should also be counted and both sets of digits checked for webbing. Extra digits are a relatively common finding and may be a family trait. The feet and ankles should be examined for talipes (clubfoot). The hips must be tested for developmental dysplasia (congenital dislocation) either by the midwife at this point or at a later examination. Two tests may be used: Ortolani's and Barlow's tests (**Box 12.1** and **Figures 12.8** and **12.9**) Ortolani's test is a test for a dislocated hip whilst Barlow's test, tests for the unstable hip which is capable of dislocation. Therefore both test should be done if both the dislocated and dislocatable hip are to be detected. This examination may be carried out by the midwife or paediatrician according to local policy. In some centres ultrasound is used, although its value in reducing late detection is unproved (Rosendahl *et al.*, 1994). Abnormality is not always present at birth or may be difficult to detect because of lax ligaments immediately after birth, so there is an argument for postponing examination of the hips until the baby is a couple of days old (MacKeith, 1995).

Box 12.1

Testing for Developmental Dysplasia of the Hips

The baby should be lying on his/her back on a firm surface. The hips and knees are flexed to 90° and the examiner holds each leg with the thumb on the inner aspect of the thigh and the middle finger over the greater trochanter.
• Ortolani's test – the leg is gently abducted and a 'clunk' is felt as the femoral head slides from its dislocated position over the posterior rim of the acetabulum into the socket. In some cases the femoral head may fail to reduce – no clunk is felt but the leg cannot be fully abducted.
• Barlow's test – starting from a position of adduction, downwards and outwards pressure is provided to dislocate the hip that is unstable. The leg is then gently abducted downwards and a 'clunk' is felt as the femoral head slides out of the acetabulum.

Back

The baby is then turned over so that the midwife can run her finger along the spine to check for absent vertebrae or swellings; dimples or hairy patches may indi-

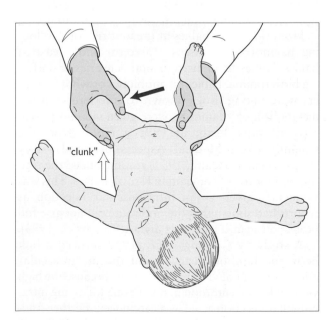

Figure 12.8 Ortolani test.

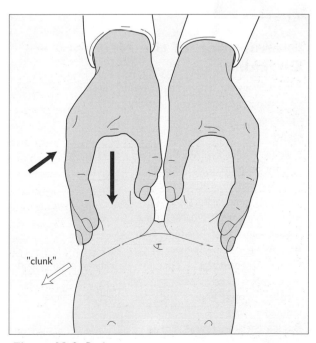

Figure 12.9 Barlow test.

cate the presence of an occult spina bifida. In non-Caucasian babies, an area of bluish pigmentation over the buttocks may be seen – known as a Mongolian blue spot, it fades as the child grows.

Auscultation of the chest, palpation of the abdomen and a neurological examination complete the full check which should be carried out on every baby within 24 hours or so of birth. Traditionally this has been done by a paediatrician or the general practitioner, but midwives and advanced neonatal nurse practitioners are now discussing whether they should take over this role (Seymour, 1995; MacKeith, 1995) in line with the recommendations of *Changing Childbirth* (Department of Health, 1993). Further training, discussion of which is beyond the scope of this book, is required for midwives who are to take responsibility for the full examination and discharge of the baby (Michaelides, 1995). Whilst in some units midwives are increasingly taking responsiblity for the full examination and discharge of babies, in others this remains the remit of the paediatrician.

Conclusion

When examination is complete, the baby is washed if warm enough and dressed or wrapped. Once practised,

the midwife is able to complete what seems at first to be a lengthy examination very quickly (**Box 12.2**).

If an abnormality is discovered it should be shown to the parents and a simple explanation given. If the midwife is unable to answer the parents' questions she should say so and assure them that a doctor will see them and the baby as soon as possible; she should then arrange for this to happen. Parents' anxieties may seem out of proportion to the size of the problem, but information rather than bland reassurance is more effective at allaying anxiety. The midwife should familiarize herself with any local policies in existence for dealing with suspected abnormalities, such as Down syndrome, where the way in which the parents are told and the timing may crucially affect how the family views the baby (Kelnar *et al*. 1995).

Vitamin K

Vitamin K is essential for the synthesis of a number of blood clotting factors – deficiency may result in a bleeding disorder known as haemorrhagic disease of the newborn. The vitamin-K dependent clotting factors are present in low concentrations at birth, but levels then fall to their lowest at 2–5 days of age. This is when bleeding is most likely to occur (Hilgartner, 1993) before levels rise again because of ingestion of vitamin K in milk and the action of gut flora. Breast milk contains very little vitamin K and breastfed babies may suffer from a late-onset form of haemorrhagic disease, in which a sometimes fatal intracranial bleed can occur.

From the 1950s babies at greatest risk of developing haemorrhagic disease (preterm and breastfed babies, babies from instrumental deliveries or suffering birth trauma, babies on antibiotics or whose mothers were taking drugs known to interfere with the metabolism of vitamin K) were given vitamin K prophylaxis after birth; in 1991 a report from the Committee on Medical Aspects of Food Policy (Department of Health, 1991) recommended the routine administration of vitamin K to all babies. This was frequently given as an intramuscular injection as reports had shown that the oral route did not give full protection against late-onset disease (Chadwick, 1993).

A study by Golding *et al*. (1992) showed a link between childhood cancer and the intramuscular administration of vitamin K, perhaps because the high vitamin K concentration in the plasma following intramuscular injection acted as a carcinogen. Further studies (Klebanoff *et al*. 1993; Ekelund *et al*. 1993; von

---

Box 12.2

Examination of the Newborn – Checklist

• *Measure*: weight, length, head circumference.
• *Assess*: colour, muscle tone, activity, cry.
• *Examine*:

Head
skull for moulding or caput,
eyes for haemorrhages, cataract,
ears for position, shape, skin tags,
mouth for cleft palate, teeth.

Skin – look for birthmarks, bruises, rashes.

Chest – apex beat, breathing pattern.

Abdomen – shape, number of cord vessels.

External genitalia – position of urinary meatus and testes (boys), urethra and vagina (girls).

Limbs – count fingers and toes, check for talipes and dislocated hips.

Back – check vertebrae, anus.

Kries *et al.* 1996) failed to replicate these findings, but publicity given to the first study led to disquiet among parents and health workers and some refusals to accept the administration of vitamin K (Croucher and Azzopardi, 1994).

Recommendations have been issued by the British Paediatric Association (BPA, 1992) for vitamin K propylaxis in infancy (**Box 12.3**); the midwife is responsible for ensuring that she adheres to the local interpretation of these guidelines, which may include obtaining informed parental consent. Midwives are only authorised to give vitamin K intramuscularly, therefore when the oral route is preferred a medical practitioner must authorise its use. The Department of Health recommends that the dose and route used in vitamin K prophylaxis are clearly recorded in the medical notes (Calman and Moores, 1992). The Royal College of Midwives produced a position paper in 1996 identifying the midwife's role in administering vitamin K (RCM, 1996).

Daily Care of the Baby

The mother is usually the baby's main caregiver – the extent to which she requires the midwife's help or teaching depends, among other things, on her state of health and previous experience with babies. The midwife may use her contact with the family as an opportunity for health education and to build up their confidence in caring for the new baby.

The baby should be examined daily for signs of illness, which entails observation of feeding behaviour, stools and urine, cry, colour and any skin lesions. A baby who is active, feeding and sleeping well and passing normal amounts of stools and urine is unlikely to be suffering from a serious illness. Conversely, a baby who is lethargic, pale, dusky, vomiting, has diarrhoea, a distended abdomen or a rash should be further examined as these may be signs of an infection or other illness.

Hygiene

The baby's face and nappy area should be kept clean, but a daily bath is not necessary – indeed, until the baby has acquired his/her own skin flora, a bath may make infection more likely. All who touch the baby should be educated to wash their hands before doing so. The eyes should not be cleaned unless they are discharging, when clean cotton wool and water are used to wipe once from inner edge outwards.

The care of the umbilicus has been the subject of considerable research (**Box 12.4**), which should underpin local policy. If the mother is to be responsible for cord care she should be shown carefully what to do and have its importance explained to her.

Box 12.3

Recommendations for the Administration of Vitamin K

• Vitamin K to be given orally to all babies within 24 hours of birth.
• Breastfed babies to receive repeat doses of vitamin K over first weeks of life.
• If the oral route is not available or is thought to be unreliable, vitamin K should be given by injection.

Box 12.4

Methods of Cord Care

After birth, the umbilical cord serves no further purpose, so the vessels fibrose and desiccate, becoming a potential site for colonization and subsequent infection. The organism most commonly associated with this is *Staphylococcus aureus*. A variety of cord-care regimes have evolved to prevent this and promote earlier separation of the cord, so removing the potential site. More recently researchers have attempted to verify these regimes and suggest a definitive plan.

Barr (1984) and Lawrence (1982) found that cords cleaned with water separated earlier than cords cleaned with spirit swabs. However, Fitzmaurice and Whiting (1993) and Bain (1994) found no differences in these two methods when used on premature babies.

Salariya and Kowbus (1988) and Mugford *et al.* (1986) showed that the use of hexachlorophane powder on the cord was associated with earlier separation, while Verber and Pagan (1993) and Allen *et al.* (1994) found that it also prevented colonization with *S. aureus*.

Feeding

Breastfeeding (*see also* Chapter 13) is promoted as the method of choice because of its advantages to both mother and baby. The midwife has a responsibility to ensure that she acquires the knowledge and skills necessary to assist the mother to fix the baby at the breast and to deal with queries and problems that she may have. Many excellent texts (*see* Further Reading) exist to help with this and groups such as the National Childbirth Trust and La Leche League offer practical training and advice to both parents and professionals.

The woman who does not wish to breastfeed should be respected in her decision and given the help she needs to establish feeding safely. Education about the preparation of formula feeds and sterilization of utensils may also be useful for the breastfeeding mother.

Weighing

From research conducted by Salariya and Robertson (1993) it has been recommended that babies are weighed daily until they gain weight. For those babies who are bottle-fed this is on the third day, and for those breastfed on the fourth day. Loss of weight during the early days was attributed to the changing patterns of stools.

Box 12.5

Information about the Baby to be Shared with Community on Discharge

• Labour and delivery details, Apgar scores, any resuscitation needed.
• Birthweight, any abnormalities.
• If vitamin K given, and route – dates for repeat doses, if appropriate.
• Method of feeding and current weight.
• Result of bilirubin check if baby jaundiced.
• Date of Guthrie or other screening tests.
• Arrangements for any further follow-up.
• Any concerns noted about the baby or mother's attitude to the baby.
REFLECTION: Consider whether your Trust's discharge documentation supplies the relevant information.

Transfer Home

Few normal term babies who have been born in hospital remain there for longer than 5 days – for many their stay is only a matter of hours. It therefore follows that the establishment of feeding and education of the family in caring for the baby takes place largely in the community. Where an integrated midwifery service exists transfer between hospital and community should be easy and 'seamless'. However, information relating to the care of the baby should be carefully passed on to the next carer (**Box 12.5**), particularly if there is a suspicion of any abnormality.

Screening Tests

Screening tests are tests carried out on a section of the population for diseases to which they may be susceptible, but of which they have no symptoms. The first neonatal examinations are forms of screening tests and their value in detecting abnormalities cannot be overestimated. To be acceptable screening tests must be sensitive enough to detect all cases of the disease, and should be cost-effective. The diseases screened for must be a significant health problem and treatment for them must be available. Therefore a limited number of diseases are suitable for neonatal screening – in the UK the conditions most commonly the subjects of screening programmes are phenylketonuria, congenital hypothyroidism, sickle-cell disease and cystic fibrosis.

One specimen of capillary blood taken on the sixth day of life is used to carry out all the tests. The midwife is usually responsible for taking the blood sample and despatching it to the test centre. She should explain the purpose of the tests to the parents, but their written consent is not normally obtained. To avoid unnecessary repetition, every effort should be made to obtain an adequate specimen the first time – practice is needed for this. The baby's heel is normally used, which should be warm and clean. A lancet, preferably an automatic type which limits the depth of insertion and reduces the pain for the baby (Harpin and Rutter, 1983), is used to puncture the heel using the sites shown in **Figure 12.10**. The foot should be held downwards, gently squeezed and released and a drop of blood allowed to form. This is then collected into a capillary tube or onto a sheet of 'blotting' paper designed for the purpose, depending on the requirements of the testing laboratory. The procedure is repeated until enough blood has been obtained. The heel is cleaned, an adhesive plaster applied and the baby given to the mother to comfort. The identification details are completed and the specimen despatched promptly.

Repeat samples are usually needed because the first was inadequate. It is important for the midwife to be aware of the anxiety caused to the parents by the need for a repeat test and for her to be able to allay this concern by an informed explanation (Polichroniadis, 1989).

Phenylketonuria

Phenylketonuria (PKU) is an autosomal recessive inherited error in the metabolism of the amino acid phenylalanine. It is caused by the absence of the enzyme phenylalanine hydroxylase, which converts phenylalanine into tyrosine. The build-up of phenylalanine in the blood leads to brain damage – incidence in the UK is about 1:10,000 with regional variations. Screening for PKU has been mandatory since 1969. Three tests are available:

1 Biochemical assay for phenylalanine within the dried blood spot. This is the most commonly used test in the UK. It is not interfered with by antibiotics.
2 The Scriver chromatography test uses liquid blood and allows identification of levels of other amino acids, some of which may also cause damage if at high levels. This test is not easily automated, so is more expensive and is the second most common test used. It is not affected by antibiotics.
3 The Guthrie bacterial inhibition test uses dried blood spots punched from the samples taken on the 'blotting' paper. The presence of phenylalanine in the blood inhibits the growth of *Bacillus subtilis* on culture medium – antibiotics given to the baby or passed in breastmilk invalidate this test. This test is used in fewer units, and there are moves within the paediatric biochemical world to abandon its use.

For the tests, the baby should have had at least three full days of milk feeds.

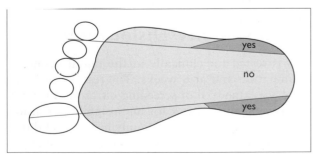

Figure 12.10 Sites for heel puncture to obtain capillary blood for screening tests.

Babies whose repeat tests are positive are seen urgently for further tests by a paediatrician who specializes in metabolic disorders; if the diagnosis is confirmed, treatment with a diet low in phenylalanine is started, which provides an excellent prognosis.

Congenital Hypothyroidism

Congenital hypothyroidism (CHT) is caused by a total or partial absence of the thyroid gland or a fault in the synthesis of thyroid hormone. The incidence is approximately 1:4000 births and if undetected or untreated mental and physical retardation occurs. Screening has been mandatory in the UK since 1980.

The low level of thyroid hormone (thyroxine, T_4) leads to greatly elevated levels of thyroid-stimulating hormone (TSH), trying in vain to stimulate the absent thyroid. The test, therefore, measures TSH levels – babies with confirmed positive results should be referred to a paediatrician immediately. Treatment is by thyroxine tablets taken for life.

Sickle Cell Disease

Abnormal haemoglobin leading to sickle-shaped red cells is an inherited condition found mainly in Afro-Caribbeans. At low O_2 tensions the abnormal cells precipitate in the capillaries, which causes acute pain, increased hypoxia, infection and anaemia. Screening is not mandatory and is only valuable in areas with a significant Afro-Caribbean population. There is no treatment for the condition, but presymptomatic diagnosis can lead to education about situations to avoid, for example, strenuous exercise, cold extremities and events where special care is needed, such as when flying or undergoing a general anaesthetic, because of the potential of these to cause hypoxia and precipitate a 'crisis'.

Cystic Fibrosis

Cystic fibrosis occurs in 1:2000 Caucasian births and is the most common inherited metabolic disorder. Mucus production, particularly by the pancreas and lungs, is affected; this leads to chest infections and malabsorption by the gut. Although there is no cure for the condition, early detection can lead to better prognosis by starting physiotherapy, enzymes and antibiotics early. Tests to detect cystic fibrosis, by measuring the pancreatic enzymes trypsin and trypsinogen, are still being developed. Screening for CF is rapidly becoming widely available so the midwife needs to ascertain whether this test is available in her area.

HEALTH EDUCATION AND HEALTH PROMOTION

In the previous section, we reviewed how abnormalities within the newborn may be detected through a system of routine screening procedures and through the daily care and observation by the mother and the caring team. Even the most minor of abnormalities in their child will create much fear and anxiety in parents. It is therefore essential that parents receive timely support and appropriate education from the caring team, as this will both alleviate their anxieties and allow them to make informed decisions. A list of some useful organisations is given in the Further Reading section.

Abnormalities on Initial Examination

Initial examination of the newborn baby may reveal skin blemishes or other minor abnormalities (webbed or overlapping toes, for instance) of no major medical significance, but which may cause apparently excessive anxiety in parents. The emphasis on screening in pregnancy and its achievements, together with society's attitudes to physical appearance and the controlling aspect of 'planning' for a baby, all lead to an expectation of perfection.

It is more common now for mothers to *assume* the baby is all right because of all the processes through which they have already passed.

Heart Problems

Most murmurs audible at the initial baby examination are 'innocent' and if heard with no other symptoms should be listened to again. If the murmurs persist, referral is appropriate. They result from turbulent blood flow through a normal heart. Innocent murmurs are short, systolic, usually only heard at one area of the chest (left sternal border) and unaccompanied by a thrill or an abnormal looking chest. Pulses are of normal intensity, the baby is pink and healthy, feeds without distress and has normal heart (100–120 b.p.m.) and respiratory rates (40–60) at rest.

A murmur that is loud (greater than 2/6), or long, or heard more widely over the chest than simply locally at the lower left sternal border requires immediate clinical review, usually a chest radiograph and an electrocardiogram (ECG), to exclude underlying organic heart disease.

By contrast, significant congenital heart disease is relatively rare (8 per 1000 babies) and may not present with an audible murmur. Routine antenatal screening can only pick up 40% of such lesions, so they may well present for the first time in the newborn period.

Even if no heart murmur is audible, heart problems can present as heart failure (breathlessness, failure to complete feeds, tachycardia) or as cyanosis either all the time or on crying or feeding. Such babies require urgent assessment as they can deteriorate rapidly, particularly if their circulation depends on the ductus arteriosus remaining open. Poor volume pulses, hepatomegaly or cyanosis on crying are all indications for immediate and urgent referral to a hospital paediatric department.

Clefts of Lip or Palate

Increasingly, these problems are detected antenatally, thus allowing parents to observe rationally and unhurriedly the results of current treatment. If presenting at birth, their appearance can shock, so careful reassurance is important. Pictures for parents of 'pre' and 'post' treatment appearances are very helpful. The baby needs a full examination to be sure the anomaly is not part of a syndrome that affects the rest of the face or other body parts.

Plastic surgery teams are being developed across the UK to provide an integrated care for these babies, which includes early help with feeding (may require a special long bottle teat or an orthodontic plate, to allow the baby to produce negative pressure in the mouth and a 'suck'). Surgery on the lip is offered at 3 months of age or earlier. This helps the baby's appearance, but also encourages palatal development. Initial palate repairs are performed at 6–9 months, but subsequent surgery may be needed. This condition is not linked to intelligence problems and most individuals will speak and function quite normally. The parents should be informed about self-help groups, e.g. the Cleft Lip and Palate Association (CLAPA).

Hip Instability/Dislocation

This is tested for clinically at the initial neonatal examination and at 6 weeks. The test is not foolproof – a large trial of screening ultrasound is now underway. Babies at risk for hip instability or dislocation include those with a family history and those who present by the breech (regardless of mode of delivery). The midwife should be aware of local schemes for screening or following at-risk babies. Splints to keep the hips abducted and flexed are the usual early management, as they allow the femoral head to sit within the acetabular cup and promote its normal development.

Talipes

Intrauterine posture, particularly if restricted (multiple pregnancy, lack of amniotic fluid, abnormal uterine shape), can result in feet which, after birth, are not held 'straight', but are either turned in (talipes equinovarus, TEV) with the toes pointing down, or out (talipes calcaneovalgus, TCV) with the heel pointing down. If the foot can be straightened to normality by gentle pulling, the condition is 'positional' and corrects spontaneously. This can be helped by encouraging the mother to move the foot 5–10 times to the 'correct' position several times daily, such as before feeds.

If the bones within the foot have developed abnormal positions, the foot cannot be pushed or pulled to a normal posture. This is 'structural' talipes and needs early physiotherapy assessment, probably splinting and possibly later orthopaedic surgery. The baby should be examined for other neurological or muscular problems.

Variations in Growth

Babies, like adults, come in all sizes. The baby's weight, length and head size can be compared to population norms using charts such as those in **Figures 12.11** and **12.12**. The solid lines refer to the 10th and 90th centiles, the outer dotted lines to the 3rd and 97th centiles. Measurements of pre-term and post-term babies should be plotted according to their due date rather than their actual date of birth.

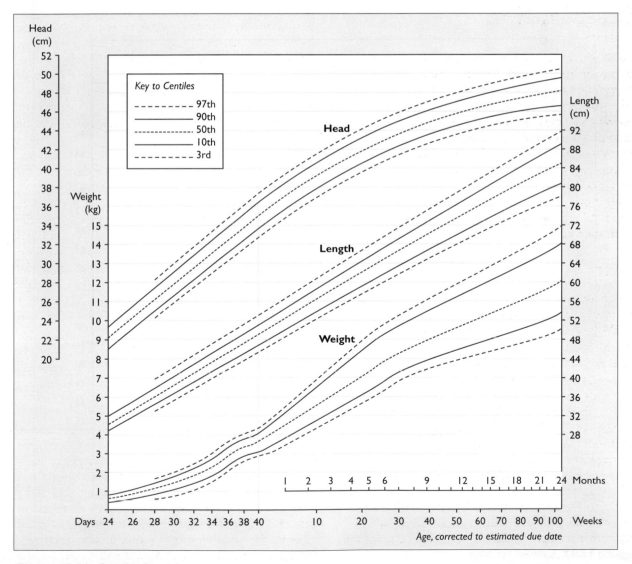

Figure 12.11 Centiles for girls.

An underweight baby may be 'growth retarded' and appear thin. Such a baby is constantly hungry, crying frequently for feeds, until growth 'catches up' to his/her 'natural' centile. During this period the baby may take 220–250 ml/kg of milk or even more, so the temptation to give early solids is strong. Another baby of the same weight may be chubby and short, with a relatively small head size. Such a baby is likely to reflect his parents' own short stature and will grow parallel to the centile of his birth.

Very large, fat babies similarly may reflect the build of their parents and grow appropriately. If the mother has diabetes or gestational diabetes, however, the baby may have been influenced by intrauterine hyperglycaemia. After birth such babies gradually fall back to their 'natural' centiles, first in weight and then in length; they may not feed particularly eagerly in the early weeks, which is normal.

Head size usually remains on the centile of birth unless the baby is growth retarded, as noted above. Deviation from this requires investigation.

The Abnormal Baby

One in every 50 babies has some abnormality, usually minor. When the abnormality is not minor, either the midwife or mother may be prepared for this. Antenatal diagnosis of some anomalies allows preparation psychologically and medically for what may need to done, for instance resuscitation and preparation for surgery

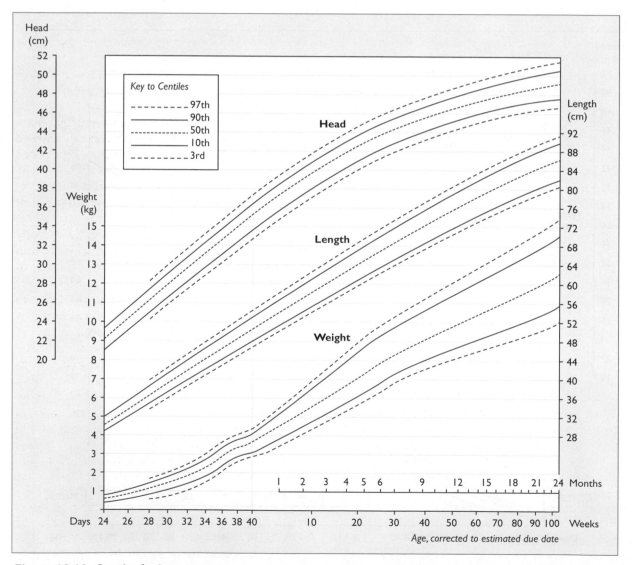

Figure 12.12 Centiles for boys.

in a baby with exomphalos or gastroschisis. 'Screening' tests do not detect all cases of a particular condition – there are always some 'false negatives'.

If a baby is born with evident signs of major abnormality, but in good condition, crying and pink, the midwife's role is to support the parents. They may or may not realize that there is a problem – an absent limb is obvious to all, but Down syndrome may not be. What needs to be said may be straightforward, but is more likely to be complex and involve the need for repeated simple explanations and the acceptance of an inevitable uncertainty about the future.

Retrospective surveys of the views of parents in these situations show that bad news is not taken in entirely. Parents may deny that they were ever told some particular point. They may often blame the bearer of the tidings.

Parents should be told important news about their baby together or with supportive friends. There should be unhurried and uninterrupted privacy and they need to be able to concentrate. The person telling them should be the most senior paediatrician available, with the midwife present. In an ideal situation this is best done out of the delivery room once the baby is old enough to have been greeted, handled and held by the parents, but within the first 24 hours. Supplementary literature is welcome, but no substitute for talking (Gosden 1994, Carr 1995).

The Baby at Home – Common Problems

General Health

Today's small and scattered families mean that most new mothers have no previous experience of caring for young babies. Literature for parents tends to stress the positive; the reality of 24-hours-a-day care, painful breasts, a constantly crying baby, laundry, the difficult in 'nipping out' of the house and anxieties about what is or is not normal can be overwhelming. The support of peers in a similar situation is extremely helpful, whether arranged formally (National Childbirth Trust) or in informal neighbourhood networks – midwives may be able to facilitate this.

Positive steps parents can take to promote their baby's health include having the baby in their room for the first weeks, attempting to breastfeed (*see* Chapter 13), stopping smoking themselves and not permitting anyone to smoke in rooms used by the

baby, and reducing or avoiding contact with the new baby by anyone with an obvious cold or virus infection.

'Cot Death'

The Foundation of the Study of Infant Deaths (FSID, 1993) produces widely available health education material for families on minimizing the risk of sudden infant death syndrome (SIDS). The rate of cot deaths in the UK fell from 1.43 per 1000 live births in 1991 to 0.78 per 1000 in 1992 following a national campaign with four main tenets:
- Place your baby on its back or side to sleep.
- Don't smoke and avoid smoky atmospheres.
- Do not let your baby become too hot.
- If you think your baby is unwell, contact your doctor.

The incidence still remains higher than in some other cultures, such as in China, so current research is studying the possible protective effects of the child sharing the parental bed (thus sleeping less deeply) or of using a soother or dummy (and promoting a non-nutritive sucking activity).

Prone sleeping (on the tummy) became customary in the UK in the 1970s. Studies subsequently showed an increased proportion of babies that slept prone among cot death victims. In the UK a study in Avon in 1990 (Wigfield *et al.* 1992) showed a fall in prevalence of prone sleeping accompanied by halving of the local cot death rate.

Maternal smoking in pregnancy has consistently been associated with an increased risk of SIDS in many studies, the risk being at least double that of nonsmokers and increasing with the number of cigarettes smoked. Passive exposure of the baby to smoking after birth has been confirmed separately as an independent risk factor in several studies.

Overwrapping has been confirmed in two case-controlled studies to be more common in cot death victims, accompanied by overheating of the baby's room. Although probably less important as an independent risk factor, overheating can interact with other factors such as infection (when parents tend to increase the amount of bedding used).

Minor illnesses are common in retrospective studies of cot death babies, although there is no evidence that they are causal. Parents may underestimate illness severity, which has led to production of information for parents, especially in the FSID *Reduce the Risk of Cot Death* leaflet (first published 1994). The 'baby check' scoring system is another method to help parents and health professionals, including midwives, assess illness severity in babies under 6 months with groups of signs or symptoms

The role of breastfeeding in cot death prevention is unconfirmed; however, breastfeeding has numerous other health benefits and therefore is to be promoted.

Care of the next infant

The care of the next infant (CONI) scheme aims to provide support with subsequent babies to parents who have had a child die a cot death. Parents are referred in early pregnancy to a trained health visitor who gives planned support before and after the birth. This may include regular weighing of the infant as an early detector of intercurrent illness, or the provision of an apnoea monitor. Conventional monitors, which detect chest movement, can provide great reassurance to families, but are of no proved benefit in the prevention of SIDS.

Nappy Rashes

Infrequently changed nappies – cloth or disposable – hot weather and the use of plastic pants promote increased contact of urine with skin. This results in production of ammonia and a chemical burn. The distribution is where urine lies against the skin, i.e. mainly at the front, avoiding groin creases and without separate 'satellite' lesions on the legs or tummy. Prevention includes avoiding precipitants and protecting the skin with any commercial barrier cream, such as zinc and castor oil cream. Nappy rash is painful, so the baby cries when he/she passes urine. Treatment involves protection of the broken skin and exposure of the skin to air in a warm, dry environment to promote healing of the ulcerated areas.

Secondary infection can occur, either bacterial or candidal. Extension of reddened skin into the groin creases and development of satellite lesions indicate this complication – specific treatment is needed. If there is candidal rash, the mouth should be treated also to prevent recurrence, e.g. miconazole gel orally and cream topically to the rash, each for 5 days.

Sticky Eyes

Ophthalmia that presents within 48 hours of birth is caused by organisms from the mother. Neomycin eye ointment for 5 days is usually effective. Gonococcal ophthalmia is rare and produces orbital cellulitis such that the eye and lids are very swollen, the eye cannot be opened and pus pours out. This requires hospital admission and frequent topical and systemic treatment. Later infections are usually staphylococcal. Chalymydial infection presents at or after 7 days and is not improved by topical neomycin. Management requires confirmation by conjunctival scrapings, topical and systemic antibiotics and referral of the mother to a department of urogenital medicine.

Sleeping and Crying Problems

There is large variability between babies in these behaviours. Most problems relate to parental anxiety and fatigue. Simple common sense, advice, demand feeding, attention to comfort and development of a bed-time routine are usually all that is required. Much helpful literature is available (Douglas and Richman, 1984). There is also a Crysis helpline (see references).

Table 12.3 Schedule of preschool immunization		
Time of birth, regardless of maturity	**All babies**	**Selected babies**
2 months	Oral polio vaccine	At birth BCG vaccine (live vaccine given intradermally over deltoid insertion)
	Tetanus	Hepatitis B immunoglobulin (if mother has anti-e antigen positivity)
	Pertussis triple vaccine Diphtheria	Hepatitis B vaccine (repeated at 1, 2 and 12 months) if mother tests positive for any Hepatitis B antigen
3 months	Repeat as above	
4 months	Repeat as above	
12–15 months	MMR triple vaccine	
Preschool	Booster of OPV and DT vaccines	

Hernias

Umbilical hernia is common, present from birth and self-limiting. Hernias that appear after birth in the groin in either sex require surgery. An irreducible hernia may become strangulated – red, hard and painful – and the baby distressed. This is an emergency requiring immediate hospital admission.

Immunization

Immunizations are of proved effectiveness in reducing the population incidence of selected diseases (**Table 12.3**), so babies should be offered immunization. Parental refusal may be based on misinformation and full discussion is warranted.

Children who are immunocompromised or who receive systemic steroid treatment should *not* be given live vaccines [oral polio vaccine (OPV), bacille Calmet–Guérin (BCG), measles–mumps–rubella (MMR) vaccine]. Inactivated vaccine is available for polio. Similarly, a double (DT) vaccine is available if parents do not wish their child to receive the pertussis component. Although intercurrent illness is a reason to defer immunization, this should not be encouraged as it produces major delays.

Developmental Screening

Screening for any condition is of two types: whole population screening, including serendipitous screening when a baby is seen for another reason; and selective screening, usually at a more intensive level and in more detail of 'high-risk' subgroups. Hospitals screen babies who have been in neonatal units specifically for growth, health and elements of development.

Any child whose parents are concerned about his/her development warrants a full examination. This includes immediate medical review of any baby aged over 6 weeks' whose parents feel he/she does not respond to sounds or does not fix visually. All children are offered formal developmental reviews, the results of which are stored in a computerized community register. These are done at 6 weeks post-term (by a doctor) looking at growth, head growth, muscle tone, head control, response to visual and auditory signals and social smile development; then again at 8 months when a distraction hearing test and a crude test of visual acuity are performed in addition to a physical examination.

Between these occasions, most babies are seen by their health visitor to be weighed, to be immunized and for the parents to be given health and nutrition advice. These opportunities should be used to ask relevant questions about developmental milestones. Developmental problems are more likely in those babies who miss 'DNA' clinic and immunization appointments, so these in particular need to be actively followed.

Neonatal Units

Of babies born in hospital, 7–10% are admitted to a neonatal unit. Work in the 1960s demonstrated the adverse effects on attachment of separating mothers and babies, so admission to a neonatal unit is now much less frequent, with 'transitional' mother and baby facilities available in many hospitals.

Major reasons for admission are asphyxia, postnatal illness such as infection, prematurity certainly below 36 weeks' gestation and abnormality precluding ordinary care. Most units try to minimize fear and separation by copious explanation, including written information, liberal or open visiting policies and provision of polaroid photographs to parents unable to visit. Social Services can often provide financial help for transport for parents whose babies are far from home. Breastfeeding can usually be facilitated by loaned pumps and help and information about expressing milk, which needs to be done 8–10 times daily to maintain supply.

Babies are allowed home when they can maintain their temperature in a bedroom environment and suck feeds adequately. This is usually at a weight of 1.5–1.8 kg and a gestation equivalent to 36 weeks or greater.

Preparation for going home includes a check on home facilities, training to replace missed parentcraft on feeding, bathing and hygiene and, often, provision of a specially trained midwife to liaise between neonatal unit and community and help in the care of the ex-premature baby at home.

MATERNAL REACTION TO THE NEWBORN

This section seeks to examine mother–infant interaction and maternal caregiving ability from the time of birth and during the early postpartum period. Until recently, it had been acknowledged that the human infant is helpless at birth and, unlike other mammals, could not even reach his/her source of nourishment without assistance. Researchers in Sweden, however, have demonstrated that newborn infants who are placed on their mother's abdomen immediately after birth and left undisturbed, will crawl to the mother's breast and begin sucking within 50 minutes if given the opportunity to do so (Lennart and O'Alade, 1990). This apart, the infant's other physical, mental, psychological and social needs at birth and in the following postpartum period require to be met by the mother or substitute caregiver. It has been said (Winnicott, 1957) that the early management of a baby is a matter beyond conscious thought and deliberate intention. It is something that becomes possible only through love.

Indeed, the human infant is dependent on others for his/her continued survival and development for several years after his birth. It must be acknowledged that the caregiving ability by parents and others is affected by cultural, social, mental, psychological and educational factors.

For many years, midwives have claimed to be able to determine a new mother's caregiving ability (for her infant) very soon after birth and during the early postpartum period. The midwife observed and loosely classified three 'types' of mothering – 'the natural mother', 'the middle of the road mother' and 'the less-than-good mother'. These deliberations were, of course, subjective opinions and the midwife kept such information personal. Only if the mother demonstrated total disinterest in her infant's caregiving and/or well-being while in hospital would the matter be reported to the paediatrician. These opinions were passed on verbally, because they are too sensitive to be written on maternal or neonatal records.

Lynch and Roberts (1977), in a retrospective study, compared birth records of abused and nonabused children. They suggested that warning signals are often given to maternity staff by those mothers who find difficulty in caring for their infant, although appropriate action does not always follow, even if or when the 'concern' is acknowledged and/or reported.

Midwives often report to the author that they had met former patients with their infants in the Hospital corridor, attending the paediatric clinic. It was of interest to note their comments when 'failure to thrive' was the known diagnosis; 'I could have told you that would happen' was the usual reaction. What had been observed by the midwife at or around the time of the infant's birth to justify this reply?

Despite progress made by medical and other sciences, many healthy infants who survive the rigours of intrauterine development, labour and delivery do not go on to enjoy a satisfactory quality of life (Salariya, 1990). Dr Henry Kempe (Kempe and Kempe, 1978), the eminent paediatrician who re-identified child abuse in the early 1960s, stated 'to provide excellent obstetric, postnatal and paediatric care in our hospitals makes very little sense if we fail to observe initial relationships between parents and their neonate, at this time.'

In 1979, a team of researchers in the USA (Gray *et al.* 1979) found that, in relation to children at-risk:

Observations by nurses of the behaviour of parents toward the newborn during labour, delivery and the first day or two of life in the nursery were as predictive as additional information gathered through a pre-natal questionnaire, pre-natal interviews and a six week follow-up evaluation.

While midwives are aware of the extreme outcomes of infant and childhood neglect and abuse, it is hoped that they might be encouraged to identify and correct some of the more subtle shortcomings of early parental caregiving in promoting good midwifery practice.

The Expert Maternity Group (Department of Health, 1993) recommend that 'providers should establish mechanisms for identifying women with more complex needs than are normally encountered.' It is hoped that maternal caregiving ability and parenting skills are essential needs which should be addressed, in the first instance, by midwives.

Infant Abilities

Despite restricted motor capabilities, the human neonate has sensory and perceptual capabilities far beyond those normally accorded (Prince and Adams, 1978). The scientific concept of the newborn infant has changed from being a conglomeration of isolated reflexes to an organism with a considerable degree of social preadaptation (Greenspan and Lieberman, 1989). Infants are born with the capacity to bond with their parents via a group of basic drives – feeding, clinging, eye gaze, touching and vocalizing (Field *et al.* 1980).

Incipe, parve puer, risu cognescere matrem. [Begin then, little boy, to acknowledge your mother with a smile.]

(Virgil's 4th Eulogy)

Smell and Taste

Human neonates, according to Morris (1991) are programmed to receive colostrum at birth and demonstrate their preference by how they suck. 'They will resist sucking salty solutions, and suck cow's milk(formula) in a different way to the way they take (expressed) breast-milk, also given by bottle' (McFadyen, 1994). Infants rely on their sense of smell to detect the pheromones a mother secretes from her breasts (Comfort, 1971) while McFarlane (1975) demonstrated that infants can recognize the odour of their own mother's milk (on breast pads) at 5 days of age.

It is said that the sense of smell in adults is 10,000 times more acute than that of taste, but whether the human mother could, if tested, recognize her infant by his/her specific smell, as do other mammals, remains to be investigated.

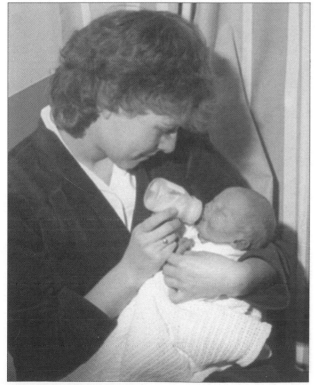

Figure 12.13 Finger holding and bottle feeding. (Courtesy of E M Salariya.)

Whether mothers are affected by the smell of their own infants may contribute to the understanding of its effect on the mother–child relationship. Some mothers (and midwives) indicate dislike of the smell of artificial milk formula, especially when bottle-fed infants are sick or 'burp' while feeding.

Research is needed to determine, along with other factors, whether a mother demonstrates less close contact (e.g. not putting the infant to the shoulder) and less cuddling of her infant compared with those who do not find the smell of artificial milk formula unpleasant (Salariya, 1990).

Grasping

A palmar grasp is usually demonstrated soon after delivery. Infants are born with the ability to finger-hold and the majority of mothers initiate the procedure at this time. Observations suggest that, while it is the mother who stimulates the infant to finger-hold, it is the infant who determines an end to the interaction. Subsequent grasping episodes are observed during infant feeding at this time, especially between the breastfeeding mother and her infant (Salariya, 1990). Several mothers have stated that they are aware of synchronization of movement between the infant's tighter grasp during active sucking and a definite relaxing of the hold during pauses in feeding. Mothers and others who bottle-feed infants should be encouraged to practice finger holding at this time. The regular skin contact at each bottle-feeding session probably compensates for the absence of skin contact automatically afforded the breastfed infant at these time (**Figure 12.13**).

Rooting

The infant, in response to a combination of stimuli, turns his/her head towards the breast in anticipation of suckling (Prechtl, 1958). These stimuli, which occur singularly or in concert, include grasping of the mother's forefinger by the infant, which in turn stimulates the infant to make 'mouthing' movements.

The specific smell of human milk identified by the infant (McFarlane, 1975) when in close proximity to the mother further exaggerates movement of the infant's lips and tongue. These 'mouthings' usually elicit a verbal response from the mother who interprets the cue as 'hunger'. The infant can be encouraged to open his/her mouth in a gaping fashion, in readiness for correct latching-on at the breast, if and when the mother touches the infant's upper lip with her nipple.

An unacceptable practice has developed in recent years, in which professionals (paediatricians, midwives and others) can be seen to substitute one of their fingers as a 'dummy' and place it in the infant's mouth during physical examination and at other times. The mothers have been very quick to follow this 'unsavoury' unhygienic practice, as have other members and friends of the infant's family.

Vision

At birth the infant's focusing distance is around 20–30 cm (Stern, 1977; MacFarlane, 1977; Brazelton and Cramer, 1991), which is the distance between the infant and mother, pupil to pupil, when breastfeeding. The object of focus becomes fuzzy if it is any closer or further away (Schaffer, 1971). Also, the infant demonstrates sensitivity to bright light by blinking, so lights should be dimmed during periods of maternal–infant interaction.

The midwife should be alert to the difference between a mother looking 'at' her infant and one who consciously makes eye contact with her infant because, as Stern (1977) has indicated, 'there is an all-important difference between looking and seeing just as there is between listening and hearing.' Even today, one may still encounter a mother who believes that her infant cannot 'see' until around 6 weeks of age.

Fantz (1961) showed that infants can tell the difference between various patterns, while MacFarlane (1977) determined that they are able to discriminate between real and 'fudged' faces, as well as between more abstract pictures, at only 4 days of age. Fantz (1961) concluded that 'some degree of form perception is innate'. Brazelton and Cramer (1991) agreed that 'a baby seems to be programmed for learning about human faces from birth.'

Gray (1958) disregarded 'imprinting' by human infants as they cannot physically follow (on foot) the moving object of imprinting, although Caldwell (1962) speculated that visual pursuit by the infant is the equivalent of 'following' in subprimate species. Scanning and searching of the maternal face are commonly reported observations during breast- and bottle-feeding, provided the infant is held in a position which makes this possible.

The professional is aware that although eye contact occurs almost automatically during breastfeeding (looking *en face*), a conscious effort must be made to facilitate this when an infant is being bottle-fed.

When one observes infants with their mothers, fathers or other caregivers (and this includes midwives) during a bottle-feeding session, it is disturbing to note how often an infant is held in a position which makes eye contact impossible.

It can be argued that an infant closes his/her eyes much of the time during a feed and so does not respond to eye-contact stimulus. Nevertheless, the bottle-fed infant opens his/her eyes periodically at this time, just as the breastfed infant does, and his/her positioning at the time of feeding should make eye contact possible. It can be postulated that if a mother and her family are made aware of verbal and non-verbal (eye contact) communication at the time of the infant's birth, they may begin and continue to interact in this way.

Roberts and Ounsted (1987) suggest 'that the time soon after the birth of a baby seems to be the time when parents are particularly receptive to help and suggestions.' Field *et al.* (1980) reported that:

> *Where a woman has herself been deprived of a stable, loving relationship within her family of origin, she, in turn, finds it difficult to provide her own child with the adequate mothering necessary for the emotional, social and intellectual needs of a young child.*

Midwives should be alert to the differences between mothers who constantly talk 'at' their infants

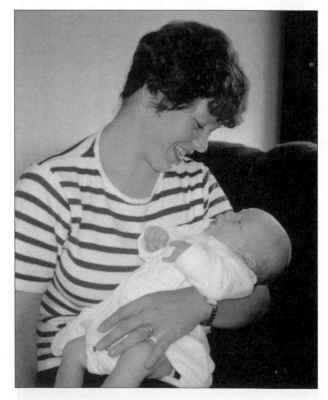

Figure 12.14 Baby mimicking mother's speech. (Courtesy of E.M. Salariya.)

in adult voice tones (for all to hear), and those mothers who engage in '*en face*' private communication with their infants. Infants who are stimulated in the latter way 'mimic' and 'converse' with the mother (**Figure 12.14**).

Infants whose mothers' caregiving ability had been assessed by midwives, using 'FIRST' score (Salariya and Cater, 1984), were followed-up at age 4–5 years. Outcomes for 30 children of 'low-scoring mothers' were compared with those of 60 mothers with 'normal or high' scores. It is of interest that although 9 out of 30 children of the 'low scores' group had been referred to speech therapy, none of the 60 'normal or high scores' group required this service (Salariya, 1987).

Hearing and Speech

The uterus is not a soundproof chamber, so the infant receives auditory stimulation throughout his/her intrauterine life. MacFarlane (1977) demonstrated that sound and vibration influenced intrauterine movement. Salariya (1990) reported that pregnant women became aware of changes in their fetuses' pattern of movement when other fetal heart rates

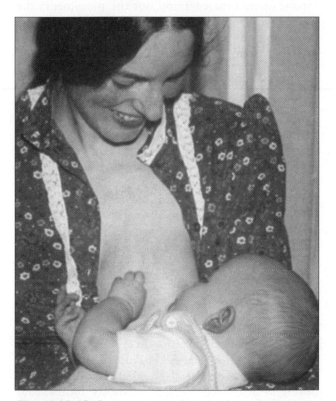

Figure 12.15 Breast massage by baby during breast feeding. (Courtesy of Medical Media Services, Ninewells Hospital and Medical School.)

were being monitored electronically, in the same ward, with the sound volume pitched at a certain level. The infant appears to prefer the tone of human voices and can discriminate between the mother's and other voices very quickly.

'Motherese', the higher and wider pitched adult speech to infants, has been reported cross-culturally, although its universality is disputed (Farnald, 1985).

The importance of pitch and tone in mother to infant and child speech should be referred to in parent education, as should the quality of what is said in conversation with the infant. The child who is shouted at in a negative, aggressive voice to 'stop doing that', 'leave that alone', 'I won't ask you again', etc., may have a very different and impoverished vocabulary by the time he/she reaches school. This should be compared with the infant whose mother is aware of the need for variable tone, the appropriate use of words and the importance of eye contact, as well as of smiling and other body language, when speaking to or listening to her infant from birth onwards.

Many argue that any short-comings in speech, language or vocabulary will be corrected by the child's attendance at nursery school, but this should not be depended upon. In a study carried out in the south of England, researchers found that children had very limited individual teacher–child communication in class, compared with that experienced by the child in conversation with his/her mother in the home (Tizard and Hughes, 1984). Knowledge about preverbal development and its relation to spoken language has grown enormously (Tait, 1987). Interactions that take place between infants and adults during the first year of life are intricate and complicated (Bruner, 1983).

Early idenfication of severe congenital hearing loss is now widely persued, helped in part by earlier and improved screening procedures by health visitors (McCormack 1983, Sancho *et al.* 1988).

Touch

The need to touch and be touched is a key primal instinct. Infants learn about the environment through touching and experience differences between hard and soft objects, as well as differences between hot and cold temperatures, from the time of birth. The observer can see how the infant explores his/her mother's breast while breastfeeding and how the mother appreciates the 'massaging' process at this time (**Figure 12.15**).

Researchers in the USA (Field, 1986) found that premature infants who were massaged for 15 minutes, three times daily, for 10 days gained weight more quickly and were discharged home 6 days earlier than a control group who did not receive this form of treatment.

Massage treatment of preterm as well as full-term infants has become routine practice in several neonatology units in the USA and Europe. Adamson-Macedo and Attree (1994), however, describe TAC–TIC therapy (Touching and Caressing – Tender in Caring) in the context of midwifery practice and are critical of:

> *The careless semantic assumption that the words 'massage', 'stroking', 'rubbing', 'patting', 'holding' and' handling' have interchangeable meanings and that this is false. They neither involve the same actions, nor produce the same reactions from babies, be they full term or preterm infants.*

Research projects in the USA and Canada support the effectiveness and safety of skin-to-skin (kangaroo) care for preterm infants (Anderson *et al.* 1986; Anderson, 1989; Hamelin and Ramachandran, 1993; Ludington-Hoe *et al.* 1994; Legault and Goulet, 1995). Parents, it is said, 'love kangaroo care'; they feel excitement, happiness and an indescribable feeling of joy. Mothers and fathers murmur quietly and sing to their infants

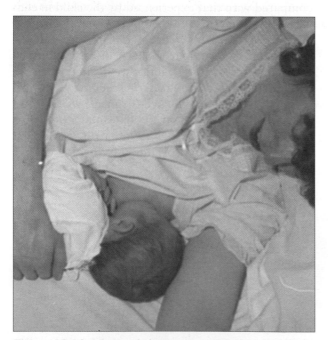

Figure 12.16 Mother–baby contact, with the baby's feet on the mother's thigh and in an 'en *face*' position. (Courtesy of Medical Media Services, Ninewells Hospital and Medical School.)

during 'kangaroo care' sessions. It is also reported that infants who receive this type of care cry less, have greater weight gain, are breastfed more successfully and are discharged home, in the care of their 'more confident' mothers, earlier. Infants demonstrate their need of skin contact when asleep in their own cot. They can be observed lying with one or both hands in close proximity to or touching their face, provided the hands are free and are not bound by blankets.

Observations during the development of an assessment tool, FIRST score, noted that the majority of mothers, when asked, were eager to have their newborn infants placed in bed beside them soon after birth (Salariya and Cater, 1984). The mother was advised that the infant's feet could be placed on her bare thigh, a modification of the total skin contact advocated by Klaus *et al.* (1972) when testing their bonding theory. It was presumed that neither the Scottish culture nor its climate favoured total skin contact at that time. After removal of the infant's blanket, the mother was invited to 'touch' her infant's foot and at once would state 'Oh dear – you are cold.'

After reassurances that this would be corrected once the infant's feet were in contact with her thigh (at the same time carrying out the placement) the mother would exclaim in a higher pitched 'motherese' and even more caring voice, 'You poor little baby – you are frozen.' This interaction offered the midwife the opportunity to discuss temperature relativity (**Figure 12.16**).

It was noted that a minority of mothers, although agreeing to have their infant's feet placed on their bare thigh, did not appear to 'enjoy' the experience. When the midwife returned to the bedside, after approximately 5 minutes, she would find that the mother had either placed the infant in the cot or was sitting up in bed with the infant (without his/her blanket) on top of the bed covers. Although the mothers were not questioned about their apparent dislike of this form of skin contact, it was not suggested to the mother that the exercise should be repeated.

This contrasted with the majority of mothers who found delight in having their infants in such close contact. Many of the mothers who breastfed continued to feed their infants in a lying position during the early postpartum period; these mothers continued spontaneously, with the feet–thigh contact as part of the breastfeeding 'procedure'. Observations by the author during or after feeding often found the mother and infant asleep. Skin contact was, however, still being maintained, even though the mother had inadvertently moved her leg, because the infant had extended his/her leg and was often making contact with only one big toe.

Midwives must be ever alert to the opportunities which present that are indicative of the individual the-oretical' and/or 'parenting skill' needs of the mother.

Before the 1970s, mothers had always cared for their infants on their 'laps'. After this time, however, a revolutionary practice developed and infants would be cared for in a more remote way. The author believes the 'new' practice evolved as a result of women beginning to wear trousers during pregnancy and in the early postpartum period. The wearing of trousers made it difficult to form a 'lap' and women were advised to place their infants on top of a suit-ably covered (blanketed) dining table while bathing or napkin changing. Very soon afterwards, changing mats became available. Unfortunately, in many instances, these mats are now placed on the floor while in use.

This 'no touch' or 'distance handling' technique was and is carried out in hospitals from the time of birth (**Figure 12.17**). Several midwives and students believed that the change was initiated 'to stop or pre-vent mothers dropping their infants'! Urgent research needs to be carried out to determine the long-term effects of 'mat' versus 'lap' caring:

• In infants deprived of close contact at these times.
• Its effect on maternal back problems, when the mat is placed on the floor during use.

Holding

Most 'mother and child' paintings demonstrate the infant being held on the mother's left side. Such 'artis-tic licence' is supported in the findings of studies by

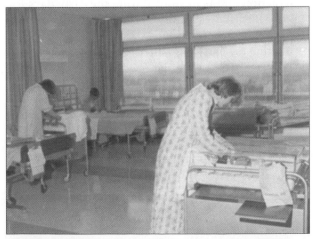

Figure 12.17 'No touch technique' during caregiving. (Courtesy of E.M. Salariya.)

Salk (1962) and de Chateau *et al.* (1978), in which 80% of mothers demonstrated 'left side preference holding' while carrying their infants.

This preference was independent of whether the mothers were right or left handed. Mothers who held their infants at the right side made less body contact with their infants and reported delay in accepting the pregnancy or the newborn infant as their own (de Chateau *et al.* 1978).

The infant receives constant, intermittent and repetitive tactile and kinaesthetic stimulation while in the uterus, from pressure changes caused by mater-nal movement and breathing (Salk, 1966). The infant demonstrates a feeling of contentment after birth, when he/she again experiences these stimuli by being held and/or carried about.

Crying

Although crying is the infant's only means of com-munication, some attention must be paid to its effect on mothers and caregivers in the early postpartum period and later. Different types of crying are recog-nizable – hunger, pain, boredom and discomfort (Brazelton and Cramer, 1991), although these are not easily differentiated in the early days after birth (Wasz-Hockert *et al.* 1968; Wolff, 1969). The mother's dilemma of learning to decipher her infant's reasons for crying can be a most distressing experi-ence (Salariya, 1990).

Mothers and caregivers may initially interpret all crying as hunger, especially with the concept of demand feeding. Bottle-fed infants were found to feed often and ingest large amounts of artificial milk for-mula from the time of birth and during the following 36–48 hours (Salariya and Robertson, 1993), but whether this was in response to crying or for some other reason was not determined. It should be remem-bered that the appetite suppressant mechanism, pre-sent when an infant breastfeeds, is absent when bottle-fed.

Midwives should endeavour to discuss infant cry-ing and enlighten the mother, father and other likely caregivers about practices known to comfort infants and alleviate the distress of infants (as well as care-givers) at this time. The crying infant upsets some par-ents more than others and some mothers are more able to soothe their infants than are others.

The practice of putting the infant to the shoulder and holding him/her ventrally (MacFarlane, 1977) as a first means of comforting the crying infant is not an automatic reaction of all mothers. Several mothers need to have the technique demonstrated, which should be done as soon as possible after the need has been identified (Salariya, 1990): **Figure 12.18**.

Midwives should not remove infants from the mother's environment to 'settle' the crying infant. All methods used to deal with crying and distressed infants, as practised by midwives, should be demonstrated or related to the mother as appropriate.

Many mothers believe that shaking the infant is a harmless way of getting him/her to stop crying (Siddal, 1994). The possible consequences of such behaviour (e.g. cerebral haemorrhage) should be imparted to mothers, along with a warning against its practice.

Midwives may question how these topics can be addressed if such opportunities do not arise in the early postpartum period. The author (as a ward sister) utilized the 'bathing demonstration' to discuss and encourage questions about parenting skills, albeit before the actual 'demonstration'.

In the past, midwives have been guilty of advising mothers to go to the sitting room to rest or smoke if and when her infant required to have some invasive examination and/or treatment carried out that was likely to elicit crying. Mothers should (from the very beginning) be encouraged to remain with their infants at these times and be encouraged to finger-hold and soothe the infant just as she (the mother) was given a hand to hold, during her time of need, in the labour suite.

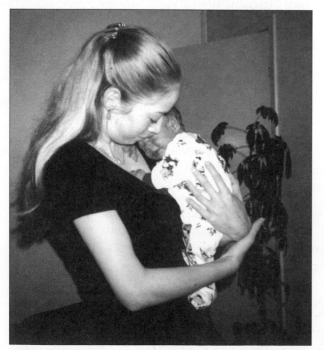

Figure 12.18 Baby at shoulder. (Courtesy of E.M. Salariya.)

Maternal–Infant Interaction and Caregiving

Maternal Attitudes and Behaviour at Time of Birth

Observations of maternal–infant interaction, by midwives and others, at and around the time of birth show very little variation between mothers in the first instance. Mothers are usually overcome by their sense of achievement and the safe arrival of their infant and there is so much information to absorb. The gender, health and weight of the infant are the questions most commonly asked immediately after an uneventful spontaneous delivery. Depending on how the mother is 'presented' with her infant, she will invariably look at the face, scan the body and stroke the limbs before returning to gaze at his/her face. The mother intermittently strokes the infant's cheek, furthest away from her, in a downwards motion, causing the infant to head-turn in that direction.

It is often reported that there is little time for parents to interact with their newborn infant after delivery in the labour room (**Box 12.6**).

Maternal Attitudes/Behaviour Postpartum

Despite repeated reminders about the 'uniqueness' of individual mothers and their infants, many similarities can be observed in relation to maternal–infant interaction and behaviour during the early days following birth. Most mothers engage in 'finger-tipping' the cot when rooming-in is practised.

During the early days after birth most mothers are totally engrossed with the needs of their infant and

> **Box 12.6**
>
> ### The Importance of Communication
>
> Midwives and other health-care personnel must not underestimate the importance of what is communicated to mothers at and around the time of delivery. Information given at this time is often remembered by the mother and her family many years after the event.

take leave of them only for short periods, to attend to their personal eating and toilet requirements. There appears to be little time afforded to socializing with other mothers. A mother spends much time 'adoring' her infant whether she/he is awake or asleep. The timid or unsure mother of yesterday very quickly gains confidence as she gets to know all the special attributes and cues of her newborn infant and begins to respond appropriately. The infant's well-being is of prime importance to the majority of mothers and everything she does reflects this priority.

A small number of mothers, however, are seen to act differently and do engage in social interaction in the smokers' sitting room regardless of whether or not they

---

Box 12.7

In 1984, an article was published that described the development of a scoring system which evolved as a method of measuring certain aspects of a mother's caregiving for her newborn infant (Salariya and Cater, 1984). The five observed factors are Feeding, Interest, Response, Speech and Touch, represented by the mnemonic FIRST. These have been combined into a numerical score. When tested for interobserver reliability the degree of agreement using the KAPPA scale (Cohen, 1968) was: Feeding, K = 0.92; Interest, K = 0.86; Response, K = 0.73; Speech, K = 0.55 and Touch, K = 0.52. The MCR FIRST score is distinguished by its simplicity of use in clinical work. The MCR FIRST score criteria booklet was given to all midwives at the study hospital. They were encouraged to examine the criteria for the appropriate scoring immediately after an observation had been carried out. Since midwives had claimed that they 'had always done this, this was nothing new', it was feared that the scoring could become less reliable if carried out from 'memory'.

Criteria

Factor	Score
(F) feeding:	0, 1 or 2.
(I) interest:	0, 1 or 2.
(R) response:	0, 1 or 2.
(S) speech + eye contact:	0, 1 or 2.
(T) touch:	0, 1 or 2.

Feeding

Score	Behaviour
0	• Mother does not give a positive answer when asked how she intends feeding her baby, i.e. breast or bottle. • If breastfeeding, the mother makes no effort to offer the breast to the baby. • If bottle-feeding, no choice of artificial formula feed is made or no interest is shown as to when the baby will be fed. • Mother overfeeds or underfeeds the baby. • Mother has no idea of the baby's feeding requirements. • Mother makes no attempt to sterilize feeding bottles.
1	• If breastfeeding the mother makes an attempt to offer breast to the baby, but may require much help and support to do so. • If bottle feeding, the mother will inquire about feeding 'regime' and at what time the baby will be fed; she may require much help and support in this. • Mother's hygiene is not good – e.g. she does not wash her hands prior to feeding the infant and is careless about sterilizing feeding bottles. • Copes with feeding and understands baby's feeding requirements.
2	• The mother recognizes and is able to satisfy the baby's feeding needs with minimal or no supervision. • Mother's hygiene is good (relative to baby and feeding).

Interest

Score	Behaviour
0	• Mother is uninterested and does not recognize the baby verbally, visually or tactually. • Mother spends much time in the dayroom – not returning to check that baby is all right. • Mother leaves the baby to be cared for by others, e.g. husband, mother-in-law, neighbours. • Mother makes no comments about baby.

(continued)

Box 12.7	**Interest continued**

1
- Mother comments about the baby's appearance – colour of hair, closed eyes, dry skin, size or behaviour, e.g. crying, fist sucking or rooting.
- Mother is concerned only about satisfactory or unsatisfactory feeding and/or sleeping patterns.

2
- Mother is generally interested in the baby's welfare and development, e.g. weight gain, other measurements, stool and urinary output, sleeping pattern.
- May inquire about attending clinics in the future or about when the community midwife or health visitor will visit.
- May be interested in vaccination and/or immunization, etc., for the baby.

Response

Score	Behaviour

0
- Mother does not react to baby crying. She persistently turns away from baby.
- Does not look at baby in cot.
- Spends much time away from cot later.
- Mother will attend to baby only if he/she cries.
- Will leave baby unattended for long periods if he/she does not cry.

1
- Mother responds to baby's crying by soothing utterances.
- She may suggest that the baby is hungry.
- Mother may spend some time away from cot, but does return periodically to check that all is well.
- Mother interprets all crying as hunger.

2
- Mother is confident in her response to baby's welfare.
- Is realistic and logical in her approach to baby's needs.
- Recognizes various cries, e.g. hunger or pain, but allows reasonable time for baby to settle after feeding changing or winding.

Speech (including eye contact)

Score	Behaviour

0
- No eye-to-eye contact attempted.
- Baby held in position which makes visual contact meaningless or impossible.
- Does not speak to the baby.

1
- Baby held in position that makes eye-to-eye contact possible.
- Mother may smile to the baby.
- She may be inhibited about speaking to the baby.
- Mother may speak 'at baby' not 'to baby'.

2
- Mother holds the baby '*en face*' and speaks to him/her.
- She generally treats the baby as if capable of understanding conversation and interpreting facial expressions.
- Mother spends time speaking to and/or looking at the baby after or between feeds.

Touch

Score	Behaviour

0
- No attempt is made to touch the baby's face, hands, body or feet.
- Minimal touching of baby (by mother) when changing napkins, bathing or feeding baby.

1
- Mother touches the baby's face, hands, body or feet.
- Mother encourages the baby to 'finger-hold'.
- 'Finger-tipping' is practised when baby is in the cot.
- Finger holding is practised at feeding time.

2
- Mother makes extended contact by touching, stroking, kissing or cuddling the baby after or between feeds.
- Mother holds baby ventrally (puts to the shoulder) allowing her cheek to touch baby's face.

smoke cigarettes (Salariya, 1986). Their infants are left unattended for variable periods while the mothers remain in the sitting room. Although these mothers may not 'report' their absences, they usually assume that 'the nurses' will oversee and attend to the infant's needs, should these arise. The same small group of mothers can also, without any apparent compassion, leave their crying infants to attend to their own 'social' needs.

This group of mothers contrasts with other mothers, in that their infants do not appear to be the centre of attraction for them. Indeed, it is believed by some of these mothers that their infants cried ' to annoy them', so they walk away from the crying infants 'to teach them a lesson'. Occasionally, some of this group initiate breastfeeding, but in the course of the first few days 'discover' endless reasons for requesting that the infant be given artificial milk formula, by bottle, before quickly deciding to bottle-feed full time.

It is of interest that newly delivered mothers who were ill or temporarily incapacitated and could not be expected to carry out physical caregiving for their infants demonstrate a keen interest in the infant's well-being and that appropriate care is being received by the infant at all times. Various other differences can be quoted (see FIRST score assessment tool, **Box 12.7**).

Parenting

Problems of behaviour in children, emotional deprivation, abuse and neglect are thought to be related to problems of parenting and may be responsible for a great proportion of morbidity in children (Liptak *et al.*, 1983):

> *The ability to parent adequately is simply not an attribute that someone does or does not have. Instead parenting is a relationship between parent and child that responds to fluctuations in other relationships.*
>
> (Reder *et al.*, 1993.)

Midwives should guard against being critical of 'less than adequate' maternal caregiving and 'insensitive mothering', as this type of mothering invariably reflects what the mother experienced as a child herself.

Factors that contribute to or detract from 'normal' interaction between the parents and their infant are:

- *Impoverished care* –if this was experienced by the mother then it is believed to affect the way the mother behaves towards her own infant (Rutter and Quinton, 1984), not only before the birth but even prior to conception.
- *Disability in the infant* – such as blindness, deafness or other congenital handicap.
- *Psychological illness or alcohol and drug abuse –*

when the mother is incapable of caring even for her own needs, and the caregiving offered to her infant is inconsistent or absent.
- *Social and other personal reasons for rejecting the newborn* – impairment or breakdown of personal relationships, lack of social support, poverty, homelessness and low maternal self-esteem.
- *Unrealistic expectations of the infant's capabilities* – that she/he should sleep for several hours after each feed and especially during the night and that the infant should, in some way, demonstrate love for his/her mother (Pugh and De'Ath, 1992).
- *Maternal self-interest* – this is demonstrated when the mother indicates directly or indirectly that the newborn infant is not expected to (and will not be allowed to) alter the mother's prepregnancy lifestyle in anyway.
- *Prematurity in the infant* – may present problems in relation to parental interaction, especially when the infant requires to be cared for in a special unit, separated from his/her mother.

Bonding

This is considered to be the one-way affection felt by a mother for her infant soon after delivery (Klaus and Kennell, 1976). The bonding concept (Klaus *et al.*, 1972) affected midwifery practice worldwide by its suggestion that bonding was something which had to occur between a mother and her newborn infant soon after birth. Failure to facilitate this within a 'sensitive' period would or could result in impaired maternal–infant relationships, it was said.

Bowlby (1969) had previously described a similar 'critical period' as being important to the attachment mechanism for imprinting in birds. Lorenz (1970) studied greylag geese from the moment of hatching and found that there was a sensitive period when they, too, would 'fix' on a moving figure. Hess (1973) supports that this theory is relevant to the human infant, although Campbell and Taylor (1980) are critical of the concept. They question the enthusiasm for early maternal–infant contact, in the hope that long-term benefits will accrue for the children who experience it. It would be of interest to know how many of you, presently reading this textbook, have 'bonded' satisfactorily, yet were separated from your mothers and cared for in the ward nursery for days after your birth.

Other researchers (Lynch and Roberts, 1977) agree, nevertheless, that the concept of 'bonding failure' can only be known retrospectively, so mothers should be given the opportunity to 'begin to know' their infants as soon as possible. Any mother who, for some reason, believes that she has not bonded during the 'critical' period, should be reassured as above.

Attachment

The process of attachment has been defined as 'an enduring and unique emotional relationship between two people which is specific and endures through time' (Kennell *et al.*, 1975). There is no scientific foundation for the belief that the biological mother alone is uniquely capable of caring for her child (Sylva and Lunt, 1994); it is suggested that this loving relationship may be carried out or shared by one or several other adults, provided that they demonstrate sensitivity, stimulation, and responsiveness.

The needs of children, on the other hand, are defined by Kellmer-Pringle (1975) and can be applied universally in different cultures and social circumstances; these are:
- Basic physical care.
- Affection.
- Security.
- Stimulation of innate potential.
- Guidance and control.
- Responsibility.
- Independence.

All these needs are as relevant to the development of good attachments as they are to the child's physical and emotional development. The essential element in the total process, however, is the quality of care offered by the parenting figures (Aldgate, 1993).

Caregiver

The role of caregiver is considered complementary to attachment and implies that the person 'is available and responsive as and when wanted, and is able to intervene judiciously should the child being cared for be heading for trouble' (Bowlby, 1977).

Neglect

'Neglecting families can drift for years beyond the boundaries of "acceptable" parenting without a systematic assessment being made of the situation' (Department of Health, 1988). Neglect implies the failure of the parent or other identified caregiver to act properly in safeguarding the health, safety and well-being of the child. Physical neglect includes nutritional neglect, failure to provide medical care or failure to protect a child from physical and social danger (Kempe and Kempe, 1978).

Parenting – The Role of the Midwife

A mother takes on the long-term responsibility for caring and cherishing a newborn child. Maternity services should support the mother, her baby and her family during this journey with a view to their short-term safety but also their long-term well-being

(Lady Cumberledge, 1993.)

Midwives are reluctant to accept that they may have a vital role to play in the assessment of maternal caregiving at such an early period in a child's life, believing that this has nothing to do with midwifery. This appears to be incongruous for the following reasons:
- A midwife is responsible for the safe care of mothers and their infants postnatally – how is the parenting ability of the mother assessed at this time?
- A midwife is responsible for teaching and demonstrating essential parenting skills – how are the mother's specific needs known in the absence of objective assessment?
- A midwife is in a privileged position (unlike any other member of the multidisciplinary team) to observe and make objective assessment of maternal caregiving throughout a 24 period in the hospital.

It is suggested that midwives should not confuse the issue of caregiving with that of love and affection, although one may be dependent on the other. The caregiving abilities and attentions of a mother towards her full-term and healthy infant cannot afford to be postponed.

Midwives should ensure that their own values and prejudices do not detract from their professional objectivity in relation to parenting.

It is accepted that cultural variations in parenting patterns exist and midwives should become familiar with these differences, in particular as they relate to the families in their areas of practice. 'Good enough parenting' is an unfortunate expression which has crept into our professional vocabulary. What exactly does it mean and how do different people interpret this? Winnicott (1986) developed the theory in the belief that no-one had or has perfect parents.

The essential feature of the concept, however, is that there is a baseline for reasonable parenting behaviour which can be identified and includes:
- Consistency.
- Adequate stimulation.
- Appropriate affection.
- Pride in child's development and achievements.
- Expectation from child of behaviour appropriate to the age and development.

Parents, it is said, who fall below this baseline endanger their children's emotional health (Aldgate, 1993). Problems of behaviour, childhood neglect and deprivation, child abuse and psychiatric disorders, which account for a great proportion of childhood morbidity, are thought to be related to parenting problems (Liptak *et al.* 1983).

Incidents of child abuse and neglect are invariably recognized retrospectively and unfortunately some believe that this will always be so. Kempe and his colleagues, however, have drawn attention to the positive value of observations of mother–child relationships made by midwives, nurses and doctors during their work in delivery and postnatal care (Gray *et al.*, 1979). Ounsted *et al.* (1982) also acknowledged the contribution of midwives' intuitive feelings while working in postnatal wards in Oxford.

Unfortunately, intuitive feelings are difficult to 'pass on' educationally and because one cannot quantify subjective data, it is not surprising that this intuitive way of carrying out such an assessment is fraught with uncertainty. Midwives' worries were said to be sometimes very general and ill defined when referrals were made about maternal caregiving concerns

(Roberts and Ounsted, 1987). It is suggested that until assessment of maternal caregiving ability is carried out by midwives more objectively, instead of subjectively, progress cannot be made. The parenting skills taught and demonstrated by midwives cannot be followed-up regarding effectiveness if individual maternal needs are not ascertained initially by some form of objective assessment (see **Box 12.7**).

Midwives are placed in a most privileged position to engender enlightenment of the newly delivered mother and her family about the infant's abilities from the time of birth. All mothers, according to their individual requirements, should receive structured information about their infant's physical, mental, emotional and social needs in relation to his/her short-term as well as long-term development. The new mother must be afforded opportunity to witness her infant's capabilities and encouragement given to ask questions and discuss appropriate interaction with her infant. Following the reduction in maternal and infant mortality and infant morbidity, Lynch and Roberts (1982) and Roberts and Ounsted (1987) suggest that a further goal of perinatal medicine should be the reduction of infant morbidity resulting from poor parenting.

KEY CONCEPTS

- Rapid cardiovascular adaptation is essential for survival.
- Adaptation is prejudiced by fetal or perinatal hypoxia.
- Bradycardia means hypoxia.
- Ventilation and oxygen are the most important parts of resuscitation.
- Any Meconium should be cleared from the airway before first breaths.
- Failure to respond to resuscitation is more likely to be caused by an inadequate airway or disconnected oxygen than by other rare problems.
- Minute-for-minute neonatal resuscitation remains the single, most cost-effective health-care measure.
- A detailed examination of every newborn baby is essential to exclude congenital defects.
- The route of administration of vitamin K remains controversial. Routine use of vitamin K is recommended by the Royal College of Paediatricans and Child Health (RCPCH) (formerly British Paediatric Association).
- Mandatory screening tests are performed to exclude some serious conditions detectable in the newborn period.
- Midwives have a responsibility to promote good maternal–infant interaction especially eye to eye contact and handling.
- The midwives role in assessing the caregiving ability of the mother is fundamental to the teaching of parenting skills and the possible determination of children 'at risk'.

References

Adamson-Macedo EN, Attree JLA: TAC–TIC therapy: the importance of systematic stroking, *Br J Midwifery* 2(6):264, 1994.

Aldgate J: Attachment theory and its application to child care. Social work – an introduction. In Lishman J, editor: *Handbook of theory for practice teachers in social work*, London and Philadelphia, 1993, Jessica Kingsley.

Allen KD, Ridgway EJ, Parsons LA: Hexachlorophane powder and neonatal staphylococcal infection, *J Hosp Infect* 27(1):29, 1994.

Anderson GC: Skin to skin: kangaroo care in Western Europe, *Am J Nurs* 89(5):662, 1989.

Anderson GC, Marks EA, Wahlberg V: Kangaroo care for premature infants ... Colombia, *Am J Nurs* 86(7):807, 1986.

Arya R, Pethen T, Johanson RB *et al.*: Outcome of low risk pregnancies. *Arch Dis Child* 75(2):97–102, 1996.

Bain J: Umbilical cord care in pre-term babies, *Nurs Standard* 8(15):32, 1994.

Barr J: The umbilical cord: to treat or not to treat, *Midwives Chron* 107(1278):224, 1994.

Bowlby J: *Attachment and loss, Vol. 1. Attachment*, London, 1969, Hogarth Press.

Bowlby J: The making and breaking of affectional bonds, *Br J Psychiatry* 130(March):201, 1977.

Brazelton TB, Cramer G: *The earliest relationship: parents, infants and the drama of early attachment*, London, 1991, Karnac Books.

British Paediatric Association: *Vitamin K prophylaxis*, Report of an expert committee, London, 1991, BPA.

Bruner JS: *Child's talk*, Oxford, 1983, Oxford University Press.

Calman KC, Moores Y: *Prophylaxis against vitamin K deficiency bleeding in infants.*

Caldwell BM: Usefulness of the critical period hypothesis in the study of filiative behaviour, *Merrill-Palmer Q Behav Devel* 8(2):229, 1962.

Campbell SBG, Taylor PM: Bonding and theoretical issues. In Taylor PM, editor: *Parent–infant relationships*, New York, 1980, Grune & Stratton.

Carr J, *Helping your handicapped child*, London, 1995, Penguin.

Chadwick J: The rationale for routine vitamin K administration, *Modern Midwife* 3(6):20, 1993.

Chameides L, Hazinski MF, editors: *Textbook of pediatric advanced life support*, Dallas, 1994, American Heart Association.

Croucher C, Azzopardi D: Compliance with recommendations for giving vitamin K to newborn infants, *Br Med J* 308(6933):894, 1994.

Cohen J: Weighted KAPPA: nominal scale agreement with provision for scaled disagreement or partial credit, *Psychol Bull* 70(4):213, 1968.

Comfort A: Likelihood of human pheromones, *Nature* 230(April 16):432, 1971.

Dear PR, Newell SJ: *Neonatology for the MRCOG*, London, 1996, RCOG Press.

de Chateau P, Holmberg H, Winberg J: Left side preference holding and carrying newborn infants, *Acta Paediatr Scand* 67(2):169, 1978.

Department of Health: *Changing childbirth: Report of the Expert Maternity Group*, London, 1993, HMSO.

Department of Health: *Protecting children: a guide for social workers undertaking a comprehensive assessment*, London, 1988, HMSO (reprinted 1992).

Department of Health: *Dietary reference values for food energy and nutrients for the United Kingdom*, London, 1991, HMSO.

DHSS: *Working together: a guide to arrangements for inter-agency co-operation for the protection of children*, London, 1988, Department of Health & Social Security London and the Welsh Office.

Douglas J, Richman N: *My child won't sleep*, London, 1984, Penguin.

Ekelund H, Finnstrom O, Gunnarskog J, *et al.*: Administration of vitamin K to newborn infants and childhood cancer, *Br Med J* 307:89, 1993.

Fantz R: The origin of form perception, *Scientific Am* 204(I):66, 1961.

Farnald A. Four month old infants prefer to listen to motherese, *Infant Behav Devel* 8(2):181, 1985.

Field TM, *et al.*: *High-risk infants and children–adult and peer interactions*, Developmental Psychology Series, London, 1980, Academic Press.

Fitzmaurice M, Whiting M: Umbilical cord care in the premature infant, *Paediatr Nurs* 5(9):19, 1993.

Fleming PJ, Gilbert R, Azar Y, *et al.*: Interaction between bedding and sleeping position in the sudden infant syndrome; a population-based case control study. *BMJ* 301:85, 1990.

Foundation for the Study of Infant Deaths: *Factfile: Research background for the advice to reduce the risk of cot death*, 1993, FSID.

Fraiberg S: Blind infants and their mothers. In Lewis M, Rosenblum L, editors: *The effects of the infant on his caregiver*, New York, 1974, John Wiley.

Gairdner D, Pearson J: A growth chart for premature and other infants, *Arch Dis Child* 46:783, 1971.

Gandy G: Examination of the neonate. In Roberton N, editor: *Textbook of neonatology*, London, 1992, Churchill Livingstone.

Golding J, Greenwood R, Birmingham K, *et al.*: Childhood cancer, intramuscular vitamin K, and pethidine given during labour, *Br Med J* 305:341, 1992.

Gosden C: *Is my baby all right?*, 1994, Oxford University Press.

Gray JD, Cutler LA, Dean JG, *et al.*: Prediction and prevention of child abuse and neglect, *J Social Issues* 35(2):127, 1979.

Gray PH: Theory and evidence of imprinting in human infants, *J Psychol* 46:155, 1958.

Gray P: *Crying baby – how to cope*, London, 1987, Wisebuy.

Greenspan S I, Lieberman AF: Infants, mothers and their interaction: a quantitative clinical approach to developmental assessment. In Greenspan SI, Stanley I, and Pollock GH, editors: *The course of life, Vol. 1: Infancy*, Madison, 1989, International University Press.

Hamelin K, Ramachandran C: Kangaroo care, *Can Nurse* 89(6):15, 1993.

Harpin V, Rutter N: Making heel pricks less painful. *Arch Dis Child*, 58(3):226, 1984.

Hess EH: *Imprinting*, New York, 1973, Van Nostrand.

Hilgartner M: Vitamin K and the newborn, *New Engl J Med* 329(13):957, 1993.

Kellmer-Pringle ML: *The needs of children*, London, 1975, Hutchison.

Kelnar C, Harvey D, Simpson C: *The sick newborn baby*, London, 1995, Baillière Tindall.

Kempe RS, Kempe CH: The abusive parent. In Bruner J, Cole M, Lloyd B, editors: *Child abuse*, London, 1978, Fontana/Open Books Original.

Kennell JH, Trause MA, Klaus MH: Evidence for a sensitive period in the human mother. In Porter R, O'Connor M, editors: *CIBA Foundation Symposium 33: Parent–infant interaction*, Amsterdam, 1975, Elsevier.

Klaus MH, Kennell JE: *Maternal infant bonding*, St Louis, 1976, Mosby.

Klaus MH, Jerauld R, Kreger NC, *et al.*: Maternal attachment: Importance of the first post-partum days, *New Engl J Med* 286(9):460, 1972.

Klebanoff M, Read J, Mills J: The risk of childhood cancer after neonatal exposure to vitamin K, *New Engl J Med* 329(13):905, 1993.

Lawrence CW: Effect of two different methods of umbilical cord care on its separation time, *Midwives Chron and Nurs Notes* 95(1133):204, 1982.

Legault M, Goulet C: Comparison of kangaroo and traditional methods of removing preterm infants from incubators, *JOGNN* 24(6):501, 1995.

Levene M, Tudehope D: *Essentials of neonatal medicine*, Oxford, 1993, Blackwell Scientific Publications.

Lennart R, O'Alade M: Effect of delivery room routines on success of first breast-feed, *Lancet* 336(8723):1105, 1990.

Liptak GS, *et al.*: Enhancing infant development and parent–practitioner interaction with the Brazelton neonatal assessment scale, *Pediatrics* 72(1):71, 1983.

Lorenz K: *Studies in animal and human behaviour*, Vol. 1, Cambridge, Mass., 1970, Harvard University Press.

Ludington-Hoe SM, Thompson C, Swinth J, *et al.*: Kangaroo care: Research results, and practice implications and guidelines ... findings of two research projects, *Neonatal Network* 13(1):19, 1994.

Lynch MA, Roberts J: Predicting child abuse; signs of bonding failure in the maternity hospital, *Br Med J* 1(6061):624, 1977.

Lynch MA, Roberts J: *Consequences of child abuse*, London, 1982, Academic Press.

MacKeith N: Who should examine the normal neonate? *Nurs Times*, 91:14, 1995.

McCormack B: Hearing screening by health visitors: a critical appraisal of the distraction test, *Health Visitor* 56(December):449, 1983.

McFadyen A: *Special care babies and their developing relationships*, London, 1994, Routledge.

McFarlane A: Olfaction in the development of social preference in the human neonate. In Porter R, O'Connor M, editors: *CIBA Foundation Symposium 33: Parent–infant interaction*, Amsterdam, 1975, Elsevier.

McFarlane A: *The psychology of childbirth*, London, 1977, Fontana/Open Books.

Michaelides S: A deeper knowledge, *Nurs Times*, 91:35, 1995.

Morris D: *Babywatching*, London, 1991, Jonathan Cape.

Mugford M, Somchiwong M, Waterhouse I: Treatment of umbilical cords: A randomised trial to assess the effects of treament methods on the work of midwives. *Midwifery*, 2(4):177, 1986.

Ounsted C, Roberts JC, Gordon M, *et al.*: Fourth goal of perinatal medicine, *Br Med J* 284(6319):879, 1982.

Polichroniadis M: Parental understanding and attitudes towards neonatal biochemical screening, *Midwives Chron* 102(1213):42, 1989.

Prectl HFR: The directed head turning response and allied movements of the human baby, *Behaviour* 13(2):212, 1958.

Prince J, Adams ME: *Minds, mothers and midwives. The psychology of childbirth*, Edinburgh, 1978, Churchill Livingstone.

Pugh G, De'Ath E: The demands of parenting. In Rogers WS, Hevey D, Roche J, *et al.*, editors: *Child abuse and neglect*, London, 1992, BT Batsford in association with The Open University.

Reder P, Duncan S, Gray M, editors: *Beyond blame: Child abuse tragedies revisited*, London, 1993, Routledge.

Roberts J, Ounsted C: Further goals of perinatal medicine. In Harvey D, editor: *Parent–infant relationships*, London, 1987, John Wiley & Sons.

Roberton N: Care of the normal term baby. In Roberton N, editor: *Textbook of neonatology*, London, 1992, Churchill Livingstone.

Rosendahl K, Markestad T, Lie R: Ultrasound screening for developmental dysplasia of the hip in the neonate: the effect on treatment rate and prevalence of late cases, *Pediatrics* 94(1):47, 1994.

Royal College of Midwives: *Position paper 13. The midwife's role in the administration of vitamin K*, London, RCM.

Rutter M, Quinton D: Long term follow up of women institutionalized in childhood: factors promoting good functioning in adult life, *Br J Devel Psychol* 18(2):191, 1984.

Salariya E, Kowbus N: Variable umbilical cord care, *Midwifery* 4:70, 1988.

Salariya EM: A study of the smoking habits and attitudes of women in a maternity unit (Scottish), *Health Bull* 44(1):22, 1986.

Salariya EM: *Maternal care-giving: a follow-up study of children at four years of age*, 1987, Midwifery Department, Ninewells Hospital, Dundee.

Salariya EM: Parental–infant interaction. In Alexander J, Levy V, Roch S, editors: *Midwifery practice, postnatal care, a research-based approach*, London, 1990. Macmillan Education.

Salariya EM, Cater JI: Mother–child relationship, FIRST score, *J Adv Nurs* 9(6):589, 1984.

Salariya EM, Robertson CM: Relationships between baby feeding types and patterns, gut transit time of meconium and the incidence of neonatal jaundice. Midwifery, 9:235, 1993.

Salk L: Mother's heartbeat as an imprinting stimulus, Trans NY Acad Sci 24(7):753, 1962.

Salk L: Thoughts on the concept of imprinting and its place in early human development, *Can Psychiatr Assoc* 11(Suppl):295, 1966.

Sancho J, *et al.*: Epidemiological basis for screening hearing. In McCormack B, editor: *Paediatric audiology 0–5*, Basingstoke, 1988, Taylor & Francis.

Seymour J: Who checks out? *Health Professional Digest* 7:8, 1995.

Schaffer HR: *The growth of sociability*, Harmondsworth, 1971, Penguin Books.

Siddall R: Danger signals (supporting families; child protection), *Commun Care* 7th May:(1015), 1994.

Stern D: *The first relationship: mother and infant*, New York, 1977, Basic Books.

Swanwick T: Normal abnormalities, *Nursing* 3(39):15, 1989.

Sylva K, Lunt I: *Child development – a first course*, Oxford, 1994. Blackwell.

Tait M: Making and monitoring progress in the pre-school years, *J Br Assoc Teachers Deaf* 11(5):14, 1987.

Tizard B, Hughes M: *Young children learning – talking and thinking at home and at school*, London, 1984, Fontana.

Verber I, Pagan F: What cord care – if any? *Arch Dis Child* 68(5):594, 1993.

Vonkries R, Globel U, Hachmeister A: Vitamin K and childhood causes. *BMJ* 313(7051):199, 1996.

Walker N, Champion R: Neonatal dermatology. In Roberton N, editor. *Textbook of neonatology*, London, 1992, Churchill Livingstone.

Wasz-Hockert O, *et al.*: *The infant cry, a spectrographic and auditory analysis*, London, 1968, Spastics International Medical Publications/Heinemann.

Wigfield RE, Fleming PJ, Berry J, *et al.*: Can the fall in Avons' sudden infant death rate be explained by changes in sleeping position?. *BMJ* 304:282, 1992.

Winnicott DW: *The child, and the outside world*, London, 1957, Tavistock.

Winnicott DW: Face to face with children. In Batty D, editor: *Working with children*, London, 1986, British Agencies for Adoption and Fostering (BAAF).

Wolff PH: The natural history of crying and other vocalizations in early infancy. In Foss BM, editor: *Determinants of infant behaviour IV*, London, 1969, Methuen.

Further Reading

Adaptation: Fetus to Infant and Neonatal Resuscitation

Dear PR, Newell SJ: *Neonatology for the MRCOG*, London, 1996, RCOG Press.

A short textbook aimed at giving an introduction to the care of the neonatal medicine.

Drife J: Reducing risks in obstetrics. In Vincent C, editor: *Clinical risk management*, p. 129, London, 1995, BMJ Publishing Group.

An introduction to the problems of risk management.

Roberton NRC: Resuscitation of the newborn. In Roberton NRC, editor: *Textbook of neonatology*, 2nd edn, p. 173, Edinburgh, 1992, Churchill Livingstone.

One chapter in the best UK textbook of neonatal medicine.

Serwer GA: Postnatal circulatory adjustments. In Polin RA, Fox WW, editors: *Fetal and neonatal physiology*, p. 710, Philadelphia, 1992, WB Saunders.

Very detailed, excellent account of neonatal physiology.

Tyson JE: Immediate care of the newborn infant. In: Sinclair JC, Bracken MB, editors: *Effective care of the newborn infant*, p. 21, Oxford, 1992, Oxford University Press.

This book systematically reviews the data available from clinical trials. It is the starting point for evidence-based practice.

Care of the Newborn

These titles offer a wide range of information for midwives – anatomy and physiology of breastfeeding and lactation, positioning, infant nutrition, maintaining lactation when separated from the infant or returning to work, breastfeeding twins and other multiples, breast milk and HIV/AIDS.

See also Chapter 13 list.

Alexander J, Levy V, Roche S: *Postnatal care*, Basingstoke, 1992, MacMillan.

Chapters 5 and 6, care of the umbilical cord and transitional care.

Akre J, editor: Infant feeding – The physiological basis, *Bull World Health Organ* 67(Suppl), 1989.

Bryan E: *The nature and nurture of twins*, Ch 8, London, 1983, Baillière Tindall.

Huggins K: *The nursing mother's companion*, Massachusetts, 1990, The Harvard Common Press.

McHaffie H, Fowlie P: *Life, death and decisions*, 1996, Books of Midwives Press.

The book contains an account of a study carried out in a neonatal unit about difficult decisions being made about babies, the agonies, complexities and conflict.

National Breastfeeding Working Group: *Breast feeding – good practice guidance to the NHS*, London, 1995, Department of Health.

Renfrew MJ, Fisher MC, Arms S: *Best feeding – getting breast feeding right for you*. Berkeley, 1990, Celestial Arts.

Royal College of Midwives: *Successful breast feeding – a handbook for midwives*, 2nd edn, Edinburgh, 1991, Churchill Livingstone.

Smale M: *The National Childbirth Trust book of breast feeding*, London, 1992, Vermillion.

Health Education and Health Promotion

Gosden C: *VIs my baby alright*, Oxford University Press

Johnston P: *Villiamy's newborn child*, London, 1994, Churchill Livingstone.

Clear guide to the baby.

Robertson NRC: *Manual of normal neonatal care*, 2nd edition, 1991, Edward Arnold.

An invaluable summary of the clinical needs of babies.

Salisbury DM, Begg NT: *Immunisation against infectious disease*, London, 1996, HMSO.

The definitive guide to indications and contradindications to baby immunisation.

Maternal Reaction to the Newborn

Corby B: *Child abuse – towards a knowledge base*, Buckingham, 1994, Open University Press.

Manolson A: *It takes two to talk. A parent's guide to helping children communicate*, Toronto, 1992, A Hanen Centre Publication. (Copies supplied by: Winslow, Telford Road, Bicester Oxon OX6 OTS.)

McFadyen A: *Special care babies and their developing relationships*, London, 1994, Routledge.

Rogers WS, *et al.*: *Child abuse and neglect*, London, 1992, BT Batsford in association with The Open University.

Schaffer R: Love, hate and indifference. In Bruner J, Cole M, Lloyd B, editors: *Mothering: the developing child*, 4th impression, London, 1982, Fontana/Open Books Original.

Sylva K, Lunt I: *Child development – a first course*, Oxford, 1994, Blackwell.

Videocassettes and Booklets

Working Party of the British Paediatric Association, College of Anaesthetists, Royal College of Midwives, and Royal College of Obstetricians and Gynaecologists: *Resuscitation of the newborn (1): basic resuscitation. Resuscitation of the newborn (2): advanced resuscitation*, London, 1996, RCOG.

Supportive Organizations

CLAPA (Cleft Lip and Palate Association), 1 Eastwood Gardens, Kenton, Newcastle, NE3 3DQ.

Crysis (helpline), BM Crysis, London, WC1N 3XX. Telephone 0171 404 5011 (sleeping and crying problems).

Foundation for Study of Infant Deaths, 35 Belgrave Square, London, SW1X 8QB. Telephone 0171 235 0965. (Room thermometers are also available from this organization at a cost of £2.50).

Nippers (premature babies groups for parents and professionals), PO Box 1553, Wedmore, Somerset, BS28 4LZ. Telephone 01934 733123.

SANDS (Stillbirths and Neonatal Deaths), 28 Portland Place, London, WS1N 4DE. Telephone 0171 436 5881.

TAMBA (Twins and Multiple Births Association), PO Box 30, Little Sutton, South Wirrall, L66 1TH.

13 Knowledge and Skills Involved in Infant Feeding

LEARNING OUTCOMES

After studying this chapter you should be able to:

- Discuss the perspective that human milk has no equivalent substitute.
- Outline the sociological factors that contribute to a mother's decision to breastfeed.
- Consider the importance of professionals exploring their own attitudes in this area.
- Identify the main constituents of breast milk that contribute to the advantages of breastfeeding for the infant.
- Define the pathological conditions against which breast milk is active.
- Discuss the anatomy and physiology that underpin effective teaching of breastfeeding by the professionals.
- Discuss research which identifies the main reasons for giving up breastfeeding.
- Specify the professional approach that responds to this research and effectively supports a woman who wants to breastfeed. **(continued)**

continued

- Consider the role of the midwife and the knowledge needed to support a mother who chooses to bottle-feed.
- Identify the research that supports the Baby Friendly Initiative and be clear about the midwife's responsibilities.

Breastfeeding practices are bound up in the cultural attitudes within a country – professionals need to be very aware of their own cultural learning, which influences their views, as well as to be sensitive to the culture of the woman. One example is the non use of colostrum by some groups, which denies the baby the protection intended and leads to mixed feeding. Turner (1994) identified 'that the mothers were unaware of the disadvantages of mixed feeding, and of the benefits of exclusive breastfeeding.' 'Culture can be seen as an inherited "lens" through which individuals perceive and understand the world that they inhabit' (Helman, 1990). This lens can provide accurate and inaccurate information, but the need to follow the accepted group practice, when it relates to something as important as childbirth or childbearing, is very strong. Just as there is a rite of passage in adolescence from child to adult, the woman makes a further transition in experiencing birth. The challenge for the professional is to understand both her/his own and another's sociological and psychological perspectives, as well as to identify the important physiological facts that should inform her/his practice.

Cows Milk versus Breast Milk

A midwife might look through her 'cultural lenses' and consider whether there is an equivalent substitute for breast milk. Minchen (1987) challenges a positive answer and her article *Instant Formula : A Mass, Uncontrolled Trial in Perinatal Care* provides important information for professionals, concerning the detrimental effects of artifical feeding.

Baby Perspective

There is increased morbidity and mortality in formula-fed infants. Cunningham (Salisbury and Blackwell, 1981) published details of the hospitalization patterns of a homogeneous middle class white US population and concluded that:

I would expect 77 admissions for illness during the first 4 months of 1000 bottle-fed infants. The comparable figure for breastfed infants is 5 hospital admissions.

There are other proved benefits of breastfeeding for babies. Preterm infants are known to be protected from necrotizing enterocolitis (Lucas and Cole, 1990). Breastfed babies are found to be less likely to be victims of cot death or sudden infant death syndrome (SIDS; Ford *et al.* 1993).

Work into the protective effects of breastfeeding against infection identified specific benefits. For example, 'Breastfeeding during the first 13 weeks of life confers protection against gastrointestinal illness that persists beyond the period of breastfeeding itself' (Howie *et al.* 1990). Babies who were breastfed for less than 13 weeks had rates of gastrointestinal illness similar to those of artificially fed infants in the remainder of their first year of life. There is evidence that total breastfeeding protects from both acute and recurrent otitis media (Duncan *et al.* 1993; Aniasson *et al.* 1994). Babies that are breastfed have fewer urinary tract and respiratory infections (Marild *et al.* 1990; Victora *et al.* 1989). The protective element continues to be explored successfully and other conditions are being found to be associated with bottle-feeding, such as insulin-dependent diabetes (Karjalainen *et al.* 1992); it is important for professionals to appreciate these. Recent work (Lanting *et al.* 1994) suggests a beneficial effect of breastfeeding on postnatal neurological development. The intellectual development of breastfed children is slightly but significantly better than that of bottle-fed children (Rojan and Gladen, 1993). Such evidence clearly states the benefits to the baby of breastfeeding.

Mother Perspective

For the mothers there is a known contraceptive effect (Howie, 1985) and there is evidence of a 'trend towards a reduced risk of breast cancer with increasing duration of breastfeeding' (Newcomb *et al.* 1994).

Midwifery Perspective

As early as 1987, Maureen Minchen looked at the claims of nutritional adequacy and equivalence for infant formula and argued that 'infant formula is unable to be humanized and is intrinsically hazardous.' The starting point for the midwife is to explore how her own attitudes have been formed, and to ask why she has come to trust a breast-milk substitute that is so inferior as to be harmful. Deficits in her knowledge may be made good by reading the articles of Minchen (1987) and Walker (1993). These articles will shock the professional who has been duped into believing cow's milk can be satisfactorily used to substitute breast milk. A baby can be intolerant of cow's milk, with a variety of reactions. Occasionally cow's milk drunk by the mother can affect the baby. Removing cow's milk products from the diet of breastfeeding women whose babies were suffering from colic was found to ease the problem in about one-third of the babies (Jakobsson and Lindberg, 1983). Work related to sensitization guides midwives not to give a single bottle of milk to an otherwise breastfeeding baby as this could sensitize the baby with serious consequences when the baby comes into contact with cow's milk later (Host, 1991).

An attitude that undermines breastfeeding could also reduce the ability to learn skills that promote breastfeeding. If there is deemed to be an equivalent alternative it is less important to succeed, and therefore easier for both the professional and the woman to give up at the first difficulty. It is essential to consider the constituents of breast milk and how they contribute to a food that actively protects the baby from infection and ensures absorption and utilization of food for energy and growth. The confidence of the woman planning to breastfeed is increased by a professional who can enthusiastically describe the anti-infection properties of breast milk and appreciate the nutritional value. It is wise for a professional to outline the benefits to the woman of breastfeeding, such as reduced risk of breast and ovarian cancer (Newcomb *et al.* 1994; Rosenblatt *et al.* 1993). Equally, it is important to understand the sociological factors that contribute to the responses of the woman and the skills of the professional.

Sociological Factors

The midwife helping a woman to feed does so within a sociological context. Her own perspective both personal and professional meets that of a woman.

Making the Choice to Breastfeed

Attitudes to feeding are formed within the family, which exists within a culture, as already discussed. Gregg (1989) explored attitudes of teenagers (sample 400) to breastfeeding in Liverpool. At the time of her research only 30–35% of babies were breastfed in Liverpool. Of these teenagers, only 70 (18% of the

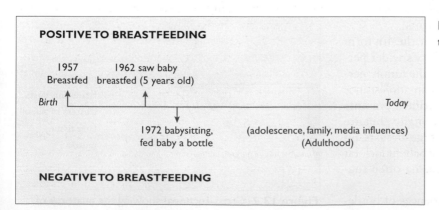

Figure 13.1 Development of attitude to breastfeeding.

sample) had been breastfed. Three-quarters thought breastfeeding was healthier and natural, but 32 (8%) thought that it was rude. Preferences about feeding were clearly formed in the teenage group.

One way for a midwife to consider the influence of her biography is to explore it through an exercise (**Figure 13.1**). First draw a line on a blank piece of paper – this is your 'lifeline'. Identify your earliest memories of feeding (see the example given). If you judge the memories to be positive to breastfeeding, place a mark and a year above the line; if negative, place it below the line. Become aware of adolescence and your peer group's response. Where were you in breast growth? Who supported or encouraged you as you grew into a woman? What were your family or house rules about nakedness? Was there a change when you reached adolescence? Consider the media influences. Each of these factors has contributed to the attitude you hold towards breastfeeding, alongside the professional knowledge you have gained. Women you care for come with similar influences and experiences that mould them. The decision as to how to feed may even be made as a child playing 'mothers and fathers' – some children lift their dresses to feed their dolls, others give a bottle! What did you do? What do your children do? This exercise will help you understand how you have formed your attitude to feeding and whether the professional knowledge has reinforced or suggested an alternative position to your family norm.

The exercise asks for a micro view of the formation of attitudes, taking the family unit, the school, peer group pressure and then the media and assessing how these impinge on the individual. This needs to be placed in the context of the geographical area in which the person grows up. A child in Scotland is considerably less likely to see a woman breastfeeding than one who grows up in the London area. Schools vary in their treatment of health subjects and family caring skills. Often these subjects are addressed in classes for the less able, for example 'home economics', and ignored for the brighter students.

Embarrassment is seemingly fixed by the 4th form (Gregg, 1989). This is related to society's wider perception of breastfeeding, as well as to the family perspective and the natural peer response in adolescence (14–15 year olds). The media sometimes presents breast images that do not relate to normality, but are surgically induced. For example, large breasts on skinny models. Athletes who are extremely fit lack fat tissue in their breasts, whereas the media often suggests the opposite.

A professional who has had experiences of bottle-feeding, both personally and professionally, may rein-force a negative attitude and indicate a lack of belief in breastfeeding. A negative attitude is powerful if developed through her own bad experience of feeding. Examples are to collude with a woman to give up when with greater skill the woman could succeed. Insufficient skill causes the midwife to blame the baby or mother – of the baby, 'He is very sleepy, he doesn't open his mouth,' or of the mother, 'She gets very nervous,' 'She hasn't got any milk,' 'She has flat nipples.' These excuses commonly mask a lack of skill. When the midwife can say 'I lack the skill to help this woman; who can I ask or how can I analyse the problem to solve it more effectively?', then she is more likely to succeed.

The undermining influences of a new grandmother can be subtle. They have clear evidence of their success, having produced either the new mother or father, and make such comments as 'You're not feeding again are you? You were never like that as a baby!' If a mother or mother-in-law has bottle-fed, she may want the daughter to mother in the same way, as it reinforces the rightness of the choice she made. Sometimes if a mother-in-law breast-fed for a short time (e.g. 3 months) she encourages the daughter-in-law to give up at this time also. Understanding of the lifeline for oneself increases awareness of others attitiudes and views. There are other factors that have also been shown to affect the duration of breastfeeding; for example, a need to return to work and lack of support from the partner (Jones *et al.* 1986; Carlson Gielen 1991).

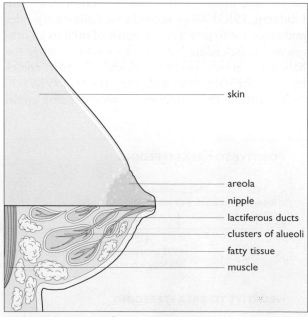

Figure 13.2 Cross-sectional showing the anatomy of the breast and the external appearance.

Biological Basis of Breastfeeding

Figure 13.2 shows the breast, which is one of two hemispherical swellings situated on the anterior chest wall between the 2nd and 6th ribs. It contains glandular, fibrous and fat tissue. Each breast is divided into segments by fibrous tissue. The glandular tissue consists of small lobes and lobules, which together are called alveoli. These are lined with the acini cells responsible for secreting the milk. Small tubules collect milk from the acini cells. These tubules widen and form lactiferous ducts which stretch to hold milk. They are made of smooth muscle that has the capacity to contract under the influence of the hormone oxytocin, which ejects the milk out of the breast. Surrounding the alveoli are myoepithelial or basket cells (**Figure 13.3**), which also form part of the duct and contract in response to oxytocin released from the pituitary gland, squeezing the milk into the ductules. The flow of milk in response to the oxytocin is called the milk ejection reflex.

Breasts are designed both to produce milk and to cause it to flow towards the baby when needed. Scientists first identified an autocrine inhibitor (**Figure 13.4**) in the milk of goats, and there is evidence that a similar protein is present in human milk, FIL (feedback inhibitor of lactation). It builds up when no milk is flowing and when the milk flows it is removed so that more milk is produced (Prentice *et al.* 1989).

Milk Production

Inhibition to the production of milk is removed after delivery and expulsion of the placenta, when the progesterone levels decline rapidly. The stimulus to both the production and flow of milk is the baby suckling. As a result of both touch and sucking, nerve messages reach the posterior pituitary gland by the hypothalamus, and oxytocin is produced. The oxytocin travels in the blood stream to the myoepithelial cells and causes them to contract. The milk is squeezed into the tubules and flows along the lactiferous ducts. To begin with, this reflex is unconditioned. Sight, sound and smell in association with sucking leads to the physiological response of milk let-down. Anxiety and stress caused by a lack of confidence can inhibit the reflex in a temporary and minor way (Akre, 1989). Later, the unconditioned reflex of milk flow being produced by sucking changes to a conditioned reflex, so that thinking about the baby can also start the milk flow. For example, when an older child is ill and refuses to drink, a mother who has stopped feeding can experience her breasts filling and milk moving as her desire for her child to drink becomes the stimulus (Akre, 1989). Sucking also triggers the message to the anterior pituitary to release prolactin. This is well described in Howie (1985) who states that 'prolactin is released in episodic fashion and ... prolactin levels reach a peak within 30–45 minutes of the start of the feed ...'. Glasier *et al.* (1984) compared the prolactin responses to suckling during day-time and night-time feeds in the same people on the same day. The prolactin response during the day was less than that at night. Such information is relevant for the mother, as it demonstrates the importance of late evening and night-time feeds.

Constituents of Breast Milk

The World Health Organization (WHO) Bulletin De L'Organisation Mondiale de la Sante (OMS) (Akre, 1989) covers breast milk composition in detail on

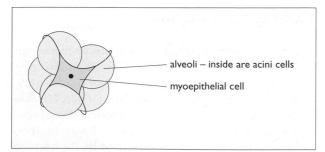

Figure 13.3 Myoepithelial or basket cells surround the clusters of alveoli, which are lined with acini cells.

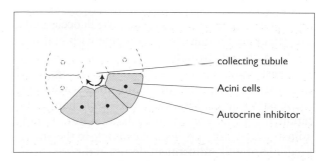

Figure 13.4 Autocrine inhibitor.

pages 25–31, including immunological qualities; also Greasley (1986) has written a seminal article which identifies the constituents. Thus, here only the most important aspects are covered. Colostrum is the early milk available to the baby and can satisfy all the nutritional needs, as well as protect with immunoglobulins and live cells that ingest bacteria. Colostrum, like the transitional or mature milk, is an excellent cleanser for the breast and also promotes healing because of its anti-infection qualities. Washing before feeding and the use of creams are not indicated because of the antibacterial properties of milk and the secretion from Montgomery's tubercles (Akre, 1989).

Constituents that contribute to the advantages of breastfeeding in infants

Colostrum or early milk, which changes to mature milk between 3 and 14 days after birth (Akre, 1989) is designed so that it does not put any strain on immature infant kidneys. The immunoglobulins (Ig) contribute by lining the gut and protecting it from bacterial and viral infection. Growth factors stimulate the infant's own immune system. Howie (1985) describes the ability of breast milk to secrete IgA in response to a pathogen that infects the mother. The pathogen enters the mother and activates B cells in Peyer's patches (gut-associated lymphoid tissue). Cells with immune activity are produced and these migrate to the breast, where IgA is secreted with a specific ability to fight the pathogen. As the milk flows the lining of the baby's gut is thus insulated from the pathogen. IgA created by the mother protects the baby from endemic illnesses of the mother's living area. A baby born at home thus has built-in defences in the mother's milk to any recent or current pathogens. This interaction with the mother's immune system appears to protect across a range of diseases and is a key advantage to the breastfed infant. In hospital, the baby is more vulnerable, as there are more pathogens, though still vastly advantaged when breastfed.

Lactoferrin in breast milk binds iron, which is a vital ingredient for the multiplication of *Escherichia coli*, for example. Colonies of lactobacilli occur in the breastfeeding mother; these compete with and thus inhibit pathogen growth.

Breast milk does not only adjust in terms of response to infection. It alters constituents according to the baby's needs. Milk for a 4-week-old baby is different from that for an older baby – human milk adjusts as the baby grows. An example in the animal kingdom of milk adjustment occurs in the kangaroo, which feeds a tiny infant from one nipple and a mature joey from another with milks designed to meet their differing needs.

Proteins

Proteins in breast milk achieve levels more than adequate for optimal growth, while providing an appropriate low-solute load for the infant's immature kidneys (Akre, 1989).

The whey:casein ratio of human milk is 80:20, which produces a softer gastric curd that reduces the stomach emptying time and helps digestion. The ratio in cow's milk is 20:80 and substitutes vary from 18:82 to 60:40 (Akre, 1989). These ratios provide a very different gastric emptying and digestive process to that of human milk.

There are many substances in breast milk that are not fully understood. For example, the amino acid taurine, which is now considered essential for human brain development and fat absorption, has only been added to artificial milk since 1984. It is not present in cow's milk (as calves have the ability to synthesize this themselves).

Fats

Just as protein substances in breast milk can aid the absorption of fat, fats themselves have a range of function in the body and are thought to be significant in the quality of the myelin laid down. It has been noted that multiple sclerosis is rare in countries where breastfeeding is common (Lawrence, 1989). The function of high levels of cholesterol in breast milk is not fully understood, but it is thought these early levels may affect the body's handling of the substance later (Akre, 1989; Hamosh, 1988). It has been suggested that dietary factors in infancy are involved in the later development of cardiovascular disease (Akre, 1989). This continues to be researched and there is increasing evidence that breastfeeding affects long-term health.

Carbohydrates – lactose

The development of the central nervous system is part of the function of lactose in breast milk; it also provides about 40% of the infant's energy needs (Akre, 1989). Lactose helps the growth of *Lactobacillus bifidus*, colonies of which (as mentioned above) contribute to inhibition of pathogenic bacteria. This occurs because the medium produced by the bacteria is hostile to the growth of other, pathogenic bacteria.

An excess intake of lactose is sometimes suspected in a breastfed infant who is irritable, unsettled and has frequent loose stools. The first response is to encourage the mother to allow the baby to finish the first breast first, thus gaining the fat in the hind milk which will satisfy, rather than giving a higher lactose intake by changing breasts early in a feed. Feeding in this way enables the baby to take a higher calorie feed in a smaller volume (Woolridge and Fisher, 1988). The baby often returns to feeding from both breasts with no return of loose stools.

Vitamins

Breast milk provides sufficient vitamins for the baby, though levels vary according to maternal diet. It is vital to give breastfed infants colostrum and later hind milk to ensure that soluble vitamins are received by the baby. Sunshine exposure of 30 minutes per week to the head and hands produces sufficient vitamin D (Specker, 1988).

Minerals

The iron in breast milk is bound to a protein that is unbound in the presence of appropriate levels of zinc and copper and the correct pH in the gut. This means that iron is absorbed very efficiently and there is no free iron available to feed pathogens such as *E. coli*. The converse is true with artificial milk, in which the iron is present as an inorganic salt and so available for pathogens. It is also poorly absorbed in this form. Zinc is another mineral associated with cellular immunity which again is present in a 'baby-gut friendly' form in breast milk so it can be fully absorbed. Even enzymes present in breast milk have their part to play as anti-infection agents – lysosyme, for example, is bacteriolytic against Gram-positive bacteria.

The complexity of breast milk can be compared to that of blood. It probably has a similar importance as a body fluid to the baby it is designed to nourish. Its anti-infection properties are the key attributes which pervade all constituents and cannot be replicated.

Tables in the WHO Bulletin (Akre, 1989) show the factors that are active against specific bacteria and viruses and make essential reading for the midwife. Breast milk, as well as being active against bacteria and viruses, also protects against some parasitic organisms; this is particularly relevant in Third World countries.

No studies have examined the growth patterns of breastfed compared with formula-fed twins (Bryan, 1983), but it is likely that the advantages of breast-feeding may be even greater for twins, especially if they have been born prematurely. Mothers should be reassured that the supply of breast milk will equal demand and that both babies will receive adequate nourishment. It is possible to breastfeed twins at the same time, but mothers will require support to help them adopt a feeding position they are comfortable with and encouragement to continue to exclusively breastfeed.

It is important for a midwife to consider how the benefits of breastfeeding in dietary and anti-infection terms can be incorporated into a discussion of choice of feeding with a mother, either prenatally or postnatally. Different cultures require different emphasis and thinking about this in advance helps a midwife be responsive (Schott and Henley, 1996).

Research into Women who give up Feeding

The key to enabling a woman to successfully breastfeed is to identify the reasons women give for stopping feeding and target these through education and support. The reasons given over the period 1980–1990 have been carefully researched by the Social Survey Division of Office of Population Censuses and Surveys on behalf of the Departments of Health or equivalent for England, Scotland and Ireland. Their findings provide a feast of information to inform the midwife (White *et al.* 1992). This report is published every 5 years with a 2-year delay.

The reasons given by women for giving up feeding have remained the same since the first infant feeding report. They vary according to the length of time for which the mother breastfed. For example, for those who breastfed for from 1 week to 4 months, more than half gave insufficient milk as their reason for stopping; 47% of mothers stopping at days 5 and 6 also gave this reason. Other reasons in order of frequency include painful and engorged breasts, baby wouldn't suck, breastfeeding took too long or was tiring.

Mothers reported that they had breastfed long enough or for as long as intended after 5 (9%) and 4 months (42%) (White *et al.* 1992). The implications for midwives are clear. The goal is to educate and support women so that they stop breastfeeding only at the point they wish, and avoid all the factors cited for discontinuing. Ideally, the latter two percentages should rise and all others fall.

Successful Breastfeeding

The function of the midwife is not only to provide the relevant knowledge for the mother, but also to identify the skills she needs and specifically enhance her confidence and autonomy. Understanding correct attachment and being able to teach it to the mother is essential.

To teach the woman, the midwife requires knowledge and understanding of the physiological processes connected with breastfeeding. This knowledge then needs to be applied so that the mother can understand what is happening.

Development of Sucking

Various anatomical areas are involved in sucking and swallowing. The lips act as an entrance to the oral cavity (which contains the gums, tongue and hard and soft palates). The pharynx contains the cricopharyngeal sphincter that leads to the epiglottis (protecting the trachea) and the oesophagus.

There are four types of reflex involved in feeding:
- The gag reflex is developed by 12 weeks' gestation and is demonstrated by fetal sucking movements seen on ultrasound scan (Carlson, 1994). It is present throughout life.
- The rooting reflex develops around 32–34 weeks' gestation and continues maturing until the baby is about 1 month post-term.
- The suck reflex also develops around 32–34 weeks' gestation (Carlson, 1994).
- The bite reflex develops much later, around 6 months of age (post-term).

The baby's tongue creates a vacuum around the breast and the gums so that a negative pressure helps to ease milk into the baby's mouth. The term baby is able to thrust his/her tongue forwards and backwards in movement against the palate, thus directing the milk down to the pharynx and oesophagus. This is clearly explained and illustrated in Woolridge's (1986) seminal paper called the 'anatomy of infant sucking.' Understanding the mechanism enables the midwife to observe correct attachment and advise a woman.

Attachment

The skill required of the midwife is to be able to teach the mother the practice of attaching the baby so that she can do it for herself. Ideally the midwife does this antenatally so that postnatally the mother is confident and can help herself effectively. *Attaching the baby for the mother* undermines the woman's confi-

dence, reduces the time she has to learn the skill for herself, decreases her autonomy and increases her dependence on the midwife. 'Hands-on' attachment of the baby by the midwife should be avoided unless there are problems; even then the amount of 'hands-on' intervention is carefully judged according to the complexity of the problem. At all times the goal of the mother achieving correct attachment unaided is integral to the midwife's intervention. The detail of this is explained later.

The main reasons given by women for stopping feeding can be avoided for the majority of mothers if the midwife transfers the skill to the mother of how to correctly attach her baby, how to recognize correct attachment and what to do if the baby is not correctly attached. Within this transfer of skill the midwife also needs to build the woman's confidence in herself as a mother and in the ability of her body to nourish her baby. None of these things can be achieved by a midwife who lacks the skill and/or holds a negative attitude to breastfeeding. To build self-confidence and self-esteem within her professional relationship requires those attributes in the midwife. Often neither breastfeeding skills nor personal development are considered essential in educating a midwife, so students limp from role model to role model, observing breastfeeding support and achieving varying levels of success in this area.

A Methodical Approach to Transferring the Skill of Attachment to the Mother (Hands Off)

This part of the Chapter is designed to help the midwife develop the skill of helping a mother to breastfeed effectively. The following list is taken from Jamieson (1995):
- Greeting and introduction.
- Listening to enable reflection on needs.
- Listening and encouraging the expression of problems and queries.
- Describing the support offered and the potential skill transfer.
- Teaching the specific skill methodically and at an appropriate pace.
- Using language and demonstration effectively.
- Confirming understanding.
- Reinforcing the skill with repetition.
- Encouraging future step-by-step autonomous use.
- Stating clear rationale for each step described.
- Giving research-based, accurate information.
- Giving consistent, coherent, non-judgemental responses that are senisitive to both the mother and the baby's individual needs and reactions.

Skill Transfer – 10 Steps to Describe the Position and Movements Made by a Midwife to Effectively Teach a Woman Baby Attachment

A midwife can show a mother using a doll (a soft toy from the cot, a hair brush sponge bag or small rolled sheet can be use to represent the baby, but it is easier to use a doll). If a midwife practices the following words and shows on herself using a doll she can explore the reality of the skill transfer for herself. The italics below indicate the words to use. Using the same words consistently helps the mother when she is practising alone and ensures the professional covers each step.

Step 1. *Hold the baby horizontal at the level of the breast facing inwards.*

Sometimes people use the words 'chest to chest'. The baby needs to be level with the breast, which will vary mother to mother. Showing on yourself without touching the mother means that you are identifying as a woman with breasts and not invading her personal space by touching her. It is an important part of transferring the skill. The hand used is the one opposite to the breast on which you wish to feed the baby (**Figure 13.5**).

Step 2. *Support your baby's head by making a shelf or platform with your hand under the ear.*

The wrist of the hand comes roughly to the neck of the baby, which means that the baby resting on the hand has freedom to extend its head (**Figure 13.6**). It is not correct to force the baby with pressure from behind its head, as such an approach creates problems for the baby and later for the mother. If you imagine you are just about to take your first spoonful of breakfast cereal when someone forces your face downwards into the bowl you will understand how forcing the baby will cause a reaction.

Step 3. *Make your breast a shape to fit your baby's open mouth.*

To do this use the hand on the same side as the breast. Make a 'V' using your thumb and forefinger. The shape is up and down to accommodate a gaping baby's mouth who is lying on his/her side (**Figure 13.7**). The breast is not lifted but held at the level it naturally

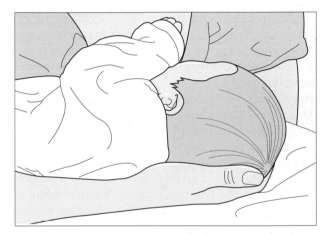

Figure 13.6 Baby attachment, Step 2. Support your baby's head by making a shzelf or platform with your hand under the ear.

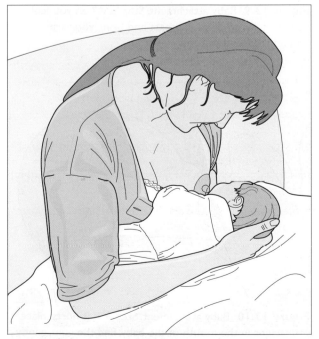

Figure 13.5 Baby attachment, Step 1. Hold the baby horizontal at the level of the breast facing inwards.

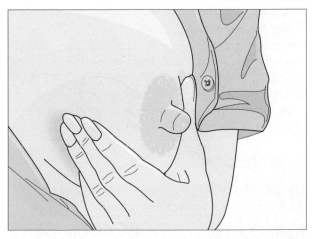

Figure 13.7 Baby attachment, Step 3. Make your breast a shape to fit your baby's open mouth.

drops to, which again varies from mother to mother. If a mother inadvertently lifts the breast , when she removes her hand the breast will drop and the baby comes off, so it is important to show her this detail.

Step 4. *Aim the nostrils at the nipple tip.*

This ensures that the most important part of the breast, the part which approximates to the bottom jaw of the baby, is well over the bottom jaw; it is the most important piece of information that is transferred to the mother and enables her to feed without pain. Discomfort occurs when the baby tries to drag the nipple and breast into the right position, sometimes repeatedly pressing on the side of the nipple and causing a burn-type mark which, without correction, develops into a crack. Alternatively, the sensitive nipple tip is repeatedly pressed against the hard palate by the tongue because insufficient breast is taken into the mouth of the baby to reach the soft palate. This results in blisters on the tip, quickly followed by cracks in the tip. Aiming the nostrils to the nipple focuses on the part of the breast that must be over the bottom jaw of the baby and helps the correct attachment (**Figure 13.8**).

Step 5. *Wait for the baby to open his/her mouth wide.* This part requires patience. It helps to explain that both are learning the skill, so the baby needs to understand where he/she is and what to do. Patience results in a baby feeling unhurried and able to learn how to fix as he/she is held lovingly in an optimal position. Speaking to the baby and telling him/her what is needed is often effective. The baby understands more than one would expect. Touching the baby's lips with the nipple lightly may encourage the baby to gape.

If a midwife considers the **conditions** necessary for learning a new skill, particularly the **environment** and the **attitude** of the support person that will enhance learning, she can then explore how this could be provided for a mother and help her in turn provide it for her baby.

Step 6. *Bring the baby to the breast.*

This prevents bending over the baby and the subsequent backache that may occur.

Step 7. *Look for signs of correct attachment.*

- *The cardinal sign has to be there is no pain.* Midwives discuss endlessly their experience of women who have pain in feeding. Sadly, their lack of skill and the inadequate support given is revealed in the position they take over this issue. Some seem not to have helped a woman effectively and some have suffered themselves, thus

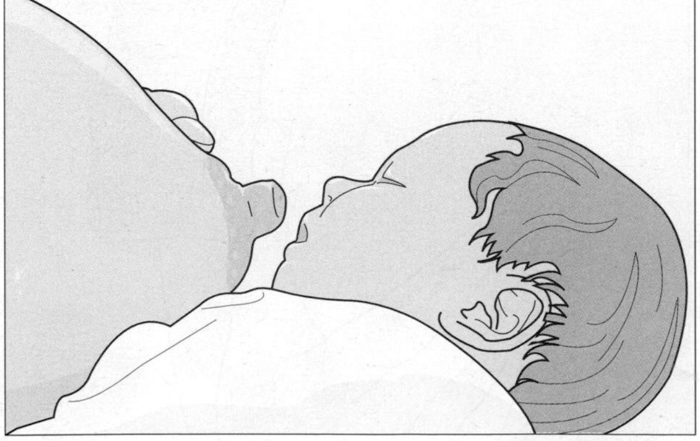

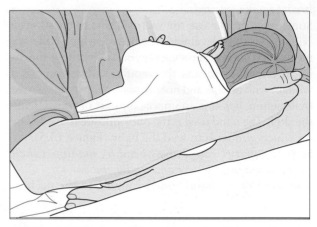

Figure 13.9 Baby attachment, Step 8. When you feel confident, let go of your breast and bring your arm around cradling the baby.

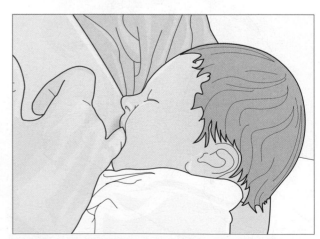

Figure 13.10 Baby attachment, Step 9. If it hurts, place your finger in the mouth of the baby, find the gum, gently press down and ease the baby away.

Figure 13.8 Baby attachment, Step 4. Aim the nostrils at the nipple tip.

confirming their belief. The amount of breast to get into the mouth varies, but pain-free feeding can be achieved and is the aim. Different sensations can accompany 'let down', such as tingling; women often describe these sensations, which quickly disappear. Understanding the affect of oxytocin on the myoepithelium and the uterine muscle is important.

- *A second sign is to look to see if the chin is pressed against the breast. There should be no shadow or daylight between the chin and the breast.* This sign means the baby has slightly extended his/her head to get on and the most important part of the breast is well over the bottom jaw of the baby.
- *A third sign is a small movement of the muscle under the skin in front of the ear, which indicates swallowing.* The mother can find this in front of her own ear with her finger tips and swallow.
- *A fourth sign is rhythmic sucking with pauses',* which indicates to the mother that the baby needs

to pause and then continue, just as we do when we eat a meal. The milk flows to the baby because of the action of oxytocin and if the flow could be seen it would have a rhythm. Sometimes when a baby comes off the breast, milk spurts from the breast in an arc and then a second arc, etc., which demonstrates the flowing pattern.

Step 8. *When you feel confident let go of your breast and bring your arm around cradling the baby.*
For some women this (**Figure 13.9**) will happen very quickly, for others it will take longer –the mother decides.

The next step is to teach what to do if attachment hurts or gives pain.

Step 9. *Place your finger in the mouth of the baby, find the gum, gently press down and when the mouth is open ease the baby away.* (**Figure 13.10**)
This approach prevents further traumatizing of the breast by the baby trying to keep hold of the breast as she/he is eased away. Just breaking the suction is not enough.

Step 10. *Speak to the baby to explain what is happening and start again.*
This encourages communication with the baby and may reduce frustration for the baby (**Figure 13.10**).

By following these steps and teaching the mother by demonstrating on yourself, she is learning how to do it for herself. You need to practise the skill and become confident using the words, so that you are consistent and the most important aspects connected with success are always shared with the woman.

Figure 13.11 shows an older baby feeding and **Figure 13.12** the correctly fixed older baby.

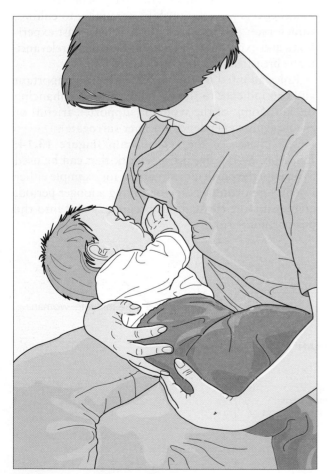

Figure 13.11 The older baby feeding.

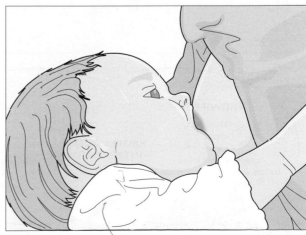

Figure 13.12 A correctly fixed older baby.

Answering Mothers' Questions on Food and Drink

Two areas to teach accurately are to guide the mother to drink according to her thirst. Her body will indicate her needs. Often women worry about their diet and its affect on the baby. To eat the diet she is accustomed to is correct. It is wise to observe the baby as occasionally foods do seem to cause some discomfort or loose stools. A mother is best placed to know. Indian babies quickly adjust to their mother's diet, which is sometimes spicy. The wisest course of action is to eat normally and observe the baby's response and not to avoid foods in anticipation of problems.

Embarrassment

Discussing with a mother her plan of where and when to feed can be helpful. A mother might know whether she would prefer to feed privately when visiting her parents or in-laws. She needs to follow whatever gives her the most comfortable feeling. Sometimes some friends have less experience and maturity than others, so she might be happy to feed in front of some and not others. Tiny anxieties about such problems can be solved early and so not develop; unresolved they can reduce confidence in the woman. It is possible for a mother to feed without anyone realizing, especially when the baby feeds easily and clothing is worn to fall loosely close to the baby. Facilities in shops and restaurants still reflect that breastfeeding is not yet the norm, but improvements are taking place. Knowing the facilities in your local area of practice is useful to women, as well as explaining how she can feed discreetly.

Effective breastfeeding support can be enhanced by using the Peplau model. The model helps the midwife explore her own attitudes within the giving of care. This is fully written up in Jamieson (1995) 'Educating for successful breastfeeding,' and provides a helpful addition to increase awareness in the midwife and enhance her skill.

Outline of a Modified Peplau Model to Help Breastfeeding Support

Peplau is a psychodynamic model which can be used to focus on the interpersonal interaction and relationship between a midwife, the mother and her family (**Figure 13.13**). The midwife is encouraged to explore her own attitudes, consider potential differences between herself and the woman, assess her own biography, responses and skills and thus relate to the woman and family more effectively. The areas the model covers are relationships pertaining to culture, values, race, preconceived ideas, beliefs, past experiences and expectations. Each of these has a relevance in the breastfeeding support relationship.

Roles adopted by the midwife are also important and can indicate to the midwife if she is enhancing the autonomy of the woman (supporter, friend) or encouraging dependency (mother surrogate).

The phases of the relationship (**Figure 13.14**; Jamieson, 1995) give a framework that can be used to analyse the particular situation, for example either briefly supporting feeding or, taking a longer period, giving support throughout pregnancy and into the postpartum period.

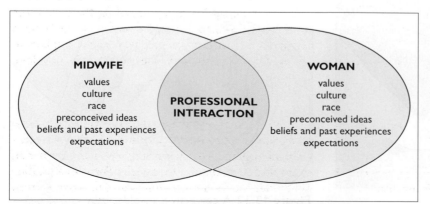

Figure 13.13 The midwife–woman relationship.

Each phase incorporates the awareness, previously stated, of attitudes and roles. Orientation is the meeting as strangers and sets the scene for future encounters. With continuity of care this has an initial importance and is then rarely used. Identification is the listening and encouraging phase: it involves clarification, comfort, consideration of goals and identification of needs and resources. Exploitation occurs as the trust within the relationship deepens and together the midwife and mother utilise the resources to meet specific needs. Advocacy will emerge within exploitation when needed. Finally, resolution is the exit from the relationship and this stage should be in the midwife's mind during all phases of the relationship, with the ultimate aim of creating autonomy for the woman. Effective resolution achieves both professional and maternal satisfaction. The phases are not linear but are utilised according to need. Reviewing goals often involves a return to the identification phase, even just before resolution.

Use of the Peplau model can enhance a midwife's ability to communicate within the midwife–mother relationship and can provide a means of reflection so that future responses can be modified and her skill increased. It promotes professional independence in a student midwife with a clear frame-work for self-assessment.

(Jamieson, 1995.)

The ability to help a mother as described in this Chapter together with application of the Peplau model enable you to develop a professional skill and independence while effectively aiding the mother. These approaches protect women from unaware, limited and potentially harmful professional interactions.

Ideas for Problem Solving

The key to problem solving is to listen and watch. The mother reveals anxieties and difficulties in what she says and does, and the baby interacts (or not!) to add further evidence. Do not be tempted to enter into the situation and, with 'hands-on', attach the baby. All this does is to delay the problem solving for later and possibly for someone else! It also reduces the confidence of the mother in her ability to breastfeed.

Position

The mother may not be holding the baby horizontal at the level of the breast facing inwards. Sometimes the baby is lying in a sunbathing position and turning his/her head to reach for the breast. Correct this by showing on you, not by touching the mother or her baby in the first instance, and explain the rationale of comfort and optimum conditions for the baby.

Timing

Sometimes the mother is simply missing the 'gape' of the baby by bringing him/her close to her breast just as the mouth is closing. This leads to insufficient breast entering the mouth and pain caused by incorrect fixing. Because she has experienced pain, the mother sometimes draws away just as the baby opens the mouth, with the same problem resulting. Teach the mother the methodical approach if she does not already know it. Position yourself on the side of the mother opposite to the breast on which the baby is trying to fix so that you can see clearly. Explain to her what you see and how she can solve the problem.

Shape of Breast

A mother sometimes shapes the breast in a horizontal wedge and tries to force it into a mouth that is a vertical oval in shape – teach her Step 3 above. Give her an example of a triangular sandwich offered to a toddler. When flat the mouth accommodates it, when vertical all the filling drops out and the toddler cannot get it

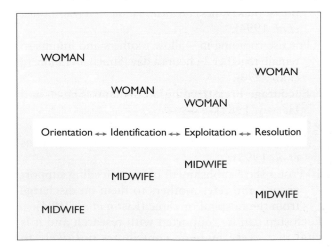

Figure 13.14 The phases of the midwife–woman relationship.

into his/her mouth. Sometimes the mother holds the breast too close to the nipple, so her finger covers the part of the breast that should be over the bottom jaw. She then tries to push the nipple into the baby's mouth. Show her Step 3 on yourself, and explain the rationale. If necessary place your hand from above, make the shape with her breast and let her place her hand from below, putting her finger on your thumb and thumb on your finger (as the hands reverse). Then you can withdraw and she will be holding the breast correctly.

Tearful Mother about to Give up

The greatest help is your belief in her, but placing your hands over her hands can be appropriate. Don't take over, but gently guide her hands so she succeeds, then withdraw your hands as soon as possible so that she is in control.

Engorged Full Breasts – Frustrated, Tense Mother and Baby!

It is possible to still share attachment by holding the baby and breast yourself, but ask the mother to 'cover' your hands so she is also holding the baby. This makes her feel a contributor and less helpless. A pillow can help give height and take some of the weight of the baby. Calm the baby first and convince her/him that all is well. If the baby knows your voice and touch this can give confidence as you help in what has been a fraught situation. As soon as possible after having helped the baby to attach, slip your hands away and allow the mother's hands to be the ones close to the baby. She is then in full charge, which will help restore her confidence.

Further Help

These are just a few of the most common problems. Helping in a consistent way increases the midwife's skills and chances of success. There are many books written on breastfeeding, but combining Henschel and Inch's *Breastfeeding – a Guide for Midwives* (1996) with Maureen Minchen's *Breastfeeding Matters* (1985) probably gives an immediate answer with a considered argument and research base. *The Politics of Breastfeeding* by Gay Palmer (1988) is also essential to understand the economic and international context of breastfeeding.

Baby Friendly Initiative

The global Baby Friendly Hospital Initiative (BFHI) was launched by the United Nations International Children's Emergency Fund (UNICEF) and WHO in New York in 1991. In the UK, because of our pattern of care, community services are also included. The initiative is designed to promote infant and child health by protecting and supporting breastfeeding. The global criteria comprise 10 steps that can be evaluated by external assessors. It is possible for a hospital to assess itself with a self-appraisal questionnaire before inviting outside assessors. The midwife's responsibility is to explore the research that supports the steps, to have a clarity about the importance of enabling breastfeeding through each step and be consistent in applying this knowledge in practice. The assessors will then note the professionals congruent care. Each step has an example of one reference to help your understanding but there are more to find.

The 10 steps are as follows:

1 Have a written breastfeeding policy that is routinely communicated to all health care staff (Garforth and Garcia, 1989).
2 Train all health care staff in skills necessary to implement this policy (Westphal *et al.* 1995).
3 Inform all pregnant women about the benefits and management of breastfeeding (Pugin *et al.* 1996).
4 Help mothers initiate breastfeeding within half an hour of birth (Ali and Lowry, 1981).
5 Show mothers how to breastfeed and how to maintain lactation if they should be separated from their infants (Righard and Alarde, 1992).
6 Give newborn infants no food or drink other than breast milk, unless *medically* indicated (Blomquist *et al.* 1994).
7 Practise rooming-in – allow mothers and infants to remain together 24 hours a day (Strachan–Lindberg *et al.* 1990).
8 Encourage breastfeeding on demand (Slaven and Harvey, 1981).
9 Give no artificial teats or pacifiers (also called dummies or soothers) to breastfeeding infants (Barros *et al.* 1995).
10 Foster the establishment of breastfeeding support groups and refer mothers to them on discharge from the hospital or clinic (Kistin *et al.* 1994).

Each step can be supported with research and it is vital that every midwife contributes positively to ensure their unit or community achieves the steps. Different countries are advancing in this at different rates, partly because some started at a higher level of breastfeeding so it is considered more the cultural norm. This initiative is an approach that benefits all countries and ultimately will benefit all babies.

Bottle-Feeding

If a mother has chosen to artificially feed, the midwife supports the mother in her choice of feeding her baby. It is important to ensure that this is an informed choice and that someone has identified for the mother the benefits of breastfeeding that relate to the immediate and future health of her baby and herself. In the future mothers, misinformed could well charge professionals with poor practice if they did not clarify and expand on the benefits of breastfeeding at the time the information was needed. Midwives would not be silent when a mother chooses a way of delivery that put her or her baby at risk. Equally, their passivity or lack of information should not allow a woman to think that artificial milk is an equivalent food to breast milk for the human baby.

In the Baby Friendly Initiative one of the 10 steps to successful breastfeeding is 'Give newborn infants no food or drink other than breast milk, unless medically indicated' (WHO/UNICEF, 1994). This indicates how important it is for the professional and the mother to consider carefully before giving artificial milk. If by our actions we collude with baby milk manufacturers, suggesting that their product is close to breast milk, we simply enhance sales of an inferior product. Breastfeeding costs professional expertise and time invested in support and education. Bottle-feeding costs less to the providers of care, but more to the mother and baby in terms of economic and health deficits. Anxiety is often expressed that the midwife might induce guilt in the mother when expressing the benefits of breastfeeding. An alternative danger is that the mother will challenge the health professionals, claiming that they failed to explain the benefits of breastfeeding to enable an informed choice to be made and/or that they lacked the knowledge and skills to solve a problem.

A route to understanding how insidious and subtle is the professional contribution in giving credence to bottle-feeding is to consider all the ways a professional might give support to artificial feeding as an equivalent alternative, without speaking!

Some examples might be ward antenatal posters, teaching aids, names of rooms or wards, cot labels, pens and pads used by professionals, position and availability of artificial milk, speed with which artificial milk is used as a supplement, demonstration to everyone antenatally or postnatally of making up an artificial feed, free samples to mothers antenatally and postnatally, literature full of advice and adverts for those with difficulty breastfeeding, creams, sprays, etc., and funded scholarships for professionals. Some of these may seem innocent to you, but trace back the motivation of the milk producer and the relationship that results with the professional.

For those mothers who do decide to bottle-feed, help and support should be given by the midwife.

Supporting Bottle-Feeding

The mother must be encouraged to hold the baby close to her own body in a cradling position. The bottle should be held at an angle that ensures there is no air left in the teat. The teat is then placed well into the baby's mouth over the tongue and the baby starts to feed.

The sucking mechanism for bottle-feeding differs gfrom that of breastfeeding (Woolridge, 1986), the baby may take some time to adapt from a normal sucking reflex to the action of stemming the flow of milk from the teat by thrusting its tongue upwards. A way to identify the two different experiences the baby has, suckling or sucking, is to suck at a teat using artificial milk or water and then compare this with an equivalent to the breast by opening your mouth wide and placing it against the pad of your hand where your thumb is and attempt to stroke the base of the thumb with your tongue (approximately corresponds to a baby with breast-tissue in its mouth). Consider how the two experiences differ.

Ways to help bottle-feeding mothers succeed

While learning to adapt to teat sucking, the baby is more likely to be seen to cough or gag as the milk flow has to be controlled by the tongue occluding the holes in the teat. Milk may also leak out of the baby's mouth, especially at the corners, which makes some sort of protection, like a bib, necessary. Normal, healthy term babies learn during the first few weeks of life, but especially during the first few days. The baby should be allowed to feed on demand with no restriction placed on either the intervals between feeds or the volume of milk. Eventually a feeding pattern emerges. Often a feeding pattern is forced by the professional or the mother, influenced by expectations and enabled by the baby's slower emptying of the stomach and reduced digestion of the milk.

These important points are explained to the mother so that she can be reassured that the baby is just learning the skill and will eventually leak less milk. Some babies never leak, but most do!

Sometimes a bottle-fed baby is not given as much contact in arms or communication time with the mother as a breastfed baby is. It is important to encourage the mother to spend time following a short feed to talk to and enjoy her baby before putting the baby to rest. A baby in light sleep appears to know whether it is held or not, often waking up as soon as the contact is lost. The danger of putting a bottle-fed baby down quickly following a feed is a loss of social loving contact for the baby. So, encouraging a time of mutual admiration to occur between the bottle-fed baby and the mother following most feeds is part of the midwife's role. Teaching that loving, secure arms communicate love and security to the baby and give a feeling of well-being is important. Allowing any and everyone to bottle-feed a baby can again give an inferior social experience for the baby. To prop a bottle in a cot is an unsafe practice and obviously isolating for the baby. Feeding and mothering are combined skills, so a midwife needs to build a woman in her ability to mother as she interacts in giving her care. Another's belief in one's ability to achieve both the skills and relationships with a new baby contributes to the ability to succeed. It is not appropriate to judge a woman who has made an 'informed choice' to bottle-feed her baby.

Winding

Winding is a subject which is often of great concern to mothers (and midwives), but in fact carries wide cultural differences – winding practices vary greatly from country to country. However, it appears to be accepted generally that bottle-fed babies get more wind, air being available in the bottle. Crying, especially for long periods, may also give a baby wind. It is probably wise to give the bottle-fed baby an opportunity to bring up wind at the end of a feed. Sometimes mothers also give an opportunity during the feed. Any position in which the baby's back is kept straight – either up against the shoulder or upright sitting on the mother's knee – can be used. The baby's back can be rubbed or patted gently if desired.

As well as understanding the differences between the sucking and winding responses of breast feeding and bottle-feeding babies, midwives need to expect other differences in babies behaviours, especially during the first few days. The size of the newborn's stomach is approximately 2.5 cm (Minchen 1985) – often comparison is made with a walnut to provide a mental picture. The stomach is designed to receive and digest small volumes of colostrum during the first 3 days of life and then mature breast milk. Therefore, should a mother choose to artificially feed her baby by a bottle, the baby's stomach often receives a much greater volume of a more indigestible milk than nature has planned. These two factors, along with the likelihood of more wind, can make the baby vomit, which causes the mother and others alarm. As midwives become more aware of the physiological responses that occur according to whether the baby is breast- or bottle-fed, they will become better placed to explain and educate bottle-feeding mothers about what to expect. Sometimes mothers and health workers misinterpret the vomiting as milk allergy or a dislike of a particularly artificial milk brand and either change brands or use soya milk, but both are usually unnecessary solutions to the problem.

Physiological Jaundice and Feeding Implications

Physiological jaundice occurs in 50% of healthy term babies and often requires no treatment nor warrants any changes to demand feeding. Jaundice reaches a peak around 3–4 days, when it can be seen as a slight yellow colour in the skin, most obviously in the sclera of the eyes and in the face. Average serum bilirubin levels around this time are 100 mmol/l (Robertson, 1993).

Treatment with phototherapy is commonly recommended if the serum bilirubin rises above 240–255 mmol/l (Oski, 1988). Once again, there is no reason why a baby should require anything other than normal demand feeding. However, the effect of the jaundice and the phototherapy lights may make the baby drowsy and thus sleep for much longer periods than it otherwise might. If this occurs it is beneficial to explain sleep states to the mother. A baby in deep sleep has regular respirations and does not move; there are no movements seen under the eyelids. In light sleep, the baby moves limbs and movements can be seen under the eyelids. The respirations vary in speed and depth. Sometimes babies make sucking movements. Recognizing these two sleep states is important as a baby in light sleep can sometimes be persuaded by handling to wake up and feed. The mother can observe and disturb the baby to feed at the optimal time.

Offering a breastfed baby supplementary feeds of either water or formula is contraindicated. If the baby is too sleepy to feed well from the breast, the mother can express her milk and give this to the baby. It is always important to encourage a woman to 'sandwich' express – that is hand stimulate the nipple followed by pump and ending with hand expression. The hand mimics the baby and stimulates prolactin production, so milk secretion is maintained. The pump alone is a poor stimulus (Howie, 1985).

Cup-Feeding

Cup-feeding is a way of offering milk to babies so that they can lap at it with their tongue. A small cup of milk is held to their bottom lip, allowing them to sample it. This is a gentle way to help a baby to feed. It is important that the milk is offered and never poured – midwives need to be shown the technique so they can do it correctly and teach women.

Cup-feeding is an alternative to bottle-feeding when giving expressed breast milk to a baby. This is useful sometimes for the jaundiced baby or the baby learning to breastfeed in the neonatal nursery when the mother is not able to be there for every feed (Lang, 1994). It can be the preferred way when a mother returns to work and leaves breast milk with the carer.

Conclusion

This chapter has indicated the importance of the midwife exploring her own biography in relation to breastfeeding, before becoming an effective supporter to women. It explores sociological dimensions which understood, enhance the midwife's skill. It has outlined the knowledge of the components of breast milk and physiology that is essential to informed practice. The description of the development of the skill of helping a woman is based on national research into breastfeeding failure and the responsiblities of the midwife in relation to the Baby Friendly Initiative are explored. The chapter emphasises throughout the importance of being a self-aware, non-judgemental and professionally skilled facilitator in all areas of infant feeding. The further reading encourages further research knowledge and socio-political awareness.

KEY CONCEPTS

- **Self-awareness and effective feeding support.** Professionals who identify aspects of their own biographies that contribute to their attitude to baby feeding are more able to give appropriate responses in their role as feeding supporters.

- **The contribution of understanding physiology in breastfeeding support.** Accurate knowledge of the constituents of breast milk and the physiology of lactation is fundamental to a professional giving adequate advice to a mother wishing to breastfeed.

- **The place of research in breastfeeding support.** Research into breastfeeding informs practice at all levels. The national research which reveals the reasons women state for giving up breastfeeding has been used to develop a methodical way to help a woman succeed with feeding.

- **Using a methodical approach effectively.** The professional transfers knowlege and skills within an aware relationship. There is a need to build the woman iin self- and mothering-confidence. The professional has to be committed to achieve satisfaction from the woman's success and autonomy with no desire for dependency.

References

Akre J, editor: Infant feeding, the physiological basis, *Bull WHO* 67(Suppl), 1989.

Ali Z, Lowry M: Early maternal-child contact: Effects on later behaviour. *Developmentat Medicine and Child Neurology*, 23:337, 1981.

Aniasson G, Alm B, Andersson B, *et al.*: A prospective cohort study on breastfeeding and ottis media in Swedish infants, *Paediatr Infect Dis J* 13:183, 1994.

Barros FC, Vitora CG, Semer TC, *et al.*: Use of pacifiers is associated with decreased breast feeding duration, *Pediatrics*, 95:497, 1995.

Blomquist HK, Jonsbo F, Serenius F, *et al.*: Supplementary feeding in the maternity ward shortens the duration of breast feeding, *Acta Paediatr* 83:1122, 1994.

Bryan EM: *The nature and nurture of twins*, London, 1983, Balliere Tindall.

Carlson B: *Human embryology and developmental biology*, St Louis, 1994, Mosby.

Carlson Gielen A, Faden RR, O'Campo P, *et al.*: Maternal employment during early postpartum period: Effects on initiation and continuation of breast feeding, *Pediatrics* 87:298, 1991.

Dick G: The etiology of multiple sclerosis, *Proc R Soc Med* 69:611, 1976.

Duncan B, *et al.*: Exclusive breastfeeding for at least four months protects against otitis media, *Paediatrics* 91(5):867, 1993.

Ford RPK, Taylor BJ, Mitchell EA, *et al.*: Breast feeding and the risk of Sudden Infant Death syndrome, *Int J Epidemiol* 22:885, 1993.

Garforth S, Garcia J: Breast feeding policies in practice – 'No wonder they get confused', *Midwifery* 5:75, 1989.

Glasier AS, McNeilly AS, Howie PW: The prolactin response to suckling, *Clinical Endocrinology* 21:109, 1984.

Greasley V: Breastfeeding in nursing – the add on, *J Clin Nurs* 3(2):63, 1986.

Gregg J: Attitudes of teenagers in Liverpool to breastfeeding, *Br Med J* 299:147, 1989.

Hamosh M: Does infant nutrition affect adiposity and cholestero levels in the adult?, *J Pediatric Gastroenterol Nutrition* 7(1):10, 1988.

Helman G: *Culture, health & illness*, 2nd edn, Oxford, 1990, Butterworth–Heinemann.

Henschel D, Inch S: *Breastfeeding – a guide for midwives*, Hale, 1996, Books for Midwives Press.

Host A: Importance of the first meal on the development of cow's milk allergy and intolerance, *Allergy Proc* 12:227, 1991.

Howie P: Breast feeding – a new understanding, *Midwives Chron* 98(1170):184, 1985.

Howie PW, Forsyth JS, Ogston SA, *et al.*: Protective effect of breastfeeding against infection, *Br Med J* 300(6)11, 1990.

Jakobsson I, Lindberg T: Cows' milk proteins cause infantile colic in breastfed infants; a double blind cross-over study, *Pediatrics* 71(2):268, 1983.

Jamieson L: Educating for successful breastfeeding *Br J Midwifery* 3(10):535, 1995.

Jones DA, West RR, Newcombe RG: Maternal characteristics associated with the duration of breast feeding, *Midwifery* 2:141, 1986.

Karjaleinen J, Martin JM, Knip M, *et al.*: A bovine albumin peptide as a possible trigger of insulin-dependent mellitus, *New Engl J Med* 327:302, 1992.

Kelnar C, *et al.*: *The sick newborn baby*, 3rd edn, London, 1995, Bailli(re Tindall.

Kistin N, Abramson R, Dublin P: Effect of peer counsellors on breastfeeding initiation, exclusivity and duration among low-income urban women, *J Hum Lact* 12(1):11, 1994.

Lang S: Cup feeding, an alternative method, *Midwives Chronicle and Nursing Notes* May:171, 1994.

Lanting CI, Fidler V, Huisman N, *et al.*: Neurological differences between 9 year old children fed breast-milk or formula-milk as babies, *Lancet* 344(12):1319, 1994.

Lawrence R: *Breastfeeding – a guide for the medical profession*, Toronto, 1989, Mosby.

Lucas A, Cole TJ: Breast milk and neonatal necrotising enterocolitis, *Lancet* 336:1519, 1990.

Marild S, Jodal U, Hanson LA: Breastfeeding and urinary tract infection, *Lancet* 336:942, 1990.

Minchen M: *Breastfeeding matters*, Sydney, 1985, Allen and Unwin.

Minchen M: Infant formula: a mass, uncontrolled trial in perinatal care, *Birth* 14:25, 1987.

Newcomb PA, Storer BE, Longnecker MP: Lactation and a reduced risk of premenopausal breast cancer, *New Engl J Med* 330(2):81, 1994.

Oski FA: Physiological jaundice, In: Avery ME, Taeusch HW jnr, (editors): *Diseases of the newborn*, Philadelphia, 5th ed, 1988, WB Saunders.

Prentice AM, Addey CVP, Wilde CJ: Evidence for local feed-back control of human milk secretion, *Biochem Soc Trans* 17:489, 1989.

Pugin E, *et al.*: Does prenatal breastfeeding skills group education increase the effectiveness of a comprehensive breastfeeding promotion program? *J Hum Lact* 12(1):15, 1996.

Righard L, Alade MO: Sucking technique and its effect on success of breastfeeding, *BIRTH* 19:185, 1992.

Robertson NRC, editor: *Textbook of neonatology*, London, 1993, Churchill Livingstone.

Rojan WS, Gladen BC: Breastfeeding and cognitive development, *Early Hum Dev* 31: 181, 1993.

Salisbury L, Blackwell AG: Petition to alleviate domestic infant formula misuse and provide informed infant feeding choice, *San Francisco: Public Advocates Inc* p. 45, 1981.

Schott J, Henley A: *Culture, religion and childbearing in multi-cultural society*, London, 1996, Butterworth.

Slaven S, Harvey D: Unlimited suckling time improves breast feeding, *Lancet* i:392, 1981.

Specker BL, *et al.*: In: Tsang RC, Nichols BL, (editors): *Nutriton during pregnancy*, St Loius, p. 268, 1988, Mosby.

Strachan Lindberg C, Cabrera Artola R, Jimenez V: The effect of early post-partum mother-infant contact and breast feeding promotion on the incidence and continuation of breast feeding, *Int J Nurs Stud* 27(3):179, 1990.

Turner G: *Factors influencing Nigerian mothers' decisions to combine breast and bottle feeding postnatally*, MSc Thesis, Brighton, 1994, University of Surrey.

Victora CG, Vaughan JP, Lombardi C: Evidence for protection by breast feeding against infant deaths from infectious disease in Brazil, *Lancet* 8 Aug:319, 1987.

Walker M: A fresh look at the risks of artificial infant feeding, *J Hum Lactation* 9(2):97, 1993.

Westphal MF, *et al.*: Breast feeding training for health professionals and resultant institutional changes, *Bulletin of WHO* 73(4):461, 1995.

White A, Freeth S, O'Brien M,: *OPCS infant feeding 1990*, London, 1992, HMSO.

WHO/UNICEF: *Protecting, promoting and supporting breast feeding: The special role of maternity services*, A joint WHO/UNICEF statement published by the World Health Organization, 1211 Geneva 27 Switzerland, 1991.

Woolridge MW, Fisher C: Colic 'overfeeding' and symptoms of lactose malabsorption in the breastfed baby; a possible artefact of feed management?, *Lancet* ii:382, 1988.

Woolridge MW: The 'anatomy' of infant sucking, *Midwifery* 2:164, 1986.

Further Reading

Henschel D, Inch S: *Breastfeeding – a guide for midwives*, Hale, 1996, Books for Midwives Press.

This text combines the basic knowledge required with a skilful experienced midwife's perspective. Dora Henschel has many years' experience of supporting women and her gentle, nonjudgmental, but expert approach is very helpful to student and qualified midwives alike.

Lang S: *Breast feeding special care babies*, London, 1996, Balliere Tindall.

A practical based book dealing wth babies requiring special care.

Minchen M: *Breastfeeding matters*, 1985, Allen and Unwin.

This is a classic text which answers both everyday and unusual queries for the midwife. The author's research base will help the midwife understand the rationale that supports teaching practices.

Palmer G: *The politics of breastfeeding*, London, 1988, Harper Collins.

This is a challenging and erudite piece of work that gives a midwife insight into the socioeconomic pressures and international politics created through feeding seen as a business.

14 *Health after Birth*

LEARNING OUTCOMES

After studying this chapter you will be able to:

- Differentiate between normal and complicated postnatal recovery through the application of a sound physiological knowledge base.
- Appraise the specific postnatal needs of individual women and their families and plan and provide care to meet those needs.
- Ensure that your practice promotes the physical postnatal health of the mother and the emotional well-being of the family.
- Apply research evidence to midwifery practice to provide effective postnatal care.
- Enable the woman and her partner to achieve satisfaction in their parenting roles. **(continued)**

INTRODUCTION

A complex series of events occurs after birth. The woman assumes a non-pregnant, parous state and embarks on the psychological adaptation to motherhood. The parents take on new roles and responsibilities as the baby is socially integrated into its new family. These changes impact upon the lives of all women and their families, who respond and adapt in individual ways.

The midwife has an important role in easing the transition to motherhood. The quality of postnatal care provided around the time of birth influences the experience of early parenthood and the confidence with which parenting skills are learnt.

In this section, the nature and organization of postnatal care and the role of the midwife in meeting the needs of women and their families at this important time in their lives are examined.

Postnatal Care

The postnatal period is defined as 'a period of not less than 10 days and not more than 28 days after the end of labour, during which the continued attendance of a midwife on the mother and baby is requisite' (UKCC, 1993).

Midwifery care during the postnatal period has traditionally been determined by the health of women postpartum. At the beginning of the twentieth century, the maternal death rate was 4/1000 births, the majority of which were caused by puerperal infection (Towler and Brammal, 1986). The puerperium, which

refers to a period of approximately 6 weeks after the birth of a baby during which time the physiological changes of pregnancy are reversed and lactation is established, was regarded as pathological and postnatal care was organized to reflect this. The Central Midwives Board specified the frequency with which women were seen and the content of visits (CMB, 1928). The latter was orientated towards the prevention or treatment of infection and demanded a high level of nursing care.

Until recently, postnatal care remained largely prescriptive, despite general improvements in women's health and the fact that maternal deaths are now rare. The frequency with which women are seen is no longer specified (UKCC, 1986) and the midwife is able to determine the nature and content of care within the postnatal period based on her own assessment of the woman's needs (UKCC, 1992). Despite this increased freedom of action, many midwives continue to work to a pre-determined routine and the emphasis remains on physical aspects of care (Murphy-Black, 1989; Marsh and Sargent, 1991; Marchant and Garcia, 1995).

In recent years, the widespread introduction of technology and moves towards hospital confinement have led to increasing consumer dissatisfaction with maternity care and a realization within the midwifery profession of the need for reform. This resulted in an extensive Government-led review of the maternity services throughout the UK. Postnatal care was concluded to be 'poorly evaluated and researched (and) delivered in inappropriate and fragmented ways' (House of Commons Health Committee, 1992, p. liv).

Policy documents that outline the future of the maternity services (Welsh Office, 1992; Department of Health, 1993; Scottish Home Office and Health

Department, 1993; Department of Health and Social Services Belfast, 1994) were published following the review. An important theme to emerge was the concept of woman-centred maternity care. This is characterized by a flexible, responsive service in which each woman receives continuity of care that takes full account of her specific physical, psychological, social and cultural needs.

A Woman-Centred Approach to Postnatal Care

The midwife makes a unique contribution to the postnatal recovery of every woman. ITo be effective, midwifery care must address the diverse, and yet specific, demands of the mother and her family. This requires effective communication with parents to identify their needs and the adoption of flexible working patterns to meet their requirements.

Womens' Expectations

Users of the maternity services value kind, supportive and knowledgeable midwives (**Box 14.1**). Continuity of care from a known professional is also important to women (Department of Health, 1993) and reduces the possibility of conflicting advice. This has long been a criticism of postnatal care and is known to worry and confuse mothers (Hillan, 1992a; Gready *et al.* 1995).

Women consistently identify the need for accurate information, skilled help and advice about breastfeeding (Hutton, 1994; Hawthorne, 1994), their own health and that of their baby (Glazener *et al.* 1993; Houston, 1994). In addition to this, they seek practical, educational and emotional support (Fichardt *et al.* 1994).

Identifying Needs and Planning Care

In the early puerperium the midwife must appraise the health and well-being of the mother, her confidence with infant feeding and the level of support available to the family. This assessment must be validated with the mother to ensure that it concurs with her perceptions, as it has been found that women often report problems that are not identified, or

recorded as such, by the midwife (Hillan, 1992b). Only when this assessment has been completed can the exact requirements, expectations and learning priorities of the mother be determined and incorporated into a plan of care. This must be sufficiently flexible to meet changing needs and priorities and it ensures that each postnatal visit has a specific purpose.

Culturally Sensitive Care

Cultural variations in childbearing exist, many of which manifest for the first time during the postnatal period. These proscriptions and practices are often based on the beliefs that labour has upset the balance of the woman's body, predisposing her to illness, and that she is in a polluted state (Horn, 1990). They are thought to hasten the mothers recovery and adaptation to a new role.

A period of seclusion for up to 40 days and minimal activity is not uncommon following childbirth to enable rest and recovery. This is at odds with the western practice of early ambulation, infant care policies and early discharge from hospital and was identified as an area of conflict by Asian women in East London (Woollett and Dosanjh-Matwala, 1990).

Women should not be stereotyped according to ethnic origin. Instead, each woman should be asked about her beliefs and childbirth practices so that the midwife can provide culturally sensitive care.

Fathers

The transition to fatherhood involves changes in role, responsibilities and relationships and is a stressful and emotional time. The extent to which each father participates in caring for his new infant will vary and may depend on the availability of paternity leave, working patterns, the care of other children and his comfort in

---

Box 14.1

Womens' Expectations

- Continuity of care.
- Consistent advice.
- Accurate information.
- Skilled help.
- Practical, educational and emotional support.

this role. New fathers report the need for continuity of information and support (Henderson and Brouse, 1991). The midwife is in a position to address these needs. Involving the father in the care of the mother and baby is likely to be important, both for his own fulfilment and the development of the family.

Midwifery Care in the Postnatal Period

Postnatal care provision is based upon a number of principles which are aimed at:
* Promoting, maintaining and restoring health.
* Facilitating the mother to care for her new baby safely and confidently.
* Ensuring a pattern of feeding that enables the infant to thrive.
* Enabling the woman and her partner to develop their abilities as parents and to achieve a valuable experience of parenting.
* Assisting the family to identify and meet its own needs and to take responsibility for its own health

The caring activities of the midwife in the postnatal period can therefore be categorized as the restoration and maintenance of health, the promotion of emotional well-being and the provision of information, education and expert practical advice.

Restoring and Maintaining Physical Health

Pregnancy and childbirth are considered to be physiological events that end normally and without complication for the majority of women (Department of Health, 1993). Similarly, by the end of the puerperium the recovery from childbirth is generally assumed to be complete. These views are perhaps over-optimistic. For many women, recovery is straightforward and becoming a mother is a normal physiological process. However, some recent studies have revealed that long-term health problems following childbirth are not uncommon (Hillan, 1992b; Glazener *et al.* 1993; Bick and MacArthur, 1995a) and may persist for many years (MacArthur *et al.* 1991).

Physical care in the puerperium should be approached against an expectation of good health, with midwifery efforts directed towards the early identification and appropriate management of health problems should they arise.

A thorough knowledge of both the physiological and psychological changes of the puerperium is essential if the midwife is accurately to appraise maternal health status and determine that a recovery consistent with expected norms is taking place. Equally important is awareness of the potential for long-term postpartum morbidity and the obstetric, anaesthetic and social factors associated with this.

Physical Examination and Applied Physiology

The way in which physical health is appraised following childbirth varies according to each woman's needs and expectations. A regular, physical examination may be appropriate for some and provides the opportunity to discuss health-related issues. However, the examination should not be carried out to a preset schedule, so each component included should be relevant to the health of the mother concerned. This is influenced by the type of delivery, the presence of risk factors for the development of complications and any reported problems. Some women may not require such a health check, but still need to be asked specifically about the occurrence of health problems.

The purpose of a physical examination is to detect complications, pre-empt morbidity and thus limit health problems. This requires knowledge of the normal parameters for postnatal recovery, which is based upon an understanding of the physiological changes that occur following childbirth and of the application of this knowledge in practice. In this Chapter, the physiology of the puerperium is therefore addressed in the context of a physical examination. Abnormal or pathological findings require the midwife to refer the woman to a doctor for appropriate treatment (Rule 40, UKCC, 1993). The process of clinical decision-making during postnatal examination is shown in **Figure 14.1**.

Physiological changes following birth

After delivery of the placenta, circulating levels of human placental lactogen, human chorionic gonadotrophin, oestrogens and progesterone fall. Human placental lactogen disappears from the maternal circulation by 2 days and human chorionic gonadotrophin by 2 weeks after delivery. Oestrogens and progesterone reach levels similar to those found during the follicular phase of the menstrual cycle by about 3 and 7 days, respectively. The withdrawal of these polypeptide and steroid hormones alters the function of all systems so that the effects of pregnancy are reversed and the woman resumes a non-pregnant, albeit parous, state (*see* Chapter 4 for the endocrine-mediated changes of pregnancy). The progress of these changes is monitored in the course of a clinical postnatal examination.

Temperature, pulse and blood pressure

Routine measurement of the temperature and pulse rate of women throughout the postnatal period is unnecessary (Abbott, 1994). The temperature is an unreliable indicator of pathology in postpartum women because it may, or may not, be elevated in the event of infection (Hibbard, 1988; Department of Health, 1991b). Furthermore, transient elevations in the temperature are normal in response to physiological changes in the uterus and the breast. Localized signs or symptoms of infection *in association with* changes in the temperature and pulse rate combine to give a more reliable indicator of a complicated postnatal recovery.

It is important for women who are at an increased risk of infection, for example following an instrumental or operative delivery, or who appear unwell on clinical examination to have their temperature measured regularly during the postnatal period. If a mercury thermometer is used, it should remain *in situ* for 4 minutes (Closs, 1987).

The pulse rate alone provides limited information about maternal condition unless the baseline is known. If maternal condition warrants recording the pulse rate, it should be counted over 1 minute.

Where pregnancy has been complicated by pre-eclampsia or blood pressure has been elevated during labour, regular recordings of the blood pressure should continue until it returns to normal limits for the woman, or the risk of an eclamptic fit has passed. Such fits are most likely within 48 hours, but can occur up to 10 days later (Novy, 1994).

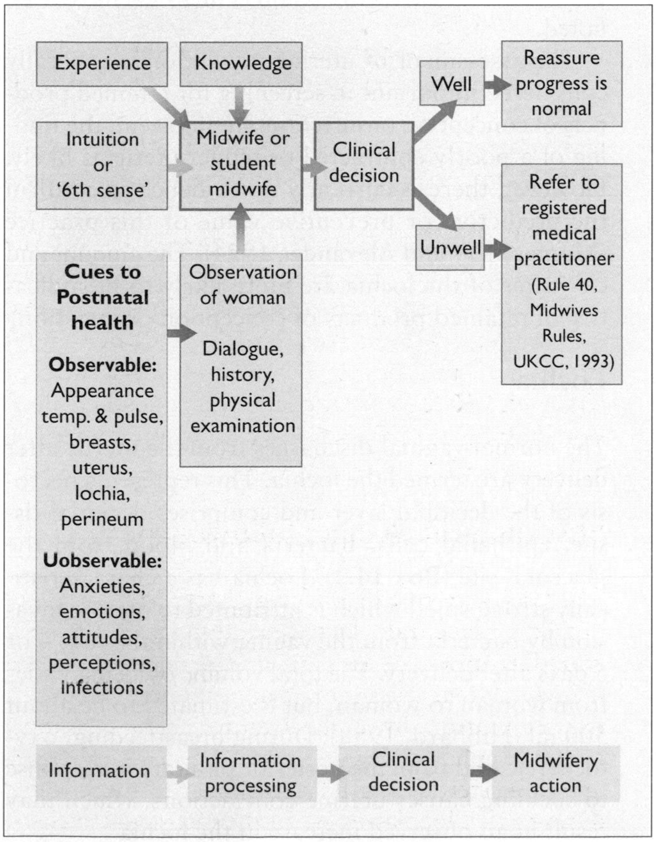

The breasts

Levels of prolactin, secreted by the anterior pituitary, rise steadily throughout pregnancy, but placental hormones inhibit the production of milk. After delivery of the placenta, concentrations of oestrogens and progesterone fall, prolactin is released and milk synthesis begins. The blood supply to the breasts increases and causes transient vascular engorgement. Milk, once produced, is stored in the alveoli and must be removed effectively by suckling for the establishment and continuation of lactation (*see* Chapter 13).

Oxytocin release from the posterior pituitary is stimulated by suckling. This causes the contraction of myoepithelial cells in the breast and the ejection, or 'let-down', of milk. Oxytocin also stimulates myometrial contraction of the uterus, which the woman may report as afterpains. These usually occur during the first 3 days of the puerperium, are more common in multiparous than in primiparous women and occur more frequently during breastfeeding. In some women, afterpains are sufficiently strong to necessitate analgesia.

The comfort of her breasts should be discussed with each mother. If a woman reports painful breasts, sore nipples or feeling unwell the breasts should be examined to ascertain the cause of the problem. Redness of a segment of the breast is suggestive of mastitis. Sore nipples indicate that the baby has been incorrectly positioned when feeding and is correctable by appropriate instruction.

Figure 14.1 The process of clinical decision-making during postnatal examination.

In the wider context, this is also an ideal opportunity for the midwife to emphasize the importance of breast awareness in order that the woman is able to detect and report subtle changes in anatomy should they occur.

Infant feeding patterns also influence the resumption of fertility. This is likely to be discussed with the woman and her partner in the context of contraception.

While a woman is exclusively breastfeeding her baby, elevated prolactin levels reduce the sensitivity of the pituitary to the effects of gonadotrophin-releasing hormone so that concentrations of follicle-stimulating hormone and luteinizing hormone remain low. The ovary is also less sensitive to the effects of these hormones. Ovulation and the return of fertility is therefore delayed.

In contrast, prolactin levels decline steadily after delivery in women who bottle-feed, reaching non-pregnant levels by 7–14 days. Menstruation and ovulation are usually re-established within about 8 and 10 weeks, respectively (Howie *et al*. 1982).

Uterine involution

Immediately after delivery, the uterus is palpable just below the level of the umbilicus. It should feel well contracted. After 24 hours, the fundus of the uterus begins to diminish progressively in height until it is no longer palpable above the symphysis pubis, by the 10–12th postnatal day. This process is termed involution. By 6 weeks the uterus has greatly reduced in weight and approximates to its prepregnant size.

This rapid reduction in uterine size is mediated by:

- **A reduction in placental oestrogens.** Oestrogen withdrawal removes the stimulus to uterine hypertrophy and hyperplasia.
- **Ischaemia of the myometrium.** The myometrium continues to contract and retract following delivery, constricting blood vessels and achieving haemostasis at the placental site. The resulting ischaemia causes atrophy of muscle fibres.
- **Autolysis of the myometrium.** During pregnancy, oestrogen increases myometrial cell size and protein content (actin and myosin). Oestrogen withdrawal after delivery stimulates proteolytic enzymes and macrophages to degrade and digest (the process of autolysis) the excess intracellular proteins and cytoplasm, resulting in an overall reduction in cell size. Connective tissue and fat are similarly engulfed, destroyed and digested by tissue macrophages.

The placental site is rapidly infiltrated by leucocytes to form a protective barrier against infection. The superficial layer of the decidua degenerates and is shed during the first week after delivery as lochia. A transient rise in temperature and leucocytosis are associated with this process. The new endometrial lining arises from the fundi of the endometrial glands in the deeper, basal layer of the decidua. This re-epithelialization process takes approximately 14 days, except at the placental site where complete regeneration can take up to 6 weeks.

The process of uterine involution is monitored by palpation of the uterine fundus. Progressive descent should occur to below the symphysis pubis by the 10–12th day following delivery.

A number of studies have failed to demonstrate an association between the rate of uterine involution and parity, type of delivery or method of infant feeding (Rodeck and Newton, 1976; VanRees *et al*. 1981; Lavery and Shaw, 1989; Wachsberg *et al*. 1994). However, positive correlation between uterine size in the puerperium and birthweight (Lavery and Shaw, 1989), increasing maternal parity (Wachsberg *et al*. 1994) and breastfeeding (Galli *et al*.1993) have been noted.

The assessment of uterine involution is generally considered important in screening for retained products of conception or infection. In this event, the finding of a poorly contracted or tender uterus is likely. However, there is currently no evidence to confirm the predictive or preventive value of this practice (Montgomery and Alexander, 1994). The amount and character of the lochia are more likely to be indicative of retained products of conception or infection.

Lochia

The normal vaginal discharges from the uterus after delivery are termed the lochia. This represents necrosis of the decidual layer and comprises decidual tissue, epithelial cells, bacteria and blood from the placental site (**Box 14.2**). Lochia has a characteristically strong smell which is attributed to uterine invasion by bacteria from the vagina within the first 4 or 5 days after delivery. The total volume of lochia varies from woman to woman, but is estimated to be about 500 ml (Hibbard, 1988). During breastfeeding, oxytocin released from the posterior pituitary in response to suckling causes uterine contractions, which may result in an observed increase in the lochia.

The woman should be asked about the amount and colour of her lochia. If there is any doubt about the quantity, the sanitary pad should be inspected. Persistent red lochia that continues beyond 10 days, the passage of clots, or lochia that smell offensive are pathological features, suggestive of retained products of conception or infection. They may also predispose to secondary postpartum haemorrhage, which is defined as excessive bleeding from the genital tract occurring more than 24 hours after, but within 6 weeks of, delivery. These findings warrant referral to a doctor and urgent investigation.

Healing of the cervix, vagina and perineum

The cervix is soft, oedematous and bruised immediately after delivery and minor lacerations to the external os are not uncommon (Cunningham *et al.* 1993). Over the first week, the cervix gradually regains its tone as the canal re-forms and the internal os closes. The external os assumes a slit-like appearance.

The vagina appears as a smooth-walled passage as a result of stretching during delivery. Rugae become evident again by the third week postpartum and tone is regained by the end of the puerperium.

Perineal tears and lacerations usually heal within a week of delivery, although the area may remain sensitive for much longer (Sleep *et al.* 1984; Sleep and Grant, 1987). Greenshields and Hulme (1993) conducted a postal survey of womens' experiences of perineal trauma and reported that the majority of women in their study (*n*= 2000) 'felt some degree of normality by the 6th week postnatally'.

The comfort and healing of the perineum or Caesarean section wound site should be ascertained by the midwife. Good hygiene is conducive to healing. Regular use of a bath or shower and bidet, and frequent changes of sanitary pad ensure that the perineal area remains clean. Perineal soreness or pain is a common occurrence (Dewan *et al.* 1993), and is frequently reported following episiotomy (Greenshields and Hulme, 1993). Only therapies of proven benefit should be recommended for the management of sore perinea; these may include the application of cooling agents such as crushed ice, witch hazel or tap water and locally applied anaesthetics (Grant and Sleep, 1989). Adequate analgesia is essential if mothers are not to be hampered by perineal discomfort.

Urinary output

A normal postpartum diuresis occurs within 24 hours of delivery in response to the withdrawal of oestrogens. Protein may appear in the urine as a consequence of autolytic changes in the uterus.

The pregnancy-induced increase in renal blood flow and glomerular filtration rate returns to normal in parallel with the reduction in cardiac output. Glycosuria induced by pregnancy disappears within the first postpartum week, at which time creatinine clearance also returns to its normal rate. Dilatation of the renal pelvis and ureters has usually resolved by the end of the puerperium, but may take as long as 3 months.

Labour and delivery can have an adverse effect on bladder function. Retention of urine can occur after epidural analgesia (Weil *et al.* 1983; Andolf *et al.* 1994) or as a direct consequence of trauma to the bladder or urethra during labour. In this event, the bladder is palpable abdominally despite the frequent passage of small amounts of urine. A sore perineum can also impair micturition. Urinary output should be discussed with the woman to ensure that she is completely emptying her bladder.

Retention of urine, catheterization during labour and a history of urinary problems during pregnancy can predispose to urinary infection. This affects approximately 12% of women postpartum (Cardozo, 1995) and can present with urinary frequency, dysuria or loin pain. The urine characteristically smells offensive.

Stress incontinence of urine after delivery, or the involuntary loss of urine in response to a rise in intra-abdominal pressure, occurs when the urinary sphincter mechanism is incompetent (Swash, 1988). The precise aetiology for this remains uncertain, but damage to the perineal branches of the pudendal nerve during vaginal delivery has been implicated (Snooks *et al.* 1984; Allen *et al.* 1990; Viktrup *et al.* 1992). An association between advancing maternal age (MacArthur *et al.*, 1991), parity (Thomas *et al.*, 1980; Wilson *et al.*, 1996) and stress incontinence has also been noted.

Box 14.2

Characteristics of the Lochia

• Lochia rubra – red in colour, consisting primarily of blood from the placental site. Lasts 2–6 days.
• Lochia serosa – pinkish-brown, comprising less blood and more decidual tissue. Persists until re-epithelialization of the endometrium is almost complete.
• Lochia alba – yellowish white, containing primarily leucocytes. May continue 4–8 weeks after delivery.

The effectiveness of pelvic floor exercises (PFEs) as treatment for stress incontinence has not been clearly demonstrated. Improvements in the prevalence of incontinence have (Ferguson *et al.* 1990; Lagro-Janssen *et al.* 1991) and have not (Sleep and Grant, 1987) been shown when daily PFEs are performed. Pelvic floor conditioning with vaginal weights has been found to improve both voluntary and reflex muscle contraction of the pelvic floor and stress incontinence postpartum (Fischer *et al.* 1996).

The woman should be informed that stress incontinence is not a normal adjunct to childbirth. If it persists as a problem beyond the postnatal period she should seek medical attention (*see* Stress Incontinence).

Bowels

As the effect of progesterone on smooth muscle diminishes, bowel motility and tone is regained. Constipation can be precipitated by perspiration loss during labour, narcotic analgesia and fluid lost during the postpartum diuresis. Food intake may also have been interrupted during labour. If a woman reports constipation after delivery, a high-residue diet, adequate exercise and good hydration are managements that may alleviate the problem. When giving such advice, the midwife should consider any dietary restrictions or cultural prohibitions on exercise. Anxieties about defecation generated by a sore perineum should be discussed. For some women, constipation does persist as a problem (*see* Constipation).

Bowel action after delivery may also be inhibited by a painful perineum, haemorrhoids that have become prolapsed and swollen during the second stage of labour or lack of privacy on a postnatal ward. Haemorrhoids may improve after the effect of straining has subsided, but some permanent damage often persists (Hibbard, 1988).

Haemorrhoids that have prolapsed after delivery can cause extreme discomfort. Local treatment with an ice pack or anaesthetic cream may provide relief. Dietary advice should be given and constipation avoided. Laxative preparations or stool-softening agents should be used with caution in view of the side effects they can produce.

Legs

Women have an increased disposition to thromboembolic disorders in the puerperium as a result of circulatory changes and the consequent increase in clotting factors. Specific risk factors for the develop-ment of this complication are increasing maternal age, obesity, operative delivery, immobilization and a previous history of thromboembolism (Department of Health, 1994). All woman should be asked if they have any swelling or pain in their legs or have noticed changes in leg temperature or colour. Women with specific risk factors for thromboembolism should always have their legs examined.

General well-being

Fatigue

Sleep patterns of mothers take on an unpredictable pattern post-delivery, with the fragmentation of sleep cycles a predominant theme (Campbell, 1986; Shaw, 1994). This, and the demands and responsibilities of a new baby, contribute to the extreme tiredness that is frequently reported (Nolan, 1995). Fatigue can adversely affect the ability to care for the baby. A priority of the midwife is to assess the mother's sleep requirements and to stress the importance of adequate rest. This may include legitimizing the need for sleep during the day, encouraging the mother to accept help if she is exhausted and suggesting that visitors, however well meaning, be restricted. Fatigue may be compounded by postpartum anaemia.

Anaemia

A reduction in the oxygen-carrying capacity of the blood is termed anaemia. It is caused by a decrease in the number of red blood cells or the haemoglobin content of the blood. Anaemic women have been found to experience more physical problems postpartum than women with a haemoglobin >10.5g dl and may therefore require more practical and emotional support (Paterson *et al.* 1994). Women with risk factors for anaemia (**Box 14.3**) should have their haemoglobin level measured postpartum. In view of the changes in plasma volume and the consequent rise in red cell count, haemoglobin and haematocrit, a haemoglobin estimation on the second day provides the most reliable prediction of postpartum anaemia (Taylor and Lind, 1981).

Diet

The midwife should advise the mother to consume a healthy, well-balanced diet. This is likely to have long-term health gains for the woman and her family. For some women, it may be necessary to detail what constitutes such a diet; this should be with due regard for the mothers culture, income, lifestyle and desire to return to her pre-pregnant weight.

Breastfeeding women do not need to modify their diet or consume additional calories to sustain lactation (RCM, 1991). However, if there is a family history of allergy, some babies may benefit from the mother's avoidance of some foods during lactation (Chandra *et al.* 1986).

Posture

The softening effects of progesterone and relaxin on joints and ligaments takes approximately 3 months to reverse, but the pelvis can remain unstable for at least 6 months (Parsons, 1995). Joint and muscle strains may occur at the time of delivery. Untreated, these can cause pain, impair movement and may result in permanent damage.

Motherhood imposes increased mechanical demands on the mother. Care is needed when lifting heavy objects at a time when the musculoskeletal system remains unstable. Correct posture is also important, particularly when feeding the baby.

The muscles of the abdominal wall are stretched considerably during pregnancy and, following delivery, may remain separated in the midline (divarication of the recti abdominis). Pelvic floor muscles are similarly stretched during delivery. A general, progressive programme of exercise reduces the risk of circulatory problems, improves posture and strengthens both abdominal and pelvic floor muscles (Gordon and Logue, 1985).

Promoting Emotional Well-Being and Providing Support

Women undergo enormous changes as a consequence of childbirth, to which a variety of psychological responses occur. These may range from short-term mood fluctuations to long-term depression. More rarely, psychosis occurs.

The emotional well-being of the mother during the postnatal period is influenced by many factors, such as fatigue, success with feeding, satisfaction with mothering, anxieties about her own health or that of her baby and the level of support available to her.

The midwife uses her knowledge about mood patterns in the puerperium and risk factors for postnatal depression to appraise the psychological well-being of the mother. It is important for the midwife to ascertain how the mother is feeling and particularly to note the expression of anxieties, tearfulness or unhappiness.

The Edinburgh Postnatal Depression Scale (EDPS; Cox *et al.* 1987) is a 10-item, self-rating questionnaire, highly specific in the detection of postnatal depression. It is generally administered 6 weeks postpartum by the health visitor, but has been found to be effective in the identification of vulnerable women 5 days after delivery (Hannah *et al.* 1992). The midwife may use this tool to screen the psychological health of all women early in the puerperium to identify those who require additional support or referral to appropriate professionals.

Support from the midwife is an essential constituent of her caring activities. It eases the complexity of learning motherhood, the responsibility of caring for a new baby and positively influences confidence with parenting activities.

Both parents may look to the professional for informational support and reassurance in respect of their own health and that of the baby. Emotional support is enhanced through contact with the midwife, who can validate and reinforce the family's methods of caring for the infant. This increases the mother's and father's confidence in their abilities, enables them to take control of the care of their baby and impacts on their satisfaction with the parenting role.

However, support from the midwife is transient and only part of the wider social support system available to the parents that consists of family, friends and lay organizations. The midwife can help the family to identify and utilize these sources. She can also facilitate comparison support by organizing postnatal groups and introducing mothers who live locally to each other. This may reduce the risk of social isolation.

Education, Information and Expert Practical Advice

The educational needs of mothers vary in relation to care of the baby. Primiparous and multiparous women have different needs, which are influenced by

---

Box 14.3

Risk Factors for Postpartum Anaemia

- Anaemia at 34 weeks gestation.
- Instrumental or operative delivery.
- Postpartum haemorrhage.
- Heavy lochia.
- Primiparity.
- 25 years of age.
- Poor diet.

the extent of support and help available from various sources. Primiparous women often require more practical information on feeding, handling, settling and looking after the new infant (Gready *et al.* 1995). Multiparous women frequently report fatigue and anxieties about sibling adjustment to the new baby. Assumptions should not be made about the level and nature of both informational and practical support required by multiparous women.

Infant feeding is an issue of immense importance to all mothers. They require information about the initiation or suppression of lactation and expert practical advice about establishing breastfeeding or bottle-feeding (*see* Chapter 13). The physiological basis for all advice should be made explicit and incorporated into infant feeding guidelines to ensure that consistent, evidence-based information is given to mothers.

The midwife should be enthusiastic about breastfeeding (Hutton, 1994) and continue to support the mother until lactation is established and she is feeding her baby confidently. Women who choose to bottle-feed their babies should similarly be supported in their decision. Advice about the preparation of infant feeds should be given at an appropriate educational level and in a language that the mother understands.

Most couples resume sexual intercourse between 5 and 8 weeks postpartum (Grudzinskas and Atkinson, 1984). Advice about contraception is required before this and the midwife is ideally placed to provide it. Accurate, up-to-date information should be given about the methods available, failure rates and possible side effects so that the couple can make an informed choice about their preferred method of contraception (*see* Chapter 3). The opportunity to discuss postpartum sexuality should also be made available.

The mother, as primary informant, must be informed of the statutory requirement to register the birth of the baby within 6 weeks of delivery (3 weeks in Scotland). If she defaults the birth may be registered by any person who was present at the delivery. The parents should also be advised of the importance of registering the baby with a general practitioner (GP).

The midwife is knowledgeable about caring for the new baby, infant feeding, family planning and many aspects of womens health and illness in the immediate postnatal period. However, it appears from the extent of reported postpartum morbidity that midwives require more information about the ongoing health problems experienced by women and the appropriate treatments. Such information is crucial if women are to be educated to anticipate and report illhealth.

The Organization of Postnatal Care

In a report by the Audit Commission (1997) hospital postnatal care received more negative comments than any other aspect of care. This was from a sample of 2375 women. Of the 13 trusts in the survey it was evident that a variety of practices existed in the organization of postnatal care. However, most women receive their initial postnatal care in hospital. Although this may not be an ideal environment for the start to family life, certain factors should be considered to ensure that care at this time is conducive to rest and prepares the mother for returning home with a new baby.

Immediate Care after Delivery

In hospital, the woman and her family should be welcomed on arrival at the postnatal ward. At the handover of care, information is required about the events surrounding labour, the type of delivery and the immediate care the mother and baby have received on the labour ward. It is particularly important to ascertain whether the placenta and membranes were delivered complete and the extent of blood loss at delivery. These factors may predispose the mother to anaemia or infection and increase her risk of postpartum haemorrhage. The mother's blood group and rhesus factor should also be noted. Should she require anti-D immunoglobulin, this must be given within 72 hours of delivery.

The midwife needs to ascertain from the mother how she is feeling. She may wish to eat, in which case a meal should be obtained for her, and she must be provided with the opportunity to rest. Palpation of the uterus is carried out to establish that it is well-contracted and the amount of lochia noted. If perineal trauma has been sustained, the midwife assesses the condition of the perineum. Analgesia or the application of a cooling agent, such as crushed ice, may be required. The mother is also asked whether she has passed urine since delivery because the adequacy of urine output must be determined, particularly if events during her labour increase the risk of urinary complications.

The mother must be informed of how to summon help if this is required and, as soon as is practicable, orientated to the ward and introduced to other mothers.

The well-being of the baby is also established (*see* Chapter 12) and the opportunity provided for the mother to feed her infant.

After birth at home, the midwife continues to appraise the health of the mother in the immediate postnatal period. The subsequent activities of the midwife are determined by the needs of the mother. Only when the condition of the mother and baby are deemed satisfactory will the midwife leave the family, ensuring that they know how to obtain help or advice, if required.

Environment

A positive and supportive environment is essential for women during the postnatal period so that their physical, emotional and educational needs can be met.

In hospital most postnatal wards are busy places, but should still be conducive to privacy, rest and sleep. The mother is encouraged to care for herself and shown how to care for her baby in an atmosphere that increases her confidence and self-esteem. Her partner and other children must feel welcome and involved in the care of the infant. Visiting should be sufficiently flexible to enable the family to celebrate the birth of their baby without compromising the need for rest.

The environment should be clean with good toilet and bathroom facilities. Comfortable chairs are important, especially for breastfeeding mothers. A choice of food should be available to meet various cultural and dietary restrictions, with additional hot and cold drinks as required.

Women who give birth at home receive postnatal care in an environment with which they are familiar. The father and other family members may also be involved in the care of the baby during the very early days of life. This assists the early integration of the baby into its new family. Help with the care of other children and household chores is essential to allow the mother adequate rest and sufficient time to spend with her baby.

Accommodation in Hospital

It is usual practice for healthy babies to remain with their mothers for the duration of their stay in hospital. This is considered essential for the development and well-being of both (Department of Health, 1993). A choice of accommodation on the postnatal ward is desirable, but may be restricted by availability. Some women prefer the relative peace and quiet of a single room as opposed to the support and companionship of other mothers in a shared room. In many hospitals accommodation is in rooms with four beds, but this can compromise privacy and unsettled babies may disrupt the sleep of other mothers.

Some women have special needs regarding accommodation in hospital. For example, deaf mothers may feel more isolated by their disability if placed with hearing mothers or they might find it reassuring that they experience similar anxieties about their new infants. A woman who has experienced a stillbirth must be accommodated where she feels most comfortable. If close proximity to other mothers and babies is disturbing, a side ward is essential. Other women may choose not to be in a single room.

Security

The safety of all mothers and babies is paramount while they remain in hospital. Various security initiatives are in place, such as electronic tagging, to minimize the risk of babies being abducted from postnatal wards. It is essential that mothers are aware of this potential danger and allow their baby to be handled only by a known member of staff, or one who is introduced to them and has appropriate identification.

Debriefing

The postnatal period provides an opportunity for reflection on the events surrounding labour and delivery. Debriefing, with both parents, has been identified as an important element in the psychological integration of the birth experience (Craggs, 1995). It is important to listen to the couple and provide appropriate information, explanations and the rationale for management. This is particularly important if emergency treatment was necessary, or the actual events were contrary to expectations. Contacts for debriefing after discharge home should also be given.

Length of Hospital Stay

Women should be free to determine the length of their stay in hospital and, as far as is practicable, return home when they feel ready to be cared for by their families and community midwife. Individual mothers vary in their needs and preferences. Those with good housing conditions and support may opt to leave hospital early to involve other family members in the care of the infant, enhance family integration and minimize family disruption. Other women with poorer social circumstances, heavy domestic responsibilities or who do not feel fully recovered from the delivery may benefit from a longer hospital stay.

A flexible, negotiated approach is important; the woman being the main person to decide when to go home. Taking control of the discharge process has been found positively to influence confidence with parenting abilities (Hall and Carty, 1993) and satisfaction with maternity care (Kenny *et al.* 1993).

The relative merits and disadvantages of early discharge from hospital have been evaluated in a number of studies (Rush *et al.* 1989). Early discharge is not associated with higher readmission rates or adverse consequences in terms of maternal or child health. Improved breastfeeding rates in women discharged early from hospital have also been reported (Carty and Bradley, 1990; Hawthorne, 1994). A planned early discharge from hospital appears to be a safe option, but is not the preference of all women.

The midwife can help a woman to decide when to leave hospital and prepare her for doing so. Consideration should be given to this during the antenatal period, so that sources of physical and emotional support can be identified. This may be available from her partner, close friends or extended family. It should not be assumed that women from ethnic minority groups always have an extended family network of support. Women with multiple pregnancies or disabilities may need to arrange for additional domestic help from the home-help service. The midwife must also provide the woman with a realistic picture of care in hospital if she is to make an informed choice about when to return home (Houston, 1994). A firm decision on the length of stay should not be made until after delivery.

Transfer Home From Hospital

When the woman and her baby are ready to return home, the responsibility for their care is transferred to the community midwife. In the majority of health districts in England, women who have had normal deliveries and who are making a straightforward recovery are discharged home by a midwife (ENB, 1993). Midwifery management of this process ensures that the ongoing needs of the mother and baby are met. A doctor is only required to discharge a mother for whom delivery or the early postpartum period have been complicated. The transfer home of healthy babies by midwives is not yet as widespread, but takes place in 49% of services in England (ENB, 1993).

Good communication throughout the transfer process is essential for a smooth handover of care. Where midwifery care is organized within a team framework, communication problems are less likely and both continuity of care and carer are more easily achieved.

On leaving the hospital, information should be given to the parents about when the community midwife will visit. A 24-hour contact telephone number must also be provided in case help or advice is required (UKCC, 1992). Most babies are transported home by car. The parents should be advised that the baby must be restrained in a car seat or carry-cot in a manner that complies with road safety regulations.

Postnatal Home Visiting

Postnatal care at home is now organized to overcome the fragmentation that was commonly seen in the past. Although different frameworks exist to reflect local needs, such as team midwifery, group practices, domino schemes and caseload management, the aim is to ensure continuity of care. The nature of caring is such that it is a developmental process (Nolte, 1992). To be effective it is therefore imperative that the carer remains constant so that the relationship has time to develop. Ideally, the named midwife to whom the woman is introduced during pregnancy (Department of Health, 1991a) should continue to care for her until the end of the postnatal period.

The frequency of postnatal visits is no longer specified (UKCC, 1986). Instead, 'each midwife is personally responsible and accountable for the exercise of professional judgement and determining appropriate practice in relation to the mother and baby. This naturally includes judgements about the number of visits' (UKCC, 1992). Postnatal visiting patterns are therefore determined by the clinical judgement of the midwife in association with the wishes of the mother (ENB, 1993). However, the Audit Commission (1997) survey of 13 units revealed that the purpose of many visits was unspecified and evidence of their effectiveness was lacking. There is evidence that selective visiting is effective (McCourt and Page, 1996), particulary when it is undertaken by one or more small groups of midwives.

The benefits of selective visiting are increasingly that women are visited according to need, so more time can be spent with women who have problems or who require extra support. Continuity of care is improved and conflicting advice minimized. Selective visiting also encourages self-care and fosters independence; women are able to demonstrate their ability to cope on the days not seen by the midwife, which has the effect of increasing confidence while simultaneously reducing anxiety.

A wide range of practice has been identified in the follow-up of mothers and babies until the 28th day (ENB, 1993). Selective visiting enables the midwife to make greater use of this facility and to see women until the end of the postnatal period. This could be an important factor in limiting the long-term morbidity associated with childbirth. However, despite the facility for midwives to organize postnatal care according to the specific requirements of each mother (UKCC, 1986, 1992), there appears to have been little real change in the actual pattern or content of postnatal visits by midwives.

Transfer from Midwife to the Health Visitor

The discharge of the mother and baby to the care of the health visitor marks the end of midwifery care. The point at which this takes place varies, but is affected by the physical well-being of the mother and baby, the successful establishment of infant feeding and confidence in parenting abilities. Readiness for this is determined by the midwife in association with the mother.

Postnatal Care

Postnatal care is important and can make an enormous difference to women. A review of all aspects of this area of care has been recommended by the Audit Commission

(Box 14.4). Whilst it is important to review care in this area, withdrawal of midwifery services should be resisted until there is evidence to demonstrate how effective the midwife is in this area of women's health. There are a number of randomised controlled trials being undertaken in the UK to try to provide the answer to this question (Henderson, 1997).

Extending midwifery care beyond the present statutory period to enable the midwife to conduct the postnatal examination could be viewed as the natural conclusion to the care initiated at the beginning of pregnancy. This is an aspect that needs considering when reviewing the future provision of postnatal care.

Summary

In this section, the physiology of the puerperium and the principles of woman-centred postnatal care are outlined. The role of the midwife at this time is determined by the specific physiological, emotional and educational needs of women and their families (**Box 14.5**). An individual approach should contribute significantly to care that is sensitive to the mother's needs, ensuring a positive experience.

Box 14.4

Recommendations for Postnatal Care

Clinicians and managers in trust should:

• Involve women in decisions about how long they will stay in hospital and the pattern of postnatal care that they will receive at home.

• Clarify the objectives and set standards for postnatal care in hospital and at home.

• Review staffing and the skill mix required to meet these objectives.

• Promote breastfeeding and monitor breastfeeding rates initially and at the time of discharge from the care of community midwives. This may require investment in the training of breastfeeding support workers.

• Develop guidelines for matching home visiting to the needs of mothers and their families.

• Compare the average lengths of hospital stay for women experiencing each type of delivery with those in other trusts, and investigate and remove administrative procedures that prolong lengths of stay.

The NHS Executive should:

• Prioritise research into effective postnatal care for mothers and babies to help the service develop cost-effective postnatal care?.

Source: Audit Commission. First Class Delivery, 1997, Oxon.

Box 14.5

Reflection on Practice

• Is a physical examination of every mother always necessary? When performed, does it always relate to the type of delivery or the presence of risk factors for complications?

• Is the postnatal ward environment in your practice location conducive to rest, comfort and privacy?

• Are all mothers given a choice of accommodation in hospital? If a policy of 'rooming-in' exists whereby babies remain with their mother at all times, is this conducive to rest and sleep?

• What measures exist to safeguard mothers and babies while resident on the postnatal ward?

• Does each mother have the opportunity to determine her length of stay in hospital?

• Do you make use of the facility to follow-up mothers until the 28th day? Could this be more widely utilized to appraise the ongoing health of the mother and infant?

• Is the postnatal examination at 6 weeks relevant to the needs of women in your care? Are ongoing health problems identified or reported at this consultation?

The midwife must ensure that the benefits of postnatal care are clearly evident. In the future, the effectiveness of midwifery input at this time will be judged in terms of increasing consumer satisfaction, reducing costs and limiting maternal morbidity. The caring activities of the midwife must therefore be relevant to the needs of every woman and her family to ensure that an optimum level of postnatal health is maintained and a satisfactory experience of parenting is achieved.

COMMON POSTPARTUM HEALTH PROBLEMS

Pregnancy is a long and very special journey for a woman ... Maternity services should support the mother, her baby and her family during this journey with a view to their short-term safety but also their long-term well-being.

(Department of Health, 1993, p. ii).
Until recently it was assumed that health problems experienced by women during pregnancy and the puerperium would resolve within about 6 weeks of delivery. Recent studies, however, have found substantial physical morbidity after childbirth and the long-term duration of much of this (MacArthur *et al*. 1991; Glazener *et al*. 1993; Garcia *et al*. 1993). It is now clear that many women are not back to normal within 6 weeks–postnatal care services need to account for this.

Widespread concern about maternity service provision in the UK prompted a fundamental review by the House of Commons Select Committee (1992, known as the Winterton Report). Little specific reference was made in this report to the health needs of women during and beyond the postnatal period, except to note the paucity of good practice. The report of the Expert Maternity Group, *Changing Childbirth* (Department of Health, 1993), emphasized the need for a woman-centred approach, continuity of care and choice, and highlighted the changes necessary to achieve this. Although the general aims apply to postnatal as well as antenatal care, the former received much less attention.

Stress Incontinence

Involuntary loss of urine arises when increased intra-abdominal pressure from coughing, sneezing or other physical activity compresses the bladder. Stress incontinence is experienced by many women and childbirth is the most common cause. It is one of the few postpartum symptoms to be well documented in the literature, but the extent of its occurrence has been established only recently. The precise causative roles of pregnancy and delivery factors are still not fully understood.

Stress incontinence is a frequent complaint during pregnancy, particularly the last trimester, when about half of primigravidae and most multigravidae are affected (Stanton *et al*. 1980). Studies of postpartum stress incontinence have documented a prevalence of 15–25% (Sleep, 1991; MacArthur *et al*. 1993a; Johanson *et al*. 1993).

Recent work has also shown that stress incontinence after delivery can persist for months or even years. A trial to compare restrictive and liberal episiotomy policies assessed stress incontinence as one of its longer term outcome measures and found that 19% of women in both trial groups (episiotomy made no difference) complained of stress incontinence at 3 months (Sleep and Grant, 1987a) and 33% at 3 years after delivery (Sleep and Grant, 1987b). MacArthur *et al*. (1993a), in a study of health problems after childbirth among 11701 women, found that 15% had stress incontinence as a new symptom, and a further 5% had recurrent symptoms. Over two-thirds of these women still had the symptom at 1 and 9 years after delivery. A subsequent study by the same group again found 22% reported stress incontinence occurring within 3 months of delivery and lasting for over 6 weeks, with 77% of these still symptomatic at 6–7 months postpartum (Bick and MacArthur, 1995a).

It has traditionally been assumed that a difficult delivery predisposes women to stress incontinence; however, more recent studies have identified which those particular delivery factors are. Investigations of childbirth-related predictors included epidemiological and urodynamic studies. Urodynamic studies, which measured changes in pelvic floor innervation after particular types of delivery, found innervation damage to be more common in multiparas, after a long second stage and the delivery of a heavier baby. One research group found an association between damage and forceps delivery (Snooks *et al*. 1984), but others found no forceps relationship (Allen *et al*.

1990). No studies found evidence of innervation damage after Caesarean section.

Epidemiological studies of stress incontinence within the general population found it occurred more frequently in multiparae, with prevalence generally rising with parity (Thomas *et al.* 1980). More specific symptom-predictors are difficult to obtain from general population surveys, without access to obstetric information. MacArthur *et al.* (1991), based on a postpartum population with symptom information from women linked to case note data, related numerous obstetric factors to stress incontinence first occurring after a nominated delivery. They showed that the proportion of women who experienced stress incontinence increased with maternal age; after the first birth 13% of women under 25 years reported stress incontinence, compared with 18% aged 25–29 years and 21% aged 30 years or over. Heavier birthweight and longer second stage were also significant predictors, again these factors showing a substantial range: 15% reported stress incontinence after delivering a baby of under 3200g, compared with 19% with weights over 3700g; and 13% after a second stage of up to 30 minutes compared with 22% after 90 minutes or longer. Instrumental delivery was not related to stress incontinence after second stage duration had been taken into account, except for a slight increase with rotational forceps. Women delivered by elective or emergency section were less likely to report stress incontinence than those delivered vaginally. Even after abdominal delivery, however, older mothers still experienced significantly more stress incontinence than younger women, although heavier birthweight only had an effect in vaginal deliveries. Asian women were less likely to report stress incontinence than Caucasian or Afro-Caribbean women, but this could be caused by reporting bias and requires further study.

Few women with stress incontinence seek medical consultation. In one general population study, symptomatic women were asked why they did not consult (Jolleys, 1988). One-half did not reply, but among responders almost one-half did not feel the symptoms posed a problem; one-quarter thought the symptoms occurred too infrequently to warrant seeking treatment and one-fifth felt that it was a normal female problem. Holst and Wilson (1988), in a New Zealand general population sample, also found that women with incontinence did not see this as abnormal, so did not consult. After childbirth, fewer than one in six women with persistent stress incontinence consult a doctor (MacArthur *et al.* 1991; Bick and MacArthur 1995a). When asked why not, the most common responses were similar; the problem was not considered bad enough or it was merely an expected consequence of childbirth.

The severity of stress incontinence has been assessed by the need to wear pads to protect against leakage. Sleep and Grant (1987a), who studied the effectiveness of PFEs, found that at 3 months postpartum 24% of symptomatic women needed to wear pads at some time, although only 6% needed them all the time. In another study by the same authors, a similar proportion of symptomatic women still required pads 3 years after delivery (Sleep and Grant, 1987b). Bick and MacArthur (1995a) showed that 47% of women with stress incontinence questioned at 6–7 months had needed to wear pads at some time since the birth. Women also rated symptom severity on a visual analogue scale (VAS), which showed that stress incontinence was not rated as severe, with more than half rating it in the lower quartile of the VAS. Yet almost one-third of the women with stress incontinence said symptoms affected their activities sporting activities, aerobics and jogging being most commonly mentioned.

One of the most common treatments for stress incontinence is PFEs (Lagro-Janssen *et al.* 1991). In a general population-based study of women aged 20–65 years presenting with urinary incontinence (defined as loss of urine twice or more per month), GP instruction in PFEs was found to be beneficial. A greater proportion of the PFE group reported subsequently being either dry or only mildly incontinent than the control group, although the study numbers, 33 per group, were small (Lagro-Janssen *et al.* 1991).

A large randomized trial of the effect of PFE instruction given immediately after childbirth, however, showed no effect on stress incontinence at 3 months postpartum (Sleep and Grant, 1987a). At the time of this study intervention in 1985, women generally remained in hospital for several days postpartum, so routinely most received daily group-based PFE instruction from an obstetric physiotherapist. The additional input for the women in the intervention group was daily individual instruction from the study midwife until hospital discharge and a health diary for the next 4 weeks as a memory aid to encourage PFE compliance. Telephone reminders were also given and on the 10th day the community midwife visited to assess PFE compliance. The lack of difference in the groups at 3 months follow-up implied that teaching PFE is not worthwhile. The authors were uncertain, however, about how different the PFE in the groups actually was, because routine PFE instruction was already substantial and a study-induced heightened PFE awareness might have enhanced teaching, generally resulting in more PFE in the control group. Although PFE after childbirth is still considered beneficial the evidence is inconclusive.

Wilson *et al.* (1992) considered whether the provision of detailed PFE instruction given to women still symptomatic at 3 months might be effective. A pilot study indicated that this could be beneficial and a larger study is ongoing.

It is certainly clear that if PFE is to have any effect it must be performed correctly and adequate advice is required to ensure this (Bo *et al.* 1988). Women are now discharged from hospital much earlier so postnatal instruction from an obstetric physiotherapist is less common, with other professionals unlikely to have taken on this role. Most women are now given no more than antenatal information and a leaflet describing the technique.

In view of the large number of women who experience long-term stress incontinence after childbirth (**Box 14.6**), its identification and treatment requires urgent review.

Perineal Pain and Dyspareunia

The majority of women who deliver vaginally experience some degree of perineal pain following delivery, usually related to the type and extent of trauma, although women with an intact perineum may also sustain painful perineal bruising or swelling. Dyspareunia (painful or difficult intercourse) and timing of the resumption of intercourse may be associated with perineal pain, but these problems can also be experienced independently.

Box 14.6

Stress Incontinence

• Stress incontinence is common after childbirth.
• Risk factors are longer second stage, heavier birthweight baby and older maternal age.
• It is a chronic symptom, but few women seek medical attention.
• Evidence as to the benefit of PFE is inconclusive.

Information on the prevalence of longer term perineal pain and dyspareunia has generally been obtained from these symptoms used as outcome measures in perineal management trials. Trial data, together with findings from observational studies, have shown that at least 10% of women experience perineal pain for longer than the immediate postnatal period (Sleep *et al.* 1984; Johanson *et al.* 1993; Klein *et al.* 1994; Glazener *et al.* 1995). Persistent dyspareunia, although less frequently studied, seems to be even more prevalent. Sleep *et al.* (1984) found it occurred in about 20% of women at 3 months postpartum and Johanson *et al.* (1993) found a similar prevalence among women who had spontaneous deliveries, followed up at 15–24 months postpartum.

These prevalences of perineal pain and dyspareunia mainly refer to women who had spontaneous vaginal deliveries, as these generally comprised the trial populations (*see* later). Studies have found greater prevalences after instrumental deliveries. Glazener *et al.* (1995) found perineal pain experienced 218 months postpartum was up to three times more common after instrumental delivery. Johanson *et al.* (1993) found no significant difference between spontaneous and instrumental deliveries for perineal pain, but significantly more dyspareunia after forceps or vacuum extraction, with over one-third of these women reporting dyspareunia 15–24 months later.

There had been little scientific evidence, but considerable dispute, about perineal management techniques, in particular the use of episiotomy, and their differential effects on the problems described above. In view of this, Sleep and colleagues evaluated the use of episiotomy where the delivery was expected to be spontaneous in a randomized controlled trial (RCT; Sleep *et al.* 1984). Restrictive and liberal episiotomy policies were developed. In the restrictive group the midwives who performed the delivery were asked to avoid episiotomy and only perform an incision if fetal indications (bradycardia, tachycardia, meconium stained liquor) warranted this. In the liberal group, the midwife was instructed to try to prevent a perineal tear. These different policies resulted in more tears and more intact perinea, i.e. fewer episiotomies among women in the restrictive policy group, but there were no differences in perineal pain at 10 days or 3 months postpartum or dyspareunia at 3 months. The only difference was that women in the restrictive group were more likely to have resumed intercourse within a month of delivery. A 3-year follow-up found similar rates of dyspareunia in the two groups (Sleep and Grant, 1987b). These researchers concluded that the rationale that episiotomies are of benefit to womens health in normal deliveries should be re-appraised.

Klein *et al.* (1994) carried out a similar trial in Canada, comparing a policy of restricted episiotomy to fetal and maternal indications with its liberal or routine use. They found that many physicians had great difficulty restricting episiotomy – 40% of those allocated to the restricted group did not change. Nevertheless, overall there were fewer episiotomies in the restricted group and, like Sleep *et al.* (1984), they found no differences at 3 months in perineal pain, urinary, sexual or other perineal outcomes between the groups.

These researchers found that episiotomy among primiparae was associated with more third-or fourth-degree tears, and in view of this and because of the difficulties involved in changing practice, a secondary cohort analysis was undertaken. For this, women were categorized into four groups according to their perineal outcome: intact; spontaneous tear; episiotomy; and episiotomy extending into third-or fourth-degree tear. Comparisons at 3 months showed that women with intact perinea had the strongest pelvic floors (as measured by perineometry), less perineal pain and attempted intercourse sooner. They were least likely to require analgesia or other perineal treatments in the first 10 days. Delayed pelvic floor recovery was found among women who had episiotomy, especially one which extended to a third or fourth degree tear. There were no differences in stress incontinence rates in the four perineal outcome groups, a finding compatible with other studies described above.

The women in this study who had intact perinea were also less likely to report dyspareunia compared with the other perineal outcome groups. The other three groups did not differ significantly from each other in the timing of first intercourse, but dyspareunia was most common with a third-or fourth-degree tear, next most common after episiotomy and less common in the spontaneous tear group. The women were also asked about sexual satisfaction at 3 months postpartum, responses being very satisfied, satisfied and not satisfied. The intact group were more likely to be very satisfied, and least likely to say they were not satisfied, with no differences between the other three groups. Like that of Sleep *et al.* (1984), the clear conclusion of this study is that episiotomy should be reserved for specific fetal and maternal indications and that the current North American practice of using episiotomy at routine and high rates should be abandoned.

In addition to the effects of perineal management and trauma on pain and dyspareunia, the effects of perineal suturing have also been examined; it was shown that the type of material and method of suturing can affect outcome.

Spencer *et al.* (1986) compared glycerol-impregnated catgut with untreated chromic catgut, in a RCT. Women whose perineum was sutured with glycerol-impregnated catgut were more likely to experience perineal pain, and at 3-year follow-up 8% of those sutured with glycerol-impregnated catgut still reported dyspareunia, regardless of whether they had given birth again. These researchers concluded that glycerol-impregnated catgut should not be used for perineal repair.

Suture material and different perineal repair techniques were compared by Mahomed *et al.* (1989) in a RCT involving 1574 women. Polyglycolic acid sutures (Dexon, Vicryl) were compared with chromic catgut for the repair of the vagina and deep perineal tissue; their use resulted in less short-term perineal pain and need for analgesia than did repair with chromic catgut. Polyglycolic acid, chromic catgut and nonabsorbable silk were compared for repair of perineal skin. No differences were found between the three groups for pain, need for analgesia and wound healing, but nonabsorbable silk was associated with delayed resumption of intercourse at 3 months postpartum.

These researchers also compared continuous subcutaneous sutures with interrupted sutures for perineal skin closure. Fewer women in the subcuticular group reported perineal pain at 10 days, although this difference was not significant. More women whose perinea were repaired with a continuous suture reported dyspareunia at 3 months, but this could be attributed to the fact that more of this group had resumed intercourse. An earlier study by Isager-Sally *et al.* (1986) showed less perineal pain following the use of continuous subcuticular suturing.

Grant (1989), in a systematic review of 14 controlled trials of perineal suturing techniques and suture materials, concluded that polyglycolic acid should be used for deep muscle and skin closure, because it is less likely to be associated with perineal pain and dyspareunia. Glycerol-impregnated catgut should not be used because of its association with perineal pain and long-term dyspareunia. A continuous subcuticular stitch is preferable to interrupted suturing because of the reduced likelihood of short-term perineal pain, with no longer term differences. The effects of the suturing skills of the operator on resultant perineal morbidity have not been examined, although this could make a difference (Enkin *et al.* 1995).

Treatments to relieve perineal pain other than oral analgesia have been assessed. Ultrasound and pulsed electromagnetic therapy do not reduce the incidence of perineal pain at 3 months postpartum (Grant *et al.* 1989), nor do different bath additives (Savlon and salt compared with no additives), although anecdotal reports from women suggest bathing does reduce pain (Sleep and Grant, 1988; Greenshields and Hulme, 1993).

The findings of studies discussed in this section show that episiotomy has no protective effect against stress incontinence, nor is it associated with less perineal pain or dyspareunia. If perineal repair is required, only suture materials associated with less pain and dyspareunia should be used (**Box 14.7**).

Bowel Problems

There are various bowel problems that women experience following childbirth.

Constipation

Constipation is most common in the first few weeks after delivery, but it may occur for longer periods. Glazener *et al.* (1995) found that 7% of their study population reported that constipation continued for more than 2 months after birth and was significantly more common after instrumental delivery. Women who complain of constipation should be encouraged to increase their dietary fibre. The use of laxatives, enemas and other bulk-forming agents has been shown to be ineffective (**Box 14.8**), with side effects of nausea, diarrhoea and abdominal cramps (Shelton, 1980); these should not be administered as a first treatment to postnatal women.

Haemorrhoids

Haemorrhoids often occur in the postnatal period, resulting from the action of progesterone on the bowel, increased varicosity from pelvic pressure and straining during the second stage. Constipation can further exacerbate the situation. Obstetric textbooks generally note that haemorrhoids can cause a great deal of pain for the first few days, but then usually resolve, although they are likely to worsen with successive pregnancies and can eventually become permanent (Hibbard, 1988).

MacArthur *et al.* (1991) found that 8% of women reported haemorrhoids as a new problem within 3 months of the delivery, and an additional 10% as recurrent or ongoing symptoms. In many cases the new haemorrhoids did not resolve quickly; 67% reported symptoms still present when questioned, 19 years after delivery. Haemorrhoids are less likely to occur following a Caesarean delivery. A heavier baby, forceps and longer second stage are all significantly associated with haemorrhoids (**Box 14.8**). There seems to be no cumulative risk to women after their first birth. Glazener *et al.* (1995) found a 15% prevalence of haemorrhoids (new and recurrent) lasting for 218 months, which were more common after instrumental delivery.

Reassurances in obstetric textbooks that haemorrhoids are short-lived, remaining unresolved only after several deliveries, are clearly misplaced. If haemorrhoids continue to be severe, surgical intervention may be necessary.

Faecal Incontinence

Those involved in the treatment of this problem have recognized that women commonly report a history of difficult childbirth. It has generally been assumed that although the underlying injury might occur at delivery, except in rare cases of third-degree tears, incon-

---

Box 14.7

Perineal Pain and Dyspareunia
• Dyspareunia may occur with perineal pain or separately.
• Instrumental delivery is a risk factor for dyspareunia.
• The liberal use of episiotomy does not reduce the incidence of dyspareunia and perineal pain.
• Suture technique and materials can affect perineal pain and dyspareunia.

Box 14.8

Bowel Problems
• Constipation can be persistent after childbirth, but medication must be used advisedly.
• Haemorrhoids are less common after Caesarean delivery.
• Risk factors for haemorrhoids are forceps, longer second stage and heavier birthweight. Postpartum haemorrhoids may become chronic.

tinence symptoms do not appear until many years later (Swash, 1993).

Few studies have examined the prevalence of faecal incontinence after childbirth. Sleep *et al.* (1984), in their trial of the effect of PFEs on urinary incontinence, reported as an incidental finding that 3% of women experienced occasional faecal loss. Most studies of this problem are very recent and have focused on the relationships between obstetric factors and both neurological damage to the pelvic floor (Snooks *et al.* 1990) and mechanical or structural damage to the anal sphincter (Sultan *et al.* 1993). Developments in investigative techniques, especially endosonography and manometry, have enabled imaging of the anal sphincters and the detection of mechanical abnormalities or injury to the external and internal sphincters. There is debate as to the relative effects of mechanical or innervation damage.

One prospective study investigated the antenatal and postnatal development of sphincter damage (Sultan *et al.* 1993). This examined women at 34 weeks gestation and 68 weeks postpartum, to investigate associations between injury and type of delivery. Of 202 women examined antenatally, 150 returned for postnatal follow-up and the 32 with structural abnormalities had a 6 months follow-up. At each assessment a questionnaire recorded symptoms of faecal urgency (inability to defer defecation for more than 5 minutes), and faecal incontinence, including incontinence of flatus. Anal endosonography showed no sphincter defects antenatally among 79 primiparae who delivered vaginally, but at 68 weeks 35% had defects. Among the multiparae, 40% had defects antenatally and 44% at postnatal follow-up. The authors suggest that anal sphincter damage is more likely following a first delivery, given that defects among the primiparae are more comparable to the antenatal incidence of defects among multiparae.

The main obstetric predictor of sphincter damage in this study was forceps delivery: 8 of the 10 women delivered by forceps had sphincter defects. No defects occurred in the five women who delivered with vacuum extraction. Sphincter defects were more common than the symptoms, so women could have abnormalities without experiencing faecal incontinence. A further study by the same group examined 26 primiparae delivered by forceps, 17 by vacuum extraction and 47 spontaneous deliveries. Defects and symptoms were again significantly more likely among the forceps deliveries. In both studies few women with symptoms sought medical consultation.

Third-degree tears involving the external or internal anal sphincter occur in 0.52% of vaginal deliveries and are known to increase the risk of faecal incontinence (Kamm, 1994). Risk factors for third-degree tear were found to be forceps delivery, birthweight of over 4kg, an occipitoposterior position at delivery and primiparity (Sultan *et al.* 1994). Of 8603 women in this study, 50 (0.6%) sustained third-degree tear, 94% of whom had at least one risk factor. Of these 50 women, 34 were interviewed and investigated further and matched for parity, age and ethnic origin with 88 controls, none of whom had ever had a third degree tear. Anal endosonography showed that sphincter defects in women with a third-degree tear were usually along the full length of the sphincter, whereas among the controls only part of the sphincter length showed a defect. Inadequate repair of third-degree tear, resulting from failure to identify the components of the sphincter, led to poor functional ability. There is concern that third-degree tears are not correctly defined by doctors and midwives, who also may have limited knowledge of their repair (Sultan *et al.* 1995).

Faecal incontinence has been described in detail because of the extreme effect it has on womens lives, yet few spontaneously report it, possibly because of embarrassment. It is not known how long faecal incontinence persists after birth or how severe it is. Much-needed studies are currently ongoing. To date, the populations on which information is based are small and, because women had to agree to have anal and perineal assessments, may not be representative. Nevertheless it is clear that faecal incontinence is a more common immediate consequence of childbirth than previously thought, is likely to occur more often after instrumental delivery and, without sensitive questioning, most women are reluctant to report it (**Box 14.9**).

Box 14.9

Faecal Incontinence

• Few studies have examined the prevalence of postpartum faecal incontinence.
• Investigative techniques have enabled detection of anal sphincter injury.
• Sphincter damage is more likely following a first delivery.
• Instrumental delivery and third-degree tears are risk factors.
• Women are reluctant to report this condition.

Backache and Other Musculoskeletal Symptoms

There are a number of musculoskeletal symptoms that can occur in the postpartum period. Backache is by far the most common of these; others occur much less frequently.

One-half of pregnant women experience backache during pregnancy (Ostgaard and Andersson, 1991; Berg *et al.* 1988). The hormonal effects of relaxin on the ligaments and altered posture to accommodate the weight of the gravid uterus are the main causes. Previous backache history and a strenuous physical occupation during pregnancy have been associated with back pain occurrence. Berg *et al.* (1988) studied pregnancy back pain in 862 women and found that almost 10% developed pain severe enough to discontinue work. They followed up the severe cases 6–12 months postpartum and found that backache persisted in two-thirds of these cases.

Backache immediately after delivery has been documented in a few studies, the results based on women questioned on the postnatal ward (Grove, 1973). Although 40% reported backache while in hospital, there was no suggestion that this developed into a long-term symptom.

Long-term backache has been documented more recently. MacArthur *et al.* (1991), in a study of 11701 deliveries, found that 14% of women reported new backache starting after delivery and lasting over 6 weeks: two-thirds of these still had backache at questioning, 19 years after the birth. Ostgaard and Andersson (1992), in a study of 817 women, examined backache prevalence during pregnancy and 12 months after delivery; 67% experienced back pain immediately after delivery and 37% of these still had back pain at follow-up, around 18 months later. Garcia and Marchant (1993) found 20% of 90 women questioned at 8 weeks postpartum had backache, and Glazener *et al.* (1993) found 20% of 1249 women had backache for 2–18 months after the birth. Bick and MacArthur (1995a) found 46% of 1278 women questioned 6–7 months postpartum reported backache within 3 months of delivery and lasting over 6 weeks; 12.8% had new backache, the remainder starting during pregnancy or previously. Three-quarters of the symptomatic women still had backache at questioning. It is clear that nontransient postpartum backache is common.

Various factors have been associated with long-term postnatal backache, in particular epidural analgesia during labour. MacArthur *et al.* (1990) found that 18.9% of women who had an epidural reported new long-term backache compared with 10.5% who did not have an epidural. This excess remained after taking into account that more women who have epidurals have difficult deliveries. The only circumstance in which there was no excess backache after epidural was in elective sections, where the woman had not laboured. The backache-producing mechanism hypothesized by these researchers was postural tensions on the musculoskeletal system from positions adopted during labour are affected by relaxin and exacerbated when mobility and discomfort-feedback are inhibited by epidural block. A National Childbirth Trust report had already noted that backache was the most frequently mentioned long-term side effect of epidurals, but this was from a self-selected group of women (Kitzinger, 1987). Other UK studies using representative samples subsequently found an epidural-backache association similar to that noted in the first study (Russell *et al.* 1993; Macleod *et al.* 1995).

In contrast to UK studies, work from the USA, found no excess backache at 2 months (Breen *et al.* 1994) or at 12–18 months postpartum (Groves *et al.* 1994) among women who had epidural deliveries. The epidurals used, however, differed from those used in the UK studies, being administered by continuous infusion and containing a lower concentration of bupivacaine mixed with an opiate, fentanyl, which allows women to remain mobile even ambulate in 70% of cases. New postpartum backache was associated with shorter stature and heavier maternal weight. Ongoing or recurrent backache was associated with a previous history of back pain, younger age and heavier weight.

Other risk factors have also been found. MacArthur *et al.* (1991; 1993a) found that Asian women had more backache than Caucasian women: 21% of Asian women reported new long-term backache compared with 14% of Caucasian women. This study found no relationship between back pain and height, and maternal weight data were unavailable.

Few studies obtained information on the severity of postpartum backache, or its effect on womens lives. Russell *et al.* (1993) included an assessment of backache type and severity to determine whether epidural–backache differed from nonepidural backache in these respects. They invited all 156 study women with backache to the hospital 12–15 months after delivery, but only 36 attended. Assessment of these 36 found pain was not generally severe and neither severity nor type of backache differed between epidural and nonepidural groups. This information, together with the lack of attendance of the remaining 120, led these anaesthetists to conclude that backache was usually not severe and did not affect daily life. Bick and MacArthur (1995a) included specific questions to women on the severity and effect of back pain and found that although backache presented daily in 40% of cases it was not considered severe by most of the women. Nevertheless, half said their backache affected activities, with lifting and general movement most commonly mentioned.

Few women seek medical consultation for their backache. MacArthur *et al.* (1991) found only 30% of symptomatic women had consulted, and a similar proportion (32%) was found in a second study by the same research team (Bick and MacArthur 1995a). In the second study, women were asked about the treatment they received. Almost half received more than one treatment type, pain-relieving medication being the most common, followed by physiotherapy. A quarter received no treatment and 10% were referred. Women who had not consulted commonly considered their backache not severe enough to warrant medical attention. Many accepted backache as inevitable after childbirth (**Box 14.10**).

Further research is needed to determine whether the epidural backache association is causal, or if other factors are present in women who choose epidural analgesia which account for the association. New epidural techniques that provide enhanced mobility are being introduced in the UK, but with little systematic evaluation of long-term or short-term effects (Howell and Chalmers, 1992). Women should be informed antenatally of the possible association between epidural analgesia and backache, allowing an informed decision about pain relief for labour. After delivery, advice on posture may limit the effects of this common symptom.

Box 14.10

Backache

- Backache is a common long-term postnatal symptom.
- Epidural analgesia has been associated with a new postpartum backache.
- Back pain is not generally severe, but may affect activities.
- Women accept backache as an expected consequence of childbirth.
- Further research is necessary to determine whether the epidural backache relationship is causal.

Headache

Headache and migraine are commonly reported in the general population, with triggers being related to many factors. A few studies documented short-term headaches that occurred after delivery (Grove, 1973; Stein, 1981). Stein (1981) studied 100 women and found that 33% reported headaches during the first postpartum week. Grove (1973), within the first 6 postpartum days, questioned 187 women who had a vaginal delivery, one-quarter of whom experienced headaches. None had received epidural anaesthesia. This work was prompted by a headache rate of 20% among women who had been given an epidural in the same hospital there was concern that this might be blamed on the epidural. The similar rates reassured the anaesthetists that it was not.

More recent studies show that women experience longer term headaches after childbirth (MacArthur *et al.* 1991; Russell *et al.* 1993; Glazener *et al.* 1993). MacArthur *et al.* (1991) found 3.6% of women reported new-onset, frequent headaches and 1.4% reported migraine within 3 months of delivery that lasted over 6 weeks. Russell *et al.* (1993) found 3.7% of women reported new post-delivery headaches that lasted longer than 6 months, and Glazener *et al.* (1995) found 15% reported headaches that lasted 2–18 months, although this included new and recurrent headaches.

Although earlier studies suggested that no excess in short-term headaches occurred after epidural, some recent evidence indicates a relationship for longer term headaches. Kitzinger (1987), in her descriptive study of women's experiences of epidurals, found 3% reported long-term headaches as side effects of the procedure. MacArthur *et al.* (1992), in a study of 11701 deliveries, showed that 4.6% of women reported headaches and 1.9% migraine that lasted over 6 weeks after epidural, compared with 2.9% and 1.1%, respectively, with no epidural. This epidural-related excess remained after taking account of confounding factors. Women delivered by Caesarean section had higher headache rates, regardless of epidural usage. In contrast, Russell *et al.* (1993) found no association between epidural analgesia and headache lasting over 6 months. Dewan *et al.* (1993) found no association, but only examined symptoms in the first 4 days postpartum. MacArthur *et al.* (1991) found that younger age and lower social class were also independent predictors of headaches, possibly resulting from additional stresses among these groups.

The severity of postpartum headaches was investigated by Bick and MacArthur (1995a); 254 (20%)

of 1278 women questioned 6–7 months postpartum reported frequent headaches (new and recurrent) within 3 months that lasted over 6 weeks, 88% of which were unresolved at questioning. Two-thirds experienced headaches several times a week, and over 50% rated them above the halfway point on a VAS. Over two-thirds said their symptoms affected activities, many having to stop and rest until the symptoms had resolved. Almost half of the women sought medical advice, a higher consultation rate than is common for postpartum symptoms. The majority who consulted received analgesics or no treatment, confirming reasons given by women who did not consult that they could self-treat with analgesics.

Postdural puncture headaches can occur within the days aft er an accidental dural puncture (Brownridge, 1983) or after spinal anaesthesia. Accidental dural puncture occurs during administration of the epidural cannula into the epidural space, when the dura mater (the membrane supporting the arachnoid mater) is inadvertently punctured, allowing the escape of some cerebro spinal fluid (CSF). In a dedicated spinal anaesthesia (increasingly used for elective section), the dura mater is deliberately punctured to administer the analgesia into the subarachnoid space. Leakage of CSF produces traction of the meninges, which leads to severe postural headache and neck stiffness, sometimes accompanied by photophobia, auditory disturbance and nausea. Fine-bore needles now used for spinal anaesthesia minimize spinal headaches (Smith *et al.* 1994), but require greater skill on the part of the anaesthetist (Reynolds, 1993). An accidental puncture during epidural administration is rare, occurring in 0.1% of cases, but because the needle is larger, CSF fluid is more likely to escape, so that a postdural puncture headache almost always follows.

Postdural puncture headaches were considered to resolve within a short time after delivery. However, MacArthur *et al.* (1993b) found longer term headache and migraine among 74 women who had an accidental dural puncture; 23% reported these symptoms, compared with 7.1% of women who had an epidural but no dural puncture, and 4.8% who had no epidural. Ten women still had symptoms at enquiry, 1–9 years after delivery. There have also been case reports of similar long-term headache symptoms after dural puncture (Scott and Hibbard, 1990).

Women who have epidural anaesthesia should be informed of possible side effects, including the risk of headache. Postnatally, women should be asked about the headaches and be told who to contact should onset occur after discharge (Stride and Cooper, 1993).

Visual Disturbances

Visual disturbances are not common, but have been reported (De Lange *et al.* 1988; MacArthur *et al.*, 1991). De Lange *et al.* (1988) found a small proportion of women, 14%, who complained of visual disturbances after spinal anaesthesia for elective section. Most symptoms were short term, but in two cases eye problems, diagnosed as pericentral ring scotomata, persisted for 1 and 4 years. MacArthur *et al.* (1991) asked women about the presence of flashing lights or spots before the eyes as part of their survey of postnatal health; 1.5% reported these as new symptoms that lasted over 6 weeks. Both general and spinal anaesthesia were significantly associated with these visual disturbances, which were unaccompanied by migraine-type headaches.

Neck and Shoulder Pain

Neckache was reported in the above study in 2% of cases, and shoulder pain in 2.2%, as new symptoms that lasted over 6 weeks. Neckache (but not shoulder pain) was associated with epidural analgesia, but only if the pain started within a week of delivery; 2.4% of women reported neckache after epidural compared with 1.6% of those who had no epidural. Neck and shoulder pains starting after birth and lasting at least 6 months were reported by 5.7% in the study by Russell *et al.* (1993), but these were not associated with epidural analgesia.

Long-term and short-term neck and shoulder pains have been associated with general anaesthesia (GA) and Caesarean section (MacArthur *et al.* 1991; Dewan *et al.*, 1993). The link is plausible, potentially arising from neck positioning to facilitate intubation, with a musculoskeletal system rendered much more sensitive by the effects of relaxin and, under GA, also unprotected by muscle tone.

Paraesthesias

Carpel tunnel syndrome (CTS) is often experienced during pregnancy, particularly in the third trimester (Wand, 1990), and other upper limb symptoms have been reported (McLennan *et al.* 1987). Carpel tunnel syndrome that persisted during the puerperium was examined in one study of 2358 women–all symptoms were found to have resolved by 6 weeks (Wand, 1990). Tingling in the hands has been associated with epidural analgesia (MacArthur *et al.* 1991) 3% of women who had an epidural reported this compared with 2.2% who had no epidural. There have also been reports of paraesthesias in the legs and buttocks after epidural anaesthesia (Kitzinger, 1987; Scott and Hibbard, 1990; MacArthur *et al.* 1992), although these symptoms are uncommon.

Pain in the Legs

Weight gain, altered metabolism and hormonal effects on the venous blood supply are factors relevant to the occurrence of painful legs during pregnancy. Varicose veins, which can be painful, often appear or worsen during pregnancy and can become permanent (Llewellyn-Jones, 1990). Apart from this, leg pain as a postpartum symptom has rarely been examined (Lee et al. 1990; MacArthur et al. 1991). Lee (1990) reviewed 12 papers that reported thromboembolic episodes during and after pregnancy, and showed that 28% of 210 women with a deep vein thrombosis were diagnosed postpartum. MacArthur et al. (1991) found that 2.1% of women reported painful legs as a new symptom, which were more common after a longer first stage (**Box 14.11**).

Asian women in the series investigated by MacArthur *et al.* (1991) seemed more susceptible generally to musculoskeletal symptoms; 31% of Asian women had one or more musculoskeletal symptom compared with 19.1% of Caucasian women. The Asian proclivity for pains and weaknesses in the arms and legs is especially large. A possible biological

explanation could be vitamin-D deficiency and associated osteomalacia. Osteomalacia is known to exist among British Asians because of dietary deficiencies and to lack of sunlight, resulting from cultural factors associated with limited pursuits outside the home, custom of dress and other lifestyle factors (MacArthur *et al.* 1993c). Further research into the effects of childbirth on the health of Asian women is needed.

Breast Problems

There are positive benefits to the health and development of infants when breastfeeding is continued to at least 4 months of age (Howie *et al.* 1990). Most women in the UK intend to breastfeed and many commence this, yet during the first 2 weeks the number who continue declines rapidly. Reasons for discontinuing breastfeeding include painful, engorged breasts and sore nipples, as well as anxiety about insufficient milk. Even if breast pain does not result in the discontinuation of feeding, the discomfort produced can be considerable and last several weeks.

Mothers should be advised as to how to avoid engorgement, which occurs when the volume of breast milk is allowed to collect in the alveoli and pressure is not relieved. Irregular feeding or incorrect positioning of the baby can result in incomplete emptying of the milk ducts, the breast becoming hard, red and hot. Various treatments have been suggested to relieve engorgement. Early trials evaluated the benefits of manual expression of breast milk, but these were also based on restricted feeding regimes with which engorgement is common (Inch and Renfrew, 1989). A small trial on the effect of placing cold cabbage leaves on engorged breasts at 72 hours postpartum did not affect engorgement, although slightly more women in the experimental group were still exclusively breastfeeding at 6 weeks (Nikodem *et al.* 1993). Controlled studies to evaluate the effects of oxytocin failed to find any benefit in relieving engorgement. Unrestricted demand feeding and correct positioning of the baby at the breast are still the most effective measures to both prevent and treat engorgement.

Mastitis, an inflammatory reaction to a blockage or pressure placed on the breast, can be infective or noninfective and is usually painful. A substantial proportion of women have no infection, but if conservative measures to relieve the blockage fail, infection can occur. Encouraging the woman to maintain breastfeeding, ensuring unrestricted feeds, can relieve

---

Box 14.11

Other Musculoskeletal Symptoms

• Postpartum headaches can be painful, occur several times a week and affect activities.

• There may be an association between epidural anaesthesia and headaches.

• Women who have epidural or spinal anaesthesia should be monitored for postdural puncture headache.

• Long-term neckache and shoulder pain have been reported after general anaesthesia.

• Asian women appear more susceptible to postpartum musculoskeletal problems.

noninfectious mastitis. Treatment for infective mastitis requires antibiotics.

Sore nipples result from incorrect positioning of the baby on the breast; this is one of the main reasons to discontinue breastfeeding (White *et al.* 1992). Gradually increasing the duration of sucking from each breast does not prevent sore or cracked nipples (Enkin *et al.* 1995). Restricted compared with unrestricted duration of feeds was not related to the occurrence of sore or cracked nipples, although significantly more mothers in the restricted group had stopped breastfeeding completely by 6 weeks. Various preparations are available to treat nipple pain, but there is no scientific evidence to justify any of these. Nor have any benefits been shown after rubbing colostrum or expressed breast milk onto the nipples, another practice traditionally thought beneficial. Nipple shields are unacceptable to most mothers, and may anyway reduce milk production.

Breast pain can also occur in women who do not breastfeed, as a result of engorgement until lactation is suppressed. The supply-and-demand physiology eventually results in the spontaneous cessation of lactation. Sometimes, however, especially following the loss of a baby, it is important to suppress lactation quickly. Pharmacological and physical measures can be adopted. Medications include bromocriptine, which reduces lactation in the first postpartum week, but has been associated with pain, engorgement and continued lactation in the longer term (Shapiro, 1984). Cabergoline is recommended as the drug of choice, as it has fewer longer term side effects than bromocriptine, although more information is necessary with regard to dosage and timing of administration for this newer drug (Enkin *et al.* 1995).

Many nonpharmacological methods have not been fully evaluated. One small trial compared fluid restriction and the wearing of brassieres, and showed that women who restricted their fluid intake reported less breast pain (Brooten *et al.* 1983). Physical methods of suppressing lactation, for example breast binding, may be more painful in the short term, but more effective in the longer term and have no side-effects.

Efforts to minimize problems should include explaining the physiological processes of breastfeeding to mothers and giving information on what to do if feeding becomes painful (**Box 14.12**).

Fatigue

Tiredness after birth is commonly regarded as normal, but depending on its duration and severity can be disabling (**Box 14.13**). It is common during pregnancy as a result of the weight of the gravid uterus and disturbed sleep patterns. With earlier hospital discharge, fatigue assessment is more important in the postpartum period, especially because of its possible connection with depression (Unterman *et al.* 1991).

Few studies have investigated postpartum fatigue. It has been examined among breastfeeding mothers (Auerbach, 1984), and the relationship between sleep disturbance and fatigue was investigated in a small sample of employed childbearing women (Lee and DeJoseph, 1992).

Gardner (1991) surveyed fatigue in a sample of 35 women who had a normal vaginal delivery, and were questioned in hospital on the second and third postpartum day and again at 2 and 6 weeks postpartum. Fatigue assessment was based on a 10-point scale (Rhoten, 1982). Mean fatigue levels at 2 days, 2 weeks and 6 weeks were 4.60, 3.96 and 3.51, respectively, indicating that the level of fatigue reduces over time, although not substantially. This study, however,

---

Box 14.12

Breast Pain

- Breast pain may lead to cessation of breastfeeding.
- Mothers must be informed about the importance of correct positioning of the baby and unrestricted feeding.
- There is little scientific evidence regarding topical preparations for sore nipples.

Box 14.13

Women's Comments

I think you should be offered vitamins or iron when you tell the doctor you are constantly tired. They say it is expected as you've just had a baby. I think I would have benefited from iron tablets, but my doctor never tested my blood.

was small and based on a population referred to as a convenience sample, so likely to be unrepresentative.

MacArthur *et al.* (1991) found that 12.2% of 11701 women reported fatigue as a new problem and 5% as recurrent or ongoing. Fatigue rarely resolved within a few weeks of delivery; 39% of the women who reported this had it for a year or more.

Obstetric factors associated with fatigue are multiple birth, a longer first stage, Entonox during labour and a postpartum haemorrhage. Older age and unmarried status were also associated with fatigue. Unmarried women, older women and those with multiple births experienced fatigue of especially long duration.

In addition to examining the prevalence of fatigue, a follow-up to this study included questions on the extent and severity of the problem and its effect on the womens lives (Bick and MacArthur, 1995a). Fatigue (new, recurrent or ongoing) that lasted over 6 weeks was reported by 41% of the sample, 80% of whom still had it 6–7 months after delivery. The greater prevalence in this study compared with the first is accounted for by the shorter time that had elapsed between birth and questioning, because fatigue is likely to be a condition that women forget over time.

Many of these women had fatigue as a daily occurrence, with few reporting it as intermittent or occasional. They were asked to rate severity on a VAS scale, and gave a mean rating of over 60. Fatigue affected physical and psychological aspects of the womens lives; 30% with fatigue said they did not feel like doing anything, whereas others mentioned specific tasks as being difficult (15%) or temper or concentration levels being affected (15%). Only 29% of women with fatigue sought medical consultation. Women who did not consult said they knew the cause of their symptom was an expected consequence of childbirth and thus there was no need for consultation.

The relationship between fatigue and PPH prompted the consideration that some symptomatic women have undiagnosed anaemia. Discharge before the third postpartum day (when haemoconcentration takes place) is common, so most women do not have a valid haemoglobin (Hb) test. A Hb check is not routinely incorporated into community postnatal care. Only 22% of women with PPH and 23% of those with a third-day Hb of <10.5g/dl had a blood test as part of their 6-week postnatal discharge examination; among those without these risk factors a blood test was even less common (Bick and MacArthur, 1995b).

Social support is an important factor that can contribute to a mothers well-being and limit her experience of fatigue, but it may not always be available (Oakley, 1992). Health professionals responsible for providing postnatal care should take social support factors into consideration when planning care (**Box 14.14**).

Depression and Unhappiness after Childbirth

Traditionally, mood disorders after childbirth have been classified as the blues, postnatal depression and puerperal psychosis, the most severe form. Postnatal emotional disorder is one of the few areas of maternal health to have been extensively investigated.

Postnatal blues are usually transient, lasting 24–48 hours, occurring between the third and tenth day and experienced by up to 80% of mothers (Riley, 1995). The mother may be upset over seemingly trivial issues (**Box 14.15**), but this rarely presents a major problem. The most serious manifestation of postnatal psychiatric illness, puerperal psychosis, is rare with an incidence of 12/1000 births, but very severe (Brockington and

---

Box 14.14
Fatigue
• Postpartum fatigue can be a long-term problem.
• Fatigue is likely to occur daily, be severe and affect physical and psychological well-being.
• A postnatal Hb check could be incorporated into the 6-week check to detect undiagnosed anaemia.

Box 14.15
Women's Comments
I wish people would give more attention to the 'baby blues', which happened to me 5–6 days after my baby was born. No great attention was paid to it and no real support was given. I was told it's just one of those things and you'll get over it. You do – but for those 2–3 days it seems like a lifetime.

Cox-Roper, 1988). It has a sudden onset and is easily recognized, the woman adopting strange behaviours, possibly hypomania, hallucinations or delusions. Psychiatric referral and treatment are essential; if diagnosed hospitalization is common. Primiparae are most at risk (Kendell *et al.* 1987).

The most commonly diagnosed postnatal emotional disorder is depression. There are differing estimates of the prevalence of depression after childbirth, varying according to the definition used and the timing of assessment, but the prevalence most commonly quoted is around 10% (Cox *et al.* 1993; Unterman *et al.* 1990). Psychiatric services recognize that many cases of depression after childbirth do not reach the threshold for referral (Brockington and Cox-Roper, 1988), others go unreported to health professionals (Unterman *et al.* 1990) and some women do not even admit feelings of unhappiness to their partner or family.

There is a current debate as to whether postnatal depression is a distinct condition, given the lack of specific definition and evidence that there is a similar prevalence in nonchildbearing women (O'Hara *et al.* 1990). Cox *et al.* (1993) compared depression in 232 postnatal women with a control group who had either not been pregnant or had not delivered a baby in the previous 12 months. The depression rate in the postnatal group was three times higher when onset was within the first month, but after this, onset declined and comparison with nonchildbearing women at 6–12 months showed no increased risk in the postnatal group.

The duration of depression after childbirth can be considerable. Kumar and Robson (1984) found 16% of 119 primiparas were depressed 3 months after delivery and 8% still depressed 4 years after birth. MacArthur *et al.* (1991) found self-reported new depression that lasted over 6 weeks in 12% of women and 5% had recurrent depression. Most cases of new depression (60%) resolved within a year. Cooper *et al.* (1988), in a study of 483 women, found that 5% were still depressed 1 year after delivery. Clearly, depression can be a long-standing problem triggered by birth for some women, although most cases resolve within a year.

Studies of risk factors of postnatal depression have produced conflicting findings. One risk factor consistently found, however, is a personal or close family history of depressive illness. Watson *et al.* (1984) showed that 60% of women diagnosed as depressed at 6 weeks postpartum had a previous personal history of psychiatric consultation. Difficulty in a woman's relationship with her partner is another consistently documented risk factor (Kumar and Robson, 1984; Watson *et al.* 1984; O'Hara, 1986).

Other factors show much less consistency. Older mothers (Kumar and Robson, 1984) and younger mothers have been found in different studies to be at risk of postnatal depression (Zajicek and Wolkind, 1978), whereas others have found no age relationship (Pitt, 1968). Excess depression has been shown to follow a first delivery (Pitt, 1968; Bridge *et al.* 1985) and among multiparas (Tod, 1964), whereas others have found no parity relationship (Cox *et al.* 1982). Being unmarried has been associated with depression in some studies (O'Hara, 1986; MacArthur *et al.* 1991), but others found no association with marital status (Watson *et al.* 1984).

Breastfeeding mothers were more depressed in some studies (Romito, 1988; Alder and Cox, 1983). In contrast, Hannah *et al.* (1992) found a positive association with artificial feeding, while Kumar and Robson (1978) and Paykel *et al.* (1980) found no relationship with type of infant feeding.

Obstetric procedures, for example induction of labour, forceps delivery, epidural analgesia and Caesarean section, have been associated with postnatal depression in some studies (Jacoby, 1987; Kumar and Robson, 1984). Maternal loss of control over the birth process resulting from the intervention is the mechanistic hypothesis proposed. Other studies, however, found no links with the obstetric interventions examined (O'Hara and Zekowski, 1988; Playfair and Gower, 1981).

Considering the varying and sometimes unclear definitions of depression used in the different studies, it is not surprising that findings vary so much. A self-complete scale, the EPDS, has been shown to be a good tool with which to screen for postnatal depression (Cox *et al.* 1987). It has been specifically designed for postpartum women, is easily administered by midwives or health visitors and takes only a few minutes to complete. It is a screening rather than a diagnostic tool – if women have high scores, then referral to the appropriate professionals is necessary.

The continuity of care advocated by *Changing Childbirth* (Department of Health, 1993) may improve midwifery recognition of depression. Women may feel more confident to admit feelings of unhappiness to a familiar midwife and awareness of behavioural or mood changes indicative of depression is more likely. The use of scales such as EPDS could help the midwife screen for depression and provide the opportunity for women to discuss their emotional well-being (**Box 14.16**).

The 6-Week Postnatal Check

The 6-week postnatal check is the final routine medical assessment and marks the end of the puerperium and the woman's discharge from the maternity services. The value of this check-up in its current form and the necessity for the examinations performed have now been questioned (Bowers, 1985; Sharif *et al.* 1993).

One main component of the 6-week check is a vaginal examination. The purpose of this was investigated by Sharif *et al.* (1993) by studying the GP records of 150 postnatal women for specific indications for a vaginal examination; genital symptoms, smear required or intrauterine contraceptive device insertion. Only 25 (17%) women had an indication, yet all 150 had a vaginal examination. Among the 125 with no indication, only six abnormalities were found, none of which were treated. The authors concluded that routine vaginal examination has no real value and should be abandoned.

Bick and MacArthur (1995b) questioned 1278 women about attendance and content of their postnatal examination. The majority (91%) attended; 93% had an abdominal and 70% a vaginal examination. Even among women delivered by elective Caesarean section, almost half had a vaginal examination. Most of the sample (84%) had blood pressure recorded, 37% had a urine test and 16% a blood test, presumably in most cases to test haemoglobin.

Uptake for the 6-week check is generally high. In the above, uptake was 91% (Bick and MacArthur, 1995b) and in a study in Oldham it was 88% (Bowers, 1985), indicating the acceptability of attending for an examination after having given birth. Some

women reported preferences for the midwife to conduct the examination. Bowers (1985) asked women if the postnatal assessment was worth attending only 17% thought that it was not.

The timing of the postnatal visit is also now being questioned, in view of the studies described earlier which highlighted the persistent nature of morbidity following childbirth. Glazener *et al.* (1993) suggested a postnatal discharge check at 3 months would be more appropriate. Sharif and Jordan (1995) suggested a visit at 2–3 weeks to discuss infant feeding, common short-term problems and contraception (the last because many women resume intercourse by 6 weeks), followed by a visit at 10–12 weeks to identify long-term morbidity.

Clearly, in its current form the postnatal check does not address the health needs of many women, yet it continues to devote time and resources to unnecessary examinations. Further research regarding the content and timing of this check is necessary (**Box 14.17**).

Implications for Midwives

Postnatal care in the days after birth has traditionally been based on various routine observations and examinations, blood pressure recording, temperature and pulse taking and abdominal palpation. A study of midwifery postnatal care by Garcia *et al.* (1994) at the National Perinatal Epidemiology Unit found that midwives performed frequent routine observations which they themselves saw little value in.

The *Midwives Rules* (UKCC, 1993) define the postnatal period as a period of not less than ten and not more than 28 days after the end of labour, during

---

Box 14.16

Depression and Unhappiness after Childbirth

- Depression is a common postnatal emotional disorder.
- Depression can be a long-term problem.
- Use of the EPDS can successfully screen for postnatal depression.
- Continuity of care advocated in *Changing Childbirth* may provide greater opportunity for identification and discussion of emotional problems.

Box 14.17

The 6-Week Postnatal Check

- Uptake for the 6-week check is high.
- The timing and content of the 6 week check should be reviewed.
- There are no apparent benefits to women's health of the routine abdominal and vaginal examinations.
- Other examinations and investigations which may detect conditions are infrequently used.

which the continued attendance of a midwife on the mother is requisite. Before 1986, daily midwifery visits were required to the tenth day. The *Midwives Code of Practice* (UKCC, 1986) dropped the specification of daily visits, and instead a midwifes role during the postnatal period was defined as ... to care for and monitor the progress of the mother in the postnatal period and to give all necessary advice to the mother on infant care to enable her to ensure the optimum progress of the newborn infant. Most health districts have allowed a policy of selective home visiting since then.

The extent to which selective visiting takes place in practice, however, is questionable. Garcia *et al.* (1994), in a questionnaire to all English health districts in 1991, found selective visiting to be variable, with minimal change in many cases. Little is known regarding how midwives determine selectivity in visiting. A pilot project in Glasgow (Twaddle *et al.*, 1993) examined the effect of midwives who followed a brief agenda that required them to plan ongoing care with each woman at the first postnatal visit. Before-and-after assessments found that significantly fewer postnatal visits were made, and there was a reduction in the number of women who saw more than three different midwives during the postnatal period. The constraints of routine and tradition have been suggested as inhibiting midwives from changing practice and providing individual care (Marchant and Garcia, 1995).

The occurrence and duration of the wide range of symptoms experienced by women after childbirth clearly highlights the need for health professionals to evaluate and review the current organization and timing of postnatal care (**Box 14.18**). Using the recommendations of *Changing Childbirth* as an agenda for change (Page, 1993), a substantial input towards the improvement of postnatal care could be undertaken by midwives as the health professionals that women have most contact with.

Once postnatal health problems have been identified, some are amenable to treatment (Garcia and Marchant, 1993). Indeed, for some women to know that they are not abnormal may do much to relieve anxiety (Trevalyan, 1994). However, many women do not initiate consultation about their problems. Some do not consider their symptoms to be serious enough, or feel that no treatment is available or that the symptom will resolve. Some are embarrassed and others feel that they should put up with things. Whatever the reasons, the result is that many women have unmet health needs for substantial periods of time following childbirth. Midwives and other health professionals need to identify the symptoms.

One possibility might be through the use of a symptom checklist, to ask about the presence of the most frequently reported postpartum problems. Women report these if specifically asked, as evidenced by the studies already described. Depending on their nature, some problems may be remediable or require GP referral straightaway. Others might require further monitoring by the midwife. A checklist could be used at the postnatal discharge check to assess more persistent morbidity and allow for follow-up treatment when necessary (**Box 14.19**).

Although recent government reports have emphasized the role and contribution of the midwife, guidance is urgently needed to enable skills and practice to be directed towards providing planned and effec-

---

Box 14.18

Women's Comments

It would be useful if the hospital provided classes where postnatal problems could be explained and dealt with more fully. There is great emphasis on health during pregnancy and the birth, but health afterwards is neglected.

Box 14.19

Implications for Midwives

• Planned postnatal care might lead to fewer home visits and greater continuity of care.
• The current organization and timing of midwifery postnatal care should be reviewed to enable identification and management of morbidity.
• A checklist could be used to ask about the presence of health problems.
• The management of maternal morbidity has important implications for the future health of women.

tive postnatal care for every mother (**Box 14.20**). The largely unacknowledged maternal morbidity which was highlighted by the House of Commons Health Committee (1992) is only marginally addressed by *Changing Childbirth*. The development of a model of midwifery care to identify postpartum health needs is required, a model which should probably be extended beyond the current 6-week period. The identification and management of health needs has implications for the future health of women and reinforces the value and contribution of the midwife to maternal well-being.

Box 14.20

Advice for Women Using the Maternity Services

The recommendations of *Changing Childbirth* are as applicable to postnatal care as to care during pregnancy and labour:

• Health problems are commonly experienced. You are not 'abnormal' if you feel your health has not recovered after giving birth. Report symptoms to your midwife, GP or health visitor.

• Discuss a postnatal care plan with your midwife to outline what advice and support you feel you would benefit from.

• Ask your midwife about local support groups.

KEY CONCEPTS

- Women require continuity of care, consistent advice, accurate information, skilled help and emotional support in the postnatal period.

- The traditional organization and content of postnatal care may not meet the needs of women after childbirth.

- The nature of postnatal care should be determined by the specific needs of each woman and her family.

- The caring activities of the midwife involve the restoration and maintenance of health, the promotion of emotional well-being and the provision of information, education and expert practical advice.

- Postnatal health has been neglected. Studies have now identified widespread and persistent morbidity after childbirth. Some symptoms can be severe and affect a woman's daily activities.

- A physical examination should detect complications, pre-empt morbidity and limit health problems. It should relate to the presence of risk factors for the development of complications.

- Health professionals must identify and manage postnatal health problems.

References

Abbott H: *An evaluation of the contribution of routine temperature and pulse rate measurements to midwives and student midwives assessments of maternal health postpartum*, unpublished MSc Thesis, 1994, University of Surrey.

Alder E, Cox JL: Breast feeding and postnatal depression, *J Psychosom Res* 27:139, 1983.

Allen RE, Hosker GL, Smith ARB: Pelvic floor damage and childbirth: a neurophysiological study, *Br J Obstet Gynaecol* 97(9):770, 1990.

Andolf E, Iosif CS, Jorgensen C, *et al.*: Insidious urinary retention after vaginal delivery: prevalence and symptoms at follow-up in a population-based study, *Gynecol Obstet Invest* 38(1):51, 1994.

Audit Commission: *First class delivery: Improving maternity services in England and Wales*, London, 1997, Audit Commission.

Auerbach KG: Employed breast feeding mothers: problems they encounter, *Birth* 11:17, 1984.

Berg G, Hammar M, Mollernielsen J, *et al.*: Low back pain during pregnancy, *Obstet Gynaecol* 71(1):71, 1988.

Bick DE, MacArthur C: The extent, severity and effect of health problems after childbirth, *Br J Midwifery* 3(1):27, 1995a.

Bick D, MacArthur C: Attendance, content and relevance of the six week postnatal examination, *Midwifery* 11(2):69, 1995b.

Bo K, Larsen S, Oseid S, *et al.*: Knowledge about and ability to correct pelvic floor muscle exercises in women with urinary stress incontinence, *Neuro Urodynam* 7(3):261, 1988.

Bowers J: *Uptake of six weeks postnatal examination by puerperal women in Oldham*. Paper submitted in fulfilment of the requirement for a BSc in Nursing Studies, May 1984, held at Royal College of Midwives Library.

Bowers J: Is the 6 week postnatal examination necessary? *Practitioner* 229:1113, 1985.

Breen TW Ransil BJ, Groves PA, *et al.*: Factors associated with back pain after childbirth, *Anesthesiology* 81:29, 1994.

Bridge CR, Little BC, Hayworth J, *et al.*: Psychometric antenatal predictors of postnatal depressed mood, *J Psychosom Res* 29:325, 1985.

Brockington IF, Cox-Roper A: The nosology of puerperal psychosis. In Kumar R, Brockington IF, editors: *Motherhood and mental illness*, 2nd edn,London, 1988, Wright.

Brooten DA, Brown LP, Hollingsworth AO, *et al.*: A comparison of four treatments to prevent and control breast pain and engorgement, *Nurs Res* 32:225, 1983.

Brownridge PR: The management of headache following accidental dural puncture in obstetric patients, *Anaesth Int Care* 11:4, 1983.

Campbell I: Postpartum sleep patterns of mother-baby pairs, *Midwifery* 2(2):93, 1986.

Cardozo L: Urinary tract problems in pregnancy. In Whitfield C, editor: *Dewhursts textbook of obstetrics and gynaecology for postgraduates*, 5th edn, Oxford, 1995, Blackwell Science.

Carty E, Bradley C: A randomized, controlled evaluation of early postpartum hospital discharge, *Birth* 17(4):199, 1990.

Chandra RK, Puri S, Suraiya C, *et al.*: Influence of maternal food avoidance during pregnancy and lactation on the incidence of atopic eczema in infants, *Clin Allergy* 16(6):563, 1986.

Closs J: Oral temperature measurement, *Nurs Times* 83(1):36, 1987.

CMB: *Rules*, London, 1928, Central Midwives Board.

Cooper PJ, Campbell EA, Day A, *et al.*: Non-psychotic psychiatric disorder after childbirth, *Br J Psych* 152:799, 1988.

Cox JL, Connor Y, Kendell RE: Prospective study of the psychiatric disorders of childbirth, *Br J Psych* 140:111, 1982.

Cox JL, Holden JM, Sagovsky R: Detection of postnatal depression: Development of the 10-item Edinburgh Postnatal Depression Scale, *Br J Psych* 150(June):782, 1987.

Cox JL, Murray D, Chapman G: A controlled study of the onset, duration and prevalence of postnatal depression, *Br J Psych* 163:27, 1993.

Craggs K: *Strengthening the psychological processes of postnatal clients*, unpublished MSc Thesis, 1995, University of Surrey.

Cunningham FG, MacDonald PC, Gant NF, *et al.*: *Williams obstetrics*, 19th edn, London, 1993, Prentice-Hall.

De Lange JJ, Stilma JS, Creeze F: Visual disturbances after spinal anaesthesia, *Anaesthesia* 43:570, 1988.

Department of Health: *The patients charter*, London, 1991a, HMSO.

Department of Health: *Report on confidential enquiries into maternal deaths in the United Kingdom 1985–1987*, London, 1991b, HMSO.

Department of Health: *Changing childbirth. The report of the Expert Maternity Group*, London, 1993, HMSO.

Department of Health: *Report on confidential enquiries into maternal deaths in the United Kingdom 1988–1990*, London, 1994, HMSO.

Department of Health and Social Services Belfast: *Delivering choice: Midwife and GP led maternity units*, Report of the Northern Ireland Maternity Units Study Group, Belfast, 1994, HMSO.

Dewan G, Glazener C, Tunstall M: Postnatal pain: a neglected area, *Br J Midwifery* 1(2):63, 1993.

ENB: *Report of the National Survey of Midwifery Practice 1991/1992*, London, 1993, English National Board.

Enkin M, Keirse MJHC, Renfrew M, *et al.*: *A guide to effective care in pregnancy and childbirth*, 2nd edn, Oxford, 1995, Oxford University Press.

Ferguson KL, McKey PL, Bishop KR, *et al.*: Stress urinary incontinence: Effect of pelvic muscle exercise, *Obstet Gynecol* 75(4):671, 1990.

Fichardt A, van Wyk N, Weich M: The needs of postpartum women, *Curationis* 17(1):15, 1994.

Fischer W, Baessler K, Linde A: Pelvic floor conditioning with vaginal weights postpartum and in urinary incontinence (German), *Zentralblatt Gynakol* 118(1):18, 1996.

Galli D, Groce P, Chia pparini I, *et al.*: Ultrasonic evaluation of the uterus during the puerperium (Italian), *Minerva Gnecologica* 45(10):473, 1993.

Garcia J, Marchant S: Back to normal? Postpartum health and illness. In Robinson S, Thomson AM, Tickner V, editors: *Research and the midwife*, Proceedings 1992, Research and the Midwife, University of Manchester, 1993,

Garcia J, Renfrew M, Marchant S: Postnatal home visiting by midwives, *Midwifery* 10:40, 1994.

Gardner DL: Fatigue in postpartum women, *App Nurs Res* 4(2):57, 1991.

Glazener C, Abdalla M, Russel I, *et al.*: Postnatal care: a survey of patients' experiences, *Br J Midwifery* 1(2):67, 1993.

Glazener C, Abdalla M, Stroud P, *et al.*: Postnatal maternal morbidity: extent, causes, prevention and treatment, *Br J Obstet Gynaecol* 102(4):282, 1995.

Gordon H, Logue M: Perineal muscle function after childbirth, *Lancet* ii:123, 1985.

Grant A: The choice of suture materials and techniques for repair of perineal trauma: an overview of the evidence from controlled trials, *Br J Obstet Gynaecol* 96:1281, 1989.

Grant A, Sleep J: Relief of perineal pain and discomfort after childbirth. In Chalmers I, Enkin M, Keirse M, editors: *Effective care in pregnancy and childbirth*, Oxford, 1989, Oxford Medical.

Grant A, Sleep J, McIntosh J, *et al.*: Ultrasound and pulsed electromagnetic energy treatment for perineal trauma. A randomized placebo controlled trial, *Br J Obstet Gynaecol* 96:434, 1989.

Gready M, Newbury M, Dodds R: *Birth choices: Womens expectations and experiences*, London, 1995, National Childbirth Trust.

Greenshields W, Hulme H: *The perineum in childbirth. A survey of womens' experiences and midwives' practices*, London, 1993, National Childbirth Trust.

Grove LH: Backache, headache and bladder dysfunction after delivery, *Br J Anaesth* 45:1147, 1973.

Groves PA, Breen TW, Ransil BJ, *et al.*: Natural history of postpartum back pain and its relationship with epidural anaesthesia, *Anesthesiology* 81:A.1167, 1994.

Grudzinskas J, Atkinson L: Sexual functioning during the puerperium, *Arch Sex Behav* 13(1):85, 1984.

Hall W, Carty E: Managing the early discharge experience: taking control, *J Adv Nurs* 18(4):574, 1993.

Hannah P, Adams D, Lee A, *et al.*: Links between early postpartum mood and postnatal depression, *Br J Psych* 160(June):777, 1992.

Hawthorne K: Intention and reality in infant feeding, *Mod Midwife* 4(3):25, 1994.

Henderson A, Brouse A: The experiences of new fathers during the first three weeks of life, *J Adv Nurs* 16(3):293, 1991.

Henderson C: Women, midwives and the health of the nation, *Bri J Midwifery* May(5):248, 1997.

Hibbard BM: *Principles of obstetrics*, London, 1988, Butterworths.

Hillan E: Issues in the delivery of midwifery care, *J Adv Nurs* 17(3):274, 1992a.

Hillan E: Short-term morbidity associated with cesarean delivery, *Birth* 19(4):190, 1992b.

Holst KY, Wilson PD: The prevalence of female urinary incontinence and reasons for not seeking treatment, *NZ Med J* 101:756, 1988.

Horn B: Cultural concepts and postpartal care, *J Transcult Nurs* 2(1):48, 1990.

House of Commons Health Committee: *Second report: maternity services*, Vol. 1 (The Winterton Report), London, 1992, HMSO.

Houston S: *Are women prepared for taking their babies home from hospital postnatally?* Unpublished MSc Thesis, 1994, University of Surrey.

Howell C, Chalmers I: A review of prospectively controlled comparisons of epidural with non-epidural forms of pain relief during labour, *Int J Obstet Anaesth* 1:93, 1992.

Howie PW, McHeilly AS, Houston MJ, *et al.*: Fertility after childbirth: Post-partum ovulation and menstruation in bottle and breastfeeding mothers, *Clin Endocrinol* 17(4):323, 1982.

Howie PW, Forsyth JS, Ogston SA, *et al.*: Protective effect of breast feeding against infection, *Br Med J* 300:11, 1990.

Hutton E: What women want from midwives, *Br J Midwifery* 2(12):608, 1994.

Inch S, Renfrew MJ: Common breast feeding problems. In Chalmers I, Enkin MW, Keirse MJNC, editors: *Effective care in pregnancy and childbirth*, Oxford, 1989, Oxford University Press.

Isager-Sally L, Legarth J, Jacobsen B: Episiotomy repair immediate and long-term sequelae. A prospective randomized study of three different methods of repair, *Br J Obstet Gynaecol* 93:420, 1986.

Jacoby A. Womens preferences for and satisfaction with current procedures in childbirth findings from a national study, *Midwifery* 3:117, 1987.

Johanson R, Wilkinson P, Bastible A: Health after childbirth, *Midwifery* 9(3):161, 1993.

Jolleys J: Reported prevalence of urinary incontinence in women in a general practice, *Br Med J* 296:1330, 1988.

Kamm MA: Obstetric damage and faecal incontinence, *Lancet* 344(8924):730, 1994.

Kendell RE, Chalmers JC, Platz C: Epidemiology of peurperal psychoses, *Br J Psych* 159:662, 1987.

Kenny P, King M, Cameron S, *et al.*: Satisfaction with postnatal care the choice of home or hospital, *Midwifery* 9(3):146, 1993.

Kitzinger S: *Some womens experiences of epidurals. A descriptive study*, London, 1987, The National Childbirth Trust.

Klein MC, Gauthier RJ, Robbins JM, *et al.*: Relationship of episiotomy to perineal trauma and morbidity, sexual dysfunction and pelvic floor relaxation, *Am J Obstet Gynaecol* 171:591, 1994.

Kumar R, Robson KM: Neurotic disturbances during pregnancy and the puerperium: preliminary report of a prospective study of 119 primiparae. In Sandler M, editor: *Mental illness in pregnancy and the puerperium*, Oxford, 1978, Oxford University Press.

Kumar R, Robson KM: A prospective study of emotional disorders in childbearing women, *Br J Psych* 144:35, 1984.

Lagro-Janssen T, Debruyne F, Smits A, *et al.*: Controlled trial of pelvic floor exercises in the treatment of urinary stress incontinence in general practice, *Br J Gen Pract* 41(352):445, 1991.

Lavery J, Shaw L: Sonography of the puerperal uterus, *J Ultrasound Med* 8(9):481, 1989.

Lee KA, De Joseph JF: Sleep disturbances, vitality and fatigue among a select group of employed childbearing women, *Birth* 19(4):208, 1992.

Lee RV, McComb LE, Mezzadri FC: Pregnant patients, painful legs: the obstetricians dilemma, *Obstet Gynaecol Surv* 45(5):290, 1990.

Llewellyn-Jones D: *Fundamentals of obstetrics and gynaecology*, Vol 1, 5th edn, London, 1990, Faber & Faber.

MacArthur C, Lewis M, Knox EG: Epidural anaesthesia and long-term backache after childbirth, *Br Med J* 301:9, 1990.

MacArthur C, Lewis M, Knox EG: *Health after childbirth*, London, 1991, HMSO.

MacArthur C, Lewis M, Knox EG: Investigation of long-term problems after obstetric epidural anaesthesia, *Br Med J* 304:1279, 1992.

MacArthur C, Lewis M, Bick DE: Stress incontinence after childbirth, *Br J Mid* 1(5):207, 1993a.

MacArthur C, Lewis M, Knox EG: Accidental dural puncture in obstetric patients and long-term symptoms, *Br Med J* 306:883, 1993b.

MacArthur C, Lewis M, Knox EG: Comparison of long-term health problems following childbirth in Asian and Caucasian women, *Br J Gen Pract* 43:519, 1993c.

Macleod J, Macintyre C, McClure JH, *et al.*: Backache and epidural analgesia, *Int J Anaesth* 4(1):21, 1995.

Mahomed K, Grant A, Ashurst H, *et al.*: The Southmead perineal suture study. A randomized comparison of suture materials and suturing techniques for repair of perineal trauma, *Br J Obstet Gynaecol* 96:1272, 1989.

Marchant S, Garcia J: What are we doing in the postnatal check? *Br J Midwifery* 3(1):34, 1995.

Marsh J, Sargent E: Factors affecting the duration of postnatal visits, *Midwifery* 7(4):177, 1991.

Mccourt C, Page L: *Report on the evaluation 'one-to-one' midwifery practice*, London, 1996, Thames Valley University.

McLennan HG, Oats JM, Walstab JE: Survey of hand symptoms in pregnancy, *Med J Aust* 147:542, 1987.

Mouritsen L, Frimodt-Møller C, Møller M: Long-term effect of pelvic floor exercises on female urinary incontinence, *Br J Urol* 68(1);32, 1991.

Montgomery E, Alexander J: Assessing postnatal uterine involution: a review and a challenge, *Midwifery* 10(2):73, 1994.

Murphy-Black T: *Postnatal care at home: a descriptive study of mother's needs and the maternity services*, Report prepared for the Scottish Home and Health Department, Edinburgh, 1989, Department of Nursing Studies, University of Edinburgh.

Nikodem VC, Danziger P, Gebka N: Do cabbage leaves prevent breast engorgement? A randomized controlled study, *Birth* 20(2):61, 1993.

Nolan M: Helping parents to adapt to parenthood, *Br J Midwifery* 3(1):23, 1995.

Nolte A: The phenomenon of caring by the midwife, *Curationis* 15(3):19, 1992.

Novy M: The normal puerperium. In: DeChernery AH, Pernoll ML, editors: *Current obstetric and gynaecologic diagnosis and treatment*, London, 1994, Prentice-Hall.

Oakley A: The changing social context of pregnancy care. In Chamberlain G, Zander L, editors: *Pregnancy care in the 1990s the proceedings of a symposium held at the Royal Society of Medicine*, Carnforth, 1992, Parthenon.

O'Hara MW: Social support, life events and depression during pregnancy and the peurperium, *Arch Gen Psych* 43:569, 1986.

O'Hara MW, Zekowski EM: Postpartum depression: a comprehensive review. In Brockington IF, Kumar R, editors: *Motherhood and mental illness*, London, Wright, 1988.

O'Hara MW, Zekowski EM, Phillips LH, *et al.*:: Controlled prospective study of postpartum mood disorders. Comparison of childbearing and non-childbearing women, *J Abnorm Psychol* 99(1):3, 1990.

Ostgaard HC, Andersson GBJ: Previous back pain and risk of developing back pain in future pregnancy, *Spine* 16(4):432, 1991.

Ostgaard HC, Andersson GBJ: Postpartum low back pain, *Spine* 17(1):53, 1992.

Page L: Changing childbirth: a renewal of the maternity services, *Br J Midwifery* 1(4):157, 1993.

Parsons C: Postnatal back care, *Mod Midwife* 5(2):15, 1995.

Paterson J, Davis J, Gregory M, *et al.*: A study on the effects of low haemoglobin on postnatal women, *Midwifery* 10(2):77, 1994.

Paykel ES, Emms EM, Fletcher J, *et al.*: Life events and social support in peurperal depression, *Br J Psych* 136:339, 1980.

Pitt B: Atypical depression following childbirth, *Br J Psych* 114:1325, 1968.

Playfair HR, Gowers JI. Depression following childbirth: a search for predictive signs, *J Roy Coll GPs* 31:201, 1981.

RCM: *Successful breastfeeding*, 2nd edn, London, 1991, Royal College of Midwives.

Reynolds F: Dural puncture and headache. Avoid the first but treat the second, *Br Med J* 306:874, 1993.

Rhoten D: Fatigue and the postsurgical patient. In Norris CM, editor: *Concept clarification in nursing*, Rockville, 1982, Aspen.

Riley D: *Perinatal mental health: a source book for health professionals*, Oxford, 1995, Radcliffe Medical Press.

Rodeck C, Newton J: A study of the uterine cavity by ultrasound in the early puerperium, *Br J Obstet Gynaecol* 83(10):795, 1976.

Romito P: Mothers experience of breast feeding, *J Rep Inf Psych* 6:89, 1988.

Rush J, Chalmers I, Enkin M: Care of the new mother and baby. In Chalmers I, Enkin M, Keirse M, editors: *Effective care in pregnancy and childbirth*, Oxford, 1989, Oxford Medical.

Russell R, Groves P, Taub H, *et al.*: Assessing longterm backache after childbirth, *Br Med J* 306:1299, 1993.

Scott BD, Hibbard BM: Serious non-fatal complications associated with extra-dural block in obstetric practice, *Br J Anaesth* 48:247, 1990.

Scottish Home Office and Health Department: *Provision of maternity services in Scotland – a policy review*, Edinburgh, 1993, HMSO.

Shapiro AG, Thomas L: Efficacy of bromocriptine v. breast binders as inhibitors of postpartum lactation, *South Med J* 77:719, 1984.

Sharif K, Jordan J: The six week postnatal visit are we doing it right? *Br J Hosp Med* 54:7, 1995.

Sharif K, Clarke P, Whittle M: Routine six weeks postnatal vaginal examination: to do or not to do? *J Obstet Gynaecol* 13(4):251, 1993.

Shaw H: *A study on the postnatal sleep patterns of Scottish primigravid women*, unpublished MSc Thesis, 1994, University of Surrey.

Shelton MG: Standardised senna in the management of constipation in the puerperium a clinical trial, *S Afr Med J* 57:78, 1980.

Sleep J: Perineal care: a series of five randomized controlled trials. In Robinson S, Thomson AM, editors: *Midwives, research and childbirth*, Vol 2, London, 1991, Chapman & Hall.

Sleep J, Grant A: Pelvic floor exercises in postnatal care, *Midwifery* 3(3):158, 1987a.

Sleep J, Grant A, Elbourne D: West Berkshire perineal management trial: three year follow-up, *Br Med J* 295:749, 1987b.

Sleep J, Grant A: Effects of salt and Savlon bath concentrate postpartum (Occasional Paper), *Nurs Times* 84:55, 1988.

Sleep JC, Grnat A, Elbourne D: West Berkshire perineal management trial, *Br Med J* 298(8):587, 1984.

Smith EA, *et al.*: A comparison of 25G and 27G Whitacre needles for Caesarean section, *Anaesthesia* 49:859, 1994.

Smith P: Postnatal concerns of mothers: An update, *Midwifery* 5(4):182, 1989.

Snooks SJ, Swash M, Setchell M, *et al.*: Injury to innervation of pelvic floor sphincter musculature in childbirth, *Lancet* ii:546, 1984.

Snooks SJ, Swash M, Mathers SG, *et al.*: Effect of vaginal delivery on the pelvic floor: a five year follow-up, *Br J Surg* 77:1358, 1990.

Spencer JD, Grant A, Elbourne D, *et al.*: A randomized comparison of glycerol-impregnated chromic catgut with untreated chromic catgut for the repair of perineal trauma, *Br J Obstet Gynaecol* 93:426, 1986.

Stanton SL, Kerr-Wilson R, Grant-Harris V: The incidence of urological symptoms in normal pregnancy, *Br J Obstet Gynaecol* 87:897, 1980.

Stein GS: Headaches in the first postpartum week and their relationship to migraine, *Headache* 21:201, 1981.

Stride PC, Cooper GM: Dural taps revisited. A 20-year survey from Birmingham Maternity Hospital, *Anaesthesia* 48:47, 1993.

Sultan AH, Kamm MA, Hudson CH, *et al.*: Anal sphincter disruption during vaginal delivery, *New Engl J Med* 329(26):1905, 1993.

Sultan AH, Kamm MA, Hudson CH, *et al.*: Third degree obstetric and sphincter tears: risk factors and outcome of primary repair, *Br Med J* 308:887, 1994.

Sultan AH, Kamm MA, Hudson CM: Obstetric perineal trauma: an audit of training, *J Obstet Gynaecol* 15:19, 1995.

Swash M: Childbirth and incontinence, *Midwifery* 4(1):13, 1988.

Swash M: Faecal incontinence childbirth is responsible for most cases, *Br Med J* 307:636, 1993.

Taylor D, Lind T: Puerperal haematological indices, *Br J Obstet Gynaecol* 88(6):601, 1981.

Thomas TM, Plymat KR, Blannin J, *et al.*: Prevalence of urinary incontinence, *Br Med J* 281:1243, 1980.

Tod EDM: Peurperal depression: a prospective epidemiological study, *Lancet* ii:1264, 1964.

Towler J, Bramall J: *Midwives in history and society*, London, 1986, Croom Helm Ltd.

Trevalyon J: *Please tell mother*, Nursing Times 90(9):38, 1993.

Twaddle S, Liao XH, Fyrie H: An evaluation of postnatal care individualised to the needs of the women, *Midwifery* 9:154, 1993.

UKCC: *The Midwife's Code of Practice*, London, 1986, United Kingdom Central Council for Nursing, Midwifery and Health Visiting.

UKCC: *Community postnatal visiting by midwives*, Registrar's Letter, London, 18th May, 1992, United Kingdom Central Council for Nursing, Midwifery and Health Visiting.

UKCC: *Midwives rules*, London, 1993, United Kingdom Central Council for Nursing, Midwifery and Health Visiting.

Unterman RR, Posner NA, Williams KN: Postpartum depressive disorders: changing trends, *Birth* 17(3):131, 1990.

VanRees D, Bernstine RL, Crawford W: Involution of the postpartum uterus: an ultrasonic study, *J Clin Ultrasound* 9(2):55, 1981.

Viktrup L, Lose G, Rolff M, *et al.*: The symptom of stress incontinence caused by pregnancy or delivery in primiparas, *Obstet Gynecol* 79(6):945, 1992.

Wachsberg RH, Kurtz AB, Levine CD, *et al.*: Real-time ultrasonographic analysis of the normal postpartum uterus: technique, variability and measurements, *J Ultrasound Med* 13(3):215, 1994.

Wand JS: Carpel tunnel syndrome in pregnancy and lactation, *J Hand Surg Br* 15(B):93, 1990.

Watson JP, *et al.*: Psychiatric disorder in pregnancy and the first postnatal year, *Br J Psych* 144:453, 1984.

Weil A, Reyes H, Rottenberg R, *et al.*, Effect of lumbar epidural analgesia on lower urinary tract function in the immediate postpartum period, *Br J Obstet Gynaecol* 90(5):428, 1983.

Welsh Office: *The protocol for investment in health gain*, Cardiff, 1992, HMSO.

White A, Freeth S, OBrien M: *Infant feeding, 1990*, London, HMSO, 1992.

Wilson PD, *et al.*: *A randomized controlled trial of physiotherapy treatment of postnatal urinary incontinence*, Proceedings of the 26th British Congress of Obstetrics and Gynaecology, Manchester, 162, 1992, Conference Proceedings.

Wilson PD, Herbison RM, Herbison GP: Obstetric practice and the prevalence of urinary stress incontinence three months after delivery, *Br J Obstet Gynaecol* 103(2):154, 1996.

Woollett A, Dosanjh-Matwala N: Postnatal care: the attitudes and experiences of Asian women in east London, *Midwifery* 6(4):178, 1990.

Zajicek E, Wolkind S. Emotional difficulties in married women during and after the first pregnancy, *Br J Med Psych* 51:379, 1978.

Further Reading

Akin V: Cultural aspects of postpartum care. In Bobak I, Jensen M: *Essentials of maternity nursing*, 3rd edn, Chapter 21, St Louis, 1991, MosbyYear Book.

This text details cultural variations in childbearing practices during the puerperium. The behaviour patterns of many non-Western societies are based on the beliefs that labour alters body balance and the woman is in a polluted state following childbirth. These are addressed in the context of diet, lactation and the activities of daily living.

Bobak I, Lowdermilk D, Jensen M, *et al.*, (editors): *Maternity nursing*, 4th edition, St Louis, 1995, Mosby Year Book Inc.

This book incorporates the cultural implications of maternity care throughout the text.

Alexander J, Levy V, Roch S: *Postnatal care: A research-based approach*, London, 1990, Macmillan Education.

This book explores the research evidence for some aspects of postnatal care and assimilates it into a framework that enables evidence-based practice.

Blackburn S, Loper D: *Maternal, fetal and neonatal physiology a clinical perspective*, Philadelphia, 1992, WB Saunders.

This comprehensive book applies detailed information about the physiological processes of pregnancy, labour and the puerperium to clinical care. The integrated approach provides a scientific basis for midwifery practice.

Chamberlain G, Zander L, editors: *Pregnancy care in the 1990s*, Carnforth, 1992, Parthenon Publishing Group.

This book presents the proceedings of a symposium held at The Royal Society of Medicine in 1990. Sixteen presentations are included, from midwives, obstetricians, GPs and consumer group representatives, which discuss how best use could be made of the professional services involved in the care of women at the time of childbirth.

Chamberlain G, Patel N, editors: *The future of the maternity services*, London, 1994, Royal College of Obstetricians and Gynaecologists.

This book presents the proceedings of a study group organised jointly by the RCOG, RCM and RCGPs, to discuss ways to take forward ideas into the future maternity service.

Cox J, Holden J: *Perinatal psychiatry*, 1994, Gaskell Press.

Kumar R, Brockington I (editors): *Motherhood and mental illness*, London, 1988, Academic Press.

These two books are essential reading for those concerned with maternal mental health. The first book describes the uses and abuses of the EPDS.

MacArthur C, Lewis M, Knox EG: *Health after childbirth*, London, 1991, HMSO.

This book presents the findings of the first large study of long-term health after childbirth. The background to the investigation is explained, and design and analysis of the study described. Separate chapters describe the onset, frequency and duration of health problems, and associations with obstetric, anaesthetic and maternal factors.

Reamy K, White S: Sexuality in the puerperium: A review, *Arch Sex Behav*, 16(2); 165, 1987.

This article provides an in-depth examination of sexuality in the puerperium. Specific reference is made to dyspareunia, episiotomy and lactation. This may be a useful resource for midwives whose advice may be sought on these issues.

15 *Adaptation to Parenthood and the New Family*

LEARNING OUTCOMES

After studying this chapter you should be able to:
- Discuss the different theories that underpin our understanding of infant development.
- Recognise the adjustments made by new parents to parenthood.
- Review the role of the midwife in supporting parents as they adjust to their new role.
- Identify the role of the family in contemporary society.
- Evaluate the development and the activity of parenting and consider the effectiveness of the preparation for parenting that you provide for couples.
- Discuss the changing role of men in childbearing and early parenthood.
- Reflect on your own beliefs and assumptions about fathers and how these may affect the service you provide.

PSYCHOLOGICAL CONTEXT OF PARENTING

The period surrounding the birth of a child is an important 'window of opportunity' for midwives to support men and women in order to promote healthy family and parent–child relationships.

Transition To Parenthood

The transition to parenthood refers to: 'the fairly brief period of time from the beginning of pregnancy through the first months of having a child' (Goldberg, 1988, p. 1). A normative developmental event, it provides an opportunity for growth for women, men and couples.

The transition to parenthood can also lead to decreased emotional intimacy and egalitarianism in roles and responsibilities between men and women (Cowan *et al.* 1985; Parr, 1996). Such mismatches in expectations and realities of men's emotional support and involvement in child care have been implicated in poor adjustment in women after childbirth (Nicolson, 1990). Emery and Tuer (1993) put forward another view. They suggest that this shift is adaptive in meeting the needs of the child: 'Views about what men's and women's family roles "ought" to be should not cloud interpretation of evidence about what they are.'

Researchers have studied the relation between parenting practice and developmental outcomes in children. This has led to an increased understanding of the importance of what transpires in the home for the developing child (Luster and Okagaki, 1993; Perris *et al.* 1994). A number of studies found that not only do mothers and fathers affect their children independently as parents, but the relationship between the parents can also have a profound influence on child development (Belsky, 1984).

So what is the evidence about what 'men's and women's family roles ought to be' that Emery and Tuer (1993) talk about? It is not the goal of this section to elaborate upon what makes a 'good' parent compared to a 'bad' one – as it is probable that 'more often than not, bad things (or good things) go together when it comes to influences on parenting', as Vondra and Belsky (1993) suggest. Neither is it to elaborate in great detail on the wide range of evidence that now exists about infant emotional development, psychological adjustment in the transition to parenthood and support for parents during this period. There is a vast literature on each of these topics, each of which deserves a separate and more complex treatment than can be afforded here.

The purpose of this Chapter is to provide a critical review of some of the key issues pertinent to expectant and new parents and their infants, in order to promote an integrative view of the early parent–child relationships and family life. The perspective taken is that the period surrounding the birth of a child is an important 'window of opportunity' for promoting healthy family and parent–child relationships. Ways in which some of this knowledge can be used to enhance the work midwives already do in supporting parents are encouraged.

Infant Development

In Western culture, birth is celebrated as the beginning of emotional life. Some theories of child development now support the view that the social and emotional life of infants begins at conception and can be influenced by events during pregnancy, birth and the early postnatal period – in which interaction with their parents only forms a part of the overall picture.

Despite lack of direct knowledge about the social and emotional life of infants, there is a wealth of literature about infancy, which McFayden (1994, p. 9) argues '... presents a somewhat confusing picture.' No single theory or model appears to describe adequately when an infant 'begins' emotionally. It is not so much a new theory of emotion or mind or new methods of study that are needed. Rather, the perspective is taken in this Chapter that existing positions need to be woven together in the light of classic and newly emerging data to develop a more integrative approach to understanding development.

McFayden (1994) provides a clear and coherent overview of contributions made by psychoanalytic theory, ethology and developmental psychology that are of direct relevance to midwives. She uses these theories (summarized below) to underpin a deeper understanding of the needs of full-term and special-care babies, especially around such important developmental issues as separation from the mother (*see also* Holmes, 1993; Jacobs, 1995).

Psychoanalytic theory

Psychoanalytic theory views human development as that of a biological organism governed by biological drives or instincts, the main aim of which is to seek pleasure. Freud (1953) considered that the organism's drive to reduce tension was through the agency of an object, most often the mother. His sexual theory of development is based on the difference between self-preservative drives (the need to be physiologically' supported by food) and sexual drives (driven to satisfy psychological needs through oral experiences, such as sucking).

Different developmental phases, or 'stages', occur during which the organism's sexual drive (or need to reduce tension) is focused on particular parts of the body:
• Oral (first year).
• Anal (second year).
• Genital or phallic stage (third and fourth year, or the Oedipal 'stage').
The main developmental task of the young child is to resolve infantile sexual feelings for the parent of the opposite gender.

Later Freud argued that the infant was born with undifferentiated 'psychic' or mental states: the id, ego and superego. Differentiation of the ego from the id was considered to gradually occur from birth, the evolution of the superego taking place with the resolution of the anxiety said to stem from the baby's perception of the mother as separate or missing. This syndrome of 'primary anxiety' was viewed as related to birth itself, the mother's absence 'reminding' the baby of the trauma of being born. A wealth of clinical literature now exists to support this idea (Share, 1994).

Object relations theory

Object relations theory is based on a modification and development of Freud's thinking. It suggests that newborns are 'undifferentiated' (i.e. cannot identify their mothers and therefore cannot demonstrate differential emotional responses to them). The relationship of the mother to baby as a whole is stressed. The quality of this mother–baby relationship either facilitates or inhibits the development of the infant's autonomous sense of self (Mahler, 1983). Klein and Winnicott (1965) focused on early mother–infant relationships and viewed the ego as present from birth. Object relations theory differs from Freud's in that it also relates to the baby's 'perceived' relationship with the 'object' (internal or intrapsychic/unconscious processes), as well as the actual external relationship.

Klein takes as her starting point of infant development 'the fear of annihilation' (Symington, 1986, p. 257). She ascribes a complex yet primitive mental apparatus to the infant from birth, believing that the baby exists from the start in a relationship with another person. The baby is considered unable to perceptualize 'mother' as a whole, who is viewed as part of that person (part object – typically as the breast or bottle). Like Freud,

Klein perceived the baby as moving through a series of phases, the 'paranoid–schizoid' and the 'depressive' positions. The main developmental task of infancy is the need to defend against anxieties from the external and internal world, representing the innate conflict between life and death instincts. This occurs through the processes of 'splitting', 'projection', 'introjection' and 'projective identification' (Mitchell, 1986; Segal, 1982). Healthy development (occurring mainly through the mother–infant relationship) is said to occur when the infant's life instinct wins its battle over the death instinct.

Winnicott (1965) concluded that in the early weeks of an infant's life a baby needs to have the mother's sole attention for healthy development (Jacobs, 1995). Evidence supporting this view is reported by Murray *et al.* (1994), who found that where mothers have postnatal depression, the immediate mother–infant relationship is adversely affected. This is seen in impaired infant feeding and infant growth, as well as in the long-term development of the child (in terms of significantly higher rates of difficulties in adjusting to school).

The study found that infant qualities and abilities influence maternal mood. Infants with poor motor control (inert and flaccid or jerky and unmodulated) sometimes make it harder for parents to achieve eye-to-eye contact and thus make it harder to relate to their infant in a meaningful way. Infants do not simply mimic their mother's behaviour, but instead they seem to develop a 'depressed' style of behaving themselves, which can remain with them throughout their life (Perry *et al.* 1995).

Unlike Freud and Klein, Winnicott (1965) believes that infants at birth do not experience the mother or her breast as separate, but view the breast as part of themselves. Like Freud, however, he viewed the infant and maternal care as a unit: 'There is no such thing as an infant.' In contrast to Klein and Freud's emphasis on defending against 'anxiety', Winnicott considered that the capacity to 'be alone', as a result of the mother's attentiveness and responsiveness to her baby, was one of the most important signs of mature emotional development.

What Winnicott meant by his famous phrase the 'good-enough mother', it was not a mother who anticipates her baby's every need and meets it almost before it has been recognized by the infant. This does not allow the baby to experience and learn to manage frustration, which does not allow the baby to grow mentally. Instead, Winnicott recognized the importance of 'reliability' and 'failure of reliability' in the mother–child relationship. The extreme opposite of total attentiveness to the infant would be total failure to notice the baby's needs, resulting in 'unthinkable anxiety' for the baby.

Recent studies have led to a review of Winnicott's ideas. Infant observation using ultrasound scans throughout pregnancy, with follow-up of the children in their homes 3–4 years after birth, has provided evidence that object-relations may begin in the womb (Piontelli, 1992). Her observation of twins found them socializing with each other at 20 weeks' gestation.

Prenatal and perinatal psychology argues that infant emotional life begins even earlier, at conception (Fogel, 1993). Hepper and Shahidullah (1994) reviewed the evidence which suggests that the behaviour of the fetus may be used to explore development of the mind. They show active use by the unborn infant of four of the main senses – auditory (hearing), chemosensory (smell and taste), cutaneous (related to pain sensation, awareness of temperature change, touch and proprioception – position of body in space), as well as visual (the sense most unlikely to be stimulated during the normal course of pregnancy).

Evidence has also been provided for fetal learning. For example, the fetus has been found to habituate to sound stimuli (essential for survival and efficient functioning, enabling the ignoring of familiar stimuli and to attend to new stimuli) as early as 24 weeks (Hepper and Shahidullah, 1994; Leader *et al.* 1982). This suggests that the mind emerges in an immature form. Stimulation received *in utero,* and the behaviour emitted, plays an important role in the development of infant emotional life (Chamberlain, 1993).

These findings support the view of Laughlin (1989) who states that: 'There exists no stage of development, prenatal or perinatal, in which the cognized environment of the child is in chaos' (p. 135). Some researchers now argue that cognitive capacities have their own foundation. That is, they are *not* built on sensorimotor experience, but are part of human endowment (Spelke *et al.* 1992).

Ethology

Ethological thinking makes a direct comparison between animal and human behaviour and development, exemplified in the notion of a 'sensitive period' in human mothers, as well as other mammals (Klaus *et al.* 1972; Klaus and Kennel, 1982). This approach views mothers as only able to 'bond' to their offspring if exposed to them during a sensitive period shortly after birth. As we see later, there is much in this approach to both commend and criticize.

Attachment theory

An important view of parent–infant interaction is provided by attachment theory. This is distinct from the concept of 'bonding', which usually refers to the parent's tie to the infant that occurs immediately after birth. The main concern of attachment theory is with the relationship an infant develops with his/her mother – with the infant's felt sense of security and separation anxiety (Bowlby, 1980; Ainsworth, 1985).

Bowlby claims that maternal deprivation (which includes even brief separations from the mother in the first 5 years of life) produces profound long-term damage. Bretherton (1991) found that in the first 3 months, mothers of secure infants respond more promptly when they cry, look, smile and talk to their babies more and offer them more affectionate and joyful holding. Mothers of less avoidant children tend to interact less, whereas mothers of ambivalent children tend to ignore their babies' signals for attention and generally tend to be unpredictable in their responsiveness. By the second half of the first year, babies classified as secure at 1 year cry less, enjoy body contact more and appear to demand it less than do those in the insecure group.

Later research, however, concludes that there is no such thing as instant attachment. Rutter (1981) suggests that the key to secure attachment is active, reciprocal interaction and the quality of the interaction, more than the quantity. This indicates a move away from simplistic event-pathology models of development. Instead, what appears to matter is not so much the separation from the mother, but its meaning and the context in which it happens.

In summary, studies have led to the general idea that by 3–4 months of age, the infant is sensitive, perceptive, conscious and perhaps even cognitive, with sufficient capacities to differentiate self from other *at least from birth (*Stern, 1985).

Developmental psychology

Not all psychologists hold the view of the sentient prenate and newborn. Traditionally, developmental psychology has sought to be more 'objective'. Conclusions about causation and outcome are drawn from observational studies and experiments. Development has classically been seen as progressing through a series of predictable stages, with the main focus on perceptual, motor and cognitive tasks. In earlier studies, there was little place for constructions of infant emotion. This has now changed, but the view taken is very different from that of other theories.

Sroufe (1996) argues that when emotions are treated as developmental constructs, an emotional reaction is said to occur when a prescribed set of circumstances elicits, with some reliability, a range of established reactions in an infant. Emotions are 'inferred' from numerous indications, rather than being identified with some single indicator.

Given the emphasis on the subjective relationship between infant and caregiver or event described by other theories, 'meaning' can be said to play a critical role in emotion. An important difference between these approaches and developmental psychology is that, for this very reason, developmental psychologists do not infer fear in the newborn – despite the presence of startle, crying, head turning or even a 'fear' face – or pleasure, as when the sleeping newborn smiles.

Sroufe (1996) argues that such reactions are not based on emotional processing of the event, but rather are 'reflexive reactions' in response to endogenous fluctuations in the central nervous system or simply reflect the intensity of parameters of external stimulation. He concludes that '*there is no subject–object relationship*' [italics added] (p. 56). This implies that meaning (the subjective relationship) has no major role in prenatal and perinatal development: 'Pain itself is not an emotion, even in later life, although it certainly may lead to anger or fear' (Izard *et al.* 1987, p. 105).

Startle and disgust are sometimes offered as examples of 'emotions' in the newborn period. Sroufe (1996) argues that the startle action is obviously a reflex and is distinguishable from a later surprise reaction. 'Disgust', where an infant wrinkles up its nose in response to a bitter taste, is also best considered a reflexive reaction:

> These newborn reactions may be prototypes for later 'genuine emotions'. They are not best thought of as emotions themselves, but as 'preemotions'.
>
> (Sroufe, 1996, p. 60.)

Developmental psychology also recognizes the importance of secure attachment in infancy. However, in contrast to psychoanalytically derived theories which argue that babies need to be emotionally contained, or 'kept in mind', by their mothers, developmental psychologists argue that the assigned role for the caregiver during the early neonatal period is to provide smooth and harmonious routines. Such an approach construes that if the quality of care is responsive and highly reliable, familiarization with the caregiver should be more readily accomplished and a sound basis laid for later interactions.

In summary, recent findings from different domains of developmental research, despite their differences, converge in finding early relationship experiences crucial to the immediate and longer term adjustment of children. Regardless of what different theories view as the key issues in infant emotional development, they have in common the importance of the period for parents. Responding to the 'perceived' emotional states and signals of the infant is the crucial issue for new parents. As the evidence shows, most theories agree that this responsivity is related to the quality of the later parent–infant attachment.

Findings need to be tempered with the knowledge of the possibility of discontinuity from childhood to adulthood. Hunter and Kilstrom (1979) identify factors that make the difference between mothers carrying their childhood experiences of abuse into their parenting role and providing adequate care for their infants. These included a supportive relationship with someone other than the abusive parent during childhood, undergoing extensive psychotherapy, a stable and satisfying relationship with a nonabusive partner, as well as with other family members and friends. In other words, individuals become more effective in dealing with emotionally demanding situations (like parenting) when personal and situational needs are met through supportive close relationships (**Box 15.1**).

Box 15.1

Parent–Infant Relationships

Studies on parent–infant relationships suggest that the crisis of the first year of life is attachment, where the infant is supposed to learn faith in people and in the environment:

• What are your beliefs about the importance of the early years for child development? Where do these ideas come from?

• How do you feel when you hear a baby cry?

• Is there anything from your own life experience (past or current) that makes listening to babies hard for you? If yes, what further support do you need for this?

• In what ways do you think 'sensitive mothering or fathering' may be difficult or not beneficial to a new parent?

• What can midwives do to encourage healthy parent–infant attachment (in fathers as well as in mothers)?

Adjustment to Parenthood

Pound (1994, p. 143) states that: 'Public concern about the current state of the family in the UK has reached what has been described as a "moral panic"'. Rather than blaming parents for current increases in family breakdown, crime and delinquency, she believes that it is important to be aware that in this modern era of small families and mobile lifestyles, few children have the experience of observing adults caring for babies or small children.

Pound (1994) reminds us that those of us in the position to support parents need to remember that the skills of parenting have to be learned afresh by each new generation. She also argues that we have to acknowledge that there is a problem – the result of the still widely held view that parenting is an innate skill and requires little learning.

In reality, the evidence suggests that parenting is a subtle and complex skill for *all* parents, and strongly influenced by a number of factors. There are no simple, universally applicable answers to these problems, but '... there is some valid knowledge and some valid direction for change' (p. 145).

Parent–infant interaction

A common factor in mothers of securely attached children is the concept of 'maternal attunement'. Sensitive mothers when interacting with their children appear to modulate their infant's rhythms, facilitating the development of the infant's sense of integrated selfhood. This process of attunement is impaired in mothers of insecurely attached infants, leading to a 'mismatch' in maternal response (Stern, 1985, 1995).

Mothers of ambivalently attached children appear to force themselves on their children when they are playing happily and ignore them when they are in distress (Holmes, 1993). Securely attached infants directly express their dependency on caregivers, consistently turning to them when threatened or needy. Infants with anxious or avoidant attachment fail to seek contact when moderately threatened and at times appear indifferent to their caregivers (**Table 15.1**). Paradoxically, more dependent infants are predicted to be more emotionally independent later.

Secure attachment is more frequent in Western Europe (70%), with 40% in Germany and on an Israeli kibbutz. Avoidant attachment is more frequent in Japan and Israel, but nonexistent in a Chinese sample. The appar-

ent stability exhibited cross-culturally in attachment behaviours is supportive of Bowlby's views of a biologically based phenomenon. Other findings consistent with this view are shown in adoption studies, where infants adopted in the first 6 months do not differ from non-adopted infants (Bowlby, 1979).

Nutritional status is also related to attachment classifications, with chronically malnourished infants accounting for a larger proportion of anxious and disorganized attachments. Attachment distributions in very low birthweight infants (singletons and twins) generally appear the same as population norms. Enormous resilience is found in normal infants raised by blind or deaf parents. The infants appear to be able to adapt to the available interaction patterns, with only some slight initial negative behaviours and delays (Rosenblith, 1992).

Mismatches in maternal responses to infant cues may, in part, be exacerbated by lack of appropriate support for the psychological issues that concern women at this time. Even before birth, maternal anxiety and negative responses to pregnancy are predictive of labour complications, prematurity and poorer relations between mother and infant (Egeland and Farber, 1984). Fathers and mothers who report frequent negative-state experiences tend to be less attentive and responsiveness to their infants. The presence of mental illness in expectant and new parents suggests that the psychological resources required for parenting may be compromised or absent altogether (Vondra and Belsky, 1993).

A crucial aspect of the way mothers negotiate their relationship with their infants centres on the quality of the couple relationship and the quality of 'complementarity' in the couple's parenting process (Diamond *et al.* 1996). Studies have found that women (St-Andre and Twomey, 1996) and men (Parr, 1996) who are better equipped to face the normal feelings of ambivalence that occur in the transition to parenthood also have the capacity to tolerate and express negative feelings in the family of origin and in current relationships. To support these processes adequately, it can be argued that midwives need to be able to tolerate expression of negative as well as positive feelings to be able to truly listen to women (Trout, 1988; Oakley *et al.* 1990; Belsky and Kelly, 1994).

Fathers

A common theme in most models of infant development is the lack of attention to the role of fathers (Biller, 1993; Marsiglio, 1995). The literature on men's adjustment to parenthood is equally scarce. This is despite evidence

Table 15.1 Types of infant attachment behavior, based on Ainsworth *et al.* 1978		
Type of attachment	**Characteristics of infant's behavior**	**Characteristics of mother's behavior**
Secure attachment	Infant is distressed by separation from mother and seeks contact with her after they are reunited, but is readily comforted and returns to absorbed play	Sensitive responsiveness to her infant's needs
Insecure avoidant attachment	May avoid the mother during reunion	Aversive to physical contact, sometimes interfering and somtimes appearing unavailable or rejecting
Insecure ambivalent attachment	Ambivalent behaviour, at times seeking proximity with the mother in a clingy way, but is not easily reassured by her, at other times resists interaction and contact	Tends to be inconsistant, insensitive and unpredictable in her responces
Insecure disorganized attachment*	Infant appears confused and apprehensive in the presence of the parents, and generally disorganised in his/her interactions	Mother thought to be suffering from some unresolved trauma, such as abuse, or the unresolved loss of an attachment figure, resulting in mother appearing frightened, or frightening to the infant

*This category was added later to cover infants whose behaviour did not fall into the first three patterns

that the same factors that make mothers important to their children make fathers important too (Lamb and Lamb, 1976).

The study of men's roles remains underdeveloped and rooted in cultural values and stereotypes, which maintain men in the breadwinner role (Hawkins *et al.* 1995). They also highlight the way in which men's lack of opportunities to get to know their babies leaves them with the legacy of having to 'remake fatherhood' (Cohen, 1989).

To develop greater equality between the sexes in terms of parenting roles, Rossi (1984) argues that studies also have to address contextual factors, such as men's employment and paternity leave. Parr's (1996) findings from a longitudinal study of 106 British couples in the transition to parenthood concurs somewhat with these findings. However, the large number of gender differences found in her study also suggests the need for a specific and unique 'Fatherhood Constellation' for men who become fathers in the 1990s.

Parr (1996) suggests that lack of clarity in delineation of gender roles, a mismatch between expectations about men's behaviour after childbirth and lack of support around the emotional, psychological and social aspects of bringing a child into the world, may have contributed to some of the findings, as Nicholson (1990) reports. Men, when given the opportunity to express how they feel, often report that they feel strongly about their role in the family and are frequently confused and distressed with the lack of support available to them (Marsiglio, 1995).

In keeping with a number of other studies, Parr (1996) found that women and men reported more need of support for the emotional and relationship aspects of the transition (**Box 15.2**), than for information about childbirth or practical aspects of baby care (Bliss Holtz, 1988).

Support in the Transition to Parenthood

Studies suggest that, in general, support for expectant and new parents affects their adjustments and the quality of the parent–child relationship (Boukydis, 1986, 1987; Luster and Okagaki, 1993; Niven, 1992; Walker, 1992). This suggests the need for parent education and support during this time to focus on couple, family and parent–infant relationships (*see* Smith, 1996).

Antenatal education in Britain is described as providing 'preparation and support for parenthood'. Most approaches focus on instructional approaches to childbirth or practical aspects of infant care (Combes and Schonveld, 1992; Pugh *et al.* 1994). Drawing on a medical perspective, the perceived role of antenatal education is often that of 'contributing to producing a happy and healthy pregnancy and baby' (Ho, 1985, p. 14). There is little evidence that this is effective in assisting adjustment to family life.

Most research on psychosocial support focuses on the psychiatric population, particularly on postnatal depression (*see* Cox and Holden, 1994). Medical models consider psychological factors as independent variables which influence women's emotional adjustments. Studies have generally investigated the influence of hormonal activity on the development of mood (O'Brien and Pitt, 1994), but the findings are inconclusive and often contradictory (Appleby, 1990; Richards, 1990). This approach has also reinforced a pathological model of experiences that surround childbirth and maintained rigid distinctions between women who have 'adjusted well' and those who have not.

Recent research acts as a valuable reminder that many of the experiences thought of as symptoms of 'poor adjustment' are, in fact, not uncommon in the general childbearing population (Barclay *et al.* 1995; Nicolson, 1995).

Box 15.2

Women, Men and Adjustment to Parenthood

Studies suggest that how women and men adjust to parenthood depends on a wide range of factors:

• In what way do you see the experience of women and men as different in the transition to parenthood?

• What factors are most important in how (a) women and (b) men cope at this time?

• How can midwives help with women's and men's adjustment to parenthood and early parenting?

• How would you rate your own ability to listen to (a) women, (b) men and (c) couples?

• What do you find easy to listen to and what do you find difficult?

• What further support do you need to be able to listen well to parents?

It has been assumed commonly that '... the secret of providing the kind of support which will enhance the coping process seems to lie in giving the client as much control over her pregnancy, labour and postnatal care needs as possible' (Ball, 1993, p. 32). Perceived 'control' is another powerful construct used widely in studies of women's adjustments (Oakley *et al.* 1990).

For women to remain aware (through less medication) and in 'active control' (of the amount of medication received), rather than to have total pain control in childbirth, is still widely regarded as the key to the quality of women's experiences. It can be argued that issues of 'control' are often overemphasized in ideas about supporting adjustment in the transition to parenthood. How women relate to 'control' may also be affected by previous experiences, such as miscarriage (Statham and Green, 1994) and social contexts of childbirth (Skinner, 1995).

Childbirth is essentially an 'uncontrollable event' (Peterson, 1981). Thus a 'learned helplessness' model would conclude that:

An overriding belief in one's own control presents two problems: it brings increased depression in its wake, and it makes meaning in one's life difficult to find.

(Peterson *et al.* 1993, p. 16.)

Women's perceptions of childbirth and the subsequent impact on adjustment have been well reported (Ballard, 1994; Charles and Curtis, 1994). Implications for the long term adjustment of the child have also been found.

This suggests that prenatal, perinatal and early postnatal health-care interventions could significantly reduce violence. However, caution is urged in interpreting such findings, as research on infancy and parenthood can be used symbolically to address the conflicts of adult life (Eyer, 1992; Trout, 1988).

Earlier research on parent–infant bonding (Klaus and Kennel, 1976) led to an 'ideology of the natural', resulting in overwhelming regret and guilt in many women. As Eyer (1992) argues: 'Women's proximity to their infants (whether they desire it or not) is still seen as a formula for preventing later problems of the child' (p. 4), and 'The requirement to give active love to their babies right after birth is a standard many women find impossible to meet' (p. 13). Eyer warns against assuming that bonding can help to prevent child abuse, raising concerns that this may '...overemphasize bonding at the cost of dealing with the complex social and emotional problems of family members' (Eyer, 1992, p. 13).

Although the existence of infant behaviours that promote proximity to the caretaker and the need for 'sensitive attunement' to infant cues for healthy infant development have been established, Rosenblith (1992) argues that interpretations of attachment behaviours that suggest the need for the sensitive attention of one continuous caretaker are biased. There is also evidence that 'sensitive mothering' is not always beneficial to all women (Woollett and Phoenix , 1991).

Why this might be so can be partly understood by revisiting some of the theories on child development reported earlier. Psychological models view physiological symptoms as dependent variables caused mainly by intrapsychic issues (within the individual; Raphael-Leff, 1991). This approach suggests that women will be psychologically troubled and less able to cope effectively with a subsequent crisis unless these issues are resolved.

This contrasts with the view taken by object relations theory (Mahler *et al.* 1975) which construes that given 'good-enough mothering' (Winnicott, 1965) (i.e. mothering which meets most of the needs of the child most of the time), there need be no unresolvable struggle or conflict when women become mothers themselves.

Feminist object relations theory (Chodorow, 1978) construes that gender identity is formed through these early mother–child relationships. Femininity represents a failure to significantly move away from the mother (hence also a greater capacity to become attached to and relate to others; Wetherell, 1995). However, there is now evidence that how a woman currently perceives her relationship with her mother has greater predictive power concerning adjustment than do the historical facts of childhood (Fonagy *et al.* 1991a, 1991b; Main and Goldwyn, 1989).

Women's adjustments have also been studied in terms of vulnerable personality styles, such as high levels of neuroticism or a negative cognitive set, low marital satisfaction and social support (Cox and Holden, 1994). Unrealistic expectations of what childbirth and parenting 'should be' may also create disappointments. These can threaten a woman's sense of competence and self-esteem, and stimulate depression.

Studies on the contribution of cognitive style to women's psychological well-being have been contradictory (O'Hara *et al.* 1982) and can be criticized for being culturally dependent. Anthropological studies on Kenyan women found no evidence of postpartum depression (Harkness, 1987), suggesting that postnatal depression may relate to Western women's experiences of the transition and Western notions of social role and identity, rather than to individual physical and psychological functioning (Barclay *et al.* 1995).

Other approaches have utilized cognitive-phenomenological theory (Lazarus and Folkman, 1984). This defines stressors as events that are appraised by individuals as threats to their present sense of well-being. Terry (1991) cites a wide range of potential stressors and construes that all women's attitudes towards childrearing change systematically as an inevitable result of becoming mothers.

Early studies were carried out at a time when women generally did not return to work after childbirth (Entwistle and Doering, 1981) and focused on the impact of working women on their children. In contrast, Parr (1996) found that women's attitudes towards childrearing did not automatically change solely as a result of becoming a mother. Parr found that over 60% of women returned to work part time by the time their babies were 6 months old. High levels of anxiety were found when the women were thinking about and planning to leave their child in someone else's care. However, separation anxiety did not appear to be a psychological issue for their partners. Why this might be so is not yet clear.

Early ideas on attachment theory (Bowlby, 1969) argue that this is because working mothers are presumed to be 'deviant'. However, evidence on women's attachment to employment being secondary to their attachment to the childcaring role is contradictory (Brannen and Moss, 1991). It has been suggested that it is how a woman views the conflicting roles of employment and motherhood that influences adjustment (Hock and Schirtzinger, 1992).

These findings suggest the need for an integrative theoretical model to explain and support women's and men's adjustment to parenthood in the late 1990s. This is in accord with Stern's (1995) view that the vast majority of women in the childbearing year are psychologically 'normal'. They do, however, have a special psychological condition, which he refers to as the 'motherhood constellation'. Parr (1996) has also identified a 'fatherhood constellation'. Both are unique organizations of mental life appropriate for and adapted to the reality of being a mother or a father in the late 1990s (**Box 15.3**).

Box 15.3

Support in Adjustment to Parenthood

Support is a key factor in the successful adjustment of men and women to parenthood:

• What different types of support are available for expectant and new parents in your area?

• What do you know about how these were developed? What view of parents, infants and family life do they encourage?

• How effective are they and how has this been measured?

• What do you think are the key features of effective parent education and support for the prenatal and perinatal period?

• How would you assess the effectiveness of any support you offer to new parents?

Implications for Midwives

Psychological support in the transition to parenthood has been shown to assist the adjustment of women and men to new parenthood (Cowan *et al.* 1985; Parr, 1996) and increase the proportion of secure parent–infant relationships (Duncan and Markman, 1988; Smith, 1996).

Midwives are often called upon to support and teach parenting as if it were merely a matter of how well a woman copes with childbirth, or a well-defined set of practical behaviours (such as feeding, bathing and other practical aspects of infant care) which are reduced to prescribed techniques. However, it is possible to see a parent who 'behaves' like a parent, but both the baby and the observer are aware that something essential is missing. Midwives are also in an unique position to support men becoming fathers.

This section provides evidence to suggest that 'Parenting is more than a sum of behaviours. It involves a commitment to nurturance' (Eldridge and Schmidt, 1990, p. 339). Parental behaviour also occurs in the context of childhood and family history, couple and family relationships and the wider social world, including work.

Although infants are equipped for growth, and poor attachment does not necessarily lead to later dysfunction, much of their early development depends on the nurturance and stimulation a parent (mother and father) optimally offers. The evidence suggest that it is unlikely

that any new parent who is caught up with their own psychological concerns has the ability to take the perspective of the dependent infant and demonstrate the patience, sensitivity and responsiveness that early parenting requires. The infant is also a source of feedback which may also guide parental behaviour and shape the parent's image of the baby as well as of themselves as parents.

The findings suggest that key issues for midwives are the need to:

• Understand that pregnancy, birth and the early postnatal period are formative experiences for both parents and their infants.

• Clarify more precisely the links between the meaning of events for women and their partners during the transition to parenthood.

• Understand the way psychological changesthat occur during this time are processed.

• Understand how these impact on parent–infant relationships and family life in general.

• Clarify the relevant type of support offered to parents during this time.

SOCIAL CONTEXT OF PARENTING

The experience of parenting consists in the adaptation to a new role identity for parents and family members. This period of adaptation and consolidation is affected by factors such as how one perceives this new role, but also by how society values it (Mercer, 1986). In Western societies there is some degree of ambiguity with regard to the status of parenting; it is held as an ideal social achievement, but in conflict with other roles, such as pursuing a career. This is particularly pertinent for women (Oakley, 1980; Ball, 1994).

Successful parenting has been equated with the well-being of children and hence of the wider society (Rutter, 1972). Enhancing the formation and consolidation of lasting new relationships in a new family is therefore a crucial goal for midwifery care.

In this section, further understanding of the nature and development of the family and the activity of parenting in Western society is provided. Various theoretical perspectives that have informed opinion and beliefs in this context are critically examined. Finally, midwifery practice is scrutinized for opportunities to enhance the adaptation to parenting, based on the real needs of individuals.

The Family

This section will address the structure and function of the family over recent history, and the gender issues arising from role divisions which exist therein. A discussion of the implications of these issues will be offered.

Form and Function – Historical Development

It is often held that the 'nuclear' family is a contemporary development in family structure, emerging as a result of socioeconomic changes, and usurping the extended family as a social unit. Contemporary social commentators, such as Anthony Giddens (1986), are critical of this view, which emerged in the 1950s and 1960s, pointing to the lack of evidence to support it.

He states that, even though the emergence of capitalism and changes in the economic base from agrarian to urban industrial occurred, the extended family did not break down. Historical sources indicate the existence of a 'nuclear' arrangement in society for several centuries. However, kinship and community networks have lost their strength over time. As the family of the past was an economically functioning unit, ties and interdependencies were inevitably more active. Laslett and Wall (1972) support this view, reinforcing the improbability of close proximity of extended families.

Giddens (1986) claims an underestimate of the complexity of change in the form of the family; previously whole families would move into employment together, the elderly and children all taking part in waged work. Only when legislation began to mitigate against child labour was a significant change brought about. He refers to the work of Laurence Stone (1977), which offers a more historically accurate view of family development since 1700. Stone refers to the 'earlier' form wherein the family consists of a couple as the nucleus with kinship ties radiating widely outwards through other family members and into the community.

In many cases, the marriage partner was chosen by others. The relationship was not based initially on romantic ties, but geared towards their function within the labour market, which could determine survival of both their offspring and dependent elderly relatives.

Relations between parents and children depended largely on the place of the family in the social hierarchy. Marriage was also a function of social position so that those at the top were concerned to ensure continued ownership of wealth and land through inheritance, whereas those at the bottom were concerned with day-to-day survival.

Living circumstances for the poor were often cramped and mean, whether urban or rural, in the eighteenth and nineteenth centuries. Large groups often lived together. It was not until the nineteenth century that housing stock, particularly in urban areas, increased, mainly in response to increasing numbers of people moving into towns for work (Best, 1971).

Segalen (1986) points out that despite this movement, kinship ties remained strong, but eventually were compromised by geographical distance and changing social circumstances. The emergence of the Victorian middle class increased earning and consuming power and changed lifestyles and attitudes – a major change that affected the breakdown in family ties.

The male head of the household became prominent as the main wage earner, so the nuclear family became the focal point for childrearing and related domestic activities – previously a shared undertaking. This 'unit' became further isolated socially; the process accelerated into the early years of the twentieth century with the result that only small pockets of communities of family and kinship networks remain, such as in East London and South Wales.

Marriage increasingly came to be based on sentiment and sexual attraction. Women began to move out of the workforce, particularly in the middle classes, some employing others to take over their domestic duties. Things remained much as they were for the poor.

Family size diminished as contraception became available and children eventually came to be seen as requiring more than food and shelter, were excluded from the workplace and education was provided. Childhood itself was beginning to be seen as a meaningful part of the developmental process towards adulthood, thus attitudes began to change.

Present Diversity – Form and Function

A common concern relating to the family of the late twentieth century is that of its apparent instability caused by high divorce rates. Segalen (1986) states that divorce is not a modern phenomenon, being common in previous centuries. Serial monogamy was common because of high mortality rates caused by poor health and living conditions. Relationships were often short in duration. Segalen (1986) extrapolates that as life expectancy is much longer now it is understandable that divorce is more common. Concern is still voiced, mainly with respect to the numbers of women alone with children.

There has been an increase in births outside marriage to one in five of all births in 1990, but 71% of these are within a stable relationship (Social Trends, 1992). There is also an increase in the remarriage rate, which may offset the divorce rate and possibly point towards a continuing trend to regard marriage as a worthwhile institution (Williams, 1989).

However, there is inevitably an increase in the formation of step families which have long been perceived as more likely to malfunction with particular problems arising for children involved. But, as Williams (1989) points out, although complex problems of readjustment are encountered in these new formations, any resultant detriment is more likely to be caused by the prevailing socioeconomic situation for that family. The implications for providing the means with which to achieve an amicable separation through policy are clear. Overall, it would seem that current trends in changing family formations may not be as deleterious as propagandists might suggest. In fact, Williams (1989) suggests that not enough attention may be paid to the parents themselves during this period of readjustment.

Fletcher (1991) suggests that the modern family's functions are commonly seen as encompassing sexual needs of the adults, the upbringing of children and the provision of a home. Although limited in its application, this general view still seems to hold even with recent changes. Despite this, the family still seems to be the target for blame for various problems in society, such as the apparent decline in morality, discipline and self-respect among young adults.

Williams' (1989) analysis states that families and how they function are very much influenced by other institutions within society. For instance, current consumerist ideologies reduce any notion of the family to a productive unit; the goal is better economic status and self-improvement, which causes a dilemma between state intervention and autonomy. He suggests that social policy should provide more real support for families who choose to follow the consumerist route. Child neglect by the working mother should be seen as a failure of the state to provide adequate childcare facilities. Increasing moral alarm continues to be expressed concerning the numbers of pregnancies that occur among teenage girls, given that this could be used as a yardstick of society's moral well-being.

It is a fact that this group do face problems concerning housing, finance and health when adapting to parenthood. Cashmore (1985) points out that when the state maintains single parents outside marriage this serves as a threat to the institution itself. Resultant poverty and hardship may be seen as deserved.

The existence of pregnant teenagers signifies the reality of teenage sexual activity within society – something to be discouraged, but for the teenagers it is and always has been an important part of identity-formation behaviour (Pheonix, 1991). The transition to parenting for these girls (or boys) is inevitably complicated by their own emotional needs in adolescence, and interferes with education and job opportunities, which may lead to fewer life chances later. However, there is no categorical proof that teenagers parent any less well than older candidates.

There is a growing number of women who choose to become mothers alone, and even more men and women who are forced into the situation by divorce or widowhood. The numbers here have increased considerably in the UK since 1970 – by 50%. It is also the case that approximately one in ten one-parent families are headed by a lone father (General Household Survey, 1991).

The overriding considerations for such families are housing disadvantages, exacerbated by recession and by falling stocks of council housing in the past 15 years. When one salary is lost to the household this inevitably presents problems for those left to maintain outgoings. Lone parents have been shown to be discriminated against in the private rented sector (Hardy and Crowe, 1991). But even when accommodation is secured, young single mothers have particular problems in securing employment (McRobbie, 1989). The fact that many lone parents remarry is perhaps an indicator of the stress lone parenting produces.

Lone parents suffer from poorer health than parents in couples (Popay and Jones, 1991), and particularly those aged 35 years and over. This may reflect the turmoil of separation and relationship breakdown and also material deprivation, even if temporary. Those who work and use childcare are not as likely to suffer from illhealth as those not working (Popay and Jones, 1988), which relates to income and lifestyle.

Provision of employment opportunities for lone parents is essential, but this means a parallel provision of childcare facilities, which is happening more slowly. However, it is true that many thousands of lone parents provide loving and suitable environments, despite the price they may pay with their health. Hardey and Crowe (1991) find that the experiences of lone women in particular are very varied – it can be seen positively with the option to remarry viewed as a curtailment of freedom; conversely the hope of remarriage is frequently expressed. But, importantly, the quality of parenting found in such situations is often consistently good, despite public rhetoric stating the reverse. In fact, Collins

(1985, in Hardey and Crowe, 1991) concludes his review by suggesting that in some cases lone parent households are less unsatisfactory than step-family groups. But overall each needs individual assessment outside the criteria set by prevailing ideologies.

It is clear that if the family is to survive into the twenty-first century intact, it must be given the resources so to do.

Sociological Theory Perspectives on the Family

The family, and how and why it functions, became a popular focus for attention in the 1960s and 1970s – in the resultant sociological discourse, various conflicting views arose. The institution of marriage and gender roles were reconsidered; feminist criticisms threw new light onto the debate.

David Cheal (1991) examines a wide variety of these analyses, warning at the outset that such theories can be subjectively biased, so provide only a limited perspective on the complexities of the family.

Nostalgia for lost unity and stability in society was predominant in the 1950s, influenced by the views of such as Talcott Parsons (1954), who persisted that the nuclear family was the most functional form given that, in Parson's structural functionalist view, this unit best met the needs of individuals in society at that time. It was small, mobile and self-sufficient, befitting an industrial economy.

Cheal (1991) criticizes this stance as simplistic, dependent on orthodox views of gender divisions of labour and implicit equilibrium within its inherent relationships, whereas reality for individuals is subjective and variable.

Feminist critics see this model as a denial of the patriarchal power dynamics necessary for this 'form' to exist (Oakley, 1985; Hall, 1992). Hall (1992) states that family life is an ideological construct that is gender based, and so needs to be deconstructed to perceive the reality. This 'monolithic model of the family' should be destroyed.

The positivist model of enquiry within sociological observation offers some insights into the causes of behaviour in a given setting, but also has its own limitations; gender issues seem to escape empirical data collection.

'Post positivism' offers greater diversity of interpretation and can be largely described under the headings of traditional, reformist, liberationist or pro-system, dependent on beliefs and ideology. It would seem wise to observe each school of thought critically.

Modern society values scientific endeavour, which can then be used for the betterment of society. Talcott Parson's (1954) model allowed for a particular understanding of the family in this context, but as the family form continues to evolve his model is becoming redundant. There is an increasing understanding of the interrelationships and a concern for dysfunctional families.

Cheal (1991) ponders the future by considering how the growth of individualism and self-responsibility will affect the family and its survival. Weakening of the motivational commitment to collective community purpose must have repercussions. Cheal (1991) reiterates that sociology is linked to biopolitics, so the underlying power relationships of class and gender must be analysed.

A family that does not conform to the currently held 'norm' is often labelled dysfunctional, so professionals can then make the interventions seen to be appropriate. Conversely, some dysfunction is considered out of bounds for outside agencies. Domestic violence is one such example, whereby it has been traditional until recent years for the police to turn a blind eye. It is women and children who take the brunt of this abuse (Kitzinger, 1992). The traditional model is decidedly unhelpful in this respect, tending to create a private and public face of the family, which can lead to situations evolving as described – domination and exploitation can occur without redress (Cheal, 1991).

Social pluralism of the 1990s has led to further variations in the form and function of family individuals, especially women, which indicates a change in established views. Standardization and diversification are occurring simultaneously. A new paradigm is needed to reflect more accurately the dynamics of interpersonal ties.

Attempts to address this are to be found in phenomenological and interactionist methodologies, which provide observations and analyses of interactions. But, again, criticisms are made concerning the lack of cognizance of gender issues in such studies. However, these approaches attempt to view experience through the eyes of individuals as far as possible, and so are more likely to incorporate the dynamic nature of a family over time.

It cannot be denied that social life implies and is based on interpersonal interaction regardless, perhaps, of the shape of vehicle for that interaction – the family. Companionship based on mutual affection will continue to provide the starting point, even if there is disorganization and subsequent reorganization – which can be complex but is not necessarily random. The realities of the world of families must be the work of sociology, not sociology imposing ideas about that reality. Thus, the plurality and rich complexity of how lives are lived requires lateral thinking and passive observation rather than deduction and theory formation.

Gender and Divisions of Labour in Family Life

Gender, as in feminine or masculine, defines one's social identity within a given culture which then dictates the function, status and value attached to gender according to the dominant ideology.

The majority of history texts tend to assume that the only gender worthy of mention is masculine. Rosalind Miles (1989), however, has graphically retold the story of the history of the world to include a feminine presence. She identifies many examples of past civilizations wherein women played a dominant social role and held economic and political power. This power was related to woman's unique ability in reproduction and giving birth – mysterious and magical events.

This power diminished, however, because of the increasing knowledge of physiology and the advent of religious cults that professed the superiority of men. This shifting paradigm usurped women's status, which thereafter declined.

Gender is expressed in accepted norms of behaviour, appearance and social etiquette, which are embedded in culture. Traditionally, 'female' is equated with characteristics such as physical weakness, emotional liability, passivity and a propensity towards caring for others. The roles which follow from this profile are inevitably servile – those of mothering, home maker and provider of emotional and physical support for others.

Conversely, masculine characteristics comprise physical strength, proactivity, decision making and are expressed as a more dominant authoritarian role in the family, being responsible for material provision but with little involvement in domestic or childcare activities (Oakley, 1985).

These commonly held stereotypes are prevalent both outside and inside the home. Masculine activities are seen as of more value in society than those undertaken by women. Housework and childcare are thereby denigrated, despite evidence of symmetry within families (Young and Wilmott, 1972).

A small number of studies have analysed the occupation of housework, such as Oakley (1974) and, more recently, Hall (1992), but although these illustrate the inequalities therein there seems little impetus for social change.

Women today have to respond to mixed messages regarding how they should best function in society. Motherhood may be unpaid, but it is still held as an ideal for woman's achievement; however, women also being drawn back into the labour market for economic and social reasons.

Such ideas about the roles of men and women are passed on to future generations through the process of socialization (Berger and Luckman, 1967). Children are exposed to role models of behaviour and attitude among adults, siblings, peers, teachers and the media – the degree to which ideas are formed regarding gender depends on the formative environment (Smith and Lloyd, 1978). The extent of the true impact of socialization as it affects adult behaviour has been questioned.

In the early and middle twentieth century, many studies undertaken inferred a biological basis for general behavioural differences (Freud 1953; Piaget 1969; Lever, 1976; Erikson 1977). These findings have been criticized by feminists, such as Carol Gilligan (1987), as androcentric. She points to, however, the wide acceptance of this 'evidence', particularly in the field of education. She reminds us that often the subjects observed were male, that the interpretation of data was undertaken from a male perspective and so caution must be applied to conclusions.

Work by McClelland (1953) showed much lower levels of success motivation in girls than in boys. These results have been variously interpreted, ranging from an innate inability or wish to succeed to Sassens' (1980) assumptions that women are more concerned to avoid the negative impact of competitive behaviour.

Mary O'Brien (1981) reverses Freud's 'envy' hypothesis to explain why many men appear to alienate themselves from the process of childbirth, claiming that feelings of redundancy after conception cause them revert to typical male gender behaviour, as dictated by the cultural norms of that society.

Such research evidence has been interpreted ideologically, leading to the reinforcement of gender roles in parenting. The ideological basis for this belief renders this assumption invalid, and unhelpful.

Parenting

This section will describe the historical development of the activity of parenting to the present day, and critically examine those factors which have been influential. Particular reference is made to the changing perceptions of children as a catalyst in this context.

The Historical Development of the Activity of Parenting and Changing Perceptions of Children

Parenting activities were carried out by a wide range of friends and relatives before the twentieth century. The focus for this role has moved increasingly towards the parents themselves, so that today many parents care for children in what amounts to social isolation.

After legislation to prevent the exploitation of children in the workplace (Best, 1971) and the more recent recognition of childhood as a distinct and important life phase, children have increasingly been viewed as having intrinsic value and specific developmental needs that are to be provided by the family, and include the enhancement of physical, social and intellectual growth. Reduction in family size serves to focus greater attention on smaller numbers of offspring who are more likely to survive than their pre-Victorian counterparts.

Parenting as a 'semi-profession' (Eyer, 1993) grew in the early and middle years of the twentieth century, informed by a growing body of pseudoscientific data, the exponents of which have become gurus in their own right; they are often men (Truby King, Benjamin Spock) and offer didactic views on how to do it.

But parenting has developed largely because of the changing perception of the needs of children through recent centuries. Early religious teaching stated that all mortals were born with original sin, thus the purpose of life was to purge that blemish to prepare for the life everlasting. Phillipe Aries (1979) describes the 'mini-adult' view of children prevalent in the sixteenth and seventeenth centuries of Europe. The eighteenth century philosopher, Locke, proposed that children could be taught to reason and were innately intelligent. However, parenting depended largely on the cultural perceptions of children and their relations with adults, and this dictated their needs. This led to the development of the myriad of customs, rites and rituals that surround birth and childhood in many societies.

Despite a prevailing Victorian romanticized view of childhood, many improvements were seen regarding poverty, illhealth and education. Reality for many was hardship and early death, but children became increasingly valued as reflected in changing attitudes. Psychological and other studies from this time on (Darwin, 1872; Gesell, 1930; Freud, 1953) and others led to changing perceptions of children, their needs and abilities.

There was concurrently a steady increase in the number of experts who professed wisdom. One famous proponent of the authoritative style of parenting was Dr F Truby King, who came to London in 1917 to set up his influential Mothercraft Training School. His ideology was that a contented, well-trained baby is more likely to become a useful, well-balanced adult in society (Humphries and Gordon, 1993). He promoted regimes of care based on discipline; feeding and sleeping to the clock; sleeping alone; potty training from birth; babies put out to air to toughen them. Crying was not responded to as this 'weakened the character', and kissing and cuddling were frowned upon.

Many women adopted this regimen in the honest belief that they were doing the best for the child, but many found that their instincts clashed with these teachings and they suffered much anxiety, guilt and confusion. King was hugely influential in childcare practices in the UK until recent decades.

But it seemed that the authoritarian model was a good 'fit' for the fast emerging smaller suburban family of post World War I Britain. Women's work, including the 'mothering', was influenced by technological advances and driven by a reliance on science. In larger, predominantly working-class families at this time, however, conditions did not allow such regimes to persist; it was common for older children to take on parenting tasks, along with relatives, neighbours and friends (Thompson, 1939).

Infant health continued to improve after World War I, mainly because of better living conditions, sanitation, food supplements and the emergence of vaccination, gathering momentum with the advent of the Welfare State in 1948.

However, alternative views were emerging based on the new ideas from psychology, which promoted a much kinder, liberal approach to childcare. The major exponent was Dr Benjamin Spock, who wrote *Common Sense Book of Baby and Child-Care* in 1946 encapsulating the new ideologies. To enjoy your baby was now 'permitted'; to kiss, cuddle and respond instinctively was encouraged. This could be interpreted as a rejection of the Freudian fears which generated the authoritative style. Humphries and Gordon (1993) offer insights into the reality of parenting before 1950. Several of their interviewees talk of their experiences with the Truby King methods; all feel angry that their own instincts were denied.

Parenting became an increasingly private function within the nuclear family. Today it can often be the case that parents, particularly women, are the sole providers of childcare, leading to loneliness, isolation and depression. Communities are fragmenting; some are reforming, but patterns of work and childcare facilities mitigate against women sharing this burden with many others. Oakley (1980) has written about the effects of such isolation; these are negative for the woman herself and potentially for the whole family. Her more recent work (Oakley *et al.* 1990) clarifies the detrimental effects of social deprivation in pregnancy exacerbated by isolation and lack of support.

A plethora of texts that advise parents exists and continues to flourish, though the pattern and tone of advice change over time, reflecting ideas hitherto described.

One of the more useful authors is Mia Kelmer Pringle (1974), who has written widely in the context of childcare. She offers a simple guide to parenting. She states that it is not useful to arrange needs in a hierarchy (Maslow, 1954), as they are interrelated and interdependent. She criticizes the sociological debate that surrounds the concept of 'mother' love (Bowlby, 1952), which has yet to state clearly the nature of the relationship a child requires to have with its caretakers. She lists a child's needs simply as love, security and a continuous dependable relationship that promotes self-approval through others. Familiar and constant caregivers provide security in which unpredictability is minimized and safety and comfort maximized. A child requires to know that it is loved. She stresses the importance of the male partner in this role, both in practical and emotional terms.

Pringle does not get caught up with the minutiae of how to parent – only principles. This point is reinforced by Newson and Newson (1963) and elsewhere, wherein patterns of childcare are observed to vary as a result of class, culture, age and other variables, but that the end result is much the same in all cases. An important issue for new parents.

The Experience of Parenting and Gender Roles

Rapoport and Rapoport (1977) state that the ongoing debates about parenting in scholarly circles are often remote from the realities of the experience, so it is necessary to find out from parents themselves what these realities are. There is limited evidence in the form of oral histories and literature (Thompson, 1939; Ross, 1993; Humphries and Gordon, 1993; Oakley, 1980), which suggests that the reality has been largely hidden, leading to the generation of myths.

Ellen Ross (1993) provides one such source of information that relates to poor women in Victorian London. For these women motherhood was inevitable, mainly because of lack of knowledge about and availability of adequate contraception. Pregnancies were frequent and

close together. Women of 35 years or older had an average of 7.6 children; 40% of these had nine or more, and only 13% had four or less.

The fatalistic attitude of many of these women is encapsulated in the phrase, 'What is fated must be', which was recorded by a midwife of the time. Women's lives were dominated by birth, childcare, death and hard toil inside and outside the home.

Humphries and Gordon (1993) offer a compilation of oral histories from individuals who were parents before 1950. They tell a very similar story to those in Ross's accounts, whereby the social expectations of marriage and motherhood proved very different in reality compared to the myth of a fulfilling experience which was potent then and still is today.

Post World War II changes in the economy of the UK brought about a rise in living standards for a large section of the population. Women who could afford not to work were actively encouraged not to; they were to be concerned with home making and mothering. However, women continued to move back into the workplace (many had never left) in the 1960s, 1970s and 1980s as attitudes and pay differentials became liberalized.

However, the prime role of women as mothers continued to be held as the ideal, a view which was based on evidence from the studies of Bowlby (1952) and Klaus and Kennell (1972). Diane Eyer (1992) offers a radical criticism of the way in which the findings of such studies have been embraced by conservative thinkers, including the medical profession. She claims that the conclusions drawn about mother–infant bonding are shot through with ideological bias, consisting in the belief that women and motherhood are synonymous. Even though Klaus and Kennell's work in particular led to the now common practice of 'rooming in', she states that this practice has been instigated under the guise of freeing women from custodial institutional practices, but is really to do with reinforcing gender stereotypes in parenting.

Medicine has been identified as a powerful profession (Illich, 1977; Foucault, 1980), which dictates normality, promotes a dependence culture and is guilty in this context of reducing the complexity of parent–infant relationships to oversimplicity.

Likewise, Bowlby's (1952) work concluded that a child's needs primarily consist of care from a loving mother, reinforcing woman's key role in parenting. But caution is needed here as Bowlby clearly states that a mother substitute is acceptable, but this rider was seldom quoted. Rutter (1972) has redressed the balance here by re-examining Bowlby's assumptions and concluding that the possibility of damaging the infant's psyche through neglect by the biological mother is fallacious.

Women remain confused as to what society expects of them in terms of the role which they should play; the conflict between that of mother versus earner persists. Oakley (1980) demonstrates the reality of parenting for women. She discusses current paradigms of women as reproducers, how the meaning of childbirth is manufactured and the problems caused by failure to address the reality of the experience.

Although the transition to motherhood is still considered a key phase in women's lives, its nature and the preparation for it have changed owing to the changes in the family as a unit hitherto described. Fewer women have direct contact with babies and children, have fewer role models and have smaller support networks. Conflict of interests between private and public functions can result in a parenthood loaded with anxiety, crises and increased dependence on professionals.

Oakley's (1980) research threw up themes such as inappropriate preparation for taking on the role of parent, and a partner who himself was not prepared and thus was not supportive. These women were more likely to succeed in their transition to parent if others perceived this shift positively. A key factor was the degree of control that the woman exercised over events that surround childbirth, which health professionals affect significantly. The most frequent experience for women is that of losing control, as shown elsewhere (Hunt and Symonds, 1995). Disillusionment was frequent due to the misfit of expectations with reality and, again, the conflict between the status of mothering and earning power. Kitzinger (1978) blames midwives for the perpetuation of this myth, by overintellectualizing about the subject. Realism must overcome idealism and some anticipatory fear is a necessary preparation.

Social policy has a role to play in terms of financial remuneration for the tasks of parenting. Changes here would be influential in altering attitudes towards this supposedly vital social role.

It is variously suggested that being a mother and being a person are mutually exclusive possibilities. This contingency must be reversed if the reality of parenting is to be accepted and undertaken successfully.

The Role of Men in Parenting

Previous sections mention gender inequalities and the focus on the female in parenting. It must be remembered that, as Raphael-Leff (1991) has stated, men have unique needs of their own during the transition to and subsequent performance of parenting, not merely as interested bystanders.

Grantly Dick-Read (1944) and others recognized the importance of mutual responsibility in parenting, but little attention has been paid to the feelings of, or preparation for, men in parenting. Humphries and Gordon (1993) offer a few insights here, which challenge the view of male disinterest. One interviewee felt he had missed out on childrearing because of the demands of work; another stayed home as often as possible to help with domestic tasks. But he admits he was an exception among his peers.

The increasing isolation of the nuclear family, better wages, cars and leisure time has meant greater opportunities for men's involvement in childcare and domestic life, so that today's 'New Age Man' is expected to participate. Contemporary parenting by men has generated a small but growing literature, often consisting of accounts of personal experiences (Jackson, 1983; Pruett, 1983; Hanson and Bozett, 1985). There is very little hard evidence for the realities of parenting for men.

Some earlier studies carried out in the spirit of the biological basis for the behaviour paradigm showed that not only did the father react physiologically to a child's cry (Lamb and Lamb, 1976), but also infants responded positively to the father (Rutter, 1972) and infants bonded equally with male and female carers – in fact, with anyone who played a regular role in their care. Keller *et al.* (1985) showed that the earlier men become involved in care the stronger these bonds became, producing high self-esteem in the subjects. So there are gains to be made all round.

But this is only so if, as Pruett (1983) and Jackson (1983) claim, society's 'sacred stabilities' based on gender role divisions are challenged. Both authors tell of their and other men's experiences of parenting, which has to be learned through trial and error because there are few role models in previous generations and few opportunities for practice.

Few studies exist of the transition to parenthood in men; one phenomenological study by Henderson and Brouse (1991) identifies such a process. They refer to social pressures on men to opt out and those individuals who wish to get involved make a 'lonely decision' to do so, with little support or guidance from any source, particularly family and friends, who appear more significant in this respect than do the health professionals.

What evidence exists in the literature seems to suggest that men's transition to parenthood is 'crisis oriented' (Roopnarine and Miller, 1985). However, this situation is changing and becoming a much more normative process – changes in family structure are bringing about modifications to traditional roles, including the emergence of the house-husband, who is yet to be fully investigated. Lutwin and Siperstein (1985) conducted interviews with such individuals who saw themselves as performing tasks equally as well as women, well satisfied with their lifestyle and felt a sense of autonomy in their role, appearing to contradict traditional views.

Much more observational data requires to be gathered to paint any accurate picture of fatherhood and its meaning in the 1990s. As Jackson (1983) points out, there is much written about fathers who are absent, deviant or dead. From what is available it must be concluded that men want to, are able to and should be given opportunities to become more involved as fathers. The paradigm of parenting which focuses on 'mothering' by women needs challenging – in the workplace, in social policy-making and in the private life of families. Somehow, as Jackson (1983) puts it, we must 'break the masculine taboo on tenderness'.

Male and female roles within parenting can no longer be polarized as they have been in Western culture if the burdens and the pleasures are to be equally shared. Paternity leave is an increasingly available option, but men need to be given reasons for opting in, for not going back to work; the culture of parenting is in need of reappraisal as much as is social policy.

Stewart (1990) proposes, from the results of his study, that mothers can be instrumental in guiding and encouraging fathers through the role transition by providing opportunities for involvement in caregiving. He observes that this involvement may not be so great with the first child, owing to society's views of who should be doing the parenting, but for practical reasons this distance cannot be easily maintained with subsequent new arrivals. So perhaps Pruett (1983) was right – women are the 'gatekeepers' of parenting.

According to Barbour (1990) fathers have made considerable headway in consolidating their position at the birth; they now need to do so in the antenatal and post-natal periods if the new family is to successfully consolidate.

Other Factors that Affect Parenting

This section briefly addresses some issues surrounding second-time parenting which need to be considered in order to make individualised care effective. Some other situations are briefly mentioned.

Second and subsequent children

It is commonly assumed that the transition to parenthood is inevitably easier the second time around. Hence, it is likely that advice and time given to such parents may well be less than that to first-time parents. Many studies of parenting are directed at first-time parents, but a study by Jordon (1989) identifies clearly that these assumptions are ill-founded, so care based on them will be less effective. Respondents in the study found the total childbirth experience different the second time, for many reasons, but mainly that having another child around affected the way in which they were able to adjust to the new baby.

Parents seemed to be just as anxious regarding their ability to care for a new baby, and needed praise and encouragement so that they could learn to trust themselves again. They needed extra help with household chores and the care of the older child. Most of all, these parents needed to be listened to by health professionals while they expressed their fears and anxieties.

Another detailed study by Stewart (1990) similarly identifies second-time parenting as stressful, but in a different way to the first time. The potential sources of stress appear to increase as the number of demands on parents grow. The effects can even cause depression in both parents.

Marital relationships are affected by the degree to which the expectations of partners' involvement meets reality. Disappointment and conflict are inevitable when a gap appears here, as was shown by Oakley (1980). Levels of conflict, however, can be reduced when couples begin to negotiate around their needs (La Rossa and La Rossa, 1981; Backet, 1982).

The first child's behaviour is a stressor, especially when it is perceived to demonstrate failure to adapt to becoming a sibling. Hence, the child is seen decreasingly as a source of positive reinforcement to the parents' esteem. This is offset by the father's increased involvement with the older child and in domestic chores. It seems reasonable to suggest that this activity by the father would be much easier to take on if he had been involved with the first child actively from its birth.

The experience is, however, perceived generally as positive; a source of family coherence despite the problems encountered.

Health-care professionals clearly need to appreciate the reality of the second and subsequent births, and the nature of the stress incurred. Appropriate care can only be given and received if assumptions are replaced by realism and a willingness to listen.

Other groups

There are other groups who are not represented well in society. These include black, disabled, drug-addicted, gay and mentally handicapped parents. Unfortunately, the remit of this chapter does not allow for a thorough exposition of their situations; suffice it to say that their needs may be very specific according to their special situations, but Mukti Campion (1995) identified some common themes.

She stresses the need for these individuals not to be measured against white, middle-class values, which predominate among health-care professionals. Variations of 'normal' need to be clearly separated from deviations. Campion (1995) points to the poor quality of research to date in which it is very hard to define exactly what quality of parenting is to be found in the aforementioned groups; the research which exists is interpreted ideologically, and so of little use in providing a true understanding. Research needs to arise from within these (deviant) groups (*sic*), but how this is to be facilitated against a background of current scientific paradigms is not clear.

Health professionals need to deconstruct old and reform new attitudes, which exclude the pathology tag attached to individuals from these marginal groups, so that at the grass roots level their real needs can be heard. We surely do not have to wait for research findings to do that.

Implications for Midwifery Practice

It has been demonstrated that to facilitate a successful transition to parenthood is one of the most important goals of midwifery care to enhance the consolidation of the new family group. The effectiveness of current practice in this context is debatable (Hillan, 1991; Page, 1993).

Midwives, like any individuals, hold a view that is made up of personal experience, cultural ideas and socialization, and these values and beliefs are altered by new experiences and an expanding theoretical knowledge base. They can be translated into stereotypes of people and situations, to enable an understanding of the world. Similarly, the process of socialization that occurs on entering a profession contributes here (Witz, 1994).

There are, therefore, many factors that influence a practitioner's philosophy of care, which, as Bryar (1995) points out, affects the quality of care given, especially if beliefs and values lead to judgemental assumptions. So, if one holds particular beliefs about how families should function and how parenting should be carried out, then those who do not conform to these values are judged as abnormal, and hence the care given may be inappropriate. Fixed ideas in relation to human social behaviour are no longer relevant.

Midwives need to critically examine their values and biases – and review and change as necessary. Developing self-awareness can be achieved if a practitioner has a real desire to make care effective.

Parenthood and its realities need to be introduced openly in discussion while the transition process is itself ongoing, so pregnancy groups or one-to-one discussion are useful in encouraging the expression of hopes and fears. How far present antenatal classes provide this is unclear, but studies by O'Meara (1993) and Hillan (1992) tend to show that there is room for improvement. Activities still seem to be based on outmoded educational methods in which midwives set the agenda and limit input from group members. This is surprising given the wealth of literature available to guide educators (Murphy-Black and Faulkner, 1988; Wilberg, 1992; Priest and Schott, 1991). Perhaps it is more to do with how midwives are selected and prepared for this role.

Becoming more familiar with one's caseload, through continuity of care, provides better opportunities for assessing individual needs. Giving information, care and encouragement to both partners, the grandparents, siblings, aunts and uncles is useful in enhancing the whole family's transition and reformation.

Oakley (1980) and Jordan (1989) offer simple clues as to how useful just listening and valuing is in fostering self-esteem, but this takes precious time which has hitherto been allocated to tasks. Time management needs to be reviewed critically to free midwives to give social and emotional care.

Similar principals apply to care given during the birth wherein the needs of partners must be met. They must not remain mere interested bystanders, as Barbour (1990) points out. The place of birth may be relevant, given that parents often feel more in control of events at home, but this is often determined by the attitude of the carer.

Midwifery in the UK is currently in danger of being accused of failing to meet the total postnatal needs of women, and therefore perhaps of families (Glazener *et al.* 1993; Ball, 1994). The statutory obligation to care has bred a certain complacency. Opportunities to enhance the transition to parenthood at a most crucial time cannot be missed or displaced by a commitment to routine physical care. Hillan (1992) urges carers to audit their own practice for meaningful outcomes, wherever the place of work.

True professional autonomy can be defined as the freedom to work in a way that is not driven by the needs of the institution, the profession or their ideologies, but by women and their families. A carer must then employ her initiative, sound knowledge and courage to make meaningful interventions. Often professional boundaries and constraints exist only in the imaginations of the carers themselves. Page (1993) describes expert care as not siting intra venous infussions or performing instrumental deliveries, but making judgements and decisions appropriately; to comfort, counsel and advise, remembering the long-term consequences of these decisions. Parenting is for life – hence the ultimate priority of midwifery care must be, 'to accompany women and their partners on their journey to parenthood' (Page, 1993, p. 24.)

Conclusion

In this section the importance of a successful transition into family life is demonstrated. It examines the family itself and discovers that, though the form may be diversifying, the function remains focused on the provision of an environment for the growth, development and nurture of children. Given the life-long commitment this means for parents, the early successful adaptation to this role is crucial.

Midwives urgently require to reconsider their role in this aspect of practice, which the medicalization and hospitalization of birth have long constrained. They need to re-examine attitudes and knowledge in this context and reaffirm their commitment to provide opportunities to meet the real needs of new and existing families. This vital aspect of the role of the midwife cannot any longer be left to health visitors, who do not have the benefit of intimate contact with families throughout the childbirth process into the early days of parenting.

Midwives must recognize this role and clearly demonstrate that this work is a hallmark of their identity, so that they can defend their right to practice in ways which only they know are appropriate, without interference or influence from outside. Midwives know midwifery – they must continue to demonstrate their commitment to expert practice in the case of the family.

Fathers – Invisible Partners?

The name given to an expectant woman is 'pregnant'; however, there is no comparable name given to the expectant father. The lack of a designated 'name' may be a reflection of the lack of attention paid to men and their experiences of pregnancy and early parenthood. The expectant father could be described as one who demonstrates an interest in the emotional and physical well-being of both the fetus and its mother. He not only assumes responsibility for parenting the child, but in the case of a first-time father undergoes a role transition with very few formal models. The health services only provide a minimal level of education and access to antenatal care to support them.

Men who undergo the transition to parenthood may experience somatic symptoms and seek medical advice more frequently where a high level of parental role preparation is demonstrated. They are often neglected by society, researchers and the maternity services, but are now becoming more of a focus of research and attention. Midwifery literature tends to concentrate on the father as provider and helper during labour. The growing attention paid to expectant fathers has been fuelled by an interest in gender role equality and a resistance to the overconcentration on the mother as parent generated by feminists (McKee and O'Brien, 1982). Rapoport *et al.* (1977, p. 35) suggest that the father is not directly important – only indirectly as a protector and provider for the mother–child couplet. However, Fein (1974) found that some men saw themselves as part of a pregnant couple and suggests that pregnancy is a psychological reality for men.

Fathers as agents and recipients of support in the postnatal period are equally neglected. There is evidence that fathers play an important supportive function within the family; however, the question of when or how to provide intervention or support for them is still unresolved.

Expectant fathers in the 1990s still feel excluded from the childbirth experience by their mates, health-care providers and society (Jordan, 1990). This suggests that the evolving process described by Jessner *et al.* (1970) is not complete and the predominant view held by society is that the expectant father is mainly a provider and helpmate to the expectant woman. In Sweden there has been an official policy to abolish gender roles for over 25 years. However, changing the paternal role has been not without problems and there has been resistance to change that has not been clearly identified (Sandqvist, 1987; Haas, 1993).

The involvement of men in the processes of child-bearing in western Europe and America is a recent phenomenon and may not be similar in all cultures. Britain is a multicultural and multiracial society, so midwives need to provide care that takes account of the language and cultural needs of their clients in order to empower them to make informed decisions about their own care (Roberts, 1996). It is equally important to avoid generalization and stereotyping, but to provide care sensitively to each individual (Schott and Henley, 1996, p. x). In this section, issues of race and culture are not specifically addressed, but providing care that is sensitive to the needs of the individual requires midwives to reflect on their own beliefs and assumptions and how this may affect the service they provide.

Couvade: As a Ritual and an Emotional State

For some men the psychological reality of pregnancy can manifest itself physically. This is described as the couvade syndrome, the most common symptoms being weight gain, toothache and loss of appetite. The term couvade has been used for centuries to describe men who demonstrate somatic symptoms related to their partner's pregnancy. Toothache and abdominal discomforts in men with pregnant wives were mentioned in the seventeenth century by Bacon and Plot (Longobucco and Freston, 1989).

Couvade is also a term used to describe rituals and roles for the expectant father common to many non-Western societies and in our own before the nineteenth century (Bedford and Johnson, 1988). The ritual form of couvade appears in preindustrial societies and consists of special observances and restrictions carried out by the expectant father (Clinton, 1987). This means that two interpretations of couvade exist, both of which relate to expectant fatherhood but have different meanings, although the symptoms of couvade experienced by some men could be caused by the absence of rituals, roles or acknowledgement of the expectant father.

A great deal of the psychological research on expectant fathers comes from the Freudian tradition and centres on abnormal responses, in which the couvade syndrome also features. It is debatable, however, whether the couvade syndrome is an abnormal reaction (Zayas, 1987). Couvade can be an indication of parental role preparation and is more common when the man's partner is anxious about the pregnancy and birth.

Expectant fathers suffer a higher incidence of colds and unintentional weight gain than nonexpectant men and fathers' health differs significantly from that of nonexpectant men during the immediate postpartum period. They suffer more emotional discomforts as well as total number of symptoms, duration and perceived seriousness of the symptoms. Expectant fathers are also more nervous, and suffer excessive fatigue and insomnia (Clinton, 1987).

Couvade could be considered the male counterpart to pregnancy, but the dynamics of the syndrome appear to vary between individuals and may be multidetermined (Klein, 1991). Most men with the syndrome do not require treatment, but the expectant father may benefit by being monitored along with his partner during the pregnancy.

Men and Parentcraft

The Royal College of Midwives stated in 1966 that 'the degree to which the modern father is prepared and indeed anxious to involve himself in his wife's pregnancy' should be publicized to dispel diffidence on the part of many fathers to become involved (RCM, 1966). Although they recommended public awareness, the RCM did not make any comments regarding the small percentage of units, only 10%, which actually made parentcraft provisions for men, nor did they comment on staff preparation to provide for this relatively new consumer of parentcraft.

Nearly 20 years after findings that men were eager to become more directly involved in their partner's pregnancy and with parenting Adams (1982) found only lip service being paid to parenthood preparation for both parents. Many educators did not invite partners to attend and 28% did not even invite them to the special fathers' evening. Many classes were still held during the day, making attendance difficult for partners who work.

There is very little published research specifically regarding parentcraft for men. They are still not recognized as prospective parents, but as helpmates and breadwinners. They have no models to assist them in taking on the role of active and involved parents and, despite the transition to fatherhood being a major life event for men, they are overshadowed by the mother. Parent education programmes have neglected to include the father as an equal partner in parent–infant interaction.

Some men feel that, unlike for women, there are few or no obvious places for them to discuss their feelings about becoming a father. They would like to become more involved in antenatal classes, but are not encouraged to attend. Some findings indicate that health-care providers see only the mother and child as their client and that men believe their presence at antenatal visits is perceived as cute or novel. They feel that they are rarely recognized or treated as parents themselves and are upset by the pervasive message that the partner's role is to support the pregnant woman and new mother. Some men perceive their own fathers as disengaged from their families, acting only as breadwinners; however, they themselves want to be a different sort of parent, but are provided with very little recognition or preparation for their new role (Jordan, 1990).

Although public opinion for nearly 30 years (Rappaport *et al.* 1977; Fein, 1970) has demonstrated a greater awareness and need for preparation for parenthood for men, this need has not been catered for by health professionals. The body of literature on fathers as users of the maternity services is growing, but the majority of the work concentrates on the intrapartum role, excluding antenatal and postnatal involvement. This does not address men's needs in preparation for their role or encourage partners to discuss transition to parenthood as a couple.

Combes and Schonveld (1992) found that men are 'missing out' on parent education. They conclude that:

Men are largely excluded from antenatal and post-natal classes, which are still not universally offered to men, and which may not address their needs.

Barbour (1990) describes the experiences of some of the men who attended parentcraft sessions that were not entirely satisfactory to them. The men found little opportunity to discuss their feelings in the classes they attended, found the content basic and were unhappy that the afternoon timing of the classes meant that few could attend.

The poor educational quality of parent education has been identified as a problem, along with the ambivalence and uncertainty among professionals about addressing men's needs as parents. However, the providers of parent education are becoming more aware of the lack of effectiveness of the classes, mainly because of the way they are organized. Lack of teaching skills has been identified by midwives and health visitors, who have also identified the need to improve the content and preparation of classes, to encourage fathers to attend and to gear the talks to what the attendees themselves want (Rees, 1982). This suggests that the professionals need more preparation for their educational role and should also evaluate the effectiveness of what they offer (O'Meara, 1993).

Men During Labour

In the 1950s and 1960s, with the move of childbirth into hospitals, the expectant father was often portrayed in the media as anxiously pacing the corridor outside the labour room, awaiting the birth from which he was excluded. It is only during the past 20 years or so that fathers have become recognized as part of the birth process; indeed, their presence in the labour ward has become almost a requisite, with midwifery and parent-craft literature focusing on this aspect, yet excluding their antenatal and postnatal role.

In the 1950s, 13% of fathers were present at the birth, but by the 1980s, 67% were present. This rise occurred mainly during the 1970s – at a time when women were requesting their partners to be present some obstetricians were also calling for an increased presence of the father at the birth (Newson and Newson, 1963; Lewis, 1986). A longitudinal survey on the father's role during labour in lay books on child care showed a change from the waiter outside the delivery room to a more active and supporting one (Wollett *et al.* 1982).

The main roles men appear to take during labour are those of supporter, coach, witness and morale sustainer (Chapman, 1991); however, men have been used as substitute carers at times of staff shortage (Keirse *et al.* 1989).

The presence of the woman's partner during labour has been found to be beneficial to the woman and aided the man's successful transition to parenthood (Pridham *et al.* 1991). In a study of the first-time father's experience of being present during childbirth, Nichols (1993) found that fathers had positive or very positive feelings about the experience, with comments such as 'glad to be with wife ... loved the experience ... excited ... gratified ... she needed me ... it was our childbirth, not hers ... overjoyed ... indescribable'. However, a significant number of fathers who had attended prenatal classes reported feeling helpless, anxious, uncertain and exhausted, finding it difficult to see their wife in so much pain, with one father reporting that 'prenatal class instructions were countermanded by labour and delivery nurses.' The men felt that the most helpful things they did to help their wives during the labour and birth were to provide physical and psychological comfort and to just be there. More negative feelings were listed by prepared fathers than unprepared fathers and Nichols (1993) concludes that the findings 'challenge the current view that prenatal childbirth education preparation is believed to contribute to a more positive labour experience for both parents.'

As the findings suggest that the labour experience may be more stressful for the prepared father than the unprepared ones, Nichols (1993) suggests that the classes may not adequately prepare them for the experience or that their needs were not met. She also suggests that as some first-time fathers find childbirth stressful, they may feel more comfortable assuming an observational rather than a coaching role, and that fathers may need more support than previously thought.

Men may therefore not be the ideal supporter and companion in labour (Hodnett, 1995). Midwives need to be aware of the pressures that may force men into a role they are not necessarily able to fulfil and should encourage couples to discuss what each of their needs are and how men see their role during labour.

Transition to Parenthood

Transition to parenthood is stressful and men need as much support as women. Transition has been described as:

> *a period of identity crisis which involves the working out of a series of changes, losses and anxieties related to the variations of one's external and internal worlds.*

(Benuvenuti *et al.* 1989.)

There is a lack of support for new fathers in the postnatal period. Men appear to have no resources or support for the early period of adjustment. Benuvenuti *et al.* (1989) quote one respondent as saying 'the first 3 weeks were a nightmare. The worst 3 weeks of our marriage.' This was not an unusual perception among their sample.

There are gender differences in the responses of new parents, in that some men find general emotional support to be most helpful, but want more material support such as paternity leave, help at work and a better salary; whereas some mothers find material support most helpful, but want more emotional support. Men appreciate other parents sharing personal experiences and advice and both parents want support for traditional gender-role enactment (Jordan, 1990). Once their partner returns to work, men experience a process of redefining roles; however, there is also a lack of role model for a dual-earner lifestyle (Hall, 1991).

Second-time parents identify both material and emotional support as most helpful during the perinatal period. They require more assistance with babysitting and household chores, general encouragement and more information about second children and parenting of two children (Jordan, 1989).

Midwives can assist men to anticipate this process of transition in the antenatal period and continue to support and guide them once the baby is born by involving them in parenting. Increasing men's feelings of competence and confidence assists fathers during the transition. Midwives should also be aware that second-time fathers may not participate as much in infant care (discussed below).

Men's Involvement in Infant Care

The relationship between father and infant is similar to the mother–infant one in that an infant can obtain competent and loving care from both parents. Lamb *et al.* (1987) suggest that parental involvement has three components. The first two are engagement or time spent in one-to-one interaction with the child and accessibility in which the parent is actively involved in one task, but will respond to the child if necessary. The third component is considered to be responsibility, which has to do with accountability for the child's day-to-day welfare and care. Although men may play varying parts in engagement and accessibility, the woman takes on over 90% of responsibility regardless of whether both the parents are in paid employment. This may alter where the woman suffers a long-term illness.

There are differences in first-time and multiple-time father's involvement in infant care and in their wives' expectations of involvement. First-time fathers assume greater responsibility for infant caretaking tasks than do multiple-time fathers. First-time fathers' behaviours are not up to mothers' expectations, but the two tend to converge over time. However, wives' expectations of multiple-time fathers are consistently higher than the fathers' actual performance and both maintain their respective positions over time (Rustia and Abbot, 1993).

Although multiple-time fathers know about infant caretaking tasks, they do not perform them in successive fathering episodes. The reasons for this are unclear, but Ferketich and Mercer (1995) suggest that after the initial transition to parenthood the birth of a second or later child leads to insignificant change in the father's personal identity. Feelings of inadequacy, fatigue, and being tied down are higher and marital happiness is lower in couples with children than in childless couples (Daglas-Pelish, 1993) and the performance of infant caretaking tasks among first-time fathers appears related to marital cohesion and satisfaction (Volling and Belsky, 1991). However Daglas-Pelish (1993) suggests that researchers have taken a narrow view on the effects of children on marital cohesion and that a broader approach should be taken to assess the impact of becoming parents.

La Rossa (1988) argues that the culture of fatherhood has changed more than the conduct of fatherhood – that is the ideologies that surround men's parenting has changed more than how fathers behave with their children. Although some fathers, particularly educated middle-income men, are assuming greater responsibility for child care, there is little evidence of a major change in fathers' caretaking activity. The unmet expectancies of women, fostered by men's promises and media images of fatherhood that their partners carry out more childcare, can cause friction within the marriage (Nicolson, 1990) and may be a result of this asynchronous social change.

One of the reasons for this lack of change may be that the transition to fatherhood binds men more firmly to the traditional breadwinner role for a period after the birth of their child, as they became the sole breadwinner for the family. Cohen (1993) suggests that although men's work role may seem unaffected when they become fathers, many men revise their commitment to their job. They began to feel more like providers when they may not have given priority to this previously, with some men expressing a wish for more involvement in aspects of parenting other than that of provider. If men are to redefine their roles they will need time and the flexible working patterns normally associated with women who work outside the home. One reason for the culture of fatherhood changing more than its conduct may be that men are not provided with the opportunities within the workplace to enable them to become more involved in infant care. However, the experiences in Sweden suggest that the matter is more complex than this.

Willinger (1993) found that men were reluctant to relinquish the provider role and that some men believed the woman should stay at home to care for the child. Although men appear to be accepting women's role as part of the workforce, some are still reluctant to accept the kind of restructuring that would enable men and women to participate equally in the workforce.

Midwives should prepare prospective parents for the changes in their lives that parenthood brings. They should explore the expectations women have of their partners' level of participation in childcare and encourage them to discuss this with their partners. Universal paternal involvement may not be achievable and may only be beneficial where it is the choice of the couple. Some women may fear the loss of traditional power over the home if men begin to participate more (Polatnik, 1974).

Men and Breastfeeding

Being separated from their mate by the baby, lack of opportunity to develop a relationship with the infant and feeling inadequate have been identified as concerns of fathers about breastfeeding (Jordan and Wall, 1990). Involving men in the decision on feeding method as well as the process of breastfeeding can improve the number of women breastfeeding, as well as the lengthen the duration of the breastfeeding episode. A high incidence of breastfeeding is found where the father strongly approves. However, it can increase feelings of helplessness and be frustrating for some fathers as they cannot participate, even though they want to (Henderson and Brouse, 1991).

Despite indications that male partners influence maternal decisions to breastfeed, clinicians and investigators have virtually ignored the male contribution to successful breastfeeding. Gamble and Morse (1993) propose that there is a need for realistic education for fathers into the realities of breastfeeding and for more outlets for fathers' negative emotions towards breastfeeding. They have identified that men compensate for being unable to feed their infants by increasing other interactions with the baby and 'catching up' once the baby is weaned. This process may take months, but men are willing to wait for the improved father–infant relationship that comes with weaning as they place the health of the infant, that is a commitment to breastfeeding, before their own needs.

Despite some negative consequences of breastfeeding for fathers, Gamble and Morse (1993) show that men are able to take constructive action that allows them to continue to support breastfeeding. Fathers may be in greater need of support than women are during breastfeeding. The use of mentors in classes to support and reassure men that father–infant relationships will not suffer long-term effects could be beneficial. Successful breastfeeding can occur with differing types of fathering styles – an awareness of this can help the midwife in providing appropriate support for differing needs.

Midwives are responsible for providing a great deal of information to prospective parents, so they should ensure that this information is accurate and comprehensive. It should address the realities of being the father of a breastfed infant, and midwives should encourage couples to explore their expectations, values and goals along with providing advice on how to breastfeed. There is a need for realistic education for fathers into the realities of breastfeeding and for more outlets for fathers to express negative emotions towards breastfeeding

Teenage and Delayed Fatherhood

Teenage fatherhood appears to be strongly linked to poor academic achievement and, to some extent, to poverty; however, young men tend to have regular contact with their children in the first year. There is a paucity of information on delayed fatherhood, other than that those men who suffer couvade are generally older, that is over 30 years old, and that their own parents were older.

Taking data from four Office of Population Censuses and Surveys (OPCS) studies of sexual behaviours of young British people between 1960 and 1990, Cartwright (1994) found that relatively few men under 20 years were identified as fathers, i.e. only 54% of the number of births to women of that age. However, Cartwright suggests that data obtained in the surveys are to some extent inaccurate or biased and proposes that one reason why so few young men become fathers in relation to their sexual activities is the high rate of termination of pregnancy in young women and so concludes that pregnancies fathered by men under 20 years are likely to end in abortion.

The characteristics of teenage fathers are approving attitudes about parenting outside marriage, early initiation of sexual activity and problems in school – teenage fathers are negatively related to educational attainment. Nord *et al.* (1992) suggest that teenage fathers are found disproportionally to have grown up in poor families.

Teachers negative assessment of their ability as well as their parent's lack of interest in their education are variables found to be strongly associated with teen fathers. Young men are less likely to marry the mothers than older men, but they tend to have regular contact with their children in the first year (Nord *et al.* 1992, Dearden *et al.* 1992).

On a positive note, those young expectant fathers who do not live with the mothers of their babies participate significantly more in antenatal activities if they use 'teenage father services'. An association with higher birthweight was also found in the babies of young men who access such a service (Barth *et al.* 1988).

In conclusion, it appears that although not many young men become fathers, those who do are likely to have education problems and are more likely to be from poor backgrounds. Offering support to these young men has benefits both for them and the baby.

Conclusion

Midwives should explore the expectant father's stresses and ways of coping with the responsibilities of fatherhood and consider providing more and better-quality preparation and encouragement for open communication with their wives. Midwives may require support and preparation for this role, either during their initial education or in the form of post-registration courses. The poor educational quality of parent education has been identified, as has the uncertainty among professionals about addressing men's needs; however, the evidence is limited and there is a need to extend the research on this topic.

Not all men wish to become involved fathers and may be happier in the provider role; however, all men have individual needs and the midwife has a role in supporting men throughout the pregnancy, birth and the postpartum period. Men's cultural background may influence the part they play in childbearing and parenting, so midwives need to be aware of these factors. Involving men in antenatal care and parenthood preparation can play a part in improving the number and the duration of breastfeeding episodes, thus directly influencing infant health. When men opt for increased paternal involvement they enjoy a richer and closer relationship with their children, but couples need to evaluate for themselves what is best for their particular personal circumstances.

Providing support for men during their transition to parenthood can benefit the men as well as their partners. To be 'with woman', midwives must be sensitive to the individual needs of all their clients.

KEY CONCEPTS

- Sociology has been instrumental in constructing myths concerning family life.
- The realities of parenting often do not equate with the expectations of parents, men and women.
- Parenting activities have been 'intellectualized', which disempowers parents and misleads professionals.
- Gender divisions within parenting are ideologically founded and currently unhelpful.
- Midwives must deconstruct stereotypes applied to care.
- Fathers play an important role within the family and require acknowledgement and support to fulfil their role.
- Couples may need encouragement to discuss their anxieties and expectations of each other.
- Providing men with information and encouraging them to support breastfeeding can increase the number and duration of breastfeeding episodes.
- Men's behaviour as expectant fathers is influenced by their cultural background and the experiences of their own fathers.
- The presence of men at the birth and their preparation for birth needs further review.

References

Adams L: Consumers' view of antenatal education, *Health Educ J* 41(1):12, 1982.

Ainsworth MDS, Blehar M, Waters E, *et al.*: *Patterns of attachment*, Hillsdale, NJ, 1978, Lawrence Erlbaum Associates.

Ainsworth M: Patterns of mother–infant attachment: antecedents and effect on development. *Bull NY Acad Med* 61:771, 1985.

Appleby L: The aetiology of postpartum psychosis: Why are there no answers? *J Reprod Infant Psycho* 8(2):109, 1990.

Aries P: *Centuries of childhood*, Harmondsworth, 1979, Penguin.

Backet K: *Mothers and fathers*, 1982, Macmillan Press.

Ball J: *Psychology of childbirth and motherhood*, London, 1993, Distance Learning Centre, South Bank University.

Ball J: *Reactions to motherhood, the role of postnatal care*, 1994, Books for Midwives Press.

Ballard CG: Post traumatic stress disorder (PTSD) after childbirth, *Br J Psychiatr* 166:525, 1994.

Barbour RS: Fathers; The emergence of a new consumer group. In Garcia J, Kilpatrick R, Richards M, editors: *The politics of maternity care*, Oxford, 1990, Clarendon Press.

Barclay L, Everitt L, Rogan F, Schmied V, Wylie A: *Becoming a mother: A grounded theory approach to women's experiences of early mothering*, Paper presented at Health Families–Healthy Children Conference, International Year of the Family, Sydney, Australia, 1995.

Barth RP, Claycomb M, Loomis A: Services to adolescent fathers, *Health Social Work* 13:277, 1988.

Bedford VA, Johnson N: The role of the father, *Midwifery* 4(4): 190, 1988.

Belsky J: The determinants of parenting: A process model, *Child Development* 55:83, 1984.

Belsky J, Kelly J: *The transition to parenthood: How a first child changes a marriage*, London, 1994, Vermilion.

Benuvenuti P, Marchetti G, Tozzi G, Pazzagli A: Psychological and psychopathological problems of fatherhood, *J Psychosom Obstet Gynaecol* 10(Suppl 2):35, 1989.

Berger B, Berger P: *The war over the family*, Garden City, 1983, Doubleday.

Berger P, Luckman T: *The social construction of reality*, Harmondsworth, 1967, Penguin.

Bernard J: *The future of marriage*, New York, 1972, World Publishing.

Best G: *Mid-Victorian Britain 1851–1875*, London, 1971, Fontana.

Bibring GL, Dwyer TF, Huntingdon DS, Valentin AF: A study of the psychological processes in pregnancy and of the earliest mother–child relationship, *Psychoanal Study Child* 16:9, 1961.

Biddle B: *Role theory*, New York, 1979, Academic Press.

Biller HB: *Fathers and families: Paternal factors in child development*, Westport, Connecticut, London, 1993, Auburn House.

Bliss Holtz J: Primipara's concern for learning infant care, *Nurs Res* 37(1):20, 1988.

Blumfield W: *Life after birth*, Shaftesbury, 1992, Element Books.

Boukydis CFZ, editor: *Support for parents and infants*, New York, London, 1986, Routledge and Kegan Paul.

Boukydis CFZ, editor: *Research on support for parents and infants in the postnatal period*, Norwood, 1987, Ablex Publishing Corporation.

Bowlby J: *Maternal care and mental health*, Geneva, 1952, World Health Organization.

Bowlby J: *The making and breaking of affectional bonds*, London, 1979, Tavistock.

Bowlby J: *Attachment and loss*, Vol. 1: *Attachment*, London, 1969/1982, Hogarth.

Bowlby J: *Attachment and loss*, Vol. 2: *Separation*, London, 1973, Hogarth.

Bowlby J: *The making and breaking of affectional bonds*, London, 1979, Tavistock.

Bowlby J: *Attachment and loss*, Vol. 3: *Loss, sadness and depression*, London, 1980, Hogarth.

Bowlby J: *Secure base*, New York, 1988, Basic Books.

Brannen J, Moss P: *Managing mothers*, London, 1991, Unwin Hyman.

Bretherton I: Roots and growing points of attachment theory. In Parkes CM, Stevenson-Hinde J, Marris P, editors: *Attachment across the life cycle*, London, 1991, Routledge.

Bronfenbrenner U: *Two worlds of childhood: US and USSR*, New York, 1972, Russell Sage Foundation.

Bryar R: *Theory of midwifery practice*, Basingstoke, 1995, MacMillan Press.

Campion M: *Who's fit to be a parent?* London, 1995, Routledge.

Cartwright A: Why don't more young men in the UK become fathers? *J Epidemiol Commun Health* 46:52, 1994.

Cashmore E: *The world of one parent families having to*, 1985, Counterpoint.

Chamberlain DB: How pre- and perinatal psychology can transform the world, *Int Prenat Perinat Psychol Med* 5(4):413, 1993.

Chapman L: Searching: expectant fathers' experiences during labour and birth, *J Perinat Neonat Nurs* 4(4): 21, 1991.

Charles J, Curtis L: Birth afterthoughts: A listening and information service, *Br J Midwifery* 2:7, 1994.

Cheal D: *The family and the state of theory*, 1991, Harvester Wheatsheaf.

Chodorow N: *The reproduction of mothering*, Berkeley and Los Angeles, 1978, University of California Press.

Clinton JF: Expectant fathers at risk for couvade, *Nurs Res* 35(5): 290, 1987.

Cohen T: Becoming and being husbands and fathers: Work and family conflict. In Risman BJ, Schwartz P, editors: *Gender in intimate relationships: A Microstructural approach*, p. 220, Belmont, 1989, Wadsworth.

Cohen TH: What do fathers provide? In Hood JC, editor: *Men, work, and family*, London, 1993, Sage.

Collins: *Sociology of marriage and the family*, London, 1985, Nelson Hall.

Combes G, Schonveld A: *Life will never be the same again*, London, 1992, Health Education Authority.

Cowan CP, Cowan PA, Heming G, Garrett E, Coysh W, Curtis-Boles H, Boles A: Transitions to parenthood: His, hers and theirs, *J Fam Issues* 6:451, 1985.

Cox J, Holden J: *Perinatal psychiatry: Users and abuses of the Edinburgh postnatal depression scale*, 1994, Gaskell.

Cronnenwett L, Newmark L: Fathers response to childbirth, *Nurs Res* 23(2):210, 1974.

Cutrona CE: Causal attributions and perinatal depression, *J Abnorm Psychol* 92:161, 1983.

Daglas-Pelish PL: The impact of the first child on marital happiness, *J Adv Nurs* 18:437, 1993.

Darwin C: *The expression of emotion in man and the animals*, London, 1872, John Murray.

Dearden K, Hale C, Alvarez J: The educational antecedents of teen fatherhood, *Br J Educ Psychol* 62(1):139, 1992.

de Chateau P: The influence of early contact on maternal and infant behaviour in primiparae, *Birth Fam J* 3(4):149, 1976.

Deutsch H: *Psychology of women: A psychoanalytic interpretation*, Vol. II: *Motherhood*, New York, 1945, Grune and Stratton.

Diamond D, Heinicke C, Mintz, J: Separation–individuation as a family process in the transition to parenthood, *Infant Ment Health J*, 17(1):24, 1996.

Dick-Read G: *Childbirth without fear*, 3rd edn, London, 1956, Heinemann.

Donovan Wl, Lewis LA, Walsh RO: Maternal self-efficacy: Illusory control and its effect on susceptibility to learned helplessness, *Child Development* 61: 1638, 1992.

Duncan SW, Markman HJ: Intervention programs for the transition to parenthood: current status from a prevention perspective. In Michaels GY, Goldberg WA, editors: *The Transition to Parenthood*, Cambridge, 1988, Cambridge University Press.

Egeland B, Farber EA: Infant–mother attachment: Factors related to its development and changes over time, *Child Development* 55:753, 1984.

Eisenberg N, Lennon, R: Sex differences in empathy and related capacities, *Psychol Bull* 94:100, 1983.

Eldridge A, Schmidt E: The capacity to parent: A self psychological approach to parent–child psychotherapy, *Clin Soc Work J* 18(4):339, 1990.

Elliott SA, Watson JP, Brough DI: Transition to parenthood by British couples, *J Reprod Infant Psychol* 3:28, 1985.

Emery RE, Tuer M: Parenting and the marital relationship. In Luster T, Okagaki L, editors, *Parenting: An ecological perspective*, Hillsdale, 1993, Lawrence Erlbaum Associates.

Entwistle DR, Doering SG: *The first birth: A family turning point*, Baltimore and London, 1981, The John Hopkins University Press.

Erikson E: *Childhood and society*, 1977, Palladin.

Everingham C: *Motherhood and modernity*, Buckingham and Philadelphia, 1992, Open University Press.

Eyer D: *Mother–infant bonding: A scientific fiction*, New Haven and London, 1992, Yale University Press.

Fein RA: Men and young children. In: Pleck JH, Sawyer J, editors: *Men and masculinity*, New York, 1974, Prentice Hall.

Ferketich SL, Mercer RT: Predictors of role competence for experienced and inexperienced fathers, *Nurs Res* 44(2): 89, 1995.

Fletcher R: *The shaking of the foundations; family and society*, London, 1988, Routledge and Kegan Paul.

Fletcher R: *Gerneral household survery*, London, 1991, HMSO.

Fogel A: *Developing through relationships – origins of communication, self and culture*, New York, 1993, Harvester Wheatsheaf.

Fonagy P: Psychoanalytic and empirical approaches to developmental psychopathology: can they be usefully integrated? *J Royal Soc Med* 86:577, 1993.

Fonagy P, Steele M, Moran G, Steele H, Higgitt A: Measuring the ghost in the nursery: A summary of the main findings of the Anna Freud Centre – University College London Parent–Child Study, *Bull Ann Freud Centre* 14:115, 1991a.

Fonagy P, Steele M, Moran GS, Higgitt, AC: The capacity for understanding mental states: The reflective self in parent and child and its significance for security of attachment, *Infant Ment Health J* 13:200, 1991b.

Foucault M: *Truth, power and sexuality*, Brighton, 1980, Harvester.

Freud S: The psychopathology of everyday life. In Strackey J, editor: *The standard edition of the complete psychological works of Signund Freud, Vol. 6, 1901*, London, 1953, Hogarth.

Gamble D, Morse JM: Fathers of breastfed infants: Postponing and types of involvement, *J Obstet Gynaecol Neonat Nurs* 22(4):358, 1993.

Gesell A: *The mental growth of the pre-school child*, 1930, MacMillan.

Giddens A: *Sociology – a brief but critical introduction*, 2nd edn, London, 1986, MacMillan Education.

Gilligan C: Woman's place in the life cycle. In Harding S, editor: *Feminism and methodology*, Ch 5, Milton Keynes, 1987, Open University Press.

Glazener, Abdalla *et al.*: Postnatal care: A survey of patients' experiences, *Br J Midwifery* 12:67, 1993.

Goldberg S: Parent infant bonding: another look, *Child Dev* 54:1355, 1983.

Goldberg WA: Perspectives on the transition to parenthood. In Michaels GY , Goldberg WA editors: *The transition to parenthood: Current theory and research*, Cambridge, 1988, Cambridge University Press.

Greenberg N, Morris N: Engrossment. The newborns impact upon the father, *Am J Orthopsychiatry* :520, 1974.

Haas L: Nurturing fathers and working mothers: Changing gender roles in Sweden. In Hood JC, editor: *Men, work, and family*, London, 1993, Sage.

Hall C: *White, male and middle class*, 1992, Blackwell Publications.

Hall JA: Gender effects in decoding non-verbal cues, *Psychol Bull* 85:845, 1978.

Hall W: The experiences of fathers in dual-earner families following the births of their first infants, *J Adv Nurs* 16:423, 1991.

Hanson S, Bozett F: *Dimensions of fatherhood*, Beverly Hills, 1985, Sage Publications.

Hardey M, Crowe G: *Lone parenting*, Hemel Hempstead, 1991, Harvester Wheatsheaf.

Harkness S: The cultural mediation of postpartum depression, *Med Anthropol Q* 1(2):194, 1987.

Harlow HF: Love in infant monkeys, *Sci Am* 22(6):64, 1959.

Hawkins AJ, Christiansen SL, Sargent KP, Hill EJ: Rethinking fathers' involvement in child care. In Marsiglio W, editor: *Fatherhood: Contemporary theory, research and* policy, Thousand Oaks, London, Delhi, 1995, Sage Publications.

Hayes N: *Foundations of psychology*, London, 1994, Routledge.

Henderson AD, Brouse AJ: The experiences of new fathers during the first 3 weeks of life, *J Adv Nurs* 16:293, 1991.

Hepper PG, Shahidullah S: The beginnings of mind – evidence from the behaviour of the fetus, *J Reprod Infant Psychol* 12:143, 1994.

Hillan E: Issues in the delivery of care, *J Adv Nurs* 17:274, 1992.

Ho E: Preparing for parenthood, *Nurs Mirror* 161(30):14, 1985.

Hock E, DeMeiss DK: Depression in mothers of infants: The role of maternal employment, *Dev Psychol* 26(2):285, 1990.

Hock E, Schirtzinger MB: Maternal separation anxiety: Its developmental course and relation to maternal mental health, *Child Dev* 63:93, 1992.

Hock E, McBride S, Gnezda MT: Maternal separation anxiety: Mother–infant separation from the maternal perspective, *Child Dev* 60:793, 1989.

Hodnett ED: Support from caregivers during childbirth. In Enkin MW, Keirse MJNC, Renfrew MJ, Neilson JP, editors: *Pregnancy and childbirth module of The Cochrane Database of systematic reviews*, London, 1995, BMJ Publishing Group.

Holmes J: *John Bowlby and attachment theory*, London and New York, 1993, Routledge.

Humphreys S, Gordon P: *A labour of love: The experience of parenthood in Britain 1900–1950*, London, 1993, Sidgwick and Jackson.

Hunt S, Symonds A: *The social meaning of midwifery*, London, 1995, MacMillan.

Hunter RS, Kilstrom N: Breaking the cycle in abusive families, *Am J Psychiatr* 136(10):1320, 1979.

Illich I: *Limits to medicine: Medical nemesis*, Harmondsworth, 1977, Penguin.

Izard CE, Hembree EA, Huebner RR: Infants' emotional expressions to acute pain: Developmental change and stability of individual differences, *Dev Psychol* 23:105, 1987.

Jackson B: *Fatherhood*, London, 1983, George Allen and Unwin Publishers Ltd.

Jacobs M: *DW Winnicott*, London, Thousand Oaks, New Delhi, 1995, Sage Publications.

Jessner L, Weigert E, Foy JL: The development of parental attitudes during pregnancy. In Anthony EJ, Benedeck T, editors: *Parenthood*, Boston, 1970, Little Brown.

Jordan PL: Support behaviours identified as helpful and desired by second time parents, *Maternal–Child Nurs J* 18(2):133, 1989.

Jordan PL: Laboring for relevance: Expectant and new fatherhood, *Nurs Res* 39(1):11, 1990.

Jordan PL, Wall VR: Breastfeeding and fathers: illuminating the darker side, *Birth* 17(4):210, 1990.

Jung C: *Man and his symbols*, New York, 1964, Doubleday.

Keirse M, Enkin M, Lumley J: Social and professional support during labour. In Chalmers I, Enkin M, Keirse M, editors: *Effective care in pregnancy and childbirth*, Oxford, 1989, Oxford University Press.

Keller W, Hildebrandt K, Richards M: Effects of extended father infant contact during the newborn period, *Infant Behav Dev* 8:337, 1985.

Kennel JH, Klaus MH: Mother–infant bonding: Weighing the evidence, *Dev Rev* 4:275, 1984.

Kitzinger S: *Women as mothers*, London, 1978, Fontana.

Kitzinger S: Birth and violence against women; Generating hypotheses from women's accounts of unhappiness after birth. In Roberts H, editor: *Women's health matters*, London, 1992, Routledge.

Klaus MH, Kennell JH: *Parent–infant bonding*, St Louis, 1982, CV Mosby.

Klaus M, Kennell, J, *et al.*: Maternal attachment; the importance of the first postpartum days, *New Engl J Med* 286:460, 1972.

Klein H: Male counterpart to pregnancy, *Int J Psychiatr Med* 21(1):57, 1991.

Klein, M: *The selected Melaine Klein*, Mitchell J (editor), London, 1986, Penguin.

Kohlberg L: A cognitive developmental analysis of children's sex role concepts and attitudes. In Maccoby E, editor: *The development of sex differences*, 1966, Stanford University Press.

Kontos D: A study of the effects of extended maternal infant contacts on maternal behaviour at one and three months, *Birth Fam J* 5(3):133, 1978.

Lamb M, Hwang, C: Maternal attachment and mother neonate bonding: A critical review. In Lamb M, Brown A, editors: *Advances in developmental psychology*, Vol. 2, Hillsdale, 1982, New Jersey.

Lamb M, Lamb J: The nature and importance of the father infant relationship, *Fam Coordinator* 25: 379, 1976.

Lamb ME, Pleck JH, Levine JA: Effects of increased paternal involvement on fathers and mothers. In Lewis C, O'Brien M, editors: *Reassessing fatherhood*, California, 1987, Sage.

La Rossa R: Fatherhood and social change, *Fam Relations* 37:451, 1988.

Lar Rossa M, La Rossa R: *Transition to parenthood: how children change families*, Beverly Hills, 1981, Sage.

Laslett P, Wall R: *Household and family in past time*, Cambridge, 1972, Cambridge University Press.

Laughlin CD: The roots of enculturation: The challenge of pre and perinatal psychology for ethnological theory and research, *Anthropologica* XXXI: 135, 1989.

Lazarus RS, Folkman S: *Stress, appraisal and coping*, New York, 1984, Springer.

Leader LR, Baille P, Martin B, Vermeulen E: The assessment and significance of habituation to a repeated stimulus by the human foetus, *Early Hum Dev* 7:211, 1982.

Leiderman P: Human mother infant social bonding: Is there a sensitive phase? In Immelmann K, Barlow G, editors: *Behavioural development*, Cambridge, 1981, Cambridge University Press.

Lever J: Sex differences in the games children play, *Soc Probl* 23: 478, 1976.

Longobucco DC, Freston MS: Relation of somatic symptoms to degree of paternal-role preparation of first-time expectant fathers, *J Obstet Gynecol Neonatal Nurs* 18(6):482, 1989.

Luster T, Okagaki L, editors, *Parenting: An ecological perspective*, Hillsdale, 1993, Lawrence Erlbaum Associates, Publishers.

Lutwin D, Siperstein G: Househusband fathers. In Hanson S, Bozett F: *Dimensions of fatherhood*, Ch 11, Beverly Hills, 1985, Sage Publications.

Mahler M: On the first three subphases of the separation–individuation process, *Int J Psychoanal* 53:333, 1972.

Mahler M, Pine F, Bergmann A: *The psychological birth of the human infant*, New York, 1975, Basic Books.

Mahler M: The meaning of development research of earliest infancy as related to the study of separation-individuation. *Inter J Psychoanal* 55:333, 1983.

Main M, Goldwyn R: *Adult attachment interview*, unpublished manuscript, Berkeley, 1989, University of California.

Main M, Kaplan N, Cassidy J: Security in infancy, childhood, and adulthood: A move to the level of representation. In Bretherton I, Waters E, editors: *Growing points of attachment theory and research*, Monographs of the Society for Research in Child Development, 50, 1-2 (Serial No 209), p. 66, 1985.

Marsiglio W, (editor): *Fatherhood :Contemporary theory, research and social policy*, London, 1995, Sage Publications.

Maslow A: *Motivation and personality*, 2nd edn, New York, 1954, Harper and Row.

McClelland D: *The achievement motive*, New York, 1953, Appleton, Century Croft.

McFayden A: *Special care babies and their developing relationships* London and New York, 1994, Routledge.

McKee L, O'Brien M: *The father figure*, London, 1982, Tavistock.

McRobbie A: Motherhood – a teenage job? *The Guardian*, 5th April 1989, p. 17.

Mercer R: *First time motherhood: experience from teens to forties*, New York, 1986, Springer Publishing Co Ltd.

Michaels GY, Goldberg WA: *The transition to parenthood: Current theory and research*, Cambridge, 1988, Cambridge University Press.

Miles R: *The women's history of the world*, 1989, Paladin.

Mitchell J: *The selected Melanie Klein*, Harmondsworth, 1986, Penguin.

Murphy-Black T, Faulkner A: *Antenatal skills training – a manual of guidelines*, Chichester, 1988, John Wiley and Sons Ltd.

Murray L: *The impact of postnatal depression on infant development*, Paper given at 9th Congress of the European Society of Child and Adolescent Psychiatry, London, 1991.

Murray L, Fiori-Cowley A, Hooper R, Cooper P: *The impact of postnatal depression and associated adversity on early mother–infant interactions and later infant outcome*, 1994.

Newson J, Newson E: *Infant care in an urban community*, London, 1963, Allen and Unwin.

Newson J, Newson E: Longitudinal studies. In Harris CC, editor: *The family and industrial society*, Boston, 1983, Allen and Unwin.

Nichols MR: Paternal perspectives of the childbirth experience, *Maternal Child Nurs J* 21(3):99, 1993.

Nicolson P: A brief report of women's expectations of men's behaviour in the transition to parenthood: Contradictions and conflicts for counselling psychology, *Counselling Psychol Q* 3(4):353, 1990.

Nord CW, Moore KA, Morrison DR, Brown B, Myers DE: Consequences of teen-age parenting, *J School Health* 6(7):310, 1992.

Oakley A: *The sociology of housework*, Oxford, 1974, Martin Robertson.

Oakley A: *Becoming a mother*, Oxford, 1979, Martin Robertson.

Oakley A: *Women confined*, Oxford, 1980, Martin Robertson.

Oakley A: *Sex, gender and society*, 2nd edn, London, 1985, Gower.

Oakley A, Rajan L, Grant A: Social support and pregnancy outcome, *Br J Obstet Gynaecol* 97:155, 1990.

O'Brien M: *The politics of reproduction*, 1981, Routledge and Kegan Paul.

O'Brien S, Pitt B: Hormonal theories and therapy for postnatal depression. In Cox J, Holden J, editors: *Perinatal psychiatry: Use and misuse of the Edinburgh Postnatal Depression Scale*, London, 1994, Gaskell.

O'Hara MW: Postpartum depression: identification and measurement in a cross-cultural context. In Cox J, Holden J, editors: *Perinatal psychiatry: Use and misuse of the Edinburgh Postnatal Depression Scale*, London, 1994, Gaskell.

O'Hara MW, Rehm LP, Campbell SB: Predicting depressive symptomatology: Cognitive–behavioural models and postpartum depression, *J Abnorm Psychol* 91:457, 1982.

Omeara C: Childbirth and parenting education – the providers viewpoint, *Midwifery* 9:76. 1993.

O'Meara CM: A diagnostic model for the evaluation of childbirth and parenting education, *Midwifery* 9:28, 1993.

OPCS: *General household survey*, London, 1991, HMSO.

Page L: Redefining the midwife's role: changes needed in practice, *Br J Midwifery* 12:67, 1993.

Parke R: *Fathering*, 1981, Fontana.

Parker R: *Split in two: The experience of maternal ambivalence*, London, 1995, Virago Press.

Parr MA: *Support for couples in the transition to parenthood*, Unpublished PhD Thesis, London, 1996, Department of Psychology, University of East London.

Parsons T: *Essays in social theory*, 1954, London, Collier MacMillan.

Perris C, Arrindell WA, Eisemann M, (editors): *Parenting and psychopathology*, Chichester, 1994, John Wiley & Sons.

Perry BD, Pollard RA, Blakley TL, Baker WL, Vigilante D: Childhood trauma, the neurobiology of adaptation, and 'use-dependent' development of the brain: How 'states' become 'traits', *Infant Ment Health J* 16(4):271, 1995.

Peterson C, Maier SF, Seligman, MEP: *Learned helplessness: A theory for the age of personal control*, New York and Oxford, 1993, Oxford University Press.

Peterson GH: *Birthing normally: A personal growth approach to childbirth*, Berkeley, 1981, Mindbody Press.

Phoenix A: *Young mothers?*, 1991, Polity Press.

Piaget J, Inholder B: *The psychology of the child*, 1969, Routledge.

Piontelli A: *From fetus to child: An observational and psychoanalytic study*, London and New York, 1992, Tavistock/Routledge.

Polatnik N: Why men don't rear children: A power analysis, *Berkeley J Sociology* 18:45, 1974.

Popay J, Jones G: Patterns of health and illness among lone parent families. In Hardey M, Crowe G: *Lone parenting*, Ch 4, Hemel Hempstead, 1991, Harvester Wheatsheaf.

Pound A: The crisis of the inner-city family, Editorial, *J Ment Health* 3:143, 1994.

Pridham K, Lytton D, Chang A, Rutledge D: Early postpartum transition: progress in maternal identity and role attainment, *Res Nurs Health* 14:16, 1991.

Pringle MK: *The needs of children*, London, 1974, Hutchinson and Co Ltd.

Pruett K: Infants of primary nurturing fathers, *Psychoanal Study Child* 38:257, 1983.

Pugh G, De'Ath E, Smith C: *Confident parents, confident children: policy and practice in parent education and support*, London, 1994, The National Children's Bureau.

Raphael-Leff J: *Psychological processes of childbearing*, London, 1991, Chapman and Hall.

Rapoport R, Rapoport RN, Strelitz Z, Kew S: *Fathers, mothers and others*, London, 1977, Routledge and Kegan Paul.

RCM: *Preparation for parenthood*, Taunton, 1966, Barnicotts Ltd.

Rees C: Antenatal classes: time for a new approach, *Nurs Times* 78(34):1446, 1982.

Ribbens J: *Mothers and their children: A feminist psychology of childrearing*, London, Thousands Oaks, New Delhi, 1994, Sage Publications.

Richards JP: Postnatal depression: a review of recent literature, *Br J Gen Pract* 40:472, 1990.

Ritter JM, Casey RJ, Langlois JH: Adults' responses to infants' varying in appearance of age and attractiveness, *Child Dev* 62:68, 1991.

Roberts G: The power of language in a bilingual community, *Nurs Times* 92(39):40, 1996.

Roopnarine J, Miller B: Transitions to fatherhood. In Hanson S, Bozett F: *Dimensions of fatherhood*, Ch 2, Beverly Hills, 1985, Sage Publications.

Rosenblith F: *In the beginning: Development from conception to age* two, Newbury Park, London, New Delhi, 1992, Sage Publications.

Ross E: *Love and toil, motherhood in outcast London*, Oxford, 1993, Oxford University Press.

Rossi A: Gender and parenthood, *Am Sociol Rev* 49:1, 1984.

Royal College of Midwives: *Preparation for parenthood*, Taunton, 1966, Barnicotts.

Rustia GR, Abbot D: Father involvement in infant care: two longitudinal studies, *Int J Nurs Stud* 30(6):467, 1993.

Rutter M: *Maternal deprivation reassessed*, Harmondsworth, 1972, Penguin.

Rutter M: *Maternal deprivation reassessed*, 2nd edition, London, 1981, Penguin.

Sandqvist K: Swedish family policy. In Lewis C, O'Brien M, editors: *Reassessing fatherhood*, California, 1987, Sage.

Sassens G: Success anxiety in women: A constructivist theory of its source and significance, *Harvard Educ Rev* 50:13, 1980.

Schott J, Henley A: *Culture, religion and childbearing in a multiracial society*, Oxford, 1996, Butterworth–Heinemann.

Seel R: *The uncertain father*, Bath, 1987, Gateway Books.

Segal H: *Introduction to the work of Melanie Klein*, London, 1982, The Hogarth Press.

Segalen M: *Historical anthropology of the family*, Cambridge, 1986, Cambridge University Press.

Share L: *If someone speaks, it gets lighter: Dreams and the reconstruction of infant trauma*, Hillsdale, London, 1994, The Analytic Press.

Skinner EA: *Perceived control, motivation and coping*, Thousand Oaks, London and New Delhi, 1995, Sage Publications.

Smith C: *Developing parenting programmes*, London, 1996, The National Children's Bureau.

Smith L: Maternal behaviour and perceived sex of infant revisited, *Child Dev* 49:1263, 1978.

Social Trends, No 22, London, 1992, HMSO.

Spelke ES, Breinlinger K, Macomber J, Jacobson K: Origins of knowledge *Psychol Rev* 99(4):605, 1992.

Spock B: *The commonsense book of baby and child care*, 1946.

Sroufe: *Emotional development: The organisation of emotional life in the early years*, Cambridge, 1996, Cambridge University Press.

St-Andre M, Twomey JE: A transgenerational conceptualisation of psychosomatic distress during pregnancy: Implications for infant mental health, *Infant Ment Health J* 17(1):43, 1996.

Statham H, Green J: The effects of miscarriage and other 'unsuccessful' pregnancies on feelings early in a subsequent pregnancy, *J Reprod Infant Psycho* 12:45, 1994.

Stern D: *The interpersonal world of the infant: Views from psychoanalysis and developmental psychology*, New York, 1985, Basic Books.

Stern D: *The motherhood constellation: A unified view of parent–infant psychotherapy*, New York, 1995, Basic Books.

Stewart RB: *The second child: family transition and adjustment*, 1990, Sage Publications Inc.

Stone L: *The family, sex and marriage in England 1500–1800*, London, 1977, Weidenfeld and Nicholson.

Stuart S, O'Hara MW: Interpersonal psychotherapy for postpartum depression: A treatment program, *J Psychother Pract Res* 4:18, 1995.

Symington N: *The analytic experience: Lectures from the Tavistock*, London, 1986, Free Association Books.

Terry DJ: Predictors of subjective stress in a sample of new parents, *Aust J Psychol* 43(1):29, 1991.

Thompson B, *et al.*: *Having a first baby: experiences in 1951 and 1985 compared*, Aberdeen, 1989, Aberdeen University Press.

Thompson F: *Larkrise to Candleford*, Reading, 1939, Penguin.

Trout M: Infant mental health: Monitoring our movement into the twenty-first century, *Infant Ment Health J* 9(3):191, 1988.

van Eerdewegh M, *et al.*: The bereaved child: variables influencing early psychopathology, *Br J Psychiatr* 147:188, 1985.

Volling B, Belsky J: Multiple determinants of father involvement during pregnancy in dual-earner and single-earner families, *J Marriage Fam* 53:461, 1991.

Vondra J, Belsky J: Developmental origins of parenting: Personality and relationship factors. In Luster T, Okagaki L, editors: *Parenting: An ecological perspective*, Hillsdale, London, 1993, Lawrence Erlbaum Associates.

Wetherell M: The psychoanalytic approach to family life. In Muncie J, Wetherell M, Dallos R, Cochrane A, editors: *Understanding the family*, London, 1995, Sage Publications.

Whitehead: *The health divide*, London, 1988, Health Education Authority.

Willinger B: Resistance and change: College men's attitudes towards family and work in the 1980s. In Hood JC, editor: *Men, work, and family*, London, 1993, Sage.

Winnicott DW: *The maturational process and the facilitating environment*, New York, 1965, International Universities Press.

Witz A: *Professions and patriarchy*, London, 1994, Routledge.

Wollett et al.: Observations of fathers at birth. In Beail N, McGuire J, editors: *Fathers: Psychological perspectives*, London, 1982, Junction Books.

Woollett A, Phoenix A: Psychological views on mothering. In Woollett A, Phoenix A, Lloyd E, editors: *Motherhood: meanings, practices and ideologies*, London, 1991, Sage

Williams P: *Family problems*, Oxford, 1989, Oxford University Press.

Young M, Willmott P: *The symmetrical family*, London, 1973, Routledge and Kegan Paul.

Zaretsky E: *Capitalism, the family and personal life*, New York, 1986, Harper and Row.

Zayas LH: Psychodynamic and developmental aspects of expectant and new fatherhood, *Clin Soc Work J* 15(1):8, 1987.

Further Reading

Campion M: *Who's fit to be a parent?*, London, 1995, Routledge.
This text gives a very broad view of mothering from differing social perspectives.

Cheal D: *The family and the state of theory*, 1991, Harvester Wheatsheaf.

Eyer D: *Mother–infant bonding – a scientific fiction*, Newhaven, 1992, Yale University Press.
A scientific fiction. This is a critical appraisal of bonding research.

Humphreys S, Gordon P: *A labour of love: The experience of parenthood in Britain 1900–1950*, London, 1993, Sidgwick and Jackson.

Jackson B: *Fatherhood*, London, 1983, George Allen and Unwin Publishers Ltd.
This is one of the few phenomenological studies of men's experiences of parenting.

Miles R: *The women's history of the world*, 1989, Paladin.

Oakley A: *Sex, gender and society*, 2nd edn, , London, 1985, Gower.

Ross E: *Love and toil, motherhood in outcast London*, Oxford, 1993, Oxford University Press.
A history of childbearing in Victorian London. It reflects midwifery care and parenting in working class women.

unit 3

Factors Influencing Midwifery Practice

16 Regulation of Midwifery Practice

CHAPTER OUTLINE

- Women's rights and expectations
- Professional accountability
- Public protection through professional regulation
- Public protection against negligence
- The right to complain
- Protection of client information
- Safe premises and working practices
- Managing the legal risk

LEARNING OUTCOMES

After completing this chapter you will be able to:

- Appreciate the legal rights of women and their families using maternity services.
- Understand the broad framework of professional statutory regulation and in particular how it applies to midwifery practice.
- Recognise the basic principles that apply to litigation, the law applying to safe premises and the use of patient information.
- Incorporate a risk management approach into your practice and to the management of the maternity services.

Legal matters can cause considerable professional anxiety. The way much of the law operates is poorly understood and constraints of the law are often blamed by health care professionals for their being forced to adopt defensive practice to protect them from accusations of misconduct, complaints or negligence. In this Chapter, the legal protection of patients and clients who receive health care is discussed, rather than the professional aspects. Also, some of the legal principles that apply are explained very briefly, although for any midwife interested in the topic further reading is essential. A short reading list is therefore given at the end. The many ethical decisions and dilemmas that face the midwife and for which the law may offer only limited answers are not described –readers are referred to an excellent supplement in the *British Journal of Midwifery* (Henry *et al.* 1996). Finally, how midwives and other health-care professionals can minimize the risk of being involved in legal or professional conduct proceedings without resort to a defensive approach to care is discussed.

Women's Rights and Expectations

Imagine you are a pregnant woman about to attend the first antenatal visit. You may know something of pregnancy, of what labour entails and something of the main elements of care you should expect. However, you certainly do not have the knowledge or skills necessary to help you safely through that pregnancy and labour. That is, of course, why you come to the health-care system and why you seek the professional help of doctors and midwives. Whatever you may know, you know there comes a point when your knowledge ends and theirs takes over. It is at that point you put trust in your carers and the system of care. You expect to receive a standard of care from professionals who have been properly trained and continue to practice safely. You expect a system that provides appropriate professional staff.

In all your dealings with the professionals, to help them devise appropriate care you tell them things about yourself and your family that you may not choose to tell anyone else. You trust that they will use this information in a way that protects the confidential nature of what you have said.

You also expect that your care will take place in a safe environment and that carers and managers of the service will provide such an environment.

You also know that, although the health service and the professional care you receive is free at the point of delivery, you have contributed financially to that care. It is paid for collectively by everyone, including yourself, through taxation. You are, therefore, the 'paymaster' of the doctor and midwives who are looking after you. So, in return for the trust that you invest in them, and in return for the salary they receive for their professional services, you expect them to be accountable to you for what they do.

However, what can you do if you believe that the staff or the health service has let down your expectations; or if you or your new baby has suffered harm because of the care (or lack of it) you have received? Very little on your own. And this is where the law plays its part in health care. Its processes, institutions and principles are designed to protect against wrong, and to offer redress if harm occurs.

Practising professionals are also answerable to statutory bodies, set up under Acts of Parliament, and must meet any codes of practice and conduct devised by these bodies. Professional regulation also has mechanisms to prevent professionals from continuing in practice when they are considered to be putting the public at risk.

Case law has developed principles to protect against the negligent actions of professionals – both case law and statute require strict confidentiality to apply to the information professionals hold about their patients and clients. Statutes require that the premises and equipment must be kept safe.

Not strictly speaking a legal process, there are complaints procedures that operate in the National Health Service (NHS), so an aggrieved patient may put a complaint to the Health Service Commissioner. Local Community Health Councils offer support and investigate complaints about the service, but not about clinical care.

Professional Accountability

Dictionary definitions of accountability variously use words such as 'responsibility', 'answerable' and 'obligation'. The United Kingdom Central Council for Nursing, Midwifery and Health Visiting (UKCC), in *A Midwife's Code of Practice*, states:

> *Each midwife as a practitioner of midwifery is accountable for her own practice in whatever environment she practises.*

(UKCC, 1994.)

Its *Code of Professional Conduct* states:

> *Each registered nurse, midwife and health visitor shall act, at all times, in such a manner as to justify public trust and confidence, to uphold and enhance the good standing and reputation of the profession, to serve the interests of society, and above all to safeguard the interests of individual patients and clients.*

(UKCC, 1992a.)

The important principles in these quotations are individual responsibility, public trust and confidence. However, in outlining the nature of the midwife's responsibility it is clear that the UKCC expects accountability to be much wider than that to the individual client. There is a clear obligation to the profession itself and to society in general.

Accountability to the Profession

A profession 'of good standing' comprises members who are skilled, knowledgeable and act consistently in the interests of their clients. Keeping up-to-date, increasing the knowledge base of midwifery through research and audit, ensuring a high standard of education and training at preregistration and postregistration levels, operating firm but fair self-regulation through a robust and open professional conduct process are all ways in which a profession retains the confidence of the public.

Accountability to Society

There may be times when matters of public policy or professional practice are not necessarily in the public interest. If they fall within the sphere of a particular profession, it may be appropriate for that profession to take action to highlight the issue or even to campaign for change. An example of this would be the work of the Royal College of Midwives, with many others, to effect a change in approach to the provision of maternity care, resulting in the Government policy *Changing Childbirth* (Department of Health, 1994). Where practices, such as female genital mutilation, occur it again may be very proper for a profession, and individuals in the profession, to take active steps to highlight it and campaign for its cessation.

Public Protection through Professional Regulation

Professional regulation defines appropriate behaviour and standards through which the public are protected, as outlined below.

The Statutory Bodies

Professions in the UK are regulated in statute as a means of public protection; in 1902, the first Midwives Act was passed. Successive Acts (for example the 1936 Midwives Act which introduced a salaried midwifery service) amended the first Act, but in its fundamentals it was retained until it was repealed with the introduction of the Nurses, Midwives and Health Visitors Act (1979).

Section 17 of the Act, which still applies to more current legislation, contains a fundamental principle of public protection – 'A person other than a registered midwife or a registered medical practitioner shall not attend a woman in childbirth.'

The 1979 Act disbanded the numerous nursing and midwifery statutory bodies that existed in the UK, creating a unified regulatory system. The new system came into force in 1983 after a period of working alongside the existing bodies. Initially, this consisted of elected National Boards for each of the four countries of the UK (which were responsible for education and training matters and the first investigation of complaints against professionals in the countries), and the UKCC, made up of representatives of the elected bodies and other appointed members. The UKCC, although not an elected body, was responsible for setting standards for education and practice, for maintaining the professional register and for framing rules for admission to, removal from and restoration to the register. To safeguard the individuality of the midwifery profession, a statutory midwifery committee was set up at UKCC and Board levels. These committees were charged with advising on all matters relating to midwifery.

After 5 years in operation, the system was felt to be unwieldy and, following a review, the Nurses, Midwives and Health Visitors Act 1992 introduced reform of the statutory bodies. The UKCC became the elected body, with up to 60 members, two-thirds of whom are elected. The remainder are appointed by the Secretaries of State for Health, for Wales, Scotland, England and Northern Ireland. The appointed members include medical and educational representatives, a system used to correct any imbalances left after the election process. Eight places are guaranteed to midwives through the election process, two midwives from each UK country. The National Boards are now executive, appointed bodies charged with the provision of training courses by approving courses and accrediting training establishments. They are smaller bodies made up of executive members (who work for the Board) and nonexecutive members appointed by the relevant Secretary of State. The midwifery committees in the countries were disbanded, but one now exists to advise the UKCC. A comprehensive description of the current structure was given in the *British Journal of Midwifery* (Henderson *et al.*) in 1995.

Regulation through Setting Professional Standards

From time-to-time the UKCC publishes rules, codes of conduct and practice (shown in **Box 16.1**), and guidance statements which outline the standards it expects of the practitioners on its register.

The *Midwives Rules* (UKCC, 1993a) and the rules on the professional conduct machinery are statutory instruments (legislation secondary to the primary Act) and therefore have parliamentary authority. The Midwifery Committee is closely involved in the formulation of any amendments to the *Midwives Rules* as well as codes of practice for midwifery.

The UKCC has published *A Midwife's Code of Practice* (1994) and the *Code of Professional Conduct for the Nurse, Midwife and Health Visitor* (1992a). Further publications elaborate on the *Code Of Conduct*, covering, for example, advertising, the exercise of accountability, record keeping, drug administration and confidentiality.

Regulation through Registration

This is, at its most basic level, the mechanism for public protection through professional regulation. The woman described at the beginning of this chapter meets registered midwives who give her professional care and support. Registration ensures for her that:

- The midwives have been educated and trained to an agreed standard before entering the register.
- They have met the ongoing requirements of the UKCC to continue in active practice (e.g. they have completed approved 5-yearly updating and have notified their intention to practice).
- They have not committed professional misconduct of such seriousness that they have had their names removed from the register.
- No midwife will put her well-being at risk.
- She may report a midwife to the UKCC if she feels the midwife has committed professional misconduct; this will be investigated and acted on appropriately.

Box 16.1

Rules and Codes that Direct a Midwife's Practice

- Midwives Rules (UKCC, 1993a; under revision at present).
- A Midwife's Code of Practice (UKCC, 1994).
- The Code of Professional Conduct for the Nurse, Midwife and Health Visitor (UKCC, 1992a).
- The Scope of Professional Practice (UKCC, 1992b).

Regulation through Professional Conduct

Anyone, NHS managers, professional colleagues, users of the service or other members of the public may write to the UKCC to allege professional misconduct.

The Council is obliged to investigate all complaints and, where it believes there is a case to answer, it will hear the case. To do this it has two committees, the Preliminary Proceedings Committee (PPC) and the Professional Conduct Committee (PCC). Both committees are made up of members of the UKCC, although to separate investigation from professional conduct hearings, members on one cannot be on the other.

Investigation

All complaints are processed by an investigating officer and passed to the PPC. This committee decides whether there is a case to answer. If there is, it refers the case to the PCC. If not, it can either take no further action or it may issue a formal warning to the professional. If it believes the health of the professional is implicated in the misconduct it can send the case to a panel of professional screeners for them to decide whether referral to the Health Committee is more appropriate. Deliberations of the PPC are conducted *in camera* and the midwife is not present. The investigating officer may ask for a statement from the midwife, but does not do so in all circumstances, particularly if the complaint is judged to be frivolous. In the latter case, the midwife is simply informed that there has been a complaint, but that it was not upheld by investigation.

Professional Conduct Committee hearings

The hearings of the PCC are held in public; the professional concerned is entitled to representation, which is often provided by a professional organization. The hearings are formal with evidence given on both sides. The Committee is first required to decide whether there has been professional misconduct. If not, the case is closed. If misconduct is proved, it then hears any evidence in mitigation and has a number of options open to it:

- To take no further action.
- To issue a formal caution which remains on record for 5 years.
- To postpone judgement until a later time.
- To refer the case to the panel of professional screeners on health grounds.

- To impose an interim suspension if for some reason the hearing is adjourned.
- To remove the professional's name from the register for a specified or unspecified length of time.

The Health Committee

Any case in which the underlying problem may be the health of the midwife can be passed to the Health Committee. It first goes to a Panel of Screeners (members of the UKCC) who look at the documentary evidence to decide whether or not the Health Committee is the most appropriate course of action.

The Health Committee sits *in camera* and is assisted by medical advisors. There are a number of courses of action it can take:

- To take no action.
- To refer the case to the PPC or PCC.
- To suspend the practitioner's registration.
- To remove the practitioner's name from the register.
- To postpone judgement.
- To impose an interim suspension if the hearing is adjourned.

To provide a robust system of regulation that offers protection to the public and a fair system for the practitioner, these regulatory mechanisms are complex and follow clearly defined procedures. It is beyond the scope of this chapter to explain them in depth, but the UKCC (1993b) has produced a very comprehensive booklet, *Complaints about Professional Conduct*, which elaborates on the structures and processes involved.

Regulation through Supervision

Unique to midwifery and introduced first in the 1902 Act, a system of local supervision is exercised over all practising midwives, whether working in or outside the NHS. Under the Health Authorities Act 1996, health authorities are designated local supervising authorities (LSA) which appoint supervisors of midwives to exercise their responsibilities. The LSA is responsible for collecting the midwives' notifications of intention to practice, for investigating any charges of professional misconduct and, if necessary, for suspending a midwife from practice pending referral to the UKCC.

The *Midwives Rules* require certain standards for supervisors of midwives. They shall be practising midwives with at least 3 years practising experience, one of which should be with 2 years of appointment, or further experience as required by the UKCC. She is also required to attend a course of instruction during the 3 years preceding her appointment and should attend further approved courses at 5-yearly intervals.

Many of the allegations of professional misconduct against a midwife are first made to the LSA, which must investigate all such claims. To do this it is advised by the supervisor of midwives. She looks at all the facts of the case, and usually asks for a written statement from the midwife to give her version of events. The LSA may ask to interview the midwife concerned before it decides whether there is a potential case of professional misconduct. If it believes there is, the LSA reports the case to the UKCC. The LSA then must decide whether to suspend the midwife from practice. To do so it considers whether the midwife's continuing practice is likely to put further women at risk. Suspension from practice only applies to practice within the boundaries of that LSA and not to other LSAs. However, a note of the suspension is made against the midwife's name on the Register until the case has been heard.

Suspension from practice must be distinguished from suspension from duty. The latter is a course of action that an employer may take as part of disciplinary action and can be carried out by the appropriate manager. Obviously, in many circumstances the midwife is both suspended from practice and from duty, but the processes are different and the former must meet the requirements of the UKCC. In particular, the LSA is required to notify the midwife in writing of her suspension, the reasons why and that she has been reported to the UKCC. Additionally, suspension from duty does not stop the midwife from continuing to practice, for example through an agency or independently.

Discussion Points

One of the central tenets of professionalism is the right of self-regulation. Thus, the majority membership of the UKCC is drawn from nurses, midwives and health visitors. For midwives this raises issues of both professional and midwifery accountability. There has been considerable midwifery opposition to the current framework, with claims that self-regulation for midwives in a body dominated by nurses cannot exist. Indeed, midwives fought the introduction of the 1979 Act. The advisory rather than executive nature of the Midwifery Committee is also questioned and together these form the basis for the current call from some parts of the profession for a return to a separate Midwives Act.

However, one school of sociological thought sees all professional regulation as a means of protecting the status of the professional against the interests of the public. Hughes (1958) wrote:

Not merely do the practitioners, by virtue of gaining admission to the charmed circle of colleagues, individually exercise the license to do things others do not, but collectively they presume to tell society what is good and right for the individual and society at large in some aspect of life. Indeed they set the very terms in which people may think about this aspect of life.

The constitution and membership of most statutory bodies tends to reinforce the concept of self-regulation rather than public protection, with very little lay representation. Although some statutory bodies, including the General Medical Council, now have lay representation, the UKCC does not. Those who support the primary role of statutory regulation as a public protection issue are beginning to argue for a deprofessionalization of the regulatory process and a strengthening of public accountability through greatly increased lay involvement.

A further view on professional regulation has been put forward by de Vries (1982):

Contrary to the beliefs of both doctors and midwives, these regulatory acts [licensure] did not result in the establishment of an independent profession of midwifery, but rather placed the midwife in a position where her autonomy has steadily declined.

Oakley and Houd (1990) claim that 'Licensing has a double message: to recognize the value of what midwives do and to limit what in future they will be able to do.' These writers suggest that far from protecting and strengthening the practice of midwifery, where statutory regulation has been introduced it tends to constrain and limit practice. Which of these arguments would you support?

Public Protection against Negligence

Negligence falls within the civil law. The aim is to provide recompense to an individual who has sustained harm as a result of another's reckless act, although, rarely, if the recklessness is deemed exceptionally serious it can become subject to a criminal prosecution.

This area of law is fairly recent, with first principles being laid down in a test case – Donoghue *v* Stevenson – in 1932. This was a Scottish case but, although the law in Scotland, England and Wales differs in many aspects, much of it that affects health care is common to all countries including Northern Ireland. In this section, the criteria that must be met if a case of negligence is to be successful are briefly explained:

• The standard of care expected of the professional against which negligence is judged.
• The rights of women to bring an action.
• The rights of the fetus to bring an action.
• Who may be liable in law.
• The limitations upon going to law.

There is nothing particularly exclusive to midwives in this area of law – indeed, much of it has been decided by cases that involve doctors. However, the recent past has seen an increase in the level of litigation and the amount of damages awarded, with maternity care one of the specialities most involved. Also, because of the independent nature of the midwife's decision making, they are as likely as doctors to be cited as a defendant in negligence claims.

Proof of Negligence

For a plaintiff (the person bringing a civil case) to be successful in a claim of negligence, the court must be satisfied that three criteria are met. If any one of these is not proved, the case fails. These are that:

• A duty of care existed between the plaintiff and the defendant.
• The defendant failed in (breached) that duty of care.
• The breach in the duty of care resulted in damage to the plaintiff.

Additionally, as the only course open to the court is to award financial recompense, if it is clear that the defendant has no financial means to meet an award, the plaintiff is likely to be advised not to bring a case.

The duty of care

In health-care cases, this is easy to prove as there is agreement that when a professional gives care to someone, a duty of care automatically exists. A midwife's duty of care to a woman is very unlikely to be contested in any case.

A breach of the duty of care

To decide whether a professional has breached his or her duty of care, the court must first come to some conclusion about the standard of care that should normally be expected in order to judge the actions of the defendant. The principles that guide this decision were laid down in another test case, Bolam *v* Friern Hospital Management Committee (1957). The judge in this case said that the applicable standard should be that which the 'ordinary competent man exercising that particular art' would accept as the standard. Thus, the standard of care given by a midwife would be judged against the standard met and recognized by other ordinary, competent midwives. To judge this standard the courts rely upon the evidence of professional expert witnesses to guide them. However, as both sides bring their own expert witnesses to testify, the judge usually has to make a decision for one side or the other on the balance of probabilities having heard all the evidence.

Many cases do not come to court for years after the event and if they go to appeal, the final judgement may take even longer. Take a look at the case in **Box 16.2**. When this case was finally considered 11 years had passed. More importantly, there were major differences in the obstetric management of such cases and doctors were more cautious about performing a 'trial of forceps'. By the standards of 1981, Mr Jordan would have probably lost. But another important principle is that the case is always judged on the standard prevailing at the time of the incident. Expert witnesses therefore must think back to the practice at the time of the incident and advise accordingly.

Although the standard expected is that of the ordinary, competent practitioner, there are many different levels of professionals who work in health care. Doctors can be house officers, registrars or consultants. Midwives can be newly qualified or highly experienced and on lower or higher clinical grades. Students work in many parts of the service and accept various levels of accountability, depending on their stage of training. In 1988 an important case clarified the legal responsibilities of professionals at different levels of competence, including those in training (**Box 16.3**).

There are a number of points to be made in this case. First, although still in a learning post, the court did not question that the houseman had done the procedure. If a person in a learning capacity has achieved a level of competence for a particular procedure he may then do it without direct supervision. If, however, he asks to have his work checked, then he has the right to expect his work to be checked competently. Finally, whatever the level of the person performing the task, the patient continues to have the right to safe and competent care. So, in this case, the health authority and the registrar were unable to avoid liability even though a junior member of staff was the one who actually inserted the catheter.

Causation

Did the breach in the duty of care case the plaintiff's damage? This is the point on which so much of the legal argument revolves. There are some cases which, by their nature, are obvious. If a person is harmed because a swab is left *in situ* after an operation, there is a clear case of negligence. But to take some of the most common maternity cases, it can be very difficult to prove that failure to act on a particular abnormal cardiotocograph (CTG) is the reason for subsequent cerebral palsy. In spite of the high-profile, reported

---

Box 16.2

Whitehouse *v* Jordan and Another (1981)

Mr Jordan, an obstetric registrar, conducted a Caesarean section following a failed attempt at a forceps delivery. The baby, Stuart, who was born in 1970, was found subsequently to have severe cerebral palsy. The case first went to the High Court where the judgement was in favour of Stuart. At the Court of Appeal, this was reversed and in a final split judgement in the House of Lords, Mr Jordan won the case.

Box 16.3

Wilsher *v* Essex Area Health Authority (1988)

A premature baby with respiratory distress syndrome was canulated by a senior houseman in order to monitor blood O_2 levels. However, he wrongly inserted the catheter into the umbilical vein rather than the artery. He asked a registrar to check its position but neither doctor noticed the error for 24 hours. The baby suffered retrolental fibroplasia.

The health authority was found liable, but in his summing up the judge found the registrar had been negligent but not the houseman. He said that the houseman was entitled to have his work checked by a competent doctor.

cases, many plaintiff's claims for damages do not succeed because of failure to prove a 'causative' link, even when it may seem obvious. This is shown in a famous non-maternity case (**Box 16.4**).

Assessment of damages

When a judge has decided that a case of negligence has been proved, he hears evidence to assess the level of damages to award. The aim is to put the plaintiff, as far as possible, in the position they would have been if there had been no negligence and to measure the cost of this in financial terms. Some cases that arise from maternity care can now attract very large amounts of damages, because of the long-term nature of the care needed to look after a damaged baby. Evidence is heard about the possible cost of ongoing health and social care and the life expectancy of the child in order to reach a final settlement. Added to this sum are the legal costs for both sides to the case.

Box 16.4

Barnett v Chelsea and Westminster Hospital Management Committee (1969)

After drinking tea in the early morning three workmen became unwell and went to a local casualty department. One was ill enough to need to lie down. The nurse called the houseman, who was himself ill and by telephone he advised that they go to their own doctors. Later that day, one of the workmen died and it was found that he had arsenic poisoning

The court agreed that the houseman had a duty of care and, by not seeing the men, had breached that duty. However, it did not uphold the claim. It found that even if the men had been seen, because arsenic poisoning was so rare, it was unlikely that a diagnosis would have been made before Mr Barnett's death. But the deciding factor was that, even if the diagnosis had been made, the hospital would not have obtained the antidote in time. The cause of Mr Barnett's death therefore was arsenic poisoning, not the negligent act of the doctor.

Who is Liable?

So far the negligent acts of the professionals have been alluded to in this chapter – midwives and doctors; indeed a general principle in law is that cases may only involve those directly concerned. However, there is an important exception. In the above case, and that of Bolam, the hospital management committee is cited as the defendant not the doctor. This is because as employers they are being held vicariously liable for the actions of their employees. The doctrine of vicarious liability developed to ensure that successful claimants have a reasonable chance of obtaining damages. Unless they are insured, people are unlikely to have sufficient money to meet damages awarded against them so the courts began to accept that employers (with greater financial reserves or insurance cover) are held liable for their employees.

Much of this complex area of law centres on an analysis of the contractual employment relationship between the apparent employer and the negligent employee. As most midwives are employees of the NHS, their NHS employer is vicariously liable for them. The NHS also explicitly indemnifies its employees for their negligent acts committed during the course of their employment. However, if a midwife undertakes any professional practice on a self-employed basis, she is held personally liable in law for that work and would be advised to hold her own professional indemnity insurance.

Employed or not employed?

Most health-care professionals are guided in at least some part of their work by clinical guidelines and employer's protocols. But what happens if a midwife fails to follow an agreed procedure? Is her employer, an NHS Trust, still liable and so indemnify her? The two following cases, although old and not relevant to health care, provide an answer to the use of or failure to follow protocols (**Box 16.5**).

In the first case the company was held to be vicariously liable whereas in the second it was not. The deciding factor lay in what the employees were employed to do. In Limpus, the driver was driving the bus even though he was doing it negligently; in the second, the conductor drove the bus and so was not at that time acting in the course of employment.

In relation to the work of midwives, the rules in operation in the case of Limpus are similar to agreed protocols and procedures in use in many situations in maternity care. Failure to adhere to a protocol may constitute negligence, but does not negate the liability of the midwife's employer. If, however, a midwife does something clearly outside her sphere of work, for example performs a Caesarean section, then the employer is not liable.

Women's Rights and Fetal Rights

To have legal recognition and therefore full recourse to the law a person must be alive. People have no rights after death, although others may sue on behalf of their estate. Until fairly recently, this also applied to the time before birth, and even now a baby only achieves full legal status after birth.

Women, therefore, have an absolute right to legal recourse for damage done to them. So does the living child. The rights of the fetus are, however, more circumscribed and have only been in existence since 1976.

Congenital Disabilities (Civil Liability) Act 1976

The thalidomide tragedy brought to the attention of the public the possibility that the actions of others can damage a fetus in such a way that its subsequent life is profoundly affected. Although the evidence against thalidomide was probably strong enough to have resulted in successful negligence claims, it was not possible to bring such cases in English Law because the damage had been done in fetal life when none of the potential victims had any legal rights. As a consequence the 1976 Act was introduced.

Even this Act does not give full legal status to the fetus. Instead, it lays down the principle that if a duty of care is owed to a pregnant woman, then her unborn child may also expect a duty of care. The fetus does not have this in its own right, but this is sufficient to enable the cases that are now brought where damage *in utero* is the main contention.

The Act also restricts the rights of the fetus to sue its parents, given that any such action would be potentially detrimental to the relationship between the child and its parents. However, there are exceptions. The child may sue its mother for negligence while driving on the presumption that she is fully insured, so that the action would then be directed at the insurance company. The child may not sue either or both parents for preconception risks, although it may sue his/her father for these if he but not the mother was aware of any risk before conception. Thus, for example, the child may sue his/her father for passing on the human immunodeficiency virus (HIV) through infecting the mother, if the father had not told the mother of his HIV status. If both parents knew of the HIV status of the father or the mother, then the child may not sue.

Women's rights versus fetal rights

Very occasionally a woman's lifestyle or actions could put the health of the fetus at risk – for example, the woman who smokes heavily or takes drugs through pregnancy. The following two cases illustrate the position taken by the law when there is a conflict between the rights of the fetus and the woman (**Box 16.6**). As the second case is not an English case it has no impact here.

In 1992 a case was heard in England which did challenge the rights of pregnant women (**Box 16.7**). Being only a High Court decision, this case does not create precedent but, like in America, there was considerable criticism of the decision. Given the strong legal misgivings expressed it is unlikely that the decision would be repeated in the UK.

There may be times when a midwife wants to give a certain treatment to ensure, as far as possible, the health of the fetus, but where the mother refuses. An example might be a woman who is about to deliver a very premature baby, but who refuses to go to hos-

---

Box 16.5

Employed or Not Employed?

Limpus v London General Omnibus Co (1862)
A bus driver used his bus to obstruct the bus of a rival company and caused damage. The company, being held vicariously liable, was sued for the damage. It, however, argued that at the time of the incident the driver was not in its employ because there was a company rule expressly forbidding such behaviour. Notice to this effect was clearly displayed in the rest room and in breaking the rule the driver was not acting as an employee.

Beard v London General Omnibus Co (1900)
In this case, involving the same company, a bus came to the end of its journey. The bus driver left the bus for a short time and while gone the conductor turned the bus around. He crashed it. In the ensuing court case the company claimed that they were not liable as he had expressly broken one of their rules.

pital. The midwife cannot force her to go to hospital and in such circumstances must just give the very best care she can.

However, the picture is very different once the baby is born. Midwives and doctors can act, transferring the baby to hospital, even in the absence of the mother's consent. If they were subsequently taken to court they could use the defence of necessity in the best interests of the child and in all probability would be successful. For additional protection, although it is not needed, application could be made to make the child a ward of court immediately on delivery and the court then orders his/her transfer to hospital. Once the immediate interests of the child have been met, care of the child is normally returned to the mother.

Limitations on Using the Law

Unlike NHS services, which are with minor exceptions free at the point of need, there are clear limitations of access to the legal system. The two main limitations are time and financial constraints.

Box 16.6

Women's Rights v Fetal Rights

Re F (*in utero*) (1988)
A young pregnant woman was a drug addict. There was some concern that she would not stay in one place and attend for antenatal care. An application was made to the court to make the fetus a ward of court, thus giving the court the power to keep the woman in one place. The application failed. The court concluded that the fetal rights could not override those of the woman to her liberty.
Re AC (1990)
This distressing American case involved a young pregnant woman who was dying of cancer. The doctors treating her obtained an order to perform a Caesarean section to save the child and went ahead with the operation, even though the woman withheld her consent. In the event both the mother and the baby died. In this case the doctors and the original court order allowed the rights of the fetus to prevail over that of the woman's expressed choice. However, there was a public outcry following this decision and the woman's estate sued the hospital. It was held, on appeal, that the decision had been unsafe and, indeed, after this the American Medical Association declared that there should be no circumstances when such a decision should be taken again.

The Act of Limitation (1980)

The Act of Limitation (1980) introduced a time limit to the start of legal proceedings – up to 3 years from the incident or 3 years from knowledge that the incident potentially caused harm. This usually places a time-limit on adults, but very different circumstances apply to children. If no-one brings a case on their behalf earlier, they are deemed to have knowledge of the event only on their 18th birthday, so the 3 year time limit applies from then – giving up to 21 years for a case to be started. Indeed, for babies who are brain-damaged, time runs without limit because they are deemed never to have knowledge of the incident, although cases are usually commenced early in the child's life by the parents or guardians.

Financial limitation – legal aid

The potential cost of legal action limits most people's access to the law. Legal Aid is very limited and means tested. The means test is rigorous and only for those with limited disposable income.

However, recently a change in the legal aid system has increased the opportunity for babies who have been harmed to seek legal redress. A baby's assets are now assessed in his/her own right rather than with reference to those of the parents. As most babies have no assets, almost all are now able to obtain legal aid, which gives increased access to the law. Although this has resulted in an increase of cases, some of which are related to events many years ago, each case heard must still met the criteria set out earlier in this section and particularly the standards of care that existed at the time must guide any final judgement.

Box 16.7

Re S (1992)
A woman in labour was found to have transverse lie with the fetal elbow protruding through the cervix. She was in danger of rupturing her uterus. On religious grounds she refused a Caesarean section and her husband supported the decision. A court ruled that the operation could be performed and it was carried out against her express consent.

The Right to Complain

If the service which is provided does not satisfy the consumer there are various mechanisms by which complaints can be addressed.

NHS Complaints Procedures

Procedures that operate in the health service are not legal mechanisms, but provide a more immediate course of action for a patient or client who is dissatisfied with the hospital facilities (for example, waiting times, catering or cleanliness) or their care. The NHS Executive issues firm guidance from time to time on how services must operate a competent complaints procedure. Each trust must have a complaints officer and complaints must be processed quickly and fairly. The patients and clients should feel they have had their complaint fully investigated and be left satisfied with the final explanation and any action the trust takes. There is an apparent relationship between the quality of complaints procedures and litigation in that it is thought some patients resort to the latter only when their complaint has not been dealt with adequately.

Community Health Councils

Community Health Councils (CHC) were set up by the National Health Service Reorganisation Act 1973 as a means of giving a public voice in the NHS. They are able to help people who are unhappy with their care by explaining the procedures and giving them support in making their complaint.

Health Service Commissioner

The Health Service Commissioners Act (1993) requires the appointment of Commissioners for England, for Scotland and for Wales. Commissioners investigate individual complaints from users of the service. The findings of any investigation are treated very seriously and the health service body held responsible is expected to implement the recommendations. Commissioners are responsible to Parliament and must publish an annual report of their investigations. Under the Act the Commissioner is now able to investigate clinical complaints.

Protection of Client Information

Health care depends considerably on what patients and clients tell professional staff. Treatments, care plans and referral to other agencies (for example, for social care) are highly dependent upon accurate physical, psychological and social histories. Health-care professionals are often in the privileged position of knowing information that a patient has shared with no-one else.

The Right to Confidentiality

Legally, information obtained in the course of professional practice is always deemed confidential and, if that confidentiality is broken, a claim of breach of confidence can be made to the courts. However, because of the cost and difficulty of bringing such claims, it is generally more common for such breaches to be dealt with through the professional conduct machinery and employment law, with the professional risking removal from the register or dismissal, or both. There are, however, some circumstances in which information can be legitimately shared:

- If the person consents to the information being shared – for example, consent to the use of the medical record for research purposes.
- On a need-to-know basis – this allows the passage of information between members of the clinical team.
- In the public interest – this is a very rare occurrence in midwifery practice, but would cover circumstances such as hearing information about a serious crime.
- Because there is a statutory duty to inform – notification of infectious diseases is an example of this.
- Because there is a court order to disclose information in connection with an impending legal action.

Any midwife who is asked to disclose information because it appears to fall into one of the above categories should, however, seek the advise of her managers. If in independent practice she should ask advice from a solicitor or her professional organization.

Rights of Access to Information

Until recently patients had no right to see the content of their medical records. If the health record was shared with the patient it was at the discretion of the health-care professional. Two statutes now give rights of access to the record with certain limitations.

Data Protection Act 1984

This Act aims to give protection to people against the improper use of personal information held on computer. It requires that anyone holding such personal information on computer must be registered and must follow principles of good practice, laid down in one of the schedules of the Act. These include that the information must be obtained fairly and legally, used only for specified purposes, be used lawfully, be adequate for the purpose and not excessive, be accurate and kept no longer than is required.

Individuals, on the other hand, have the right to see information kept about them on computer. The Act applies to all information and therefore to any computerized records generated in clinical practice.

In health care this created an anomaly, giving rights to patients whose records were computerized but denying these rights to those whose records were still manually created.

Access to Health Records Act 1990

This anomaly was corrected with the 1990 Act, which gives rights of access to manual as well as to computer health records.

Restriction on access

Both Acts allow for information to be withheld if it might cause serious harm to the physical or mental health of the person or any other individual, or where it might reveal the identity of another person. Where an application has been made to see the medical record, the health professional concerned must be consulted. The professional makes a decision on whether disclosure will cause harm and advises accordingly. The person making application must be informed if any information has been withheld.

A small but important requirement of the Act is that information when disclosed must be in a form which is understandable to the person. If it is not, it is returned to the professional to further interpret the notes. It would, however, be more sensible to make records in the first place that are generally comprehensible – for example, by avoiding abbreviations as far as possible and by writing legibly.

Safe Premises and Working Practices

Both employees and those who use services and premises of others have the right to be protected in a safe environment and that working practices and processes be carried out as safely as can reasonably be expected. Two Acts of Parliament are intended to safeguard these expectations.

Health and Safety at Work Act 1974

This stringent legislation requires that all measures are taken to protect people during the course of their work. The Act requires employers and employees to take all action required to maintain a safe working environment. Additionally, the employer must take all reasonable steps to ensure the safety of nonemployees using the premises. This clearly extends the protection to patients and clients.

Compliance with the requirements of the Act is monitored by the Health and Safety Executive (HSE). The HSE has considerable powers, as the Act allows criminal proceedings to be instigated against organizations or individual people if there is blatant and continuing noncompliance or if an incident has been so serious that it warrants prosecution.

The Occupiers Liability Acts 1957 and 1984

These Acts confer a responsibility on those who own premises to maintain them in a safe condition for those who are on the premises. This applies to the safe condition of the premises, furniture and any equipment. The Acts protect the rights of people who are on the premises either lawfully or unlawfully (e.g. trespassers). Although this applies to health service premises and any health service body has policies in place to ensure reasonable safety, which the staff must follow, these Acts are of particular importance to midwives in independent practice who use their own premises in the course of their work. It is possible to display a disclaimer against damage to property (e.g. cars are parked at the owner's risk), but any disclaimer against personal injury is considered null and void.

Product Liability

Much health care depends on the use of equipment, some of which is highly complex; the safety of patients and staff can depend on its safe operation and use. There can be circumstances when such equipment is made unsafe because of the way it is used. It may not be serviced according to manufacturer's instructions; it may be wrongly wired into the electrical supply. Clearly these are the responsibility of the service, which is found liable for any resulting damage.

However, modern equipment is very complex, so hospitals and professionals may not have the skills or knowledge necessary to assess the safety of the equipment in use. In 1985 a European Directive placed liability for defective equipment on the manufacturer in the first place; this principle was introduced into UK law in the 1987 Consumer Protection Act. It protects the user and supplier of products (for example, drugs are included) that are found to be faulty due to the manufacturer. It is therefore important for product users or suppliers to keep a record of the product manufacturers. That may sound simple – a CTG machine has its manufacturer's name on it. But what about a circumstance when a prescribed drug is wrongly manufactured and harms a patient. The patient's drug bottle does not necessarily have a manufacturer's name on it. If the end suppliers of products cannot trace the manufacturer they then may be held liable. Pharmacists therefore have very clear processes for tracing back prescriptions to the batches of drugs they have bought. If an independent midwife supplies a drug to a client and cannot trace back to her supplier, she also could find herself liable. This is a very good reason for keeping a clear record of where she has obtained all her supplies, for drugs or any of the equipment she uses.

Managing the Legal Risk

Although professional regulation and legal rights and processes are in place to protect the users of services, there are many ways in which the professional can protect against the risk of litigation, while at the same time enhancing public protection. Using the principles described in this chapter should help midwives to reflect on ways to assure and increase safety margins for their clients. A particular challenge would be for groups of midwives and their managers to develop a risk-management strategy – the following topics give a framework for this.

Standards of Care

First and foremost, all the law and the public can expect is that the professional reaches the standard of the ordinary competent professional. This means, of course, keeping up-to-date, practising according to research-based findings and meeting currently acceptable standards of care. Questions for particular consideration are:
- What are the prevailing standards?
- How can we ensure all midwives meet these?
- What audit measures might be introduced into everyday practice to ensure standards are being met?

Using Protocols

Protocols, based on current research and information on clinical effectiveness and used by all staff to guide the care they give, can serve to minimize error and assure agreed standards of care. Beth Israel Hospital in the USA found that strict adherence to agreed protocols resulted in a marked reduction in obstetric litigation (and a subsequent reduction in professional indemnity payments). There can be considerable antipathy to this approach in that it is seen as curtailing clinical freedom. If, however, all professional staff who are expected to follow the protocols are involved in their production and the protocols reflect current research and are sufficiently flexible where research is inconclusive to allow considered deviation, they are usually found to be acceptable. In the Beth Israel Hospital (personal communication, 1993), it was possible for the clinicians to deviate from the protocols, but they had to make a full record of the decision they had taken in the notes; these notes were regularly peer-reviewed by a multidisciplinary group that included doctors and midwives.

Monitoring Practice

Regular audit of case notes and audit meetings to discuss both difficult and straightforward cases allows for a review of decision making and gives early warning of falling standards. It is particularly important to look at random samples of straightforward cases to pick up on potential problems before something happens.

Identifying Risk Activities

Some areas of clinical practice are more prone to or favour successful litigation. These include CTG interpretation, the interpretation of meconium staining, decisions on referral to medical aid and resuscitation. Regular and persistent training in these areas should be undertaken by all professional staff involved. The training should simulate what goes on in clinical practice, for example, running practice resuscitation or presenting midwives and doctors with CTG traces for them to make decisions on what action to take. Publications such as *CTG Made Easy* (Gauge and Henderson, 1992) give examples of CTG traces and discuss the action needed and the reported outcomes of the cases; these can be invaluable if incorporated into regular training sessions

Keeping Records

One of the most common reasons why health bodies find it difficult to defend claims is because they do not have sufficient evidence. Clinical records often omit important information, although at the same time they often contain a welter of comparative trivia. It can be difficult to ascertain the time sequence of events, particularly if recordings of events are made separately. This can present problems in trying to match up the notes made on a CTG recording or those made in midwifery notes with those made in the medical record. The introduction of a single set of maternity notes may minimize this problem, but is still reliant on the professional who writes a record in the first place. Clinical records should be made contemporaneously, should be legible, should accurately reflect the clinical situation, should record all clinical decisions and the reasons why they were taken, should record all relevant times accurately and should be signed. They should pay particular attention to anything that deviates from the expected. Where problems have arisen, a contemporaneous statement of all salient information should be made and filed with the notes.

Very often when being assessed for legal purposes, records fall very short of these minimum requirements. Earlier in this ß, it is explained that the time interval between an incident and a subsequent court case can be very long. In such circumstances, unless the case is very unusual, the professional does not remember any of the details and the court is likely to accept the plaintiff's version. However, courts are very likely to accept the contemporaneously made records of the professional as the most accurate version if they are complete and comprehensible.

Managers should therefore consider introducing standards for record keeping and then carry out a regular audit of samples of notes to check they continue

to meet the standard set. Additionally, all midwives should follow the guidance given by the UKCC on record keeping (UKCC, 1993c).

As accurate notes often act as potent evidence for the defence of a case, it cannot be stressed enough that an 'aggressive' approach to standardization and competent standards is perhaps the single most important action a unit can take to defend an allegation of negligence when it has not in fact taken place.

Responding to Complaints

There is some evidence that people turn to litigation, particularly if their claim is small, because they have not been satisfied with the working of the complaints procedure. To minimize this possibility complaints should be processed quickly and the system should be understandable. People should feel they have had adequate opportunity to put their complaint and should feel satisfied with any action taken.

Maintaining a Safe Environment

Strict adherence to the requirements of the Health and Safety at Work Act 1974 goes a long way to protect all people – staff and patients. Managers, along with trade union officials, should ensure that regular safety audits are performed. All adverse incidents should be reported and regularly reviewed to see if there are any worrying trends – these should be investigated and appropriate action taken.

Adverse incidents involving medical equipment should be reported to the Medical Devices Agency so that a national picture of potential defects or misuse of equipment can be spotted and correcting action taken. Similarly, doctors should report all adverse and unexplained drug reactions. To help do this, a doctor needs to be informed by a midwife of any drug reaction she thinks may have occurred.

Summary

The way the law operates to protect the public receiving health care has been discussed. The chapter has also referred to the way in which midwifery practices is regulated by the UKCC. It has been suggested that it may be helpful for midwives to develop a risk management strategy to protect the public and at the same time to protect themselves against litigation.

KEY CONCEPTS

- Women who use the maternity services have a right to be kept safe and not to be harmed by the service, by equipment or other products used in their care or by those who are looking after them.

- The aim of statutory professional regulation is to provide professionals who have reached a satisfactory level of training and continue to practice to currently acceptable standards.

- The UKCC with National Boards exercise this process of statutory regulation by setting standards and rules for education and practice and by operating a professional register. For midwives, in particular, local supervising authorities and their supervisors of midwives ensure that this happens at the local level.

- In the field of general law, the civil law of negligence offers the opportunity for redress to anyone injured as a result of the negligent actions of others.

- Women have the right to confidentiality subject to certain exemptions. Following the Data Protection Act and Access to Health Records Act they may, with some exceptions also have access to their medical records.

- Statute protects the users of premises, requiring buildings to be maintained in a safe manner and providing sanctions where they are not.

- Manufacturers are held to be liable for all products, including those used in health care, which are faulty due to manufacturing processes, thus placing a responsibility for safe manufacture of goods and redress in cases where damage has been sustained.

- Balanced against these rights, professionals can take a risk management approach to litigation which, on the one hand ensures high standards of care and on the other high standards of evidence should litigation be threatened.

References

The cases used in this chapter are referenced according to the law reports in which they appear. If any reader wants to read the full facts of the cases and their judgement, the law reports are referenced using the following standard abbreviations:

- A – Appeal (United States).
- AC – Law Reports, Appeal Cases.
- All ER – All England Law Reports.
- H & C – Hurlestone and Coltman.
- QB – Queens Bench.
- WLR – Weekly Law Reports.

Barnett v. Chelsea and Kensington Hospital Management Committee [1969] 1 QB 428, [1968] 1 All ER 1068, [1968] 2 WLR 422.

Beard v. London General Omnibus Co. [1900] 2 QB 530.

Bolam v. Friern Hospital Management Committee [1957] 2 All ER 118, [1957] 1 WLR 582.

Department of Health: *Changing childbirth: the Report of the Expert Maternity Group*, London, 1994, Department of Health.

De Vries RG: Midwifery and the problem of licensure. In *Research in the sociology of health care*, Vol. 2, Greenwich, 1982, Jai Press Inc.

Donoghue v. Stevenson [1932] AC 562.

Gauge S, Henderson C: *CTG made easy*, London, 1992, Churchill Livingston.

Henderson C, Roch S, Hunt SC, McDonald KS, McCausland R, Page L, Thomas M: Supplement on statutory bodies, *Br J Midwifery* 3:4, 1995.

Henry C, Marsh BJ, Siddiqui J: Supplement on ethics in midwifery, *Br J Midwifery* 4:2, 1996,

Hughes EC: *Men and their work*, Glencoe, 1958, The Free Press.

Limpus v. London General Omnibus Co. [1862] 1 H & C 526.

Oakley A, Houd S: *Helpers in childbirth: midwifery today*, Copenhagen, 1990, Hemisphere Publishing on behalf of WHO Regional Office for Europe.

Re AC. District of Columbia Court of Appeals [1990] 573 A 2d 1235.

Re F (in utero) [1988] 2 All ER 193.

Re S [1992] 4 All ER 649.

UKCC: *The code of professional conduct for the nurse, midwife and health visitor*, London, 1992a, United Kingdom Central Council.

UKCC: *The scope of professional practice*, London, 1992b, United Kingdom Central Council.

UKCC: *The midwives rules*, London, 1993a, United Kingdom Central Council.

UKCC: *Complaints about professional conduct*, London, 1993b, United Kingdom Central Council.

UKCC: *Standards for records and record keeping*, London, 1993c, United Kingdom Central Council.

UKCC: *A midwife's code of practice*, London, 1994, United Kingdom Central Council.

Whitehouse v. Jordan [1981] 1 All ER 267, [1981] 1 WLR 246.

Further Reading

For those readers who want to read further on health service law in general or the law relating to midwifery in particular, the following are recommended.

Jenkins R: *The law and the midwife*, Oxford, 1995, Blackwell Science.

This book relates legal principles to everyday midwifery practice as well as highlighting current debates and controversies. As well as legal principles that related directly to care, it additionally covers employment law, the legal system and the legal basis for health care.

Kennedy I, Grubb A: *Medical law; Text and materials*, London, 1994, Butterworth.

This very comprehensive textbook covers all aspects of medical law. It gives the case reports and relevant judgements, providing a detailed commentary on their relevance and applicability to practice and health care provision.

Mason D, Edwards P: *Litigation, a risk management guide for midwives*, London, 1993, Royal College of Midwives.

This short booklet describes the main principles of negligence as it relates to midwifery practice. It then considers ways in which midwives and midwife managers can minimize the risk of successful litigation against them and their employer.

17 Maternity Policy and the Midwife

LEARNING OUTCOMES

After studying this chapter you should be able to:

- Place current developments in maternity policy into an historical context.
- Discuss the various influences on the policy making process.
- Understand how different organizational structures influence midwifery practice.
- Demonstrate how professional ideologies affect policy and practice.
- Debate the advantages and disadvantages of professionalism.

The control and management of birth is an important issue for any society. As Margaret Stacey (1988, p. 259) noted: 'Reproduction is a crucial area which reveals starkly the relations between health care and the dominant social values.' Throughout the twentieth century, there has been a lively debate about the choice and control women have over the care they receive and the roles and responsibilities of the professionals involved.

How do policies emerge? Both local and national maternity policies are influenced from a variety of directions, including the reports of government committees, Royal Commissions, professional bodies and campaigns by pressure groups. In this chapter, three themes are explored. First, maternity policies and how the resulting organization of maternity care has affected the division of responsibilities of professional groups. Second, the impact this had on midwives' autonomy and third the extent to which midwives have been able to influence events.

Twentieth-Century Maternity Policy (1900–92)

State involvement with maternity care increased from the turn of the century, following registration of midwives in 1902; midwives had fought hard to be included in the 1911 National Insurance Bill, to enable women to have a choice of midwife or doctor. The Maternal and Child Welfare Act in 1918, precipitated by the World War I, increased the number of midwives in local government salaried service, although this provision was always patchy, and enshrined a medical model of care (Peretz, 1990). The difficulty of making a living from independent practice was perennial, so by the early 1930s independent midwives represented about 50% of the 15,000 midwives in practice (Fox, 1993).

Both midwives and general practitioners (GPs) were competing for work in a declining market, caused by a falling birth rate and an increase in the institutional confinement rate, from 15% in 1927 to 40% by 1940 (Lewis, 1980, p. 120). Robinson (1990) suggests this trend was caused by three factors:

- First, the removal of the stigma of poor law hospitals in 1929 by placing them under local authority control.
- Secondly, working class women covered by national insurance now had free access and were demanding admission to the voluntary hospitals.
- Thirdly, obstetricians were advocating hospital confinement because it would reduce maternal mortality, which showed no sign of decreasing below 5/1000 live births (compared with 0.11/1000 in 1990). Indeed, the rate did not begin to drop until the introduction of sulphonamides in the late 1930s and of blood transfusions in World War II.

It is important to note that this trend reflected the preference of many women at the time, although some wanted a hospital birth because they were told it was safer, this was only part of the cause. Before 1920, women's organizations were calling for hospital beds to accommodate those in poor home circumstances, stressing the need for rest, privacy and running water. Furthermore, the greater availability of pain relief in hospital was a great attraction for middle-class women. In 1939 only 0.5% of home deliveries used analgesia because of the restriction by the Central Midwives Board (CMB) on midwives' use of pain relief (Lewis, 1980).

It is important to note that a 100% hospitalization rate was not inevitable before World War II – it was assumed by obstetric consultants and the government that home confinements would continue, mainly because of the cost implications. For example, in 1936 a salaried domiciliary National Maternity Service was established, its strength being flexibility, continuity of care and subsidized care. As Peretz (1990) points out, provision varied and relied heavily on charitable help; if a woman or her husband were part of the National Insurance scheme then she would receive a 30 shilling maternity benefit. For example, in 1939 the hospital was an expensive option, costing £4 a week, whereas a midwife could be engaged for between 10 and 25 shillings in some places and the General Practitioner for £2 (Lewis, 1980).

By the end of World War II the institutional confinement rate had risen to 54% and, with the introduction of the NHS, the consultant-led service expanded at the expense of Local Authority services (*see* Dingwall *et al.* 1988; Honigsbaum, 1979, 1989). It also destroyed the economic basis of independent midwifery as it was now cheaper for women to go to hospital than stay at home (Ministry of Health, 1953, p. 125).

The biggest growth in hospital delivery took place between 1963 and 1972, when the rate went from 68.2% to 91.4% (Oakley, 1984a, p. 215). Public pressure for hospital maternity services had grown and obstetric knowledge and methods had classified more pregnancies as high risk (Lewis, 1990). By 1959, the Cranbrook Committee was doing little more than following the prevailing trends in recommending provision for a 70% hospital confinement rate (Ministry of Health, 1959). The committee had reached its target based on a perceived demand from women for a hospital confinement and the prevalence of 'avoidable' deaths in the home.

By 1970, the Peel Committee (DHSS, 1970) advocated a 100% hospitalization rate. The committee was dominated by obstetric expertise, which aimed to secure resource allocation for a policy already agreed upon within the profession. The main grounds for this recommendation were that the rate was already moving in that direction and that hospital birth was safer. As Macfarlane (1985) pointed out, the evidence in support of this view was doubtful, but it wasn't until 1971 that Cochrane made a blistering attack on the dubious causal correlations that had been drawn between maternal mortality and increasing hospitalization, latterly borne out by other research (Russell, 1982; Macfarlane, 1985; Tew, 1977, 1978, 1985, 1990; Campbell and Macfarlane, 1987).

The 1970s saw an upsurge of interest in the costs of perinatal handicap and perinatal health. This culminated in the publication of the Second Report of the Social Services Committee on Perinatal and Neonatal Mortality – the Short Report (Social Services Committee, 1980). This report was concerned with the wide variations in perinatal and neonatal mortality within Britain and internationally. Although it identified the social and medical factors associated with high perinatal mortality, it assumed that social factors could be compensated for by 'well-applied medical intervention'. Thus, electronic fetal monitoring for all deliveries, a 50% increase in obstetric consultants and a 100% increase in neonatal intensive care cots were advocated.

It is important to note that the concerns with reducing perinatal, infant and maternal mortality rates throughout the twentieth century focused specifically on medical interventions. The Ministry of Health had always been resistant to the view that maternal mortality was part of the larger issue of women's health. In an analysis of the politics of the Short Report, Russell suggested that:

> An oversimplification of the inter-relationships that exist between the social and medical factors related to perinatal mortality has justified an almost exclusively medical or individualistic focus and has resulted in the exclusion of socio-economic factors from the general debate.
>
> (Russell, 1982, p.306.)

Impact on Midwifery Autonomy

As a result of the above policies, by the early 1980s the sphere of practice of midwives had been constrained in three key areas – clinical practice, licensing and education.

Practice

Firstly, the midwife's relationship with a pregnant woman changed in a fundamental way. She now went to her GP and not the midwife as the first point of contact with the maternity services. Furthermore, whereas previously the community midwife gave most of the care throughout pregnancy, calling on other professionals when needed, obstetricians and GPs were now involved in routine care (Oakley, 1984a).

The work of hospital midwives also became increasingly specialized; for example, in 1969 75% of midwives were giving total continuity of care during the hospital stay, i.e. the same midwives provided antenatal, labour and postnatal care to women on one ward. By 1979 this had fallen to 36% (Robinson *et al.* 1983), partly because of the introduction of centralized delivery suites. Some midwives were providing continuity of care through domino schemes, where the community midwife provided antenatal and postnatal care and delivered the baby in hospital, but this provision was patchy (Campbell and Macfarlane, 1987, pp. 51–52). These changes curtailed the freedom to use clinical judgement, unused skills grew rusty and midwives became increasingly concerned about the erosion of their role (RCM, 1977).

From the early 1980s onwards the role of the midwife in the provision of maternity care was the subject of several government and professional reports (Social Services Committee, 1980; RCOG, 1982). It was concern with the erosion of this role that prompted the DHSS to fund a survey to examine the role and responsibilities of the midwife (Robinson *et al.* 1983).

In 1979, 60 health districts were randomly selected from the Regional Health Authorities in England and Wales. Questionnaires were sent to all midwives and obstetric medical staff in each district, and to a sample of health visitors and GPs. Of the midwives, 78% returned the questionnaire.

Results showed that, despite being qualified to do so, midwives only played a minor role in antenatal care and that care was duplicated by doctors. During labour, although the majority of deliveries continued to be supervised by a midwife, her decision-making responsibilities and freedom to exercise her clinical judgement had been eroded by the introduction of policies and guidelines.

The report concluded that resources were being wasted because midwives' skills and training were being underused and care was being duplicated and fragmented. Furthermore, newly qualified midwives were unable to develop and maintain clinical expertise and lacked job satisfaction.

Since then, these findings have been substantiated by other studies (DHSS, 1984; Garcia *et al.* 1985), practising midwives (Towler, 1982), representatives of statutory (CMB, 1983) and professional bodies (Ashton, 1987), and parliamentary committees (Social Services Committee, 1980) all expressed concern at the continued underuse of midwives' skills.

At the same time, the incidence of obstetric intervention that began to rise in the 1960s rose sharply in the 1980s (Macfarlane and Mugford, 1984), reflecting maternity units 'active management of labour' policies, although still unproven in efficacy (Chalmers, 1978). Although these might have been confined to high-risk deliveries, research has had little success in predicting risk (Oakley, 1984a, pp. 220–1), so pregnancy and childbirth became only 'normal in retrospect'. This followed the medical profession's tendency to intervene in cases of uncertainty (Scheff, 1968) and in areas at high risk of litigation (Ennis *et al.* 1991). The result was that, in practise, the midwife had been transformed into an obstetric nurse with limited autonomy, 'she is responsible for her own action within a framework of rules defined by modern obstetric practice' (Dingwall *et al.* 1988, p. 171).

Licensing

Other developments highlighted midwives' dependency on the state to license their activity. The Nurses, Midwives and Health Visitor's Act of 1979 abolished the CMB and replaced it with the United Kingdom Central Council for Nursing, Midwifery and Health Visiting (UKCC). This brought midwives under the same legislation as nurses, but many midwives felt this replaced medical control with that of nurses (*see* the letters in the *Midwives Chronicle* of 1978). These developments in the 1980s prompted a campaign, initiated by the Association of Radical Midwives (ARM), for a new Midwives Act (Hardy, 1990; Cronk, 1990; RCM, 1991b). The campaign was characterized by debates among midwives about whether they should use their energy to strengthen existing legislation within the 'nursing' body or to make claims to be separate from nursing (Cardale, 1990).

Education

New education proposals, such as *Project 2000* (UKCC, 1986) which moved nurse training into higher education, also considered midwifery as a nursing specialism (RCM, 1986). Midwives successfully kept control over their education and the number of 3-year direct entry courses for those without a nursing qualification rose. But midwifery schools were being incorporated into higher education, which resulted in fears about losing control over the educational process (Kent and Maggs, 1990). At National Board Level in England the replacement of specialist midwifery education officers with generalists against the wishes of the midwifery committees fundamentally challenged

the professional monopoly that midwives had established in the 1902 Act. (*Note:* Specialist midwifery officers continue to exist in Scotland, Wales and Northern Ireland.)

The New Midwifery Professional Project

Dingwall *et al.* (1988) argued that midwifery emerged in the twentieth century within the context of specific social and economic conditions. This united the provision of a cheap service for the poor with the desire of some middle-class women to establish female control over childbirth. They suggest this alliance kept the ideology of a midwife as an independent carer alive during the twentieth century, while in practice the economic and clinical sphere of midwifery practice was being eroded (Fox, 1993).

The sphere of midwifery practice had always been defined by medical men; it increased during the twentieth century as the boundaries between normal and abnormal pregnancies and births were redefined. There had also been continuing concern expressed by midwives that their traditional remit had been eroded by an increasing medical dominance of birth since the 1960s (Robinson, 1990). Partly in response to these events, but also influenced by feminism and an altruistic empathy with consumer unhappiness about their experience of childbirth, midwives began to develop their new 'professional project' to regain occupational autonomy (Sandall, 1995).

Professional projects have been defined in the sociological literature as strategies developed by an occupation to achieve a monopoly over the provision of certain skills and competencies in a market for services (Witz, 1992, p. 5). The tactics that an occupation uses are called professional strategies and the process is called professionalization.

By the late 1970s the critique by midwives of these changes in maternity care reflected the impact of feminism on midwifery and the formation of an alliance between midwives who were unhappy with their subordinate role and women who wanted more control over their experience of birth. Feminist writing validated midwifery as a career for women (Ehrenreich and English, 1973; Oakley, 1976), and several feminists entered midwifery because of their feminism (Weitz, 1987).

In response to these developments, ARM was

formed in 1976 to express concern about the erosion of the midwife's role and the resulting poor quality of care offered. Originally started as a study and support group for student midwives, ARM evolved into a political action group, both in alliance with organizations in the maternity rights movement and with the professional bodies.

The aims of ARM contained important new constructions of the midwife–woman relationship that aimed to return to women both choice and control over the processes of pregnancy and birth. To provide complete continuity of care was seen as the best way of empowering midwives and extending the boundaries of midwifery autonomy and thus empowering women (Flint, 1981). There is the assumption here that to empower midwives then empowers women. What evidence is there for this and what happens in practice?

Support for ARM from most midwives was limited. Midwives sampled in a survey at the time (Weitz, 1987) were happy with their role, thought that midwives had not become obstetric nurses, were not constrained by hospital policies, felt little concern about their training or that fragmentation of care had deskilled midwives. In consequence, only about 50% supported a change of the system to give continuity of care. They found the label 'radical' and notions of feminism alienating and feared stigmatization at work. Weitz found significant differences in educational backgrounds of the two groups, with radical midwives having more education and many being direct-entry midwives who had not trained as nurses. ARM activists surmised that the difference was caused by 'the emphasis on conformity, obedience, and medical ideas about childbearing that underlay British nurse training' (Weitz, 1987, p. 88).

More recent strategies of ARM addressed these issues by members becoming active in mainstream professional organizations, moving into teaching, research and managerial posts and as a consequence being able to advance their proposals onto the professional and political agenda.

For example, in 1986 ARM published *The Vision*, a draft proposal for the future of maternity services, which proposed a radical change in the division of labour (ARM, 1986). It argued that midwives should be responsible for about 80% of normal births, that 70% of midwives should work in community-based group practices, be independent practitioners contracting services into the NHS and give continuity of care in conjunction with teams attached to consultants; and that women should have a choice in the manner of their delivery (Flint, 1986).

A year later, a RCM (1987) discussion document also proposed community-based midwifery care, including midwife-controlled beds, and recognized that there was some doubt as to the assumption that the safest place of delivery was in a consultant unit. By 1989, in a response to the White Paper *Working for Patients* (Department of Health, 1989b), ARM was proposing group practices of midwives, who would contract for services with the new purchaser health authorities, emphasizing the improved outcomes (Flint *et al.* 1989) and cost effectiveness of midwifery care, along with consumer demand for the service (ARM, 1989).

As such, these proposals could be seen as a professional strategy (Witz, 1992) because they promised increased occupational autonomy, challenged three sets of power relations in the arena of work, management and medicine, and appealed to the state to legitimate such change.

This strategy was developed by the self-proclaimed 'think tank' of the midwifery profession and then taken up by more conservative elements as part of the struggle for survival of the midwifery profession in Britain in the mid 1970s and 1980s (**Box 17.1**). The success of the ARM campaign is seen by the extent to which the government's report *Changing Childbirth* reflects its principles (Department of Health, 1993a).

Box 17.1

The Vision (ARM, 1989) as a Professional Strategy

• **By establishing direct client access** to midwives and providing continuity of care throughout pregnancy, birth and the postnatal period, midwives become established as the key professional in maternity care. This challenged the traditional hierarchical division of medical and/or midwifery labour.

• **By providing continuity of care** to all women in a geographically defined area regardless of risk categorization, midwives challenge the traditional demarcation boundaries between medicine and midwifery – both in challenging the definition of 'normal' and in demanding direct access to clients and direct referral rights to consultants of the midwives' choice.

• **By proposing that midwives set up in their own practices** and contract their labour to the new purchaser health authorities, they challenge the managerial and medical domination within the NHS.

Government Concerns

The midwifery 'professional project' may also have been successful, because it agreed with government concerns. At this time the government sought to challenge unacceptable professional power (DHSS, 1983), shift acute services into the community (Department of Health, 1989a) and emphasized the rhetoric of consumer choice (Department of Health, 1989b; Department of Health, 1991; Department of Health, 1992; Department of Health, 1994). It also coincided with the neoliberal view concerned with restricting consumer choice (Green, 1988). These concerns are all reflected in the key themes of the Changing Childbirth report (Department of Health, 1993a; Box 17.2).

Policy Background

Efficiency and cost constraints

From the early 1980s, the government was concerned to keep health costs down; one of the major ways to do this was to increase emphasis on the cost-effectiveness of care (NAO, 1990). Economic assessments in Britain (Mugford, 1990), USA (Annandale, 1989) and Canada (Romalis, 1985) were beginning to provide evidence that centralization of maternity units was not as cost-effective as previously thought.

Concerns about escalating costs and equitable resource allocation led to financial restraints by the Labour government in 1975 (DHSS, 1976). But it was only after 1979 that a shift in philosophy and a coherent ideology were applied to many areas of welfare policy; these had the elements of market mechanisms, competition, individual choice and minimal state provision (Flynn, 1989). After the Griffiths Report (DHSS, 1983), general managers were given the responsibility to ensure the efficient use of resources and from

---

Box 17.2

Key Themes in Changing Childbirth (Department of Health, 1993a)

- Consumer-led care responsive to local needs.
- Accessible and appropriate care.
- Efficient and effective care.
- Shift to community-based care.
- Provides value for money.

1984 onwards there were increasing calls for professional and managerial accountability within the NHS, accompanied by greater financial restraints.

The implementation of the NHS reforms (Department of Health, 1989b) took these earlier initiatives further. Central to this managerial revolution was the relationship between management and medicine. The freedom to incur expenditure by the medical profession was being challenged as managers sought more control over what doctors did. These elements created a climate in which it was valid for the politicians, public and media to question the effectiveness and efficiency of medical care.

Effectiveness of care

Accompanying the concern with escalating costs were doubts about the contribution that high-technology scientific medicine was making to health. For example, a report from the World Health Organization (WHO) described the adverse impact of increasing medicalization of childbirth on perinatal and maternal morbidity (WHO, 1986). Furthermore, the first systematic meta-analysis of research in the fields of reproductive medicine and maternity care was published in 1989 (Chalmers *et al.* 1989). Reviews of the evidence on safety and the place of birth suggested that planned home birth in a low-risk pregnancy had a better perinatal outcome than an equally low-risk pregnancy delivered in an obstetric unit (Tew, 1977, 1978, 1985, 1990) or at least a similar outcome (Campbell and Macfarlane, 1987).

Consumers and the cultural critique of medicine

The assumption that the increased use of technology was responsible for a decline in mortality rates had been questioned in general medicine (Mckeown, 1976), and specifically in obstetrics (Cochrane, 1971; Tew, 1977,1978; Chalmers and Richards, 1977). The early feminist literature was polemical, intentionally political (Arms, 1975; Haire, 1972) and critical of the medical model imposed on pregnancy and birth; it accused medicine of sustaining patriarchy and challenged the legitimacy of the professional's authority (Ehrenreich, 1978).

Although doubts were expressed about obstetric practice in the academic literature in the 1970s, (Richards, 1975; Oakley, 1980; Macintyre, 1977), it was the consumer organizations, such as local Community Health Councils (CHC; Robinson, 1974), the National Childbirth Trust (NCT) and the

Association for Improvements in Maternity Services (AIMS) that played a key role as activists in this debate around childbirth (Durward and Evans, 1990; Kitzinger, 1990). These were followed up by media and parliamentary interest, which resulted in the government commissioning Ann Cartwright's (1979) survey of women's experiences of maternity; this found that women were very unhappy with the way that hospitalization of birth and active management of labour dehumanized their experience.

These studies enabled women to speak for themselves. Women complained about impersonal care, lack of continuity of carer and long waiting times (Reid and McIlwaine, 1980), and about the unnecessary use of interventions and lack of explanation in labour (Cartwright, 1979; Oakley, 1980). As Chalmers (1978) pointed out, obstetricians are particularly vulnerable to lay criticism as pregnant women are less willing to adopt the sick role (McKinlay, 1972).

Winterton Report

Concern about the underuse of midwifery skills continued to be an issue in the 1990s. For example, following the National Audit Office report (NAO, 1990) and Committee of Public Accounts report (1990) on the maternity services and the strong interest of some members, such as Audrey Wise, the government ordered a review of the maternity services. The backbench Health Committee of the House of Commons (chaired by Nicholas Winterton) terms of reference were:

> To enquire into maternity services to determine the extent to which resources and professional expertise are used to achieve the most appropriate and cost-effective care of pregnant women and delivery and care of newborn babies.
>
> (House of Commons, 1992.)

After taking extensive evidence from 400 submissions for 10 months, the report highlighted three major themes:

- The need for continuity of care.
- The desire for women to have more choice.
- The right for women to have control over their own bodies at all stages of pregnancy and birth.

(House of Commons, 1992, p. xiii, para 38.)

Where previous inquiries tended to focus on mortality [i.e. The Short Report (Social Services Committee, 1980)], this time the Health Committee stressed that central to the inquiry was the management of normal pregnancy and birth. Thus it supported a move from medicalized birth and fragmented care to a woman-centred approach with an emphasis on increased choice

and control. It was felt that continuity of carer, primarily in midwifery-led settings, would be the best way to achieve this. It drew attention to the changes required in the roles and responsibilities of midwives and doctors. It also finally drew attention to the importance of the social context of pregnancy and birth, particularly the impact of poverty, and expressed concern over inadequate maternity benefits and maternity leave for working women. The broad principles of the recommendations are summarized in **Box 17.3**.

These recommendations, announced in March

Box 17.3

Main Recommendations of the Winterton Report

- That the relationship between the woman and her caregivers is recognized as being of fundamental importance.
- That schemes should be set up enabling women to get to know one or two health professionals during pregnancy who will be with them during labour and delivery, whether at home or in hospital, and who will continue the care of the mother and baby after birth.
- That the majority of maternity care should be community based and near to the woman's home; and that obstetric and other specialist care should be readily available by referral from midwives or GPs.
- That those GPs who wish to provide a continuum of care throughout pregnancy, labour and the puerperium should be able to do so; and that their training should equip them to do so.
- That women needing intensive obstetric care within the NHS should also be able to enjoy continuity of care and carer, so far as is possible.
- That within a hospital environment women should be able to exercise choice as to the personnel who will be responsible for their care.
- That the woman having a baby should be seen as the focus of care; and that the professionals providing that care should identify their needs and develop arrangements to meet them which are based on full and equal co-operation between all those charged with her care.
- That proper attention should be paid to the needs of the baby, with particular regard to skilled resuscitation at birth, examination for abnormalities and the encouragement of breastfeeding.

House of Commons Health Committee 1992. Maternity Services, para 384, chaired by Sir Nicolas Winterton, HMSO.

1992, were seen as a milestone in maternity policy by consumer groups and midwives in particular. For the first time an independent committee at national level had focused on whether women were receiving the kind of service they wanted.

The Government Response to the House of Commons Report

In response to the Health Committee report, the Government established a departmental task force to address wider issues in the organization of care (Department of Health, 1992), which set up, for example, a national study of team midwifery (Wraight *et al.* 1993) and of midwifery-led and GP-led units (Department of Health, 1993b). The survey of midwifery-led and GP-led units found 100 units in England, either community-based stand-alone units or within a district general hospital. The report expressed preference for units to be sited within a hospital. It was recognized that midwives who worked in these units needed regular updating in skills such as neonatal resuscitation, siting intravenous drips and ventouse delivery.

It was recognized that the policy of care during childbirth needed review and a Clinical Standards Advisory Group was set up to give advice on the care of women in normal labour. The Clinical Standards Advisory Group reported in 1995 on a survey of clinical guidelines in a sample of hospitals in Great Britain. They also conducted a prospective study of 5000 'low-risk' births in primigravidae. The findings confirmed the high intervention rates in normal labour, particularly the high episiotomy rate (46%), and concern was expressed over the significant regional variations of interventions in labour.

Finally an Expert Maternity Group was established to 'review policy on NHS maternity care, particularly during childbirth and to make recommendations. The group was chaired by Lady Cumberlege, Parliamentary Under-Secretary of State for Health, and its members consisted of midwives, obstetricians, GPs, paediatricians and lay representatives.

Cumberlege Report

The report of the Expert Maternity Group, *Changing Childbirth* (Department of Health, 1993a) laid out three key principles of maternity care. Whereas the Winterton Report (House of Commons, 1992) provided a highly detailed overview and philosophical framework for the future of maternity services, the Cumberlege Report was an action document for change.

The fundamental principle that underpins all the proposals in *Changing Childbirth* is that the woman and her baby are at the centre of all planning and provision of maternity care. It identifies three principles that should be the foundation for a woman centred service (**Box 17.4**).

This was initially reduced to a consultative paper until January 1994, when the NHS Management Executive (NHSME, 1994) told all regions, districts and trusts to review their maternity services and develop a strategy to implement the recommendations (**Box 17.5**), which would be evaluated by their progress within the next 5 years towards the 10 key indicators of success outlined in the report (**Box 17.6**).

Changing Childbirth was welcomed by midwives, consumer groups and the National Association of Health Authorities and Trusts (NAHAT, 1993). But the responses made by the Royal College of Obstetricians and Gynaecologists (RCOG) focused on two areas of disagreement. The concept of the lead professional, which implied the exclusion of the obstetrician from normal pregnancy, and the assertion that home confinement is a safe alternative to hospital (RCOG, 1993).

The report endorsed the value of continuity of carer and stipulated a greater role for midwives in proposing that women with uncomplicated pregnancies should be offered complete antenatal, intrapartum and postnatal care from a small group of midwives, with referral to obstetricians when necessary. It also confirmed that there is no clear evidence that home birth is less safe

---

Box 17.4

Key Principles of Good Maternity Care

• **That the woman must be the focus of maternity care.** She should be able to feel that she is in control of what is happening to her and able to make decisions about her care, based on her needs, having discussed matters fully with the professionals involved.

• **Maternity services should be readily and easily accessible to all.** They should be sensitive to the needs of the local population and based primarily in the community.

• **Women should be involved in the monitoring and planning** to ensure that they are responsive to the needs of a changing society. In addition care should be effective and resources used efficiently.

Department of Health: Changing Childbirth, London, 8:1993a, HMSO.

Box 17.5

Changing Childbirth Recommendations

• Women should be fully involved when decisions are made about their care. They should have a choice regarding the professional who will lead their care and should, if they wish, carry their own case notes. They should be kept fully informed on matters relating to their care (Department of Health, 1993a, p. 13).

• Every woman should have the name of a midwife who works locally, is known to her and whom she can contact for advice. She should also know the name of the lead professional who is responsible for planning and monitoring her care. Within 5 years, 75% of women should be cared for in labour by a midwife whom they have come to know during pregnancy (Department of Health, 1993a, p. 17).

• A woman with an uncomplicated pregnancy should, if she wishes, be able to book with a midwife as the lead professional for the entire episode of care including delivery in a general hospital (Department of Health, 1993a, p. 18).

• Antenatal care should be provided so as to maximize the use of resources. It should also ensure that the woman and her partner feel supported and fully informed throughout the pregnancy, and are prepared for the birth and the care of their baby (Department of Health, 1993a, p. 22).

• Women should receive clear, unbiased advice and be able to choose where they would like their babies to be born. Their right to make that choice should be respected and every practical effort made to achieve the outcome that the woman believes is best for her baby and herself (Department of Health, 1993a, p. 25).

• When emergency services are required by the woman or her baby at or around the time of birth they should be of the highest standard that can be achieved in the circumstances (Department of Health, 1993a, p. 28).

• Women should have the opportunity to discuss their plans for labour and birth. Their decisions should be recorded in their birth plans and incorporated into their case notes. Every reasonable effort should be made to accommodate the wishes of the woman and her partner, and to inform them of the services that are available to them (Department of Health, 1993a, p. 31).

• A woman who gives birth in hospital should be able to return home, as far as is practicable, when she feels ready. Once home, she should be supported by her midwife, knowing that the GP is available if medical advice is necessary. The pattern of support should be appropriate to the woman's needs and planned in consultation with her (Department of Health, 1993a, p. 34).

• GPs who wish to provide maternity care should receive appropriate training and encouragement to do so. Midwives and GPs should work in partnership in the best interests of the woman (Department of Health, 1993a, p. 37).

• The part which the midwife plays in maternity care should make full use of all her skills and knowledge, and reflect the full role for which she has been trained (Department of Health, 1993a, p. 39).

• The knowledge and skills of the obstetrician should be used primarily to provide advice, support and expertise for those women who have complicated pregnancies (Department of Health, 1993a, p. 41).

• The role and training of senior house officers working in obstetrics should be designed primarily to equip them with the skills and knowledge that they will require in order either to provide a full range of maternity services working as GPs, or to continue their education and training to become obstetricians (Department of Health, 1993a, p. 43).

• Users of maternity services should be actively involved in planning and reviewing services. The lay representation must reflect the ethnic, cultural and social mix of the local population. A maternity services liaison committee should be established within every district health authority (Department of Health, 1993a, p. 47).

• Information about maternity services should be provided in a form appropriate and accessible to women (Department of Health, 1993a, p. 49).

• Regular monitoring of the uptake of services should take place to identify those women who are least likely to seek care and use the service to their full advantage. A strategy should then be developed to ensure that services are accessible to those women (Department of Health, 1993a, p. 52).

• Women with disabilities should have full access to services and have confidence that their needs are fully understood (Department of Health, 1993a, p. 54).

• All women should have the opportunity to be fully involved with their care (Department of Health, 1993a, p. 56).

• Staff should have received training to enable them to support all women with different needs so that they can use the service to maximum advantage (Department of Health, 1993a, p. 58).

• Within a period of 5 years providers should be able to demonstrate a significant shift towards a more community-oriented service (Department of Health, 1993a, p. 60).

• The views of women who use the service should be regularly monitored and services adjusted to reflect their needs (Department of Health, 1993a, p. 62).

• Clinical practice should be based on sound evidence and be subject to regular clinical audit (Department of Health, 1993a, p. 64).

• New patterns of service should be designed to allow evaluation of both their effectiveness and their acceptability to women using the service (Department of Health, 1993a, p. 65).

• The service provided must represent value for money and the cost and benefits of alternative arrangements assessed locally (Department of Health, 1993a, p. 67).

Department of Health: Changing Childbirth, London, 1993a, HMSO.

Box 17.6

Ten Key Indicators of Success

(1) All women should be entitled to carry their own notes.

(2) Every woman should know one midwife who ensures continuity of her midwifery care – the named midwife.

(3) At least 30% of women should have the midwife as the lead professional.

(4) Every woman should know the lead professional who has a key role in the planning and provision of her care.

(5) At least 75% of women should know the person who cares for them during their delivery.

(6) Midwives should have direct access to some beds in all maternity units.

(7) At least 30% of women delivered in a maternity unit should be admitted under the management of the midwife.

(8) The total number of antenatal visits for women with uncomplicated pregnancies should have been reviewed in the light of available evidence and RCOG guidelines.

(9) All front-line ambulances should have a paramedic able to support the midwife who needs to transfer women to hospital in an emergency.

(10) All women should have access to information about the services available in their locality.

Department of Health: Changing Childbirth, London, 70:1993a, HMSO.

than hospital for women with uncomplicated pregnancies (Department of Health, 1993a, p. 23).

Both the Short Report and *Changing Childbirth* acknowledged the evidence, but did not take any action concerning the wider socioeconomic context of childbirth. For example, the Short Report recognized the association between poverty and an increased perinatal mortality rate (Social Services Committee, 1980, p. 158) and assumed that obstetric intervention could compensate for adverse social circumstances (Russell, 1982). Although the Winterton Committee had expressed concern about the financial needs of parents living in poverty and made recommendations about benefit levels (House of Commons, 1992, paras 121–51), while acknowledging the effects of poor nutrition and poverty, the Cumberlege Report had no remit outside NHS care and contained an assumption that social support and increased choice and control on the part of women may partly compensate for poverty (Streetly, 1994).

In December 1994 a survey of the eight regional health authorities in England showed progress towards

the indicators of success as illustrated in **Figure 17.1**. By July 1995, almost £1.5 million had been awarded to 38 new initiatives, but the most difficult areas to change have been those that involve a shift in roles and responsibilities of the professionals and those to achieve continuity of carer.

Figure 17.1 shows that there are two areas that have the lowest levels of achievement (ENB, 1995, pp. 21–2). The first is in shifting responsibility from doctors to midwives, where the best region achieves 28% for the target of 30% of women who see a midwife as the lead professional (20% nationally). The second is in providing intrapartum continuity of care, where the best region achieves 26% for the target of 75% of women knowing the person caring for them at delivery (15% nationally). The low level of achievement in these areas is demonstrated by the work of Henderson (1997) in the West Midlands. However, the data from her research regarding progress towards the indicators actually demonstrate a worrying regression in most areas (**Figure 17.2**) when compared with the ENB West Midlands data of 1994. Possible reasons are highlighted by Henderson, but it must be remembered that these indicators, like other NHS performance indicators, are also open to misinterpretation.

Continuity of Care

The literature on the maternity services contains a recurrent theme of the need to have a more 'humanized service'. As early as the 1960s there was enough concern to issue a policy statement called 'Human Relations in Obstetrics' (Ministry of Health, 1961). The distress caused to a woman by seeing as many as 20 different professionals during her pregnancy and meeting a stranger for the birth has been documented by lay and professional groups through the 1980s (Kitzinger, 1981; Boyd and Sellars, 1982; RCOG, 1982; Parents, 1986; RCM, 1991a).

Continuity of care by the midwife was seen as a desirable 'ideal' way to overcome these problems, but as being too difficult to achieve in practice (Social Services Committee, 1980, para 292). The Maternity Services Advisory Committee (1982, para 1.10) went further and recommended the use of midwives in a more independent capacity, and were aware of the 'numerous consumer complaints about the so-called impersonal nature of care in hospitals, where maternity services are now concentrated.'

Continuity of care was conceptualized by women

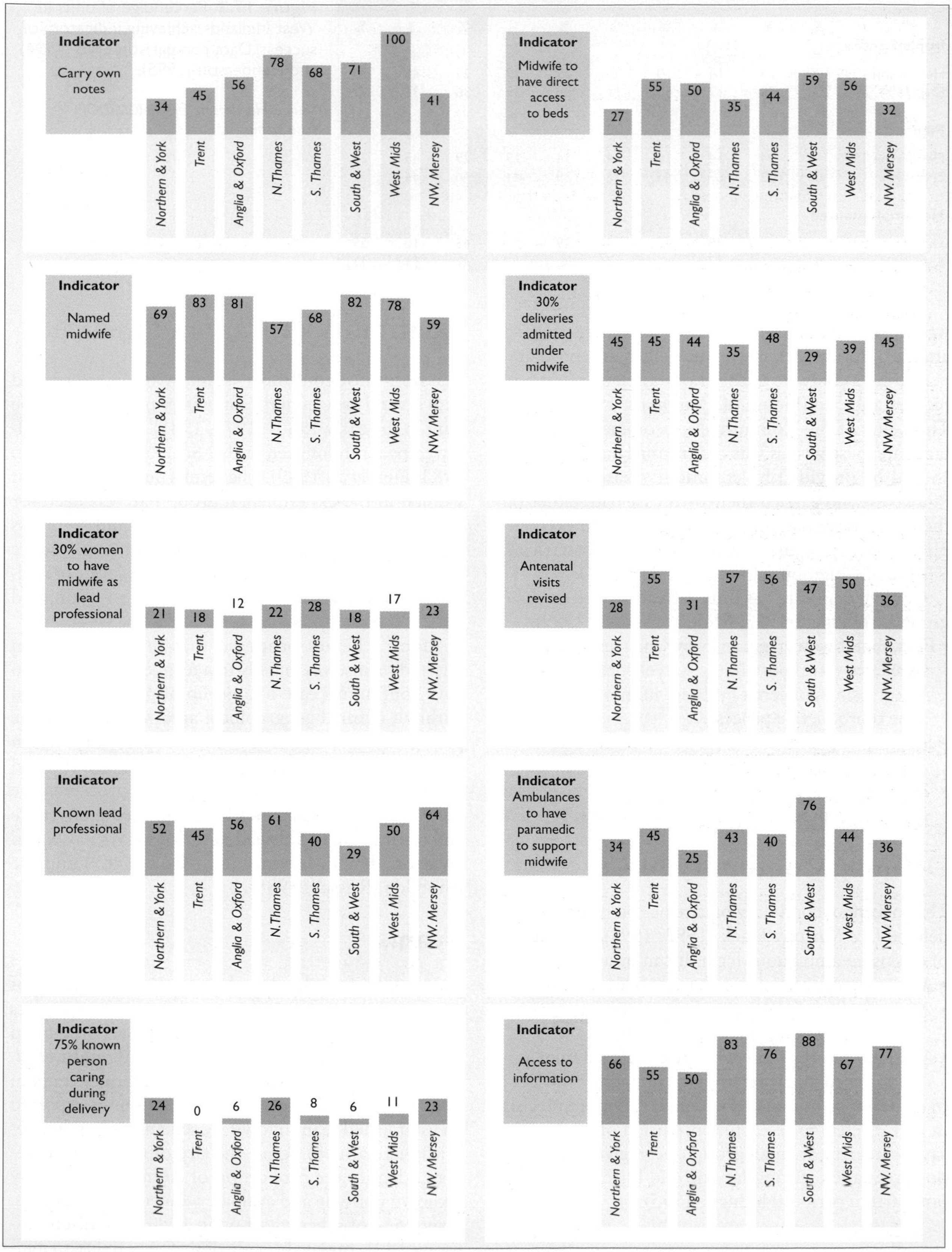

Figure 17.1 Percentage of maternity services within each region that meet the criteria set within the indicators of success as at December 1994. From NAHAT Briefing No. 92 (ENB, 1995).

Indicator	1	2	3	4	5	6	7	8	9	10
	%	%	%	%	%	%	%	%	%	%
Implemented										
Henderson 1995	100	24	14	10	0	19	29	29	48	33
ENB 1994	100	78	17	50	11	56	39	36	36	77
Planned										
Henderson 1995	–	14	14	10	24	14	19	29	43	29
ENB 1994	0	22	67	44	72	39	44	44	44	22
Not Implemented										
Henderson 1995	–	–	48	48	33	29	24	43	10	29
ENB 1994	0	0	17	6	17	6	17	6	11	11

Figure 17.2 Percentage of units in West Midlands achieving indicators of success. Data comparison ENB (1994) and Henderson (1995).

Source: Henderson, 1997, RCM/DOH scholarship.

who gave evidence to the Health Committee as being attended during their pregnancy, birth and postnatal period by a midwife with whom a relationship had been established (House of Commons, 1992, p. xiii). Thus, one of the Committee's recommendations to facilitate these wishes was that routine maternity care should be provided by community-based teams of midwives who carried their own caseload, either on their own responsibility when women had no complications, or in association with an obstetrician (House of Commons, 1992, para 219, 344).

Continuity of care has thus been advocated on three grounds (Hodnett, 1995; Middlemiss *et al.* 1989):
- First, that if women get to know and trust a few staff well, they are more likely to feel confident about expressing concerns and feel in more control of the reproductive process.
- Second, midwives are more likely to provide more sensitive care.
- Third, there is some evidence to suggest beneficial effects on pregnancy and birth outcome.

Defining Continuity of Care

The concept of continuity of care has been very poorly defined (*see* Murphy Black, 1992, 1993). Continuity of care is an ambiguous term. It can mean:
- A stated commitment to a shared philosophy of care.
- A strict adherence to a common protocol for care during pregnancy and/or childbirth.
- A system whereby those who are discharged from hospital are routinely referred to community services.

In contrast, 'continuity of caregivers' is more precise, in that it refers to the actual provision of care by the same caregiver or small group of caregivers throughout pregnancy, during labour and birth, and in the postpartum period (Hodnett, 1995).

Continuity of Care in Practice

The notion of continuity of midwifery care started with several articles in the midwifery press by Caroline Flint in the early 1980s (1979, 1981). These were followed by a randomized trial at St Georges Hospital in 1983 (Flint *et al.* 1989). The results demonstrated that women in the experimental group had less need for analgesia or oxytocin, shorter labours and were less likely to have a baby with a 5-minute Apgar score below 8. The study also reported greater levels of midwife and maternal satisfaction and an estimated 20–25% reduction in cost.

Many schemes proposed that pregnant women referred themselves initially to a team of midwives who gave continuous care to a group of pregnant women within a defined geographical area regardless of the pregnancy outcome. The midwives give total care on their own responsibility if the woman is healthy and in association with an obstetrician if problems are identified. These schemes had high media coverage and teams were established in various ways in Oxford (Watson, 1990), Bloomsbury (Kroll, 1989) and the Rhondda (Russell, 1988).

Teams

Team midwifery developed to increase continuity of carer and the current pattern of maternity care has been mapped by the Institute of Manpower Studies on behalf of the Department of Health (Wraight *et al.* 1993). This national survey of all maternity units in England and Wales found that 37% of units reported an established team midwifery scheme, but only one-third were able to define the size of their team caseload, identify the proportion of women delivered by a known midwife and evaluate women's views of care. Over 25% of schemes set up in 1990 were discontinued in 1991, mainly because of unacceptability to midwives, failure to increase continuity of care and inadequate staffing. Three models were identified in the survey:

- Hospital teams.
- Community teams.
- Combined hospital and community teams.

There was insufficient data to estimate the comparative costs of each model.

In the absence of an agreed definition of team midwifery the report listed five key indicators for the 'genuine' teams, which they defined as:

- No more than six midwives in a team.
- Defined caseload.
- Total continuity from booking to postnatal period.
- Midwives working in hospital and community depending on the woman's needs.
- At least 50% of women delivered by a known midwife.

Wraight *et al.* (1993) found only 14 teams that fulfilled these criteria, all based in the community; their findings confirmed Watson's (1990) earlier study of team midwifery in Oxford – that the reality of continuity of care is much more difficult to achieve than by simply reorganizing midwives into teams.

Apart from the difficulties of implementing new ways of working in the way that was intended, there is limited evidence as to what continuity of care means in practice to midwives and women (Lee, 1994) and some evidence that continuity does not automatically equate with good-quality care (Reid and Garcia, 1989).

A woman's experience of team continuity may vary significantly from 'getting care from known caregivers at crucial times' (Garcia, 1995, p. 96). Garcia's review of the evidence concerning women's views of continuity indicates that although continuity of care matters to most women, its importance depends how the question is asked – to focus on continuity may neglect other aspects of care that are equally important.

Caseloads and Group Practices

Caseload midwifery has been defined in an NCT policy statement (Hutton, 1995) as the way forward to achieve real continuity of carer. When a midwife carries a caseload she is the primary provider of care during pregnancy, birth and the early postnatal period for an agreed number of women. For most full-time midwives this would be 35–40 women per year. She provides care whether the women are in the community or hospital and refers to the appropriate colleagues and social agencies. Each midwife has a reciprocal arrangement with a partner to ensure holiday and sickness cover and her partner meets all the women on her list. Midwives who carry a caseload may form a group

practice to provide support and peer review (*see* Flint, 1993; Page, 1995). So far there has not been a complete evaluation of caseload midwifery or group practices, although interim evaluations suggest higher levels of continuity of care and maternal satisfaction are achieved and marginally lower intervention rates (Centre for Midwifery Practice, 1995).

Implications for Doctors

From reading the literature on professions, one would expect a certain amount of opposition to midwives reasserting their control over the birth process; indeed, the proposals for continuity of care schemes have been seen as a threat to the 'obstetric team' (Howie, 1987). The initial response of the medical profession to the *Changing Childbirth* recommendations was a perceived threat to obstetric demarcation boundaries and contained a justifiable critique of the inadequate research evidence to justify radical change (Dunlop, 1993). The result was an overemphasis on the safety of home birth (RCOG, 1993) and debates about the respective roles, responsibilities and competencies of midwives and obstetricians. For others, there was a recognition that choice and safety were not mutually exclusive (Anderson, 1993) and they supported the new policy on the grounds of rationality, expediency and cost effectiveness. As in 1902, there were simply not enough doctors to provide care to all women (Lilford, 1993).

Debate about the respective roles of midwives and medical staff is not a new phenomenon – much discussion of maternity care in the twentieth century has focused on this issue. There is no dispute that obstetricians should be responsible for the care of women with complications, but there has been a lack of clarity as to where 'normal and abnormal' boundaries are drawn, with a tendency to regard the process as a trajectory with pathological potential (see Kitzinger, 1990, p. 152). Similarly, there is an even greater lack of clarity and more duplication between GP's and midwives' roles (Robinson, 1985).

The relations between doctors and midwives have traditionally been highly charged and antagonistic (Donnison, 1988). There has been a contested sphere of each occupation's legitimate area of concern and many disputes crystallize around the normal–abnormal boundary, with each occupation constructing competing models of birth. One assumes birth is a normal physiological process unless proved otherwise and the other assumes every birth is potentially abnormal until over. This is in the context of the obstetric profession having altered its perspective on its role in childbirth during the twentieth century from it being an art to a science (Cartwright, 1979; Oakley, 1984a; Arney, 1988). As a result, Schwarz (1990, p. 57) argued that 'the active management of childbirth by consultant obstetricians led to a redistribution of interprofessional responsibilities.'

The early studies of midwife–obstetrician relations in Britain found that, although midwives made a claim to be practitioners in their own right, this was rarely recognized in practice. Walker (1976) found that midwives strongly held the view that they must work as a team, since the woman's needs were paramount. As a result midwives, like nurses (Stein, 1967) developed strategies to avoid overt conflict, which Green *et al.* (1986) called 'hierarchy maintenance work'.

Green *et al.* (1986) found that increasing interpersonal contact between midwives and consultants (by replacing the three-tier structure of consultant, registrar and senior house officer with a two-tier system of senior house officer and consultant), resulted in greater midwife autonomy, and in better relationships with the consultants, but 'the power of the consultants to determine the details of the labour ward working means that their attitudes are crucial.' Annandale (1987) also found that midwives working in an American free-standing birth centre (which had an explicit philosophy of patient control and natural childbirth) were still constrained by the obstetric policies and protocols of the back-up hospital. Thus, consultant obstetrician support for innovations in maternity care still appears to be an essential element for a successful programme.

The boundaries that have traditionally marked medicine and midwifery are breaking down in response to the 'new deal' in junior doctors hours (NHSME, 1991), the increased specialization of care and changes in medical education (COPMED, 1995; GMC, 1993; Department of Health, 1993c). The initial response of most hospitals to staffing shortfalls has been to identify particular tasks that can be delegated to midwives from junior doctors; for example, perineal suturing, intravenous cannulation and examination of the neonate (Audit Commission, 1995). Harvey (1995) argues that as a result of this 'upskilling', midwives' work has been intensified for no increase in remuneration or social prestige, as well as increasing the possibility of more childbirth interventions (Rothman, 1982). Whether 'upskilling' results in greater midwifery autonomy depends upon existing power relations in the workplace.

General Practitioners

There has been a long history of economic competition between midwives and GPs for their patients (Dingwall *et al.* 1988). The GP's role in maternity care has declined throughout the twentieth century. In 1927, 85% of deliveries were under the care of the GP, which has fallen to less than 6% in England and Wales in 1988 (Smith, 1990). The participation by the GP at the time of birth continues to decline and many feel their skills are limited and would support the midwife as the key professional present at 72% of births (Flint, 1990). Those GPs actively involved in intrapartum care have sought an alliance with midwives to form pressure groups, but not without acrimony on both sides (*Midwifery Matters*, 1990).

Thus, it seems that political and economic circumstances have combined to shift the roles and relationships of professionals involved in maternity care to give midwives more responsibility and autonomy; taken together these changes have far-reaching implications for the delivery of care.

Implications for Midwives and Midwifery Practice

It is important to remember that the concept of 'professional' carries an ideological load' (Salvage, 1988) – within midwifery the concept of professionalism is popular and has informed strategic thinking. It has also been assumed that professionalization is a desirable goal, but this may not be so. Thus, for Salvage professionalism is as much about 'pursuing the narrow interests of a particular group as it is about improving health care' (Salvage, 1988, p. 100). Oakley (1984b) too has argued that the current obsession for professional status may be counterproductive at a time when there is a lack of public confidence in the professions in general. Noting the increasing assertiveness by 'consumers' of health care, she suggests that an alliance with women would be more fruitful in gaining occupational and consumer satisfaction, especially as the importance of social and emotional support to maintain health is being formally recognized (Oakley *et al.* 1990).

Lastly, one of the major effects that the pursuit of professional status has had is to reinforce existing gender and class divisions within an occupation. As Abel

Smith (1960) suggested, the search for professional status by the 'lady' midwives in the 1900s was more an expression of antipathy to those recruited from the working class. Historical evidence suggests that one result of the professionalization process in midwifery (Heagerty, 1990; Leap and Hunter, 1993; Sandall, 1995) has been an increase in divisions along the lines of race (King Edward's Hospital Fund for Nursing, 1990), class (Carpenter, 1993; Robinson, 1992) and domestic commitments (Robinson, 1993).

This antipathy has continued towards midwives who either cannot pursue full-time work (because of children) or who operate outside the norms of practice independently; for example, the disciplinary control of independent midwives (Drife, 1988; Demilew, 1989; UKCC, 1988), including the withdrawal of their practice insurance by the RCM (Van de Kooy *et al.* 1996), the discrimination against women with children who attempt to train as midwives (Braun, 1990), the downgrading of midwives who return to work part-time (Sandall, 1990) and the reluctance to implement job sharing (McDowall, 1990).

The exclusion of women with domestic commitments generally has been legitimized by the perception that such women have a less than full-time commitment to their work (Lorber, 1985) and replicates findings from other studies of women in the NHS (Davies and Rosser, 1986; Mackay, 1989; Equal Opportunities Commission, 1991). But professional strategies have always relied on the single woman's or man's career path – this emphasis has disadvantaged those women who cannot pursue a full-time career (Davies, 1990).

This notion of gendered jobs and gendered organizations was explored by Acker (1990, p. 179) who argues that 'the concept of a job assumes a particular gendered organization of domestic life and social production.' Thus, the gendered notion of a job is modelled on the full-time male career pathway. Female career pathways that require career breaks and part-time work are seen as a nuisance and disadvantage (Davies, 1995) and the associated benefits rarely recognized (Warwick, 1995).

Providing continuity of carer requires a radical change in the way that many midwives work, in terms of increased flexibility and the impact of regular on-call work on midwives' personal lives (Jackson, 1995). For midwives who are setting up continuity of carer schemes, the issue of job sharing presents contradictions in a work organization pattern that may require flexible shifts, being on-call and full-time commitment. Of all midwives, 53% are estimated to have dependent children (Buchan and Stock, 1990) and the number of midwives who work part-time has increased in the past 5 years to approximately 44% in 1993 (Department of Health, 1995).

This issue is of particular importance to an occupation in which many of the carers, having experienced birth and childrearing themselves, could potentially have much to bring to their work. A recent case study of midwives who work in teams and group practices found that midwives who carry their own caseload find it easier than midwives who work in teams to combine a family life with providing continuity of care. The midwives who worked part-time simply carried a smaller caseload. Caseload midwives had more control over how they organized their working day and found it far easier to negotiate appointment times with the women in their caseload than when covering a team caseload (Sandall, 1996).

Robinson's longitudinal study of midwives' careers (Robinson, 1993; Robinson and Owen, 1994) suggests the possibility that midwives with domestic responsibilities may be excluded from the potentially higher status and higher paid work. A recent national survey of midwifery found inconsistencies in the grading of salary scales and the development of two tiers of midwives, those who could work flexibly and those who were limited to shifts and part-time work (Stock and Wraight, 1993; Lewis, 1995). How can you reconcile the provision of equal opportunities for midwives to work part-time or job share with the provision of continuity of care?

Burnout

There is a suggestion that providing continuity of care results in increased autonomy that improves job satisfaction (Shoham and Carmel, 1989; Robinson and Owen, 1994; Hundley *et al.* 1995). But there is also evidence of increased stress in midwifery generally (Carlisle *et al.* 1994). Stock and Wraight (1993) found that midwives were trading off increased autonomy and job satisfaction with greater intrusion into their personal lives and increased demands for flexible work hours. Some evaluations of team midwifery have confirmed that some midwives felt 'burnt out' by the stressful on-calls, poor sick cover and interprofessional conflict (Watson, 1990); there has been concern that the introduction of new models of midwifery care may drain midwives (Currell, 1990).

For example, although midwives working in a midwife-led unit reported increased satisfaction with work, they felt that they would not be able to sustain the work rota in the long term (Turnbull *et al.* 1995).

Some of these midwives shared the characteristics identified in a survey of American midwives who suffered 'burn out' – of being young and qualifying in the previous 5 years (Beaver *et al*. 1986). On the other hand, one of the most important factors in increasing job accomplishment and reducing the risk of burnout is to have a personal caseload rather than a team caseload. This is because one of the main sources of job satisfaction is to provide continuity of care to women. Midwives who work with a team caseload find their work very fragmented and as a result frustrating, as they rarely saw 'women' through their pregnancy to birth and the postnatal period (Sandall, 1996; Brodie, 1996).

Implications for Women's Choice and Control

Sociologists have used the medical-dominance viewpoint to explain the hospitalization of birth and active management of labour (Cartwright, 1979; Tew, 1990), which resulted in the loss of control by and alienation of women. Thus, there was a focus in sociological research on the notion that women and obstetricians have 'competing ideologies of reproduction', where women see pregnancy and birth as a normal process over which they should exert active control and in which medical intervention should only occur in exceptional circumstances, and where obstetricians see it as a potentially pathological event to be controlled and managed (Comoroff, 1977; Graham and Oakley, 1981; Nash and Nash, 1979).

There are theoretical and methodological difficulties in researching consumer views of medical care, as Locker and Dunt (1978) have identified. Reid and Garcia (1989, p. 137) and Mason (1990) discuss the specific difficulties of obtaining women's views at the time of birth. These views also change over time; the answers given depend on where the women are being questioned, by whom and the form of question. Interpretations of reported satisfaction are also difficult to analyse, as alternatives are difficult to envisage and service users tend to prefer the familiar (Porter and Macintyre, 1984).

A prospective study of 825 women (Green *et al*. 1990) found that what was important to women was to feel in control – the more interventions a woman had, the less in control she felt, but only when she believed they were unnecessary. The MORI poll reported in *Changing Childbirth* stated that 72% of women would like the option of a different type of care, 22% said they would like a home birth and 44% said they would like a midwife-led domino delivery (Department of Health, 1993a, p. 23).

The conclusion to be drawn is that women have different views depending on their level of education, class, and race (which is only just beginning to be explored; *see* Phoenix, 1990). One theme that does appear to come through consistently from all the studies of consumer views is the lack of information, explanation and communication, bearing out a conclusion of Cartwright's that 'working-class women, like middle-class ones, want to be informed, but they are less successful in obtaining information (Cartwright, 1979, p. 115; *see also* Jacoby, 1988, for a more detailed study).

Since the early 1970s concern has been expressed about shortcomings in the nature of consultations concerned with reproduction (Doyal and Pennell, 1979). Shapiro *et al*. (1983) found women did not receive all the information they wanted from their obstetrician, yet there was an absence of conflict and a high level of satisfaction. It is suggested that the encounter is subtlety manipulated by the obstetricians in a way that keeps issues off the agenda and women 'unaware that their interests have been set aside' (Shapiro *et al*. 1983, p. 145).

Sociological research in obstetrics has attributed much of women's passivity and inability to take an active role in decision making because high-status male providers control the information flow and structure the physical encounter (Oakley, 1980; Comoroff, 1977). Thus Annandale (1987) hypothesized that female midwives would enable women to be more in control of their birth. But in reality the need to emphasize normality to prevent events transgressing obstetric norms tended to motivate midwives' practice behaviour and inhibit women from raising anxieties about complications, resulting in them not being consulted about decisions made during labour. As Kirkham (1987) concluded, one of the reasons midwives fail to provide women with information during labour is that they themselves are unhappy with the policies that they are required to implement in the management of care.

It has been assumed that because midwifery is a female-dominated occupation, midwives will guard the rights and interests of women and give a more holistic, empathetic and egalitarian style of care, which will thus ensure choice and control for women (Page, 1993; House of Commons, 1992). But this assumption needs to be critically examined as there is little evidence to support it. Lorber (1985) found that external structural factors influence professional behaviour regardless of gender and others have highlighted how organizational factors can curtail or enhance the giving of woman-centred care by midwives (Annandale, 1987; Kirkham, 1987; Green *et al.* 1986).

In thinking about midwifery it is important to recognize that at least three different types of interests are at stake:

• The interests of midwives as people.
• The interests of midwifery as a profession.
• The interests of midwifery as a service (interested in the health and well-being of mothers and babies).

It is often assumed that an improvement in one will bring about improvement in the others, but this is often not true – De Vries (1993) demonstrates how the interests of midwives can be directly opposed to those of women. As Freidson (1970) wrote in relation to the medical profession, the motive of professionalization as an explanation of changes in health care should not be underrated.

For example, Benoit's (1994) study of Canadian midwives argued that although midwives shared gender status with women, they had to contend with the dilemma of balancing professional self-interest with the concerns of women. Furthermore, evidence from the Netherlands suggests that Dutch midwives face similar problems in combining a private life with a job that requires total dedication and continuous availability (Benoit, 1991). Indeed, midwifery could be characterized as a 'greedy profession', i.e. where great commitment, loyalty, time and energy are required (Coser, 1974; Segal, 1986), but where the rewards are great.

The issue of whose interests are served is explored further in relation to nursing by Oakley (1984b) and Salvage (1988), who both suggest that the struggle to achieve professional status (in terms of a male-dominated paradigm as a professional model) may reproduce the unequal power relationship that already exists between the medical profession and many patients. Oakley suggests that a feminist-inspired model of partnership with users of services [as in *Changing Childbirth* (Department of Health, 1993a)] is the way forward and both Stacey (1992, p. 257) and Davies (1995) elaborate on what a client-centred paradigm of professional partnership and practice may begin to look like, such as:

• A profession with an independent voice th... advocate on behalf of its clients.
• Greater lay involvement in midwifery education and regulation of practice.
• Sharing knowledge with women and their families and acknowledging the special skills that other groups have to offer.
• Relationships of greater equality with women, both at an individual level and at an organizational level.
• A profession that prioritizes equal opportunities for midwives who wish to job share or work part-time.
• A profession that acknowledges the needs of all midwives in establishing sensible working hours and practices.

Summary

The ideology of continuity of care reasserts control over the heart (in a metaphorical sense too) of the practice of midwifery. Thus, midwives claim a discrete sphere of knowledge and expertise, legitimized by a desire for a more equal partnership with women in an area where medical care has been criticized. Current attempts to develop professional status are dependent on state mandate, funding and political expediency (Declerq, 1994). The interest shown by the British government in the cost-effectiveness of midwife care and the alliance that midwives have forged with consumers may well enable this particular professional project to be successful.

However, midwives need to remember that what a woman very often wants is a trusting supportive relationship with one or two midwives who will be with her through her pregnancy, birth and the postnatal period, who will support her, be her advocate 'within the system' and enable her to be more assertive in making sure her needs are met (Gready *et al.* 1995). There is a danger that a profession aiming to increase its autonomy and sphere of practice may lose sight of the ideology of continuity of care. Midwives should be aware of the implications for themselves individually and for the women they care for in pursuing this particular path. What needs to be remembered is that neither midwives nor women are homogeneous groups about whom generalizations can be made. So does this new way of organizing care empower midwives, women, both or neither?

KEY CONCEPTS

- To understand current and future developments in maternity policy, it is important to be aware of the historical context.

- Policy-making is not based on the weight of the evidence available, but is often influenced by political considerations and pressure groups.

- Historically, the organization and delivery of maternity care has affected the autonomy of midwifery practice.

- The attempts by midwives to regain their role, culminating in *Changing Childbirth*, can be seen as a new midwifery professional project.

- This project has been successful because it is a partnership between women and midwives that fits in with various interests of the state.

- This process of professionalization can have costs for midwives as individuals and may not be in women's best interests.

- The empowerment of midwives does not necessarily result in increased choice and control for women.

References

Abel Smith B: *A history of the nursing profession*, London, 1960, Heinemann.

Acker J: Hierarchies, jobs, bodies: A theory of gendered organisations, *Gender Soc* 4(2):139, 1990.

Anderson M: *Changing Childbirth*, commentary 1, *Br J Obstet Gynaecol* 100:1071, 1993.

Annandale EC: Dimensions of patient control in a free standing birth centre, *Soc Sci Med* 25(11):1235, 1987.

Annandale EC: The malpractice crisis and the doctor–patient relationship, *Soc Health Illness* 11(1):1, 1989.

ARM: *The vision – Proposals for the future of the maternity services*, Ormskirk, 1986, ARM.

ARM: Working for mothers and babies, *ARM Magazine*, 42, 1989.

Arms, S 1975 Immaculate Deception, Bantam Books, New York.

Arney WR: *Power and the profession of obstetrics*, London, 1982, University of Chicago Press.

Ashton R: Interview, *Midwife, Health Visitor, Community Nurse* 23(17):292, 1987.

Audit Commission: *The doctors tale: the work of hospital doctors in England and Wales*, London, 1995, HMSO.

Beaver RC, Sharp ES, Cotsonis, GA: Burn-out experienced by nurse midwives, *J Nurse-Midwifery* 31:1, 1986.

Benoit C: *Midwives in passage: a case study of occupational change*, St John's, 1991, ISER Press.

Benoit C: Paradigm conflict in the sociology of service professions: Midwifery as a case study, *Canadian J Sociol* 19(3):303, 1994.

Brodie P: *Australian team midwives in transition*, contained in the Proceedings of the International Confederation of Midwives 24th Annual Congress, 26–31 May 1996, Oslo, Norway.

Boyd C, Sellars L: *The British way of birth*, London, 1982, Pan Books.

Braun J: *Sex discrimination against student midwives*, MIDIRS Information Pack Number 15, December 1990, MIDIRS, Bristol.

Buchan J, Stock J: *Midwives careers and grading*, IMS Report 201, Brighton, 1990, Institute of Manpower Studies, University of Sussex.

Campbell R, Macfarlane A: *Where to be born? The debate and the evidence*, Oxford, 1987, National Perinatal Epidemiology Unit.

Cardale P: Breaking away, *Nurs Times* 86(28):68, 1990.

Carlisle C, Baker G, Riley M, Dewey M: Stress in midwifery: a comparison of midwives and nurses using the work environment scale, *Int J Nurs Studies* 31:1, 1994.

Carpenter M: The subordination of nurses in health care: towards a social divisions approach. In Riska E, Wegar K, editors: *Gender, work and medicine; women and the medical division of labour*, London, 1993, Sage.

Cartwright A: *The dignity of labour? A study of childbearing and induction*, London, 1979, Institute for Social Studies in Medical Care.

Centre for Midwifery Practice: *An evaluation of one-to-one midwifery practice*, Interim Report, 1995, CMP, Thames Valley University, London.

Chalmers I: Implications of the current debate on obstetric practice. In Kitzinger S, Davis J, editors: *The place of birth*, Oxford, 1978, Oxford University Press.

Chalmers I, Richards M: Intervention and causal inference in obstetric practice. In Chard T, Richards M, editors: *Benefits and hazards of the new obstetrics*, London, 1977, Spastics International Medical Publications.

Chalmers I, Enkin M, Keirse MJNC: *Effective care in pregnancy and childbirth*, Oxford, 1989, Oxford University Press.

Clinical Standards Advisory Group: *Women in normal labour*, London, 1995, HMSO.

CMB: *The role of the midwife*, Suffolk, 1983, Hymns Ancient and Modern Limited.

Cochrane A: *Effectiveness and efficiency*, London, 1971, Nuffield Provincial Hospitals Trust.

Committee of Public Accounts: *Thirty Fifth Report, Maternity Services, House of Commons Sessions, 1989-90*, HC 380, London, 1990, HMSO.

Comoroff J: Conflicting paradigms of pregnancy: managing ambiguity in antenatal encounters. In Davis A, Horobin G, editors: *Medical encounters: The experience of illness and treatment*, London, 1977, Croon Helm.

COPMED: *SHO training: tackling the issues, raising standards*, London, 1995, Committee of Postgraduate Medical Deans.

Coser L: *Greedy institutions: patterns of undivided commitment*, New York, 1974, Free Press.

Cronk M: Midwifery: A practitioners view from within the National Health Service, *Midwife, Health Visitor Community Nurse* 26(3):58, 1990.

Currell R: The organisation of midwifery care. In Alexander J, Levy V, Roch S, editors: *Midwifery practice, antenatal care, a research based approach*, Basingstoke, 1990, Macmillan.

Davies C: *The collapse of the conventional career*, English National Board Project Paper 3, London, 1990, ENB.

Davies C: *Gender and the professional predicament in nursing*, Buckingham, 1995, OUP.

Davies C, Rosser J: *Processes of discrimination: a study of women working in the NHS*, London, 1986, DHSS.

Declerq E: A cross national analysis of midwifery politics: six lessons for midwives, *Midwifery* 10:232, 1994.

Demilew J: *The struggle to practice, a sociological analysis of the crisis within the British midwifery profession*, unpublished MSc, London, 1989, University of South Bank.

Department of Health: *Caring for people: Community care in the next decade and beyond*, Cm849, London, 1989a, HMSO.

Department of Health: *Working for patients*, Cm555, London, 1989b, HMSO.

Department of Health: *The patients charter*, HPC1, London, 1991, HMSO.

Department of Health: *Maternity services, Government response to the Second Report from the Health Committee, session 1991-2*, Cm2018, HMSO, 1992, London.

Department of Health: *Changing childbirth, Report of the Expert Maternity Group*, London, 1993a, HMSO.

Department of Health: *A study of midwife- and GP-led maternity units*, 1993b, NHS Management Executive, London.

Department of Health: *Hospital doctors: training for the future*, The report of the working group on specialist medical training, London, 1993c, Department of Health.

Department of Health: *The patients charter, maternity services*, London, 1994, Department of Health.

Department of Health: *Health and personal social statistics for England*, London, 1995, HMSO.

De Vries R: A cross national view of the status of midwives. In Riska E, Wegar K, editors: *Gender, work and medicine*, London, 1993, Sage, pp. 131–146.

DHSS: *Report of the Sub-Committee on Domiciliary and Maternity Bed Needs*, Chairman, Sir John Peel, London, 1970, HMSO.

DHSS: *Sharing resources for health in England*, Report of the Resource Allocation Working Party (RAWP), London, 1976, HMSO.

DHSS: *NHS management inquiry*, DA, 83 38, Chairman Mr R Griffiths, London, 1983, HMSO.

DHSS: *Study of hospital based midwives*, A report by Central Management Services, London, 1984, DHSS.

Dingwall R, Rafferty A, Webster C: *An introduction to the social history of nursing*, London, 1988, Routledge.

Donnison J: *Midwives and medical men: A history of interprofessional rivalries and women's rights*, London, 1988, Heinemann.

Doyal L, Pennell I: *The political economy of health*, London, 1979, Pluto.

Drife JO: Disciplining midwives, a better system is needed, *Br Med J* 297:806, 1988.

Dunlop W: *Changing Childbirth*, commentary 2, *Br J Obstet Gynaecol* 100:1072, 1993.

Durward L, Evans R: Pressure groups and maternity care. In Garcia J, Kilpatrick R, Richards M, editors: *The politics of maternity care: Services for childbearing women in twentieth century Britain*, Oxford, 1990, Clarendon Press.

Ehrenreich J, editor: *The cultural crisis of modern medicine*, New York, 1978, Monthly Press.

Ehrenreich B, English D: *Witches, midwives and nurses: A history of women healers*, London, 1973, Glass Mountain Pamphlet No 1 Compendium.

ENB: *Developments in midwifery education and practice: A progress report*, London, 1995, English National Board.

Ennis M, Clark A, Grudzinskas JG: Change in obstetric practice in response to fears of litigation in the British Isles, *Lancet* 338(8767):616, 1991.

Equal Opportunities Commission: *Equality management: Women's employment in the NHS*, Manchester, 1991, EOC.

Flint C: A team of midwives: a continuing labour of love, *Nurs Mirror* 149(20):16, 1979.

Flint C: Continuity of maternity care, part 1–5, *Nurs Mirror*, 2/12/81–22/12/81, 1981.

Flint C: A radical blueprint, *Nurs Times* 82(1):14, 1986.

Flint C: Aiming for the stars, *Nurs Times* 86(48):66, 1990.

Flint C: *Midwifery teams and caseloads*, London, 1993, Butterworth–Heineman.

Flint C, Poulengeris P, Grant A: The 'know your midwife' scheme – a randomised controlled trial of continuity of care by a team of midwives, *Midwifery* 5:11, 1989.

Flynn N: The new right and social policy, *Policy Polit* 17(2):97, 1989.

Fox E: An honourable calling or a despised occupation: Licensed midwifery and its relation to district nursing in England and Wales before 1948, *Soc Hist Med* 6:2, 1993.

Freidson E: *The profession of medicine*, New York, 1970, Dodd, Mead, & Co.

Garcia J: Continuity of care in context, What matters to women? In Page L, editor: *Effective group practice in midwifery: Working with women*, Oxford, 1995, Blackwell.

Garcia J, Garforth S, Ayers S: 'Midwives confined?' Labour ward policies and routines. In Thomson A, Robinson S, editors: *Research and the midwife*, Conference Proceedings, London, 1985, University of London, Kings College.

GMC 1993 Tomorrow's doctors, London, GMC.

Graham H, Oakley A: Competing ideologies of reproduction: medical and maternal perspectives on pregnancy. In Roberts H, editor: *Women, health and reproduction*, London, 1981, Routledge and Kegan Paul.

Gready M, Newburn M, Dodds R, Gauge S: *Birth choices, women's expectations and experiences*, London, 1995, National Childbirth Trust.

Green D: *Everyone a private patient*, London, 1988, Institute of Economic Affairs.

Green JM, Kitzinger JV, Coupland VA: *The division of labour: Implications for staffing structure for doctors and midwives on the labour ward*, Cambridge, 1986, Child Care and Development Group, University of Cambridge.

Green JM, Coupland VA, Kitzinger JV: Expectations, experiences and psychological outcomes of childbirth: a prospective study of 825 women, *Birth* 17(1):15, 1990.

Haire D: *The cultural warping of childbirth*, New York, 1972, International Childbirth Association.

Hardy B: Emancipation for midwives, *Midwife, Health Visitor Community Nurse* 26(11):433, 1990.

Harvey J: Up-skilling and the intensification of work: the extended role in intensive care nursing and midwifery, *Sociol Rev* :765, 1995.

Heagerty BV: *Class, gender and professionalisation: the struggle for British midwifery, 1900-36*, unpublished DPhil, 1990, Michigan State University (lodged RCM library).

Henderson C: *Changing childbirth and the West Midlands region 1995–1996*, A Report of the Royal College of Midwives/Department of Health Visiting Scholar, London, 1997, Royal College of Midwives.

HMSO: *Women in normal labour*, London, 1995, Clinical Standards Advisory Group, HMSO.

Hodnett ED: Continuity of caregivers during pregnancy and childbirth, Review No 0762, *Cochrane database of systematic reviews*, Oxford, 1995, Update Software.

Honigsbaum F: *The division in British medicine, a history of the separation of general practice from hospital care 1911–1968*, London, 1979, Kogan Page.

Honigsbaum F: *Health, happiness, and security, the creation of the National Health Service*, London, 1989, Routledge.

House of Commons: *The Health Committee Second Report: Maternity services*, Vol. 1 (Chairman N Winterton), London, 1992, HMSO.

Howie PW: The future role of midwives, *Br Med J* 294:1502, 1987.

Hundley VA, Cruickshank FM, Milne JM, Glazener CMA, Lang G, Turner M, Blyth D, Mollison J: Satisfaction and continuity of care: staff views of care in a midwife managed unit, *Midwifery* 11:163, 1995.

Hutton E: *Midwife caseloads*, NCT Policy Statement, London, 1995, NCT.

Jackson K: Changing childbirth: Encouraging debate, *Br J Midwifery* 3(3):137, 1995.

Jacoby A: Mother's views about information and advice in pregnancy and childbirth: Findings from a national study, *Midwifery* 4:103, 1988.

Kent J, Maggs C: *An evaluation of pre-registration midwifery education in England: A research project for the Department of Health, Working Paper 1, research design*, Bath, 1990, Maggs Research Associates.

King Edward's Hospital Fund for London: *Racial equality: the nursing profession*, Equal Opportunities Taskforce, Occasional paper No 6, London, 1990, King Edward's Hospital Fund for London.

Kirkham M: *Basic supportive care in labour: Interaction with and around labouring women*, Unpublished PhD thesis, Manchester, 1987, Faculty of Medicine, Manchester University.

Kitzinger J: Strategies of the early childbirth movement: A case study of the National Childbirth Trust. In Garcia J, Kilpatrick R, Richards M, editors: *The politics of maternity care: Services for childbearing women in twentieth century Britain*, Oxford, 1990, Clarendon Press.

Kitzinger S: *Change in antenatal care*, A report of a working party, London, 1981, NCT.

Kroll D: Team approach in Bloomsbury, *Midwives Chron* 102(1220):305, 1989.

Leap N, Hunter B: *The midwives tale: An oral history from handywoman to professional midwife*, London, 1993, Scarlet Press.

Lee G: A reassuring familiar face? *Nurs Times* 90(17):66, 1994.

Lewis J: *The politics of motherhood: Child and maternal welfare in England*, 1900–1939, London, 1980, Croon Helm.

Lewis J: Mothers and maternity policies in the 20th century. In Garcia J, Kilpatrick R, Richards M, editors: *The politics of maternity care: Services for childbearing women in twentieth century Britain*, Oxford, 1990, Clarendon Press.

Lewis R: Standing up for midwives: Introducing the RCM's employment affairs committee, *Midwives* 198(1285):54, 1995.

Lilford R: Midwives to manage uncomplicated birth; a proposal worth supporting, *Br Med J* 307:339, 1993.

Locker D, Dunt D: Theoretical and methodological issues in sociological studies of consumer satisfaction with medical care, *Soc Sci Med* 12:283, 1978.

Lorber J: More women physicians: will it mean more humane healthcare? *Soc Policy* 16(1):50, 1985.

Macfarlane A, Mugford M: *Birth counts*, London, 1984, HMSO.

Macfarlane A: Statistics and policymaking in the maternity services in England and Wales, *Midwifery* 1:150, 1985.

Macintyre S: The management of childbirth: a review of the sociological research issues, *Soc Sci Med* 11:477, 1977.

Mackay L: *Nursing a problem*, Milton Keynes, 1989, OUP.

Mason V: *Assessing women's views of maternity services*, London, 1990, HMSO.

Maternity Services Advisory Committee, *Maternity Care in Action*, PtI 1982, PtII 1984, PtIII, London, 1985, HMSO.

McDowall J: Working in tandem, *Nurs Times* 86(28):72, 1990.

McKeown T: The role of medicine: Dream, mirage or nemesis?, London, 1976, Nuffield Provincial Hospitals Trust.

McKinlay JB: The sick role – Illness and pregnancy, *Soc Sci Med* 6:561, 1972.

Middlemiss C, Dawson A, Gough N, *et al.*: A randomised study of a domiciliary antenatal care scheme: maternal psychological effects, *Midwifery* 5:69, 1989.

Midwifery Matters (47): 1990; Letterspage.

Ministry of Health: *Chief Medical Officer's report for 1952*, London, 1953, HMSO.

Ministry of Health: *Report of the Maternity Services Committee*, London, 1959, HMSO.

Ministry of Health: Central Health Services Council, Standing Midwifery and Maternity Advisory Committee, London, 1961, HMSO.

Mugford M: Economies of scale and low risk maternity care: What is the evidence? *Maternity Action* 46:100, 1990.

Murphy Black, T 1992 Systems of midwifery care in use in Scotland, Midwifery, 8,113-124.

Murphy Black T: *Identifying the key features of continuity of midwifery care*, Report prepared for the Scottish Home and Health Department, Nursing Research Unit, Edinburgh, 1993, Edinburgh University.

NAHAT: *NAHAT's response to Changing Childbirth*, The report of the Expert Maternity Group, London, 1993, National Association of Health Authorities and Trusts.

NAHAT: *Briefing*, January, No. 92, Birmingham, 1996, NAHAT.

NAO: *The Maternity Services: Report by the Comptroller and Auditor General*, No. 297, London, , 1990, HMSO.

Nash A, Nash JE: Conflicting interpretations of childbirth, *Urban Life* 7(4):493, 1979.

NHSME: *Junior doctors: The new deal*, London, 1991, HMSO.

NHSME: *EL949 Woman-centred maternity services*, Leeds, 1994, Department of Health.

Oakley A: Wise woman and medicine man: Changes in the management of childbirth. In Mitchell J, Oakley A, editors: *The rights and wrongs of women*, London, 1976, Penguin.

Oakley A: *Women confined: Towards a sociology of childbirth*, Oxford, 1980, Martin Robertson.

Oakley A: *The captured womb: A history of the medical care of pregnant women*, Oxford, 1984a, Basil Blackwell.

Oakley A: The importance of being a nurse: What price professionalism? *Nurs Times* 80:24, 1984b.

Oakley A, Rajan L, Grant A: Social support and pregnancy outcome, *Br J Obstet Gynaecol* 997:155, 1990.

Page L: Changing childbirth, *MIDIRS Midwifery Digest* 3:4, 1993.

Page L: *Effective group practice in midwifery: working with women*, 1995, Blackwell Science.

Parents: BIRTH, 9000 mothers speak out, birth survey results, *Parents Magazine* 92, 1986.

Peretz E: A maternity service for England and Wales: Local authority maternity care in the inter-war period in Oxfordshire and Tottenham. In Garcia J, Kilpatrick R, Richards M, editors: *The politics of maternity care: Services for childbearing women in twentieth century Britain*, Oxford, 1990, Clarendon Press.

Phoenix A: Black women and the maternity services. In Garcia J, Kilpatrick R, Richards M, editors: *The politics of maternity care: Services for childbearing women in twentieth century Britain*, Oxford, 1990, Clarendon Press.

Porter M, Macintyre S: What is, must be best: a research note on conservative or deferential responses to antenatal care provision, *Soc Sci Med* 19:1197, 1984.

RCM: *Evidence to the Royal Commission on the NHS*, London, 1977, RCM.

RCM: *Report of the Royal College of Midwives on the role and education of the future midwife in the United Kingdom*, London, 1987, RCM.

RCM: *Comments by the RCM on UKCC Project 2000: A new preparation for practice*, London, 1986, RCM.

RCM: *Delivery*, No. 6:4, London, 1991a, RCM.

RCM: RCM Commission on legislation relating to midwives, *Midwives Chron* 104(1245):295, 1991b.

RCOG: *Press release*, London, 6th August and 28th October 1993, Royal College of Obstetricians and Gynaecologists.

RCOG: *Report of the RCOG working party on antenatal and intrapartum care*, London, 1982, Royal College of Obstetricians and Gynaecologists.

Reid M, Garcia J: Women's views of care during pregnancy and childbirth. Chalmers I, Enkin M, Keirse MJNC: *Effective care in pregnancy and childbirth*, Oxford, 1989, Oxford University Press.

Reid M, McIlwaine G: Consumer opinion of a hospital antenatal clinic, *Soc Sci Med* 14A:363, 1980.

Richards M: Innovation in medical practice: Obstetricians and the induction of labour in Britain, *Soc Sci Med* 9:595, 1975.

Robinson J: Consumer attitudes to maternity care, *Oxford Consumer* May, 1974.

Robinson K: The nursing workforce: Aspects of inequality. In Robinson J, Gray A, Elkan R, editors: *Policy issues in nursing*, Milton Keynes, 1992, OUP.

Robinson S: Midwives, obstetricians and general practitioners: the need for role clarification, *Midwifery* 1:102, 1985.

Robinson S: Maintaining the independence of the midwifery profession: A continuing struggle. In Garcia J, Kilpatrick R, Richards M, editors: *The politics of maternity care: Services for childbearing women in twentieth century Britain*, Oxford, 1990, Clarendon Press.

Robinson S: Combining work with caring for children: Findings from a longitudinal study of midwives' careers, *Midwifery* 9:4, 1993.

Robinson S, Owen H: Retention in midwifery: Findings from a longitudinal study of midwives careers. In Robinson S, Thomson A, editors: *Midwives' research and childbirth*, Vol. 3, London, 1994, Chapman and Hall.

Robinson S, Golden J, Bradley S: *A study of the role and responsibilities of the midwife*, NERU Report 1, London, 1983, University of London, Kings College.

Romalis S: Struggle between providers and recipients: the case of birth practices. In Lewin E, Oleson V, editors: *Women, health and healing*, London, 1985, Tavistock.

Rothman B: *In labour: Women and power in the birthplace*, London, 1982, Junction Books.

Russell C: The know your midwife scheme in the Rhondda, *Midwifery Matters* 36:14, 1988.

Russell J: Perinatal mortality: the current debate, *Soc Health Illness* 4(3):302, 1982.

Salvage J: Professionalisation – or struggle for survival? A consideration of current proposals for the reform of nursing in the United Kingdom, *J Adv Nurs* 13:515, 1988.

Sandall J: Do nurses with children want to return to work? *Senior Nurse* 10(8):9, 1990.

Sandall J: Choice, continuity and control: Changing midwifery towards a sociological perspective, *Midwifery* 11:201, 1995.

Sandall J: Midwive's burnout and continuity of care, *Bri J Mid* 15:106, 1997.

Shapiro MC, Najman JM, Chang A, Keeping JD, Morrison J, Western JS: Information control and the exercise of power in the obstetrical encounter, *Soc Sci Med* 17(3):139, 1983.

Scheff TJ: Negotiating reality: notes on power in the assessment of responsibility, *Social Probl* 16:3, 1968.

Schwarz EW: The engineering of childbirth: A new obstetric programme as reflected in British Obstetric Textbooks, 1960–1980. In Garcia J, Kilpatrick R, Richards M, editors: *The politics of maternity care: Services for childbearing women in twentieth century Britain*, Oxford, 1990, Clarendon Press.

Segal M: The military and the family as greedy institutions, *Armed Forces Soc* 13:1, 1986.

Shoham Y, Carmel S: Autonomy, job satisfaction and professional self image among nurses in the context of a physicians strike, *Soc Sci Med* 28:12, 1989.

Smith L: Is there a future for general practitioner obstetricians?, *Assoc Gen Pract Maternity Care Newsletter* 2:2, 1990.

Social Services Committee: *House of Commons, Second Report from the Social Services Committee on Perinatal and Neonatal Mortality*, Paper 663-1 (Chair: Renee Short), London, 1980, HMSO.

Stacey M: *The sociology of health and healing*, London, 1988, Unwin Hyman.

Stacey M: *Regulating British medicine: The General Medical Council*, Chichester, 1992, Wiley.

Stein L: The doctor/nurse game, *Arch Gen Psychiatr* 16:699, 1967.

Stock J, Wraight A: *Developing continuity of care in maternity services: The implications for midwives*, Brighton, 1993, Institute of Manpower Studies, RCM.

Streetly A: Maternity care in the 1990s, *Health All 2000 News* 26:14, 1994.

Tew M: Where to be born? *New Soc* 1:120, 1977.

Tew M: The case against hospital deliveries. In Kitzinger S, Davis J, editors: *The place of birth*, Oxford, 1978, University Press.

Tew M: Place of birth and perinatal mortality, *J Coll Gen Pract* 35:390, 1985.

Tew M: *Safer childbirth? A critical history of maternity care*, London, 1990, Chapman and Hall.

Towler J: A dying species: survival and revival are up to us, *Midwives Chron* 95(1136):324, 1982.

Turnbull D, Reid M, McGinley M, Sheilds N: Changes in midwives attitudes to their professional role following the implementation of the midwifery development unit, *Midwifery* 11:110, 1995.

UKCC: *Project 2000: A new preparation for practice*, London, 1986, UKCC.

UKCC: *Council statement relating to the case of Jilly Rosser, 12/9/88*, in MIDIRS information pack number 9, November 1988.

Van de Kooy B, Gledhill A, Coyle A, Brailey S, *et al.*: 'Free speech' midwives insurance, *Midwives* 109(1298):62, 1996.

Walker JF: Midwife or obstetric nurse? Some perceptions of midwives and obstetricians of the role of the midwife, *J Adv Nurs* 1:129, 1976.

Warwick C: Midwives and maternity leave, *Maternity Action* 67:6, 1995.

Watson P: *Report on the Kidlington midwifery scheme*, Oxford, 1990, Institute of Nursing.

Weitz R: English midwives and the Association of Radical Midwives, *Women Health* 12(1):79, 1987.

Witz A: *Professions and patriarchy*, London, 1992, Routledge.

World Health Organization: *Having a baby in Europe*, Geneva, 1986, WHO.

Wraight A, Ball J, Seccombe I, Stock J: *Mapping team midwifery, A report to the Department of Health*, IMS Report series 242, Sussex, 1993, Institute Manpower Studies.

Further Reading

Allison J: *Delivered at home*, London, 1996, Chapman & Hall.
A study of the work and life of district midwives from 1948 to 1972 in Nottingham.

Harrison S, Pollitt C: *Controlling health professionals : The future of work and organisation in the NHS*, Milton Keynes, 1994, Open University Press.
Offers an analysis of British health policy since 1979 with an emphasis on the impact of policy changes on healt professionals.

Hunt S, Symonds A: *The social meaning of midwifery*, Basingstoke, 1995, Macmillan.
An ethnographic study of a labour ward which attempts to understand the culture, work practices and strategies of midwives.

Johnson T, Larkin G, Saks M: *Health professions and the state in Europe*, London, 1995, Routledge.
Explains and illuminates the specific relationship between health professions and the state. Provides an overview of the current situation in eight European countries.

Riska E, Wegar K: *Gender, work and medicine: Women and the medical division of labour*, London, 1993, Sage.
A critical assessment of the division of labour in medicine and other health professions, sets current practice within its historical and international context.

18 Consulting Consumers of the Maternity Services

LEARNING OUTCOMES

After studying this chapter you should be able to:

- Identify the three levels at which consumer organizations operate.
- Describe the new developments occurring within consumer organizations.
- Analyse the role of consumer organizations at both national and local level.
- Discuss the problems facing consumer representatives on Maternity Services Liaison Committees.

The recognition afforded the consumer in the mid-1990s is increasing and, with it, a growing power to establish their own stamp on the evolving shape of the National Health Service (NHS). While consumer organizations have no statutory powers, lying structurally outside the NHS, they do have increasing influence. Maternity Services Liaison Committees (MSLCs), although not yet developed into a solid channel of consumer communication, hold the potential to do so.

In this chapter, two forms of consumer voice, consumer organizations and MSLCs, are discussed. First, the activities of consumer organizations within the maternity services are reviewed, their role, activities and the difficulties they face outlined, and the issue of those they do not serve addressed. It is argued that these organizations fulfil a number of roles for the consumers, and

that the growing sophistication of consumer organizations is apparent in their use of a number of channels for consumer feedback to policy makers. Second, the work of MSLCs is reviewed; these provide a significant nonstatutory channel of consumer representation – at the time of writing they hold the potential to develop stronger consumer representation within the NHS. The terminology needs a brief analysis, for while some speak of pressure groups, others prefer to write about consumer or voluntary organizations. Here the term 'consumer organization' is adopted, as one hopefully less contentious than some. Although the language used herein implies that consumers are female, all consumer groups are very welcoming to male partners – many men become involved with their local consumer groups.

Consumer organizations in the maternity services

preside over a diverse set of issues associated with pregnancy and childbirth, so generalizations should be made with caution. Durward and Evans (1990) argue that all function as advocacy agencies, in other words to support and promote the needs of a particular group; others suggest, however, that channelling individuals concerns and needs into specific areas may, in fact, blunt the 'cutting edge' of perhaps more publicly visible activities.

Such organizations have existed since the 1970s, although a few organizations are older – the National Childbirth Trust (NCT, originally the Natural Childbirth Association) dates back to the 1950s while the Association for the Improvement of the Maternity Services (AIMS) was set up in 1960. The majority were set up in what has been termed 'the self-help decade', the 1970s (Robinson and Henry, 1977). Examples are numerous, thus MAMA (Meet-a-Mum Association) was founded in 1979 by Esther Ranzen and *Woman* magazine, TAMBA (Twins and Multiple Births Association) was 18 years old in 1995 and the Maternity Alliance, an organization with a broader remit, began in 1980; SATFA (Support Around Termination For Abnormality), one of the newer organizations, was set up in 1988.

There is little analysis of the role and impact of consumer organizations within the maternity services, although more generally there has always been debate over the consumer voice within the NHS. To locate the discussion more closely to activity in the field of pregnancy and childbirth, contact was made with a sample of consumer organizations, literature from the organizations reviewed and a sample of representatives interviewed. Interviews were also carried out with a sample of user representatives involved with MSLCs. Notes were written up and all quotations reported within this chapter relate to these interviews. A detailed analysis of all aspects of consumer organizations is not presented, but key features of their work are covered. Further research is certainly required to understand the role of these organizations in greater depth.

Consumer Organizations in the 1990s

Democracy, participation and consumerism are central tenets of an NHS in the 1990s. The introduction of *The Patient's Charter* (Secretary of State for Health, 1991), consolidated the shift in political rhetoric. But while consumer involvement in the NHS is a relatively new development its roots may be traced back several decades in maternity care, certainly to the late 1960s and early 1970s, when consumers spoke out against the trend towards inducements of convenience (Stacey, 1988). While sociologists highlighted the role of medicalization in the maternity services (Oakley, 1980), earlier still general concern about professional accountability had been voiced. Consumers have always had the possibility of redress for complaints by approaching their MPs or through the formal complaints machinery, although its effectiveness has been questioned (Klein, 1973). The creation of Community Health Councils (CHCs) in 1974 gave consumers a structured and controlled mechanism by which to voice their opinions and concerns about the NHS. In so doing CHCs opened up the areas on which consumers could have opinions and, according to Klein and Lewis (1976, p. 153), 'It has widened the political arena within which discussions about the allocation and use of NHS resources take place.' The meaning of concepts such as consumer participation in the NHS, however, is still under scrutiny – commentators have pointed out that consumer involvement is not a fixed entity, but exists along a continuum of participation (Lupton *et al.* 1995).

Many, but not all, maternity organizations deal with *problems*, although the nature and type of the cause can vary. Many are concerned with difficult emotional situations which, it is argued (Robinson and Henry, 1977), are either poorly managed by the NHS or ignored, such as problems which arise around a termination for fetal abnormality (SATFA), a stillbirth or infant death [SANDS (Stillbirth and Neonatal Death Society)]. The mere existence of a group can make the condition more difficult to ignore, thus the Toxoplasmosis Trust, founded by a couple whose daughter has congenital toxoplasmosis, has raised the public profile of this formerly little known condition. Literature from the Miscarriage Association that cites a personal statement from a distressed parent is indicative of why women (and their partners) turn to such organizations:

> ... the inability of the medical profession to provide me with any information or explanation as to why this terrible thing had happened.

While some organizations deal with problems during pregnancy, others are concerned with circumstances that arise after childbirth. Perhaps it is not surprising to find a support group for those with postnatal depression (MAMA), or for those with twins or multiple births (TAMBA), the latter not a 'problem' in itself but a situation which research has indicated brings its own difficulties, and in which tiredness, isolation and depression may last (Garel and Blondel, 1992). Crysis was set up for parents whose infant cries endlessly.

These organizations can take many forms, and their shape has evolved to fit their function and ethos. The NCT, easily the largest of these organizations, is 'concerned with education for parenthood'. As an organization aimed at providing support and information to childbearing women, it is a truly national organization with, in 1993, 381 branches across the country and a membership of 52,000. Although not a 'single-cause' organization, it was set up in 1956 as the *Natural Childbirth Association (NCA)* to promote the ideas of Grantly Dick Read (Kitzinger, 1990). A central theme of the NCA was to establish a more general awareness about the processes of birth, and to encourage knowledge and confidence in childbearing women. By the 1960s the Trust had set up its own structure of antenatal classes and had begun to promote breastfeeding through counsellors; like other similar organizations, the NCT is still emerging into a form appropriate to the 1990s.

Most of the organizations are registered as charities – although this may provide benefits, they are restricted under charity law not to act as campaigning organizations nor to become involved in political lobbying. AIMS is one of the few noncharities, and can describe itself as a 'campaigning pressure group'. Although a relatively small organization, it maintains a high profile within the maternity services, with regional contacts who 'spearhead local and national campaigns'. AIMS is run by voluntary workers and funds are raised almost entirely from donations and publications. Its workers have managed to sustain a prickly mid-way position, working alongside but not always with professionals. AIMS tends to focus upon concerns over technology (induction, electronic fetal monitoring, episiotomy, routine use of ergometrine plus oxytocin in labour, rising Caesarean rates), 'rights' of mothers (for example, fathers admitted to labour wards, right of mother to choose position of birth, access to records) and the availability of choice for women at all stages of pregnancy and childbirth (for example, place of birth, practitioner).

The Maternity Alliance is a London-based organization of a different kind, not fitting the conventional model. Indeed, it may not necessarily perceive itself to be a consumer organization in the traditional sense – for example, it has a number of subgroups but no regional network. The Maternity Alliance takes a wider remit than most groups, working with the broad aim of putting pregnancy into a social setting. This means that, unusually among consumer organizations in this area, Maternity Alliance tackles maternity legislation, benefits and rights, and legal issues to do with employment. It has, then, a professional advocacy role along with other organizations less immediately associated with maternity care, such as the Child Poverty Action Group.

The fact that three of the most influential organizations in the field of maternity care are so different in terms of focus and structure underlines the point that consumer organizations do vary considerably. The majority of these are national, providing links across the UK. The work they carry out is complex, however, and most provide not only a range of services, but also function at a number of levels (**Table 18.1**). To begin to appreciate the breadth of work undertaken, three levels of functioning are discussed, at national, local and individual level.

Table 18.1 Structure and Functions of Consumer Groups	
Levels	**Functions**
National	Co-ordination of organization, consultation, policy making, responding to government papers or other initiatives, fundraising, research, liaison with other organizations, newsletters, publications, conferences, publicity
Local	Local fundraising, running clubs, groups/subgroups, newsletters, education (schools, etc.), study days, conferences, networking, publicity
Individual	Phone calls, letters, individual contacts, networking

Consumer Organizations at a National Level

Klein, an experienced commentator on health-care developments, is clear that the growth of such organizations should not be taken as an indication of a general desire to become involved with determining future health-care policy. However, the evidence today is very much that consultation at policy level is increasingly accepted as one of the tasks of consumer groups and, indeed, is an involvement that many foster. Consumer representatives may now be a part of the NHS planning process, sitting on Trust Boards and Health Authorities as nonexecutive members. Although the review of MSLCs (*see* later) raises serious questions about the effectiveness of the consumer voice, it is difficult to dismiss the success of consumer representation on higher level committees, at minimum to note progress by their presence and at most to influence government reports – most recently, and importantly for the discussion in this chapter, the Winterton Report (House of Commons Health Committee, 1992) and Expert Maternity Group (1993 – The Cumberlege Report), both of which made explicit comments on the contribution of consumer organizations.

While many agencies have always put pressure not only on the professions but also on the state (Robinson and Henry, 1977), what emerges today is a more complicated relationship with government, with some organizations playing a more proactive role. Writing about exactly this issue, the editors of the *British Medical Journal* note:

> No longer patient [patients], these sophisticated consumers and their agents are challenging the unique authority of doctors and insisting on a greater role in clinical decision-making.
>
> (Morrison and Smith, 1994, p. 1099.)

It has not always been so. Over the decades a series of influential Government Reports directed the maternity services in ways almost diametrically opposite those of known consumer wishes [for example, the Peel Report 1970 or The House of Commons Social Services Committee (1980 – The Short Report)]. In the latter report the recommendation of a 50% expansion in consultant grade obstetricians and gynaecologists over the following 5 years, combined with a lack of recognition of the value of midwives' contribution to low-risk births, lowered the morale of many, including those who worked in consumer organizations (which had limited input only to the Committee). Indeed, Tew (1990) maintains that it was as a direct result of the Short Report that the Maternity Alliance was formed. Research within the field of maternity care emphasized

consumer dissatisfaction with the services, noting the powerlessness felt by many consumers and the difficulty of achieving their wishes when lines of communication were not clear and lay–professional interactions were sometimes profoundly unsatisfactory (Macintyre, 1984; Oakley, 1993; Reid and Garcia, 1989). Despite formal consumer representation and a decade or more of research highlighting a range of consumer dissatisfactions it was not until the 'paradigm change' of the 1990s that the gulf between consumer research and official pronouncements appeared to be diminishing. By that time, the health services were undergoing a series of cutbacks and restructuring, so the balance between the consumer and the provider had shifted. Today consumer groups have become an integral part of the consultation process.

The shift in thinking – and rhetoric – was first in evidence with the 1992 House of Commons Health Committee Report (1992 – the Winterton Report). The Report notes early on that the focus of inquiry is 'normal birth' and places at the top of the agenda 'continuity, choice and control' of the situation by women. Although it could be argued that at one level this is political rhetoric, the committee received written and oral evidence from a number of consumer organizations. At the time *Local Voices* (NHSME, 1992; *see* below) had recently been published – the importance of consulting the consumer was emphasized not only by consumer groups, but also by some enlightened professional staff.

When it became known that the government was to form an Expert Maternity Group under the leadership of Baroness Cumberlege, representatives from the NCT lobbied the Department of Health to enquire about consumer representation and proposed the chair of the NCT as someone who was both experienced and respected in the field by consumer organizations. As such, it was understood that she would be the consumers representative rather than that for one specific organization. Formal written evidence by the main consumer organizations was also sent to the Committee.

Changing Childbirth, the resulting report from the Expert Maternity Committee (1993), extended the push for woman-centred services developed in the Winterton Report, arguing that:

> Consumer groups should play an active role in assessing services on behalf of the women using them, and work with purchasers and providers to bring about change.
>
> (Expert Maternity Group, 1993, p. 6.)

The Report explicitly acknowledged the contribution of consumer organizations, while the role of the Maternity Alliance in relation to disabilities was also noted. Because the impact of consumer organizations is not always easy to measure, markers such as this are received with particular pleasure.

Ham (1992) notes that traditionally consumers of the services have been less well organized than the producers, but that now 'a variety of consumer groups are active in the central policy-making system and that many of the groups are consulted on a regular basis by government.' As one representative said, 'We used to be much more reactive, much more passive, not actively lobbying and some of the key members were a bit afraid of being seen to be politically active.' The Maternity Alliance has regular meetings with civil servants, while many of the organizations' representatives reported being asked to respond to draft documents. This could be a straightforward matter on which the organization had a clear policy. On the other hand, it might require more extended reading and research to formulate the group's response. Such responses take up an organization's time and resources, and for this reason one representative was concerned about the increasing demands of this nature on her organization. 'The moment I'm getting very cosy with (central government) I think, hello, we're not being very efficient here.' Retaining distance from government allows a more critical stance, which has positive features.

Consumer consultation comes in a number of forms; another example can be found within Scotland where the Clinical Resource and Audit Group/Scottish Management Executive Group (CRAG/SCOTMEG) Working Party for the Maternity Services prepared for their policy document rather differently, by drawing in both individual consumers and consumer groups at several stages of consultation. After a literature review of consumers' views (Reid and McMillan, 1992) and a study of women's views (Bostock, 1993) a baseline document was drawn up to delineate the service of the future. The Working Party held a series of roadshows around the country, including representatives of local branches of consumer organizations, who were also represented on the Working Group (CRAG/SCOTMEG Working Group on Maternity Services, 1995). The policy review which arose from such elaborate consultation, *Provision of Maternity Services In Scotland* (Scottish Office, 1993) set the stage for the Scottish Health Boards by producing a detailed set of recommendations.

Fundraising must appear in any discussion of consumer organizations, simply because it is a dominant aspect of their work, as funds influence not only the number of staff an organization can employ but also dictate the extent of their activities. Charities in the UK are pressured from all sides; increasing unemployment,

competition from the National Lottery, cutbacks in the budgets of local government and Health Authorities may all serve to threaten their annual income. More frequent mentions in the media, better publicity and an increase in the number of consultations combine to make demands on organizations which, in terms of staffing, are often very small indeed. The majority of organizations work with part-time administrators, part-time secretarial help and volunteers who work whenever other commitments allow. Small wonder that one representative described her organization as 'a tiny bunch of low-paid workaholics'.

Patrons, by the nature of their celebrity status, contribute to raising the profile of such organizations; the literature of these organizations confirms that many have a well-known name to head the list of patrons. Fundraising has turned into a juggling act: 'We mainly rely on membership subscriptions, various grants from the Department of Health, and we also apply to Trusts and companies, so there's various sources helping us at the moment, and small donations from our members.'

As one newsletter acknowledged: 'In this climate, [the organization] has also suffered. Lack of donation and having to go for many months without a fundraiser, has shown in our financial situation ...' This particular organization subsequently employed an enthusiastic fundraiser.

While annual reports reflect donations from a range of organizations, often representing a personal interest of the firm or agency, recurrent grants are much sought after. The Department of Health contributes to a number of English-based charities by providing funding for projects; examples are often in the form of training for staff or ways of improving their services, but even this was reported to create its own stresses – 'it's a constant battle to keep thinking up projects'. Publications are increasingly a source of income generation. Most organizations now offer a range of leaflets, the sales of which contribute substantially to the organization's funds. Indeed, selling information and publicizing the organization are twin ventures, with organizations also offering posters, envelope labels, Christmas cards and car stickers. Despite such creativity, the major problem remains the lack of certainty of funding for future years, leading one representative talking about funding to conclude 'Oh it's hell!'

A few organizations also felt that the nature of their cause made it inherently more difficult to fundraise. For example, the SATFA representative noted that termination and disability were both topics which were controversial, while CHILD, too, felt that their cause was unfashionable and so fundraising was additionally difficult for them.

One might anticipate intense competition for funds between organizations. This hypothesis was only partially confirmed in the interviews ('It can be awkward', 'It used to be quite extraordinary, the lack of co-operation within the voluntary sector'). Instead, representatives stressed the good links with at least 'neighbouring' organizations, where there may be opportunities to share study days and hence resources. Good working knowledge of other organizations, too, promotes a better service for members and there seems to be little problem in referring an individual to an organization more relevant to the enquirer's needs.

The Maternity Services Group now exists within the arena of the maternity services, the purpose of which is 'to share information and promote areas of mutual concern.' An informal group, its membership represents the major organizations within the field. Regular meetings offer the opportunity to discuss issues on a number of policy and practical levels, to share new research findings, discuss potential action (although not necessarily joint action), ask advice and offer help. The meetings are portrayed by all as ones of mutual trust and respect, and their existence suggests a contrary hypothesis, that in times of need sharing is a more positive way forwards than competition. The group is now serviced by a member of the Changing Childbirth Implementation Team (CCIT) from the NHS Management Executive (NHSME), and because of this the group has direct links to central government.

Broadening their roles: science and research

Although all consumer organizations are committed to providing their members with information, the newsletters and leaflets suggest a public which is now more than ever interested in understanding the science of the situation, the research debates within the field. Today's consumer operates with a different understanding of the boundaries around 'consumer knowledge', many believing that they have a right to understand the scientific evidence upon which professionals act. Much of the literature provides the reader with a key to relevant medical terminology, while some go further, setting out medical debates about the situation (for example, the Miscarriage Association provides detailed information about the various theories of miscarriage).

One of the newer roles of consumer organizations has been their involvement with research. In the past, consumer organizations were happy to support research on relevant topics and this continues, with newsletters carrying notices about a research project, implicitly (or sometimes explicitly) encouraging members to co-operate with the project. A good example of the newer approach comes from AIMS, one of the broad-based organizations which has long-tackled scientific issues as a matter of course. The newsletter provides analyses of research findings, research articles reprinted and a section which carries research abstracts. In recent years consumer organizations have become more involved in the research process in a number of ways and, although this relationship is in its infancy, it seems likely that the research role will become more important.

Bringing in consumer organizations as consultants on a research project is now seen more often. The Midwifery Development Unit (MDU) study based in Glasgow drew on the Local Health Council (LHC, Scottish version of a CHC) and NCT for advice when setting up the project (Turnbull *et al.* 1995). The MDU used the QAMID model (quality assurance model for midwifery, a World Health Organization model; Holmes *et al.* 1996) to set up the job specifications for midwives who worked in a randomized controlled trial in which a small group of them provided care for women throughout pregnancy, delivery and postnatally. The project team invited representatives from LHCs and the NCT to meet with staff in QAMID meetings to discuss setting standards for care (for example, what was reasonable to expect in the way of continuity). The meetings were reported as helpful for both parties, for staff to listen to consumer wishes but also to present the practicalities of research and practice to consumers, who are not always aware of the constraints under which staff work.

While the MDU project brought in consumer organizations at a specific stage of the research, another innovatory project used the NCT as a major channel for recruitment of women, thereby involving the organization more centrally in the whole study. The MAIN study ['multicentre randomized controlled trial of alternative treatments for inverted and nonprotactile (flat) nipples in pregnancy'] was set up by the National Perinatal Epidemiology Unit at Oxford using a pioneering methodology whereby women were recruited either through midwives working in nine centres in England, or through the NCT network (Renfrew and McCandlish, 1992). Recruitment was not easy and the analysis of the project makes interesting reading, for Renfrew and McCandlish (1992) noted the competing cultures of a research project and a voluntary organization, the latter being run at a local level by volunteers who faced many incompatible demands on their time.

Some would argue that including consumers in

research is simply an act of political correctness, and that consumer organizations should not necessarily be committed to aid research spearheaded by professionals who are paid to do it. If this is the case, to initiate their own research project is perhaps the logical next stage for an organization. A handful have become involved in projects. Along with a number of other studies funded by CCIT, the NCT ran a successful project to assess the impact of *Changing Childbirth* (the *Choices* project), while *Through the Maze* (funded by the King's Fund Centre) is a guide directed towards information services and self-help groups on research-based evidence on aspects of pregnancy, birth and early parenthood. More recently the NCT, now large and specialized enough to have appointed a research and policy officer, prepared a successful application for a large-scale research project funded by the North Thames Regional Health Authority, winning out over more experienced researchers in so doing; this was, as they said, 'a first for us and a sign of our growing experience, confidence and professionalism in the research field but also in terms of how we work.'

Local Activities

'The groups are the heart of the organization' is a sentiment that many would echo. Most organizations operate with similar structures, namely a head office to carry out policy and decision-making tasks, respond to formal enquiries, oversee the local groups and co-ordinate fundraising. On the second tier lie the local groups, although the scope and number of these varies across the different organizations. The NCT, for example, fulfils many of its roles at this level, providing a national network of antenatal classes, and a postnatal support system across the UK. The scale of these activities is evident from the 1993 statistics, with 642 registered antenatal teachers covering 10,448 couples and 1507 individual women at the antenatal classes, while 438 postnatal co-ordinators and 211 specialist groups operate postnatally. MAMA, a far smaller organization, nevertheless reports more than 70 groups in existence, the Miscarriage Association has 67 groups with a membership of 11,500. Others now offer a range of groups so that the parent can select the one whose experience most mirrors their own. TAMBA, to give one example, offers five support groups directed towards families who have had a multiple birth but with differing circumstances or outcomes, namely supertwins, a special needs group (infants with hand-

icap), a one-parent family group, an infertility support group and a bereavement support group. It is clear that not all regions necessarily have an active membership all the time, but the level of local activity is impressive and must surely answer any doubts as to the importance of the role of consumer organizations.

Although newsletters are produced from head office they fulfil a number of functions at the local level (some organizations in fact produce more than one newsletter, each going to different subgroups; for example, NCT's *RepRap* for user representatives on other committees, or TAMBA's *Bulletin* for the 'health and education' group). The networking function, linking the activities of the local groups, is central as the newsletter provides members with contact addresses and news of the local clubs, as well as sharing the distinctive philosophy of the organization. TAMBA's newsletter provides short, jokey articles from 'twin club' newsletters from around the country as well as a more serious 'regional round-up' which lists the representatives and activities of the 12 regions, which include Scotland, Northern Ireland and 'overseas'.

A further article from the same newsletter on running a twins club emphasizes the importance of the Association's role in bringing together parents with shared experiences: 'Clubs exist for MUTUAL support' (original caps, Scarr, 1995). With rarer events, such as twins and multiple births, Scarr emphasizes both the value of such an organization and also the difficulty in keeping a local club with sufficient members active. 'Clubs such as my own which serve a smaller population and a local maternity unit may only have one expectant family at a time' (Scarr, 1995, p. 20). The MAMA annual report illustrates the range of local activities in the previous year:

> 80% of the groups meet at least once a week, 67% in their own homes, the remainder in a local venue; more than 50% organize evening meetings, 78% of the groups organize regular social meetings but 55% of the groups also organize talks or demonstrations by professionals, and 84% also organize outings for the children.
> (MAMA Annual Report 1993/94.)

Not all organizations work in this way; one notable example is SATFA, which does have a local network, but not 'branches', and it operates more centrally than most. SATFA has a London office which acts as a clearing house, and although there is a national support network and befrienders around the country, their names are not published and callers are directed through the London office. The reason for this is twofold. First, termination is both a controversial and an emotive issue, so many may not wish to have their name widely advertized or approached by 'anyone and everyone'. Second, the executive felt that considerable harm could be done to an enquirer being given an out-of-date address or phone number. There were reports of this delaying contact being made with someone from the organization (at a time when a day or a week could be especially important); the preferred strategy of channelling all enquiries through the central office is to avoid this occurrence.

The supportive nature of local activities is, of course, intrinsic to such groups through the therapeutic act of talking; 'through identifying and sharing problems, experiences and attitudes of others ... members of self-help groups begin to help themselves' (Robinson and Henry, 1977). For a bereaved couple or first-time mothers wishing to meet together postnatally, talking to others with a shared experience forms the core activity essential to the continuance of the local group. Support may be offered through one-to-one contacts (discussed below), social activities such as 'open house' or coffee mornings or evenings.

Part of the group work is to allow the consumer not just to talk about the event but to encourage her (and her partner) to express feelings about the situation. Emotions are recognized by such organizations as being 'naturally' associated with pregnancy and childbirth, and the problems that arise from these events. Publications describe common emotions experienced by women and their partners, thereby legitimating them for others; women undergoing miscarriage, for instance, may feel 'loss, guilt, helplessness', as may their partners while women told they are expecting twins may find it 'brings mixed emotions; on the one hand excitement ... on the other apprehension' (the personal accounts, poems and letters recorded in the newsletters, too, testify to the importance of this aspect of the experience). Becoming involved with women's emotions is a difficult task for professionals, not least because the pattern of work at the antenatal clinic or on the ward may prohibit such involvement. But while professional support may well be offered, the effectiveness of sharing emotions with others who have undergone the same experience cannot be challenged.

Local groups have a developing educational function, too. All groups are committed to the provision of information to their members and, as we have seen, this is done in an increasingly sophisticated manner. The newsletters provide examples of the range of activities in which members may educate themselves about the issue addressed by the organization. Study days, conference and 1-day meetings are a further way of keeping group members up-to-date with research in the area, as well as facilitating meetings with local health-service professionals. Others noted local work with educational establishments, going into schools and colleges to give talks (and special student packs for school pupils undertaking projects on the topic are available).

One-to-One Contact – The Essence of Consumer Organization's Work

The one-to-one contact with members represents the essence of these organizations. The Miscarriage Association argues the need:

> When I lost my baby they said it happens to one in five pregnancies. But when I came out of hospital there was no one to talk to. I felt I was on my own.

Stories emphasize successes – in *A mum's story* a phone call to a group member offers salvation for a depressed mother, 'She was there, someone to listen and to hear what I had to say ...' Personal contact represents the reason many people join such an organization and it is important for continuing membership that the service be seen as successful from the user's perspective.

Thus considerable effort is placed in making key individuals contactable; many organizations offer 24-hour phone lines and the possibility to talk to someone day or night. TAMBA advertizes a 'twinline, unique confidential and listening service, 7 PM to 11 PM weekdays and 10 AM to 11 PM weekends', suggesting a complicated on-call rota similar to those of other organizations. Because of restricted working hours, central offices sometimes provide only a recorded message, but always provide alternative numbers for 'instant' availability of individuals ready to talk with advice and support. The extent to which both telephone and letters are received provides some indication of the workload of these organizations. Although data are not always precise, it is worth quoting a few figures. SATFA reported receiving between 7000–8000 calls in 1995, while the Central Office of the Miscarriage Association receives an average of 300 letters and calls a week, a figure which had trebled over the previous year. With its postnatal breastfeeding support network, NCT records 621 counsellors and a total number of 101,350 breastfeeding support contacts in 1993.

Continual contact with grass roots members is a two-way process, for the giving to members is counterbalanced by the ability of members to keep the 'executive' in touch. Consumer organizations, unlike business organizations, do not usually operate (only) with long-term plans that create an inflexible set of goals to be achieved during the year; one reason is that the uncertainties of funding may operate against long-term plans, but secondly the more flexible and democratic structure allows greater input from the grass roots. Thus, they rely more heavily on their membership to raise with them the important issues to be tackled. The frequent telephone and personal contact with the membership constitutes an important way of ascertaining the problems and concerns of the membership (for example, problems with a particular hospital).

Consumer Organizations – Who Joins?

Thus far a fairly uncritical view of consumer organizations is offered – lack of studies hinders any alternative approach. Their structural position outside the NHS precludes them from formal audit procedures, and questions such as how effectively do they work can only be answered obliquely. That voluntary agencies have their roots in the nineteenth century philanthropic tradition is, however, well recognized and thus the criticism that consumer organizations are, in the main, run by and for middle-class women is not new. One of the very few studies of consumer representation carried out 20 years ago confirmed the middle-class nature of such membership. Klein and Lewis (1976) reported from their sample of 3796 CHC members in England and Wales various striking differences in terms of membership of voluntary organizations and social class. They found a 10% membership of no voluntary organizations for the middle-class sample (professional and managerial groups), which contrasted with 29% of the 'blue-collar' group. On the other hand, 41% of the middle-class sample were members of three or more voluntary organizations, contrasted with 25% of the 'blue collar' group.

Is the same still true? There is little evidence that most consumer organizations have a membership representative of the general population in terms of ethnicity or social class. The NCT President, Eileen Hutton, in the 1994 *Annual Review of the Trust*, indicated that a more accessible NCT was one of the goals of their 3-year plan:

At present we recruit mainly from the middle classes, but in all honesty, we know little about

the needs of many pregnant women and mothers in Britain. We have little to offer people in Britain's less advantaged housing estates, for example, or people from different ethnic minorities.

(NCT Annual Report, 1994.)

Problems encountered by disabled women and women who do not conform to the majority sexuality, for example, are seldom addressed by any organization.

The question of 'who are local people?' was seen as one worth asking in *Local Voices*, a document prepared in 1992 by the NHSME. Noting that there was more than one public, the document highlights the groups seldom included in consumer participation, namely the 'silent voices', those who are house-bound, disadvantaged, not represented by groups (NHSME, 1992, p. 8). The document is seen as innovative in recognizing that consumer involvement should take a number of different forms and advocates a wide array of means, such as focus groups, rapid appraisal, telephone hotlines, one-to-one interviews, as well as the more established means of voluntary organizations and CHCs.

There are costs involved in running or being involved in local groups in terms of travel to meet new members and telephone calls, or in providing secretarial services for the group (one Chair of an organization reported that she had always worked without pay, funding her work and the organization by carrying out paid work in other areas). *Local Voices*, too, mentions the need to provide support for such organizations by providing grants, reimbursing costs and so on. There is no question that such support would be appreciated, but to suggest that improved funding might essentially change the representativeness of organizations, i.e. that economic reasons are withholding the greater involvement of ethnic minority women and women from working-class backgrounds, offers a rather superficial analysis.

Costs are usually repaid where possible, but there are other factors which may inhibit a broader membership. Coffee mornings and get-togethers imply a confidence about sharing your house and your experiences with others, and although the 'cause' is the uniting factor, the ability to feel part of a group implies other shared factors associated with a lifestyle. Thus one can imagine that single parent or lesbian mothers (for instance) might feel less comfortable with a group where the talk brings in the partner's involvement. The tenor of the newsletters, too, is to encourage members to become involved with their local groups. One newsletter urges:

If you're to become known as a group, a) put

posters up in your local baby clinics, b) talk to your health visitor, c) get in touch with the area health authority, d) get all the publicity you can. Another introductory leaflet is exemplary, explaining the necessity to be organized, to arrange financial matters and to encourage a social side of the group's activities. While the advice is sound, many might shy away from such assertive behaviour which requires at minimum some knowledge of health-service organization and an ability to generate publicity.

There is little doubt that black and ethnic minority women are likely to face less favourable treatment in the NHS than are middle-class or white women (Phoenix, 1990). On certain issues (for example, screening, family planning) there has been some interest in communicating with black and ethnic minority women. A number of CHCs (especially in East London) have worked with race and class issues; in *Listen with Mother*, an important book in this field, Khawaja (1996) discusses the particular needs of women from minority communities.

On the whole, however, agencies and consumer organizations do not address these concerns. It has been left to city-based groups who represent different cultural categories to redress the balance. Not all specifically focus upon the maternity services – some are concerned with abusive practices of black women, some are actively campaigning and information organizations, while others deal specifically with health issues (Phoenix, 1990). The African Association for Maternal and Child Care International and London Black Women's Health Action are both London-based organizations that serve local communities and are involved in improving the maternity services in their area; one can find examples of groups that attend to the interests of their women at a local rather than a national level in all the major cities.

Other groups of mothers are similarly neglected. The Maternity Alliance and NCT, almost alone, have addressed the specific concerns of disabled women. ParentAbility, a network organized by the NCT, is one of the few support groups to focus upon pregnancy and parenthood for disabled women and their partners. O'Farrell (1996) and Glendinning (1996), in two separate chapters in *Listen with Mother* (Doods *et al.* 1996), stress the need to think about practical issues (transport, physical access, Braille, funding for expenses) as well as noting concerns which also affect able-bodied women, e.g. confidence to participate and understand the process (*see* the discussion on MSLCs below). AIMS, notably, works with pregnant women in prison.

Formal Mechanisms of Consumer Involvement – Community Health Councils and Maternity Services Liaison Committees

The first part of the chapter discusses consumer organizations which, it is argued, have an expanding role in relation to consumer feedback to the NHS. Formal channels of feedback exist, however. CHCs in England and Wales are 'the official voice of the consumer'; although they have emerged from the series of health-service reforms intact, their central role has been challenged. Incidentally, differences exist between England and Scotland with regards to both CHCs (LHCs) and MSLCs, those in England both being more active and more advanced than those in Scotland (Jones *et al.* 1987).

Although a complaints procedure has been in place since 1948 (Klein, 1973), a formal mechanism for the community as opposed to the individual has existed since 1974, when CHCs were first established in England to represent the interests of local communities in the NHS. Unlike MSLCs, which have not yet gained statutory powers, CHCs were set up with statutory responsibilities, including legal requirements to respond to consultation documents. Ascertaining the work of CHCs nationally is difficult as much is unpublished, although results from a funded study (Lupton *et al.* 1995) provide a wider information base than before and stress the *types* of roles CHCs have played in consumer participation. They have a wide remit, not restricted to maternity services, which Lupton *et al.* (1995) typify as five types:
• Health Authority (HA) partners.
• Consumer advocates.
• Patients' friend.
• Independent arbiters.
• Independent challengers.
These demonstrate a continuum from working alongside and with their HA to a position of strong independence. Many will have come across CHCs as supporters of campaigns against the closure of local maternity hospitals, or involved with ascertaining consumers views about the maternity services locally;

Here, however, we discuss in rather more detail

MSLCs which focus specifically upon the maternity services. The idea of MSLCs was first described in a report of the Maternity Services Advisory Committee (MSAC, established in 1982). One of the key recommendations was that every District Health Authority (DHA) set up an MSLC, with representation of:

> ... *all professions involved as well as lay maternity service users (with) the agreement of generally applicable procedures and the monitoring of the effectiveness of these procedures as they apply to the individual woman.*

(Department of Health, 1982, Part 1, para 1.13.) The inclusion of lay representation was, according to Lewison's (1994) excellent review, a major innovation and one which the chair of the MSAC had to fight for.

Subsequent Government reports have supported the existence of MSLCs, the Winterton Report for example, recommending an increase of lay membership because they were not providing 'women using maternity services with a fully effective channel to influence the shape of those services' (House of Commons Health Committee, 1992, para 171). It is becoming common practice for local NCT branches and CHCs to have formal representation on bodies involved in planning maternity services. 'Such representation is warmly welcomed, and we hope it is a practice which will be adopted in areas where this is not yet happening ...' (Expert Maternity Group, 1993, p. 47). Despite such apparent support, both the Winterton and Cumberlege reports failed to make their existence a statutory requirement of HAs and Health Boards; Lewison, writing nearly 10 years after their founding, surveyed the evidence for the success of MSLCs and found that 'there is scant hard evidence about the effectiveness of MSLCs' (Lewison, 1994).

A number of surveys indicate that the majority of HAs in England have set up such Committees, although the studies underline the variability of the Committees, not all of them having lay representatives, some lacking direction and being dominated by local health professionals 'unwilling to take seriously the views of the consumer representatives' (Lewison, 1994, p. 3). At the time of writing feelings are strong but hopes not always high:

> *Mine's a mess! They're not statutory bodies, when they've been mentioned it's rather vague and they are open to huge misinterpretation and this has led to a lot of abuse. Sometimes there's genuine misunderstanding, other times more wilful. They didn't want them to succeed.*

The innovatory nature of MSLCs has also been noted by participants, 'it's breaking new ground in the whole

health service', but the lack of terms of reference has lead to considerable variation across the country. From the beginning the shape and form of the committees were left unspecified and therefore open to being shaped at a local level. MSLCs exist not only without terms of reference, but also without a specific location within the NHS structure and without a clear route to progress. Although this may be a transient state, it is nevertheless a difficult time for enthusiastic lay representatives who are keen to take forward certain issues. In one area the MSLC was abandoned by their HA because of pressure put on them by lay representatives who felt that the Committee had been ineffectual and dominated by certain professional groups. The Committee was described as:

> *Very top heavy ... the only time they turned up was if there was something interesting, like a hospital closure ... at other times it was often just rubber stamping things that were decided elsewhere.*

In this HA, the lay representatives were in the process of forming a maternity users forum which would work directly with consumers and would link straight to the commissioner of the health authority. Whether they are able, as they hoped, to invite onto the committee the health professionals as observers is not known, but the initiative underlines the frustrations experienced by some lay representatives.

In Scotland, development of MSLCs has been less far advanced and the Scottish Office (1993) policy document published the same year as the Expert Maternity Group's Report made no mention of MSLCs. A 1994 Scottish Needs Assessment Programme (SNAP) document proposed that MSLCs should be linked directly to purchasers and a Health Board chair, although the door has been left open for a user representative to take over, 'consideration needs to be given to the advantages of a user representative as chairperson since the key focus of the Committee's work will be to promote the development of a service responsive to users' needs' (SNAP, 1994). No figures exist for the number of MSLCs that exist in Scotland.

A Royal College of Midwives postal survey of MSLCs in all UK DHAs and (Scottish) Health Boards carried out in 1992 confirmed that they were by then widely set up and with a range of professional representatives – all MSLCs had representatives from obstetricians, paediatricians, general practitioners (GPs), midwives and general management (unpublished study cited in Lewison, 1994) **Table 18.2** provides the findings from the study.

Findings from a more recent study (Maternity Action,

1995) carried out by Greater London Authority Community Health Council (GLACHC) reported themes now familiar, with about half of the committees having lay chairs some of whom were also non-Executive members of district or family health service authorities. The remaining chairs were split between being purchaser-based and provider-based chairs, with meetings held on hospital sites. The trend towards more user chairs is confirmed by CCIT who are in the process of building up a data base on MSLCs.

CCIT are also currently drafting guidelines for MSLC committees, which are to cover how the committees work and their scope, with a list of common difficulties faced by such committees. One commentator was hopeful that such guidelines 'would have a knock-on effect and especially if they were endorsed by the Royal Colleges, would have an impact in Scotland'. An earlier set prepared by the NCT argued for either a lay chair or 'a nominee of the purchasing authority'; and that 'the MSLC should submit not only a national report to the DHA on the state of maternity services and their own activities, but also to set its agenda in consultation with the DHA', thus declaring their allegiance very firmly with the purchasing authority. The importance of this was spelled out by someone who had worked on a successful committee:

The only thing that can give clout is the purchaser's money, one of the reasons that our (MSLC) is effective is that we've always had an executive director looking after us, making sure the minutes were OK, doing the agenda jointly with the chair ... she knew what was possible and what wasn't, and also making sure that relevant things from the health authority enters the agenda.

Some MSLCs have been exploring other ways of involving users, such as setting up a subgroup for users sometimes with the chair of MSLC in attendance. Such a subcommittee taps grass roots views and allows women who could or would not wish to move onto the main committee to become involved in the consultation process.

Some of the problems that face consumer representatives on MSLCs are practical. Lewison (1994) reports, albeit at an anecdotal level, that it is often difficult for users to put items onto the agenda or even to gain a place on an MSLC, while committees may also meet at times less convenient to consumers. Many highlighted the problem of allocating greater responsibility to lay members with no additional support. As one said, 'You're setting them up to fail.' Lay representatives have often been recruited from the NCT which has provided support, expenses and a newsletter (*RepRap*) to inform user representatives on outside committees about relevant developments. Without that support other lay representatives reported feeling lost and GLACHC correctly identified:

It is questionable whether lay members always feel able to speak out in such situations, particularly where the chair is a consultant or provider representative.

(Maternity Action, 1995).

Another difficulty faced by consumers has been that of the 'style' of the work, sitting on a committee alongside purchasers and providers with considerably more experience of such work. Here gender politics (women

Table 18.2 Royal College of Midwives Survey of MSLCs (1992)	
Group	**Percentage**
DHAs and Boards with an MSLC	88%
MSLCs with consumer representation	92%
MSLCs with a CHC representative	82%
MSLCs with a NCT representative	58%
MSLCs with two or more consumer representatives	44%
MSLCs meeting on three or more occasions during the year	63%
MSLCs meeting once or not at all	4%

Reproduced with permission of Royal College of Midwives

users, often a high proportion of male purchasers and providers) compounded the professional–lay distinctions. One solution, obvious in retrospect, was that both sides should be socialized into this new form of committee work, with an 'increasing recognition for the need for training, which needs to be directed at both health professional and consumers' (Kelson, 1995, p. 38).

A breakthrough has been to secure funding for training for users representatives on MSLCs (and indeed other committees) through the creation of the GLACHC Changing Childbirth Project (funded by CCIT). GLACHC piloted a training scheme which provided skills-based training for existing and potential lay members of MSLCs in the Greater London Area. Following on from the project's apparent success (the evaluation had not been completed at the time of writing) the NCT was awarded further funding from the Department of Health (and overseen by CCIT) to broaden the training to include assertiveness, structure and function of the NHS, discussion about policy, research and practice, and something on commissioning; the pilot schemes are to be tested in several centres in England and the project team to devise a representative's resource pack to support the training and also as a stand-alone resource (the *Voices* project). This project is currently ongoing and is exploring ways of interesting a wider range of individuals in consumer involvement through MSLC participation; it is also concerned with exploring, through discussion, issues which groups sometimes neglected in this process (e.g. Asian women's group) would like to see brought to the committee table.

There is as yet insufficient information to comment on the scope of MSLCs. Some reportedly deal with potential or impending hospital closures, unsatisfactory waiting lists and other 'traditional' concerns of users. However, consumers are affected by a range of issues more closely allied to clinical practice, even though it has been argued, 'consumers can never know what professionals do' (Klein, 1995, p. 199). The line which defines the limits of lay concern is not clearly drawn and the extent to which, through MSLCs, consumers could challenge professionals about procedures and practices in the maternity services is not fully tested. This is a path along which some consumer organizations have already trodden, notably NCT with their *Through the maze* project and AIMS in querying professional practice, particularly in relation to routine technological procedures and the justification for certain research projects.

One unusual, but successful, MSLC started an 'effective care' project which looked at clinical policy; it took three interventions which were clearly identified on the Cochrane database and assessed where and whether they were being carried out in the DHA in which the MSLC was based. The study found that there was sometimes a mismatch between written policy and practice, the latter tending to reflect changes faster than the former. This kind of exercise is important for a number of reasons and, as one member reported, it 'gave lay members a handle on the clinical issues in the way they had not had before, and in many instances the providers really welcomed the opportunity to discuss differences ...'

Conclusion

Finally, the future – pessimism or optimism? Despite the activity of consumer organizations in the maternity field there are many commentators who argue that the contribution of the consumer remains token, whether the focus is on formal representation (CHC), MSLC or informal through consumer organization. Klein and others (Klein and Lewis, 1976) have argued that consumers are effectively consigned to comment on a limited set of issues.

On the other hand, it is argued here that there is a closer link between public policy and consumer wishes. Consumer input into NHS planning is increasing, whether through consumer organizations or the MSLCs; with both these channels, boundaries are expanding and groups are becoming more 'professional' in their skills and more able to have dialogue with professional groups. More than ever before, problems with such dialogue are being explicitly identified and are in the process of being addressed.

Midwives have, until recently, been concerned to maintain their own professional strengths so their support for the consumer voice has been less in evidence. Surely critical to the future is a clearer alliance between consumers and midwives, in which the strengths of the consumer organizations are more explicitly recognized by midwives. The consumer voice within the maternity services should be seen by all as one which challenges, but also one which has a close investment in the future.

KEY CONCEPTS

- Consumer groups function at a number of levels, from national to individual.

- Consumer groups are becoming involved with research projects, some of their own making.

- Some groups of consumers are more difficult to make contact with and it is important to be aware that those who are more silent have views as well.

- Consumer groups need the support of professionals as well as consumers (professionals also consume).

- Consumer groups may contribute to the creation of new health policy.

- There is a growing awareness that consumers on MSLCs may need to learn new skills to function effectively as representatives; professionals may well also need to learn new skills, to interact with consumers.

- Midwives are potentially great allies for consumers and may well be members of the same consumer groups, or work with consumers on an MSLC.

- MSLCs function with a range of professional and consumer representatives; however, they are not structurally linked into the NHS.

References

Bostock Y: *Pregnancy, childbirth and coping with motherhood: what women want from the maternity services*, Edinburgh, 1993, The Scottish Office CRAG/SCOTMEG Secretariat.

CRAG/SCOTMEG Working Group on Maternity Services: *Antenatal care*, Edinburgh, 1995, HMSO.

Department of Health: *Maternity care in action*, Part 1, London, 1982, HMSO.

Doods R, Goodman M, Tyler S: *Listen with mother, consulting consumers of maternity services*, Cheshire, 1996, Books for Midwives.

Durward L, Evans R: Pressure groups and maternity care. In Garcia J, Kilpatrick R, Richards M, editors: *The politics of maternity care*, Oxford, 1990, Clarendon.

Expert Maternity Group: *Changing childbirth*, London, 1993, Department of Health.

Garel M, Blondel B: Assessment at 1 year of the psychological consequences of having triplets, *Hum Reprod* 7:729, 1992.

Glendinning C. Researching the needs of disabled parents: 2. In Doods R, Goodman M, Tyler S: *Listen with mother, consulting consumers of maternity services*, Cheshire 1996, Books for Midwives.

Ham C: *Health policy in Britain*, 3rd edn, London, 1992, Macmillan.

Holmes A, McGinley N, Turnbull D, *et al.*: A consumer-driven quality assurance model for midwifery, *Br J Midwifery* 10:512, 1996.

House of Commons Health Committee: *Second report: Maternity services*, The Winterton Report, London, 1992, HMSO.

House of Commons Social Services Committee: *Perinatal and neonatal mortality; second report from the Social Services Committee, 1979–1980*, The Short Report, London, 1980, HMSO.

Jones L, Leneman L, Maclean U: *Consumer feedback for the NHS – a literature review*, London, 1987, King Edward's Hospital Fund for London.

Kelson M: *Consumer involvement initiative in clinical audit and outcomes*, London, 1995, College of Health.

Khawaja R. Researching the needs of women from minority groups. In Doods R, Goodman M, Tyler S: *Listen with mother, consulting consumers of maternity services*, Cheshire, 1996, Books for Midwives.

Kitzinger J: Strategies of the early childbirth movement: a case-study of the National Childbirth Trust. In Garcia J, Kilpatrick R. Richards M, editors: *The politics of maternity care*, Oxford, 1990, Clarendon.

Klein R: *Complaints against doctors*, London, 1973, Charles Knight.

Klein R: The politics of ideology vs. the reality of politics: The case of Britain's national health service in the 1980s, *Millbank Memorial Fund Q J* 62(1):82, 1984.

Klein R: *The new politics of the National Health Service*, London, 1995, Longman.

Klein R, Lewis J: *The politics of consumer representation: a study of community health councils*, London, 1976, Centre for Policy Studies.

Lewison H: *Maternity Services Liaison Committees – a forum for change*, London, 1994, National Childbirth Trust.

Lupton C, Buckland S, Moon G: Consumer involvement in health care purchasing: the role and influence of the community health councils. *Health Soc Care Community* 3:215, 1995.

Macintyre S: Consumer reactions to present-day antenatal services. In Zander L, Chamberlain G: *Pregnancy care for the 1980s*, London, 1984, Royal Society of Medicine.

Maternity Action: *Roundabout*, 68:11, 1995.

Morrison I, Smith R: The future of medicine, *Br Med J* 309:1099, 1994.

NHSME: *Local voices, the views of local people in purchasing for health*, London, 1992, Department of Health.

Oakley A: *Women confined*, Oxford, 1980, Martin Robertson.

Oakley A: *Essays on women, medicine and health*, Edinburgh, 1993, Edinburgh University Press.

O'Farrell J. Researching the needs of disabled parents: 1. Doods R, Goodman M, Tyler S: *Listen with mother, consulting consumers of maternity services*, Cheshire, 1996, Books for Midwives.

Peel Report: *Domiciliary midwifery and maternity bed needs: The report of the standing Maternity and Midwifery Advisory Committee*, London, 1970, HMSO.

Phoenix A: Black women and the maternity services. In Garcia J, Kilpatrick R. Richards M, editors: *The politics of maternity care*, Oxford, 1990, Clarendon.

Reid M, Garcia J: Women's views of care during pregnancy and childbirth. In Chalmers, I, Enkin M, Keirse M, editors: *Effective care in pregnancy and childbirth*, Oxford, 1989, Oxford University Press.

Reid M, McMillan M: *Review of consumer views of maternity care*, Clinical Resource and Audit Group Working Party Paper, Edinburgh, 1991, NHS in Scotland.

Renfrew M, McCandlish R: With women: new steps in research in midwifery. In Roberts H, editor: *Women's health matters*, London, 1992, Routledge.

Robinson D, Henry S: *Self-help and health; mutual aid for modern problems*, London, 1977, Martin Robertson.

Scarr R: Running a club, *Twins, triplets and more* 6:2, 1995.

Scottish Office: *Provision of maternity services in Scotland*, Edinburgh, 1993, Scottish Office.

Secretary of State for Health: *The patient's charter*, London, 1991, Department of Health.

SNAP: *Increasing choice in maternity care in Scotland: Issues for purchasers and providers*, Glasgow, 1994, Scottish Forum for Public Health Medicine.

Stacey M: *The sociology of health and healing*, London, 1988, Unwin Hyman.

Tew M: *Safer childbirth; a critical history of maternity care*, London, 1990, Chapman and Hall.

Turnbull D, McGinley M, Holmes A, *et al.*: *The establishment of a midwifery development unit based at Glasgow Royal Maternity Hospital*, Edinburgh, 1995, Scottish Office.

Further Reading

There are very few books which directly address the issues that surround consulting with consumers.

Changing Childbirth Implementation Team: *Maternity Services Liaison Committees*, London, 1996, NHS Executive, Department of Health.

This publication is free from the Health Literature Line, 0800-555-77. Its purpose is to provide advice on ways in which MSLC's can work effectively, taking account of the wishes of local women.

Doods R, Goodman M, Tyler S, editors: *Listen with mother, consulting consumers of the maternity services*, Cheshire, 1996, Books for Midwives.

This is perhaps the most accessible book and very relevant. Chapters within it report not only on whom to consult but make very excellent suggestions about how to consult consumers, an issue which is not dealt with in full detail herein.

Jones L, Leneman L, Maclean U: *Consumer feedback for the NHS - a literature review*, London, 1987, King Edward's Hospital Fund for London.

Although this is a somewhat older book, it is still useful; it reviews the different channels for feedback, feedback appropriate to hospital and community, methodology and special groups. It concludes with complaints procedures.

NHSME: *Local voices, the views of local people in purchasing for health*, London, 1992, Department of Health.

This is a key reference for those interested in the topic. It offers much practical advice on how to consult consumers, emphasizing the difficulties of obtaining views of those consumers and groups of consumers who are less accessible.

19 Developing Midwives for Practice

LEARNING OUTCOMES

After studying this chapter you should be able to:
- Identify your current knowledge, experience and competence.
- Develop a model of your 'ideal' midwife.
- Understand how competence develops over time.
- Prepare a personal action plan for professional development and career progression.

The transition from student to autonomous, accountable midwife practitioner is likely to be one of the most challenging times in a midwife's career. Without careful planning and the formulation of a personal strategy there is a danger that one's career pathway will be haphazard, uncoordinated and the student vision for effective midwifery practice will become lost in the busyness of the world of work. This chapter is designed primarily to assist the student who is nearing course completion to plan effectively for an exciting career in midwifery. It is hoped that others will find it equally helpful.

In the first part of the chapter, the nature of professional knowledge and competence and how to describe the competence necessary to register as a midwife is examined. Following on from this is a dis-

cussion of some of the paradoxes likely to be encountered during midwifery practice. The third section is concerned with the development of professional knowledge, competence and expertise through education. Finally, there is a summary of the career pathways open to practising midwives.

However, before embarking upon a discussion of professional competence it is useful to consider what might be expected of an autonomous professional. Walker (1996) suggests that truly autonomous midwife practitioners are those who practice at an advanced level. This contrasts with the expectations of health-care workers who, at level 2 National Vocational Qualification, are expected to have some autonomy (NCVQ, 1991). Eraut (1994) questions whether one's autonomy is influenced by the degree of subordination to others, which adds weight to Walker's suggestion. Historically, the ideology of professionalism lies in the importance accorded to the professional knowledge base and the control invested in the expert practitioners themselves (Goode, 1969). In this sense professional autonomy implies the creation of boundaries and having and exerting power to protect one's territory.

This philosophical notion does not sit comfortably with woman-centred midwifery care in which control should be given to women and midwives work in partnership with women and members of other professions. Perhaps a more appropriate understanding of professional autonomy for midwives is the freedom invested in them to act on behalf of women and to provide total care for childbearing women. This freedom is not, however, without limits (UKCC, 1993). Midwives need to be conversant with UKCC rules, codes of practice and conduct (UKCC 1992a, 1992b, 1993, 1994) to know when they are free to take decisions, when their own judgement is sufficient and when they need to involve others. The findings of the EME (Effectiveness of Midwifery Education) project (Fraser *et al.* 1997) suggest that being autonomous and free to make decisions is highly stressful. It is easier to follow rules, not freedom, and to feel able to blame others if something goes wrong. Chamberlain (1993) found some midwives used guidelines as though they were rules and ended up constraining the role of the midwife and hence the quality of care given to mothers.

The following therefore intends to provide some guidance on the transition from the somewhat protected world of the student midwife to the challenging world of autonomous midwifery practice and to challenge all midwives to consider:

Where am I now, where will I be and what will I have done for childbearing women and the midwifery profession by the end of my career?

Competence for Practice

The targets of *Changing Childbirth* (Department of Health, 1993) and similar reports relating to the maternity services in Wales (Welsh Office, 1992), Scotland (Scottish Home Office and Health Department, 1993) and Northern Ireland (DHSS, 1994) make it even more imperative that midwives are educated and assessed as competent to provide the care that childbearing women expect. Although UKCC Rule 33 (UKCC, 1993) specifies the required outcomes

of programmes of education that lead to admission to Part 10 of the register, it has been suggested that there is a need to define explicitly what is meant by professional competence (Worth-Butler *et al.* 1995). Before a midwife can exercise accountability she/he must have the ability to take decisions and act upon them. Effective decision-making assumes an acceptable level of knowledge supported by research, essential skills and values. It has been argued that students can only be assessed as having achieved the requirements for competent practice if there is an agreed model of competence in midwifery (Worth Butler *et al.* 1994).

Models of Competence

Page (1993a) suggests that, 'the midwife of the future must balance competent and effective clinical care with a sensitivity to the significance of birth as a life event.' This suggests a two-fold approach, that is clinical skills combined with in-depth knowledge alongside personal qualities such as empathy. The preliminary findings of the EME project, commissioned by the English National Board (ENB; EME Evaluation Project, 1993–1996) identified a tentative three-dimensional model (Fraser *et al.* 1995). It emerged from this study that the midwife needs to integrate a whole variety of abilities to account for the influence of context and time. Each of the three dimensions are closely interlinked (**Figure 19.1**). One or more dimensions might

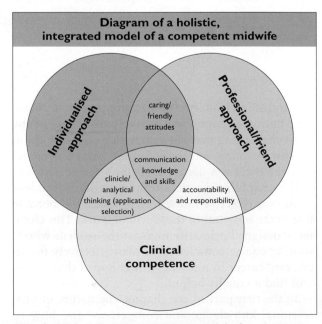

Figure 19.1 A holistic integrated model of a competent midwife (Source: Fraser *et al.* 1995).

be more dominant at any one time to account for a woman's needs at that moment. Writers such as Wilkins (1993), Hutton (1994) and Fraser *et al.* (1996) found that many women are looking for qualities such as friendship in their midwife, one dimension that is not an outcome anticipated in statute (UKCC, 1993). These findings help to demonstrate the value of constructing and using models in midwifery practice (**Box 19.1**), without which there can be a tendency to stress one element to the neglect of others. A woman might find childbirth a very negative experience if her carer is cool and distant, even though knowledgeable, clinically very capable and ensures her birth plan is implemented.

Models, however, are of no use if they are not referred to or are not acceptable to the practitioners concerned. Reflecting upon our own experiences, suggests Schön (1987), as well as on models and ideas put forward by others, can enable midwives to produce their own model of the midwife they think mothers would like them to be (see **Box 19.1**).

Box 19.1

Developing a Model of Competence

One way to do this is to use personal construct laddering as described by Kirkham (1995). In the example (**Figure 19.2**) arising from Kirkham's research she illustrates a 'construct ladder' produced by a midwife 'she would like to be'. By reflecting upon experiences, the midwife was able to differentiate positive and negative aspects and explore her belief systems.

• Use this 'laddering' process to consider why each concept is important to you.

• Reduce each concept, step-by-step, to basic values.

• Reflect upon past experiences to identify which side of the ladder was most evident.

• Consider the model in **Figure 19.1** and decide whether you have deficits in your abilities and take action to develop these.

Kirkham, 1995.

Figure 19.2 One person's personal construct of the 'ideal' midwife ('the midwife I would like to be'; Source: Kirkham, 1995).

Construct	Opposing concept
Listens and observes Can be quiet with women	Talks too much Nervous of silence and of losing control of the conversation
Picks up cues, areas of concern for the woman	Gives expert advice, but misses cues
Helps the woman to open up to specific issues she is worried about	The woman's worries are not elaborated
Plans care with the woman, specific to her needs	Plan of care initiated by the midwife

As our experiences change so might our beliefs and values. It is therefore useful to repeat the construct laddering exercise at stages throughout our careers, to increase our understanding of responses to different events.

Conflicts about Competence

Although a model or definition of competence should facilitate agreement about 'fitness for practice' and eligibility for registration, there can be conflicts about what constitutes 'fitness for purpose' to undertake the work demanded by employers. By recognizing the potential areas of conflict, students are in a better position to address these issues and take positive action before completing their preregistration midwifery education programme. In the literature, professional competence is usually conceptualized in terms of potential to carry out a role effectively (Eraut and Cole, 1993). However, the student approaching registration needs to be aware that some employers might favour a reductionist approach to competence, such as that adopted by the NCVQ (1986). These qualifications require there to be evidence that the award holder has performed each activity in the check list, successfully and satisfactorily. This emphasis on performance to fulfil an employment function (Jessop, 1991) implies an expectation that newly qualified midwives are able to carry out the full range of skills likely to be drawn upon in midwifery practice. This view takes no account of the amount of practice required to achieve competence or of the mental processes or personal qualities necessary to ensure that performance is appropriate and effective. Although students are known to be critical of the 'number counting' to achieve the requirements in the EC Midwives Directive (European Council, 1989), it does ensure that they must have had reasonable opportunities to practice. This minimum amount of 'practice' that has to be guaranteed for eligibility to register (UKCC, 1993) gives Trusts good reason to expect 'fitness for practice' when employing recently qualified midwives.

Although newly qualified midwives might feel they have had sufficient supervised practice to be trusted to take responsibility for a woman's care, their new midwife colleagues might be less trusting. This perceived lack of trust can undermine confidence, but Handy (1995) argues that confidence and trust have to be earned and cannot be ordered. He suggests that we 'need to prove our capabilities and it takes time if people don't know us' (Handy, 1995, p. 126). This situation is more likely to be encountered when the midwife moves away from her/his training institution.

Recently qualified midwives could find themselves in the situation described by Handy (1995) in which they feel overprotected because the team of midwives does not know them or their capabilities. Conversely, there could be those who expect the midwifery education programme to equip new carers for every eventuality and to have tested them in all possible situations. This takes no account of the need to develop knowledge and abilities over time, nor of the importance of experiential wisdom. The majority of midwives are likely to assume that because student midwives have been immersed in 'normal' midwifery they will have sufficient experience to be able to identify when something is 'not quite right' and ask for a second opinion. Achieving the right balance between doing it oneself and seeking advice can be quite difficult.

It has been found that some midwives have unreal expectations of the abilities of newly qualified mid-wives (Fraser, 1994; Maggs and Rapport, 1995; Fraser *et al.* 1997). This inevitably has an adverse effect on their confidence. It is possible that assumptions as to ability are made, based upon each midwife's own education and training – which might be viewed nostalgically. These midwives may fail to appreciate that 'understanding of the context, a sense of priorities, awareness of alternatives, and an ability to predict the consequences of various courses of action' take a long period of time to develop (Eraut, 1990, p. 184).

Recognizing that these conflicts about competence exist and realizing that the protective environment of the education institution is to be exchanged for the role of the autonomous midwife practitioner are first steps in the preparation for transition from student to effective carer. The next section provides some guidelines to assist with this transition

Adapting to Change

It is important to recognize that midwifery is a profession in which there are no concrete answers for every situation, so being autonomous means that on reflection we can also, at times, be wrong. To recognize this is vital. Mistakes are or should be tolerated, provided one learns from them, but too many mistakes erode confidence, particularly if they are mistakes which put the life and/or health of the mother and baby at risk.

Box 19.2

Developing Competence

Consider your model of a competent midwife and ask yourself the following questions:
• What competencies and/or abilities do midwives have that I have not yet achieved?
• Which of these competencies am I most likely to need when practising in:
– community settings,
– hospital settings,
– all settings?
• How crucial is it for me to develop these competencies before registration and/or before working in a team or other settings?
• Where can I achieve these competencies?
• Can I create my own learning opportunities or do I need assistance?

			Table 19.1 Mapping Competence Deficits and Developing an Action Plan		
Element of competence	How crucial	Most likely setting	Potential learning opportunities	Assistance/support needed	Date when achieved
IV injections	Need to be knowledgeable and dextrous	Hospital	Simulation	Personal Teacher	
Blood transfusions	Need to be knowledgeable and able to set up an IVI quickly Need actual experience if possible	Hospital	Look up procedures Knowledge Care for woman	Self Self Ask midwives to call me	
Catheterization	Essential	Hospital School	Revise knowledge Simulation Real practice	Self Self-skills lab Assessor midwife	
Assertiveness	On-going improvement	School Scenarios Hospital	Teachers and peers Increase knowledge Be prepared to challenge if have evidence	 Self-reflection Midwives assessment	
Decision making	On-going improvement	Community Hospital School and practice	Alternate visits with midwife Ask midwife to let me undertake care and tell her my decisions first Case studies	Report back to midwife, discussion and reflection Discussion and reflection with midwife Teachers, midwives, peers	
Confidence	Essential mothers have confidence in me Essential colleagues trust me	Practice School	Identify knowledge deficits and remedy Practice and feedback	Self-assessment Mentor assessment	

One common mistake is to have excessive optimism or unreal expectations of our abilities. It is therefore essential to engage in reflection and self-assessment to identify what has been learned, what needs to be learned before the end of the course and where and how the necessary learning opportunities can be created or grasped. A SWOT (strengths, weaknesses, opportunities, threats) analysis has been found by some to be a useful exercise. It does, however, have limitations. Although identifying strengths and opportunities is a positive strategy, being asked to specify weaknesses and threats can undermine confidence. Learning is a continuum and therefore everyone has learning needs. The activity described in **Box 19.2** may be a more helpful alternative to a SWOT analysis.

Creating a map of incomplete competencies can be a useful way of developing an action plan to achieve them. The examples in **Table 19.1** illustrate some of the deficits cited by one group of students who were approaching course completion.

Paradoxes in Midwifery Practice

One way in which practitioners might be able to cope more effectively with the transition from student to midwife, or when changing jobs, is to accept that paradox is a feature of our lives. Those who are able to learn to use paradoxes and make sense of them are those who will find life more liveable, as Handy says:

Life will never be easy, nor perfectible, nor completely predictable. It will be best understood backwards, but we have to live it forwards.

(Handy, 1995, p. 18.)

Most people in the developed countries have come to expect a 'perfect' outcome from every pregnancy, but it is not that easy to predict. This sense of knowledge with hindsight was part of the reason for the move to 100% hospital confinement and urgency felt by some to manage labours actively (O'Driscoll and Meagher, 1980). Women have challenged the assumption that hospitalization and active management are the safest options. Trusts are required to develop strategies to achieve the woman-centred vision supported in all four UK countries. The three 'C's in the reports from these countries provide a useful framework to consider some of the paradoxes midwives need to face as part of their everyday practices – choice, control and continuity.

Choice

Choice itself is a paradox because the freedom to choose implies the freedom to make a wrong choice. As a midwife teacher expecting my first baby I thought I was well-enough informed to make sound choices. On reflection I believe I chose wrongly, but as there is not the opportunity to re-run events with different interventions I will not know for certain. How, then, can the new midwife enable women to make informed choices? The Informed Choice Initiative leaflets (MIDIRS and the NHS Centre for Reviews and Dissemination, University of York, 1996), should provide an invaluable source of information both to women and the professionals who care for them. Unfortunately, Henderson (1996) cites evidence that many Trusts have chosen not to purchase them. With such a tremendous information explosion it has been recognized that practitioners do not have immediately all the answers to a woman's questions. What is important is that midwives seek out the information and provide evidence for the women in a usable form. These information leaflets and other resources such as the Cochrane Library, The Midwives Information and Resource Services (MIDIRS) and The Midwifery Research Database (MIRIAD) leave midwives with little excuse not to provide women with the most up-to-date current knowledge on which to base their choices for care.

Control

Wang (1995) and Lawson (1995) suggest that women must be empowered to feel in control of their pregnancy and labour, but empowerment can be a misused and abused term. How much control do women want? Does empowerment also imply the ability to disempower if we do not like the choices a woman wants to make. Midwives might themselves feel the paradox of control when they are expected to be both more autonomous and yet more of a team, or when the NHS appears to be more delegating and yet also exerts more control. Control and power can be liberating and yet constraining; how, therefore, does the new midwife know the extent of her power to influence? Page (1993a) asserts that we can only find

power if we believe in what we are doing, are skilled, knowledgeable and committed to midwifery and the needs of childbearing women. It is particularly important to find a balance between what we can and must do, grasping opportunities that will make a difference for childbearing women. It is easy to hide behind rules and regulations, but while some control is necessary it is essential to take the initiative when required and demonstrate 'passion aligned with reason' (Page, 1993b, p. 83). The questions in **Box 19.3** can help us think about the proper balance between procedures and flexibility, provided that at all times the safety of mothers and babies is the prime goal.

Continuity

It is said that continuity of carer avoids duplication of care and conflicting advice, and increases women's satisfaction (Department of Health, 1993). In spite of this there is evidence that such change is being implemented slowly in some parts of the country (Beckmann, 1996). Perhaps one of the problems is failure to consider the paradox of time. Although we have more aids to save us time and we live longer, we never seem to find enough time. Midwives frequently have family responsibilities which make demands upon their time. An important challenge for midwives is to consider the balance of time needed to provide continuity of care for women and continuity of family life and friendships. Just as much planning is needed to balance time once qualified as to balance

---

Box 19.3

Balancing Choice and Control

A woman is expecting her second baby in January, her first baby having been delivered by forceps for fetal distress. The little girl is now 2 years old and the family lives in a 'yurt' (tent-like dwelling) in a farmer's field. The parents want their second baby to be born at home. The yurt is the sleeping accommodation, it has a solid floor. Cooking and toilet facilities are provided in a nearby van. The team midwives are divided about supporting this family in their choice of place of birth.

• Consider your immediate response to this request.
• In the light of research think about the reasons that the team midwives might have for their passionately held but different views.
• How would you seek to resolve the issues?

activities when a student. It can be easy to 'make time' for things we want to do and suggest there is 'not enough time' for others. If new midwives are not to lose their vision of meeting the challenges of changing childbirth it is essential not to become socialized into conforming to the norms of an organization (Giddens, 1993) that has no vision for the future of midwifery practice and uses lack of time and resources as an excuse.

Developing Knowledge and Competence

Perhaps one of the most important decisions or concerns following registration as a midwife is the first job (Maggs and Rapport, 1995). For some, choice is limited because of family commitments, but for those free to travel it is important to choose a 'learning organization' as described by Argyris and Schön (1978). In such an organization there is evidence of reflective practice, innovation and a willingness to learn from experience. Personal experience has found that critical, analytical competent students who move to organizations that are resistant to change stagnate or fail to push the profession and midwifery care forwards. The power of socialization and adaptation to the norm of the majority should not therefore be underestimated. It is likely to take greater determination and initiative to push midwifery forwards if developing knowledge and competence is not made an important priority by the organization.

Preceptorship

From April 1993 the UKCC determined that a 4-month period of support and preceptorship is essential for all newly registered practitioners and those who return to practice. The need for preceptors for midwives was initially challenged, but after additional clarification that it 'should not in any way influence the grade the practitioner is employed in, as they are still accountable' (UKCC, 1995) preceptorship has been widely accepted as a good practice. There is no suggestion that a newly qualified midwife is not equipped to take on the full responsibilities of a caseload, but the transition from student to autonomous carer can be stressful and support is likely to be needed (Maggs and Rapport, 1995; Fraser *et al.*). The preceptor should ensure that excessive responsibilities are not given to the inexperienced midwife and recognize that competence is progressive rather than achieved once and for all. Eraut (1994) suggests that time and speed in professional work are important aspects when considering a carer's 'fitness for purpose'.

One element of a midwife's role that students might have limited opportunity to practise is to manage time effectively when competing demands are encountered. Students generally have the luxury of concentrating on one task at a time or caring for only one woman during a shift. The ability to prioritize and handle competing demands effectively is learned over time and, argues Benner (1984), is normally experientially developed. The preceptor therefore has a vital role in offering feedback and advice to the new midwife. Eraut (1994, p. 149) describes this development of professional expertise as 'the link between speed and mode of cognition.' The top row of **Figure 19.3** illustrates the distinction between instant, rapid and deliberative ways of analysing a case or situation. There is then a period of decision making which follows a similar pattern. Finally, the bottom row illustrates Eraut's (1994) interpretation of the work of Schön (1987). Eraut (1989, 1990) has also argued that during a typical day at work a professional is likely to make many more rapid decisions than deliberative, but is also required to change actions in response to unforeseen events. These actions must be communicated effectively. Given the demands made upon professionals, deliberation in the workplace could be squeezed out unless it is specifically scheduled into the day's work. The preceptor therefore has a responsibility to the midwife to develop the discipline of regularly reflecting upon performance, even though formal assessment is no longer required.

		speed	
analysts	instant recognition	rapid interpretation	deliberative analysis
decision	instant response	rapid decisions	deliberative decisions
action	routinized unreflective action	action monitored by reflection	action after a period of deliberation

Figure 19.3 The link between speed and mode of cognition (Source: Eraut, 1994).

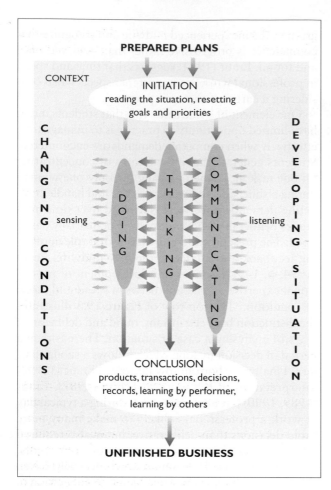

Figure 19.4 Activities during a performance period (Source: Eraut, 1994)

| Box 19.4 |

Goals for the Period of Preceptorship

The following suggested goals could form the basis of negotiating an action plan with your preceptor:

• Develop confidence in decision making.

    Action:

• Become more independent of support and advice.

    Action:

• Learn and practise skills.

    Specifically:

• Extend competence over a wider range of situations and contexts.

    Action:

• Develop expertise in responding rapidly or deliberately through correct reading of situations.

    Reflection and feedback

This reflection should also include drawing upon the expertise of more experienced colleagues to add to the quality of the learning process.

Eraut (1994) also describes a model of a typical performance period to illustrate the resetting of goals and priorities based upon the correct reading of situations (**Figure 19.4**). As midwives try to offer women more choices for care they could face situations such as being in the middle of an antenatal clinic when a woman phones to say she is in labour. A whole range of factors need to be considered before appropriate actions can be taken. Of importance for the new midwife is to understand that being able to do this effectively comes with experience, so the time of preceptorship needs to be used effectively to build upon student learning. The formulation of goals and development of an action plan enables the preceptorship to be used efficiently and systematically (**Box 19.4**).

Post preceptorship

Once the formal period of support is complete new midwives have the same responsibilities as all their colleagues to continue with their personal and professional development. The local institution that provides midwifery education programmes should continue to be an important source of advice; in England the approved midwife teacher has a specific role in providing for the continuing education needs of midwives. In addition, the designated Supervisor of Midwives should collaborate with the Head of Midwifery Education to provide suitable educational events and be available to help midwives 'evaluate their practice, identifying areas for development and the means by which expertise can be maintained and strengthened' (Mayes, 1995, p. 35). There has always been a statutory requirement for midwives to attend a refresher course every 5 years to assist with the updating process, but from April 1995 the requirements for statutory refreshment changed and now include nurses as well.

Statutory requirements for maintaining registration

Before the UKCC PREP (Post-Registration Education and Practice) legislation coming into force, midwives had to select National Board approved refresher courses to comply with statute. This provided a quality control mechanism to ensure that the refresher activities were appropriate for the needs of midwives. Under the new legislation the responsibility for ensuring appropriateness rests with the practitioner. Furneaux (1995, p. 34) advises practitioners or midwives to check whether the continuing professional education events are 'appropriate and cost effective, meet contract specifications and ... evaluated for fitness for purpose.'

However, midwives do not necessarily have to attend formal education events and the following highlights the specific requirements under PREP:

- Maintain a personal, professional profile which demonstrates that you have retained and developed your professional knowledge and competence.
- Undertake the equivalent of at least 5 days of study during each 3-year registration period. The study must be relevant to your practice and the UKCC has defined five categories that it believes cover all appropriate areas of practice:
– reduce risk, e.g. health problem identification, protection of individuals, health promotion and screening,
– care enhancement, e.g. developments in practice, standard setting, empowering women,
– patient, client and colleague support, e.g. counselling, leadership, supervision,
– practice development, e.g. exchange visits, personal research and study,
– education development, e.g. teaching and learning skills.
- Complete a 'Notification of Practice' form, giving details of your qualifications and area of practice, when renewing your UKCC registration. This is in addition to the midwives' annual 'Notification of Intention to Practise'.
- Submit your profile for audit if requested.

Profiling

There is a vast array of commercially produced profiles on the market, but it is not necessary to purchase one of these. A ring binder and a set of dividers can be more useful as the file can be ordered in your own style and entries can be word processed more easily. There are many advantages in maintaining a personal, professional profile, but it does need to be regularly added to and updated otherwise it ceases to be useful (*see* Critten, 1996).

Advantages
- Could be used for nonstandard entry to courses or for credit towards a course (advanced standing).
- Readily available curriculum vitae for job applications.

- Personal development through reflection.
- Systematic self-assessment and educational guidance.
- Assists long-term planning.

Items to include in the profile
- Personal details.
- Summary of academic achievement.
- Summary of professional education.
- Summary of employment and career history.
- Record of each learning activity undertaken to meet the UKCC requirements for 5 study days.
- Record of all other professional development.
- Action plan for maintaining and developing professional knowledge and competence.
- Section for certificates, testimonials.
- Section for evidence to claim accreditation of prior learning (APL) or accreditation of prior experiential learning (APEL).

APL and APEL

APL is often possible when applying for courses which have elements that might have been done elsewhere. If the course matches and there is evidence of equivalence, then exemption from certain units or modules might be given. APEL is more complex. For example, a carer may have undertaken specific work which appears to equate to the demands of an element of a longer course. The course leader cannot, however, just accept the midwife's word that she/he has done this piece of work. It is necessary to demonstrate the underpinning knowledge and understanding of any relevant research associated with the work, explain what has been learned from doing the work and how it was assessed or evaluated. Evidence of authenticity, relevance, appropriate depth and breadth and recency are required before credit is likely to be awarded. For those who consider registering for a recordable qualification, such as the ENB Higher Award, then APL and APEL form an important component as repetitive learning should be avoided. Claims for credit are cross-checked against outcomes of the programme.

ENB Framework and Higher Award

In an endeavour to enable midwives to plan their continuing professional development, the ENB has produced a framework to assist with the planning process. For those who wish to achieve a professionally focused academic award, the Higher Award is an English National Board recordable qualification.

The Framework

The ENB Framework was designed following a research study concerned with analysing the training needs of nurses, midwives and health visitors (ENB, 1991). The key characteristics were identified as representing the key areas of knowledge, skill and expertise which all practitioners should have. The framework provides a systematic way for midwives to identify their professional development needs. It also promotes reflection upon practice as individuals self-assess whether they have achieved the learning outcomes listed for each characteristic of health care practitioners. Obviously, these outcomes are generic in nature, so the midwife needs to adapt them to the sphere of practice of the midwife. The adaptation of the 10 key characteristics in **Box 19.5** may provide useful page headings for a midwife's portfolio of evidence.

Higher Award

Institutions have developed a variety of ways in which midwives can demonstrate eligibility for the ENB Higher Award and a University Degree. It is important to appreciate that it is a Higher Award in the field of midwifery, so there must be evidence of development as a midwife practitioner. Credits from a pre-registration programme have only partial currency. The midwife who presents a portfolio of evidence for the Higher Award must demonstrate an increased knowledge and understanding of theories and research that underpin midwifery practice and show how this has made a difference to their care of mothers and babies.

Although it is possible for many of the learning outcomes of the Higher Award to be demonstrated through APL or APEL claims, because the ENB Award is combined with a university award, the regulations of the awarding institution have to be met as well. A total of 360 credits are required for an Honours Degree, as illustrated in **Box 19.6**.

In some instances there is a limit on the number of credits that can be counted from an APL or APEL claim. Most universities appear to accept credit accumulation and transfer (CAT) from the preregistration programme for Level One. That is, 120 Level One CAT points are the equivalent of the first year of an undergraduate degree programme. Claiming credit at Level Two (standard required during the second year of a degree programme) is extremely variable between universities, so it is worth finding out what the rules are for a particular institution before making a formal application. As most degree classifications are based upon the standard of work achieved in the third year, many institutions are reluctant to allow credits to be transferred at Level Three. This is because the university expects their external examiner to be involved in the assessment of degree level work and to agree the final classification. In this way each university believes it can safeguard its own standards. It is likely, therefore, that midwives who would like to register for the ENB Higher Award and University Degree will have to do at least one-third of their programme with the awarding university. There are,

---

Box 19.5

A Framework for Continuing Development

Use the following headings to create a page in your portfolio of evidence:
1. Professional Issues and Autonomous Practice.
2. Midwifery Expertise and Evaluation of Care.
3. Research.
4. Team Working.
5. Innovation and Management of Change.
6. Health Education/Promotion.
7. Teaching and Assessing.
8. Communication.
9. Management/Decision Making.
10. Using Information Technology.

• On each page, review your abilities and identify your priorities for continuing education.

• When you have identified your priorities for development, look to see whether there are appropriate modular programmes accessible to you that would fill the gaps in learning to meet women's needs more effectively.

• Discuss with your supervisor of midwives the sort of activities that you could participate in.

Box 19.6

Credits required for Honours Degree

A total of 360 Credits are needed for an Honours Degree:
• 120 Credits at Level One (equivalent to the first year of a full-time 3-year undergraduate degree programme).
• 120 Credits at Level Two (equivalent to the second year of a full-time 3-year undergraduate degree programme).
• 120 Credits at Level Three (equivalent to the third year of a full-time 3-year undergraduate degree programme).

however, exceptions – university regulations are specific to each university and its individual programmes.

As more midwives are undertaking degree-level programmes that lead to registration, it is becoming less appropriate to offer the Higher Award at first degree level. For this reason some institutions now offer the Higher Award at Masters level for experienced midwives. Again the professional portfolio is an essential source of evidence to demonstrate the midwife's potential to learn and succeed at Masters level. It is likely, however, that diploma, first degree and masters courses will continue to be available for the reasonably foreseeable future to meet the varying needs of midwives.

Career Pathways

The UKCC (1994) has described two levels for practitioners to achieve beyond registration. The first of these, specialist level practice, is not relevant to midwives because, at the point of registration, they must have achieved the outcomes prescribed for specialist practitioners. Midwives are, however, included in the level of advanced practice and it is suggested that preparation for this must be at Masters level. Sisto and Hillier (1996) argue that advanced practitioners must be experts themselves and will also need to draw upon the expertise of their colleagues to act as a catalyst to influence the development of midwifery practice at the organizational level. This view is not held by all midwives (Editorials, 1996). There are some who see advanced practitioners as those with all-round clinical midwifery expertise and the intellectual and interpersonal skills to advance their practice. Alternatively, others would appoint advanced practitioners if they have particular skills and expertise in an area such as high dependency intrapartum care. Some midwives expect advanced practitioners to be a sort of expert midwife consultant, but with a non-hierarchical function, such as a supervisor of midwives who is not a manager. It is likely that the debate surrounding advanced practitioners will continue, especially as trusts may formulate very different job descriptions. Each midwife no doubt has her/his own perspective, but it is still essential to weigh the arguments and plan for one's own future development. Many academic awards in midwifery are now available through taught programmes, distance learning programmes and research degrees. Selection of continuing education activities needs to be made alongside the career pathways being considered as long-term goals.

Expert practitioner

This could possibly be an experienced midwife who leads a team or a group practice of midwives, as well as having a case load. Alternatively, a midwife could become an expert in a particular area of practice, such as in ultrasound or fetomaternal medicine, or a core hospital staff team member who has responsibility to provide advice and support to colleagues when a woman requires particularly complex care.

Midwife researcher

Although all midwives must use research effectively in their practice, it takes time to develop research skills. It is therefore essential that some midwives spend a significant part of their time undertaking research and helping to develop research skills in colleagues. A common misunderstanding is that researchers are experts in all fields, from randomized controlled trials to ethnographic or naturalistic studies. This is rarely the case, so what is important is for there to be a variety of expertise among midwife researchers so that appropriate skills and methodological approaches can be drawn upon as necessary.

Midwifery education

To pursue a career in education, midwives must be experienced practitioners (at least 3 years full-time equivalent) and have been involved in teaching and assessing students in midwifery practice areas. To be accepted onto an approved course for the preparation of midwife teachers, applicants must be graduates and have studied midwifery at a higher level. Although most midwife teachers are now employed by universities, they are also likely to hold an honorary contract to continue to practise as midwives. Although some midwife teachers carry a caseload, Chesney (1995) has developed this further and includes students as her co-lead professionals.

Midwifery supervision

Supervisors of midwives have an important statutory responsibility to promote and safeguard the health and well-being of mothers and babies. The preparation of a supervisor's programme is a distance learning programme with tutor and/or counsellor and supervisor and/or mentor support. Each supervising authority provides guidelines for effective supervision in their geographical area – midwives are normally nominated for this role by their own supervisor of midwives.

Management

Midwives who demonstrate expertise in management may wish to become midwifery managers or managers of the maternity services. It is, however, essential that some midwives follow a general management career pathway so that the specific needs of mothers and babies are not omitted when Trust Boards engage in strategic planning.

Conclusion

Although these five major career pathways appear mutually exclusive, many midwives combine these areas of expertise. Examples include lecturer–practitioner, researcher–clinical expert, supervisor–manager and an integration of all these for work overseas. This chapter begins with a consideration of the challenge of change from student to midwife. It ends with the challenge for every practising midwife to have a vision for the future so that opportunities are grasped to develop and advance your practise. This needs to be done in collaboration with colleagues, to encourage and take them with you so that at the end of your career you can look back and reflect on the difference you made for childbearing women.

KEY CONCEPTS

- The transition from student to autonomous, accountable midwife practitioner is challenging and exciting, but requires planning to enhance development as a midwife.

- Professional knowledge and competence develop over time – supporting and learning from and with each other and from childbearing women is essential to advance midwifery practice; it does not imply a loss of autonomy.

- Midwives need to integrate a whole variety of abilities to account for the influence of context and time; constructing a model of competence can help avoid emphasis in one area to the neglect of others.

- Midwifery practice situations at times requires intuitive responses which draw upon prior knowledge, experiences and adaptability. Deliberative reflection 'out of the action' needs to be scheduled in or it can be squeezed out.

- Career pathways need to be planned to assist in the selection of appropriate education events and practice-based learning opportunities.

- A regularly updated personal profile enhances the learning process, as well as being a statutory requirement.

References

Argyris C, Schön D: *Organisational learning*, London, 1978, Addison-Waley.

Beckmann C: Guide to maternity services, *Changing Childbirth Update* 5:13, 1996.

Benner P: *From novice to expert: Excellence and power in clinical nursing practice*, Menlo Park, 1984, Addison-Wesley.

Chamberlain M: Strategies used by midwives for teaching their skills to midwifery students. In: *International Congress of Midwives 23*, International Congress Proceedings, Vol. 1: p. 375, Vancouver, 1993 International Congress of Midwives.

Chesney M: Midwife teacher carrying a caseload: a personal account, *Br J Midwifery* 3(12):661, 1995.

Critten P: *Developing your professional portfolio*, Edinburgh, 1996, Churchill Livingstone.

Department of Health: *The report of the expert maternity group: Changing childbirth*, London, 1993, HMSO.

DHSS: *Delivering choice: Midwife and GP led maternity units*, Reports of the Northern Ireland Maternity Units Study Group, Belfast, 1994, HMSO.

Editorials: What constitutes an advanced practising midwife? and What is an advanced midwifery practitioner? *Br J Midwifery* 4(4):174, 1996.

ENB: *Framework for continuing professional education for nurses, midwives and health visitors: guide to implementation*, London, 1991, ENB.

ENB: *Creating lifelong learners: partnerships for care*, London, 1994, ENB.

Eraut M: Initial teaching training and the NVQ model. In Burke JW, editor: *Competency based education and training*, pp. 171–185, Lewes, 1990, The Falmer Press.

Eraut M: *Developing professional knowledge and competence*, London, 1994, The Falmer Press.

Eraut M, Cole G: *Assessing competence in the professions*, Sheffield, 1993, Employment Department.

European Council: Midwives Directives, EC Council Directive 89/594/EEC Article 27 Chapter 5, *Official Journal of the European Communities* L341/28, 1989.

Fraser DM: *Evaluation of the non-midwifery placements in a three year pre-registration midwifery education programme*, unpublished MPhil thesis, Nottingham, 1994, University of Nottingham.

Fraser, DM, Murphy RJL, Worth-Butler M: *Second Interim Report of the EME Evaluation Project to the English National Board for Nursing, Midwifery and Health Visiting*, unpublished report, Nottingham, 1995, University of Nottingham.

Fraser DM, Murphy RJL, Worth-Butler M: Developing a model of competence in midwifery: The consumer's perspective, *Br J Midwifery* I4(11): 576, 1996.

Fraser DM, Murphy RJL, Worth-Butler M: *An outcome evaluation of the effectiveness of pre-registration midwifery programmes of education (the EME Project)*, Final Report to the ENB, London, 1997, ENB.

Furneaux N: Achieving professional empowerment through education. In *ENB midwifery educational resource pack 2.5*, London, 1995, ENB.

Giddens A: *Sociology*, Cambridge, 1993, Polity Press.

Goode WJ: The theoretical limits of professionalization. In Etzioni A, editor: *The semi-professions and their organisation*, pp. 266–313, New York, 1969, Free Press.

Handy C: *The empty raincoat. Making sense of the future*, Reading, 1995, Arrow Books Limited.

Henderson C: Prioritising the priorities: is there a choice? *Br J Midwifery* 4(3):117, 1996.

Hutton E: What women want from midwives, *Br J Midwifery* 2(12):608, 1994.

Jessop G: *Outcomes, NVQs and the emerging model of education and training*, London, 1991, The Falmer Press.

Kirkham M: Using personal planning to meet the challenge of changing childbirth. In *ENB midwifery resource pack 1.3*, London, 1995, ENB.

Lawson M: Building partnerships with women and their families, In *ENB midwifery resource pack 2.6*, London, 1995, ENB.

Maggs C, Rapport F: *Getting a job and growing in confidence*, A report to the Department of Health, Bath, 1995, MRA Limited.

Mayes G: Supervisors of midwives How can we facilitate change? In *ENB midwifery educational resource pack 5.4*, London, 1995, ENB.

NCVQ: *The National Council for Vocational Qualifications: Its purposes and its aims*, London, 1986, NCVQ.

NCVQ: *Criteria for National Vocational Qualifications*, London, 1991, NCVQ.

O'Driscoll K, Meagher D: Active management of labour, London, 1980, WB Saunders.

Page L: Redefining the midwife's role: changes needed in practice, *Br J Midwifery* 1(1):21, 1993a.

Page L: Midwives hear the heartbeat of the future. In *Keynote Addresses, ICM 23*, International Congress, 75-86, Vancouver, 1993b, London, 1993, ICM.

Schön D: *Educating the reflective practitioner: towards a new design for teaching and learning in the professions*, San Francisco, 1987, Jossey-Bass.

Scottish Home Officer and Health Department: *Provision of maternity services in Scotland–- a policy review*, Edinburgh, 1993, HMSO.

Sisto S, Hillier D: Advanced midwifery practice: myth and reality, *Br J Midwifery* 4(4):179, 1996.

UKCC: *The scope of professional practice*, London, 1992a, UKCC.

UKCC: *Code of professional conduct*, London, 1992b, UKCC.

UKCC: *Midwives rules*, London, 1993, UKCC.

UKCC: *The future of professional practice – the council's standards for education and practice following registration*, London, 1994, UKCC.

UKCC: *Registrar's letter*, March, 1995, UKCC.

Walker J: The need for ten key characteristics. Editorial, *Br J Midwifery* 4(4):177, 1996.

Wang M: Communication and negotiation, the consumer's view. In *ENB Midwifery resource pack 2.3*, London, 1995, ENB.

Welsh Office: *The protocol for investment in health gain*, Cardiff, 1992, HMSO.

Wilkins R: *Sociological aspects of the mother/community midwife*, unpublished PhD thesis, Surrey, 1993, University of Surrey.

Worth-Butler M, Murphy RJL, Fraser DM: Towards an integrated model of competence in midwifery, *Midwifery* 4(10):225, 1994.

Worth-Butler M, Murphy RJL, Fraser DM: Recognising competence in midwifery, *Br J Midwifery* 3(5):259, 1995.

Further Reading

Although many very appropriate texts could be offered to those readers who want further reading to guide and stimulate their thinking and professional development, the following are particularly recommended.

Bryar R: *Theory for midwifery practice*, London, 1995, Macmillan.

This book provides as an analysis of the contributions made by theorists from an international perspective, but ensures a grounding in midwifery practice. The summaries and activities are helpful whether or not the reader is doing an assessed midwifery course.

Critten P: *Developing your professional portfolio*, Edinburgh, 1996, Churchill Livingstone.

This ring binder contains a self-contained module plus Reader in the PDQ Series (Professional Development for Quality Care). It provides very comprehensive information on many aspects of professional development and competence as well as clearly designed exercises. For those who have limited access to a well-resourced library or education department, it provides a well-structured, directed learning resource for the self-disciplined practitioner.

Palmer A, Burns S, Bulman C: *Reflective practice in nursing*: The *growth of the professional practitioner*, Oxford, 1994, Blackwell Science.

Although specifically related to nursing, this book has practical application to midwifery, provides student, mentor and education perspectives and is a useful additional text to supplement the much quoted Donald Schön.

NHSE: *Testing the vision: A report on progress in the first year of 'A vision for the future' April 1993–April 1994*, London, 1994, Department of Health.

A report from the Chief Nursing Officer to Parliamentary Under Secretary of State (Baroness Cumberlege) on progress in nursing, midwifery and health visiting since the launch of The Vision. *Especially good in relation to individualized nursing and midwifery care, clinical practice and research. 5 catagories laid out as:*

- *quality, outcomes and audit;*
- *accountability for practice;*
- *clinical and professional leadership, research and supervision;*
- *purchasing;*
- *education and personal development.*

20 *Interpersonal Skills*

LEARNING OUTCOMES

After studying this chapter you should be able to:

- Recognize those factors besides language which you use to communicate.
- Consider what you're trying to communicate, and how it is perceived by others.
- Evaluate your listening skills.
- Express your thoughts and ideas more clearly.
- Demonstrate an awareness of understanding, empathy and counselling techniques.
- Recognize factors which enhance or impede communications.
- Discuss the application to midwifery practice of effective interpersonal skills.

Interpersonal skills are the means by which people communicate with each other. They involve more than just talking and listening. The term 'interpersonal skills' is used frequently, without the meaning being fully understood. Scan the careers section of any newspaper and you find that good 'interpersonal skills' are required for a range of positions, from salespeople to receptionists.

What the potential employer is trying to ascertain is whether an applicant can communicate well and put people at ease. The midwife must possess much more complex and sophisticated skills than this, as she must be able to perform both these tasks, interpret subtleties in language and understand. The midwife uses a complex mix of skills, including effective listening, skilful use and recognition of language and using and observing subtle aspects of behaviour, known as body language. These skills enable the midwife to understand, interpret and communicate, and so foster the development of a midwife–client relationship that is caring, nurturing and supportive.

Throughout their careers, midwives find themselves

working in many different environments. Sometimes they form midwife–client relationships that are long-lasting as they care for women and their families through many pregnancies and over many years.

These relationships may develop slowly and evolve over time, as do relationships with colleagues and other professionals. However, there are always situations in which a midwife is called upon to care for a woman she has never met, such as when called to an emergency. In such an instance, the midwife–client relationship needs to be developed quickly, which requires complex and sophisticated skills. Hunt and Symonds (1995) noted how quickly midwives who work in a delivery suite could form relationships with labouring women whom they had not previously met. In such cases, midwives appear to possess advanced interpersonal skills. Consider observing the midwife(s) with whom you work. List those skills and techniques that you consider enhance or diminish the relationship between midwife and client [referring to Hunt and Symonds (1995) may help you to identify these techniques].

New entrants to the midwifery profession already have interpersonal skills. As they are mature adults with unique life experiences they already possess many of the personal qualities described earlier, such as compassion, caring, listening, language, communication and skills.

Many disciplines, including linguistics, counselling and teaching, have attempted to understand the processes involved in interpersonal skills. Many of these areas overlap so the student midwife will benefit from examining a range to develop his/her own unique and effective style. In this chapter, current theories on interpersonal skills are examined. These may assist the midwife to understand why sometimes the best intentions at communication fail to produce the desired results.

Apart from survival, which requires communication with others to maximize safety and food production, interpersonal skills also enable socializing and socialization: i.e. the processes through which individuals learn the rules and 'norms' of their society. Each individual belongs to many communities – family, racial, work, religious and/or special interest groups. Behaviour and communication may be of a different type and level, depending on the culture of the group. The midwife has to become skilful at recognizing, understanding and respecting cultural differences between women. She can then adapt her communication skills in a flexible way, to facilitate the midwife–client relationship.

Communication is also a vehicle for power, especially when linked to knowledge. Facial expression and body language can maintain the power differential and make communication between mothers and midwives a hierarchical discourse. In this chapter, the influence of power and status on interpersonal skills is explored further, as is how midwives may inadvertently send and/or receive mixed messages. In some aspects of midwifery it is necessary for communication to be used to empathize with the woman, when the skills are those of caring, nurturing and supporting the mother, whereas at other times the mother may need the midwife to be her advocate and be powerful for her. These varying roles require different approaches from the midwife, so if she understands the diversity of interpersonal skills and their effect on those around her, she can select the most appropriate mix for each situation.

Body Language

Human beings were communicating with each other long before they developed sophisticated spoken languages. Archaeological study shows that primitive humans shared food and cooking utensils, and lived together in small communities, probably depending upon each other for food and protection. To do this they must have communicated. They possibly depended on facial expression, eye contact, body movements (posture, attitude, signing or pointing and other gestures) and touch to convey messages such as danger, hunger, pain; and emotions such as fear, love, happiness and sadness. This form of communication is still used today, for example in situations where people cannot speak the language, such as travelling abroad. The skills described are complex and are often termed 'body language', as they can be as subtle and sophisticated as any spoken language. Imagine that you are in a situation where no-one can understand your language. Try to convey your need for a lavatory or a bank! Note your feelings and any techniques that you could employ. This could be useful to remember if you are caring for a woman who does not speak your language.

Actions

Anthropologist Desmond Morris (1989) has studied human body language. He subdivides body language into five categories of actions:

- Inborn actions are those we do not have to learn. Morris (1989) states:

  People all around the world perform a rapid eyebrow-flash action when greeting. The eyebrows are momentarily raised and then lowered. Even though it does not provide conclusive proof, the global distribution of this facial movement strongly suggests that the action is inborn.

- Discovered actions are those we discover for ourselves, such as arm folding.
- Absorbed actions are those we acquire unknowingly from our companions – gestures and postures that may be group-specific or culture-specific.
- Trained actions are those we have to be taught, such as winking.
- Mixed actions acquired in several ways, such as leg-crossing which is a discovered action, but as women grow older they may be taught that one way is more 'feminine' than another and so the action becomes modified.

Not everyone agrees with Morris's view. The issues are pertinent to the 'nature versus nurture' debate. In other words, how much of human behaviour is learned and how much is inherited or instinct? Anthropologists, psychologists and sociologists have various theories on this topic so the student midwife will find further reading in this area of great interest.

In describing absorbed actions, Morris (1989) implies that people are like sponges that absorb all behaviour. He does not allow for choice, yet some actions are 'chosen' in the sense that we deliberately imitate someone whom we admire and respect (a role model), whereas other actions are ignored. We may also become conditioned to perform some actions under certain circumstances, similar to a reflex action, such as returning a smile. The smile is one of the first conditioned responses that humans learn – midwifery students will have ample opportunity to observe the processes by which new mothers teach their infants to smile on cue!

It is particularly important to note that different cultures and subcultures have different body languages. Some actions can have more than one meaning within a culture. For example, we generally understand a 'thumbs-up' may signify 'yes' or 'OK', yet anyone who undertakes deep-sea diving quickly learns that underwater it means you wish to return to the surface! Some actions are specific to one culture and inappropriate in another culture. Gestures are a good example of this. Using the thumb and forefinger to form a ring is a gesture with only one meaning in Britain – 'OK'. Yet Morris (1989) describes many meanings for the same gesture, one of which in Greece or Sardinia is an obscene insult. It would be prudent for midwives to remember this when caring for women from cultures different to theirs, as gestures that we may perform almost unwittingly could have deleterious effects.

Once an awareness of body language has been developed, the midwife may apply these skills to gain insight and understanding of the women she cares for. Besides developing the midwife–client relationship, understanding body language can assist the midwife in anticipating women's needs.

Experienced midwives can often tell if a woman is in established labour or not by just looking at her, or whether the cervix is fully dilated and the second stage of labour imminent. How can they do this? They are observing subtle changes in the woman's body language – her posture, the position she 'naturally' adopts, the sounds she is making, her facial expression, her breathing or other actions such as toe-curling. Subtle changes in any of these can signal to the midwife that a woman is advancing in labour, and so allow the midwife to offer additional care and support before the woman asks. This is interpreted by women as sensitiveness in the midwife – the ability to judge what the woman wants before she knows that she wants it! It is interesting to note that a similar 'sensitiveness' has been observed in some new mothers, as when the mother anticipates the baby's needs before the baby resorts to crying (Bell and Ainsworth, 1972). It is suggested that their babies appear more content and cry less.

It may be useful at this point to consider the expectations that the client has of the midwife before they meet, as body language plays an important part in forming first impressions.

Most women expect a certain standard of professional behaviour, as we expect certain standards from other professionals. For example, we expect a solicitor to be polite, welcoming, knowledgeable and have time to listen and advise on our problem. The woman expects similar behaviour from her midwife. If the midwife appears to be short of time, brusque and avoids eye contact, the relationship can be strained.

In your role as midwife, you will be conscious of modifying your behaviour to suit the task(s) you are to perform. The midwife can use appropriate body language to convey to the woman that she is attentive and approachable. She can do this by relaxed body posture, good eye contact, smiling, use of head nods, etc., and as the relationship develops your personal style becomes apparent to the woman.

The midwife must be aware that some body language can be interpreted as overfamiliarity. She needs to develop a relationship with the woman, but must remember that at first she is a stranger. This must be taken into account when considering the appropriateness of touch. There are occasions when it is appropriate to touch a woman and it can assist the formation of the relationship, but on other occasions touch may be misinterpreted and/or unwelcome. This may be a particular problem for the male midwife, who may fear his actions will be misinterpreted if he does not match the woman's idea of a midwife (Flint, 1986).

The midwife during her work must necessarily invade a woman's 'personal space', yet we all know how uncomfortable it feels when someone invades ours. This physical touch should be undertaken with care, kindness and consideration of the individual woman's reaction and with her permission.

Besides the immediate effect on the individual, body language can have wide-reaching effects if particular behaviours are imitated by the individual. For instance, in communicating with her infant, the new mother draws upon examples of mothering taken from many role models she may have met, such as her own mother, sister or friends, television or even the attitude and actions of the midwife.

The midwife who perfects the art of body language unconsciously teaches by example, as the new mother observes how the midwife communicates with the baby by the way she handles and smiles at the newborn. This may also be apparent during the pregnancy, as the midwife cares for the woman or gently palpates the fetus in the abdomen.

Body language is such an integral part of our communication style that we often don't think about it or its effect on other people, while being very aware of other people's body language and its effect on us. Sometimes a person's body language can appear to contradict what they are saying, e.g. the midwife who appears anxious while reassuring a woman that all is well. The midwife could, in fact, be anxious about going off duty on time, but because she is unaware of her own body language she conveys a confusing message to the woman she is caring for; this may cause unnecessary anxiety. In such instances, we convey mixed messages and appear insincere.

It can be seen from the example above how important it is for midwives to develop an awareness of their own body language. The good communicator develops the art of body language so that it enhances and compliments the spoken word.

Language and Communication

In discussing language and communication it is important to consider culture. New students to midwifery are fortunate to be, in a sense, in the same position as pregnant women. That is, they are 'outside' the culture of midwifery. This affords them the opportunity to study the professional subculture within midwifery from an objective viewpoint.

Sociologists describe culture as:

...the way of life of members of a society. Culture includes the values, beliefs, customs, rules and regulations which human beings learn as members of a society.

(Haralambos, 1987.)

Each profession has a subculture that distinguishes the professional group from mainstream society – midwifery is no exception. As can be seen from the above quote, culture involves ones' values, beliefs, customs, rules and regulations. All these factors permeate communication. A common feature of human societies, which often differentiates cultures and enables us to identify one culture from another, is language. Midwives must understand and use language effectively if they are to become excellent communicators, but can the 'culture' in hospitals and in the midwifery profession affect midwives' attempts to communicate with women?

Using ethnographic research methods (in which one studies familiar activities as though they were strange or unfamiliar) Hunt and Symonds (1995) conducted a study of midwives who worked in a delivery suite. They made some illuminating observations of midwives communicating with women. Specifically, they noted that the midwives addressed women in labour using 'endearing' terms – 'Well done, girlie', 'Good girl', 'Love', 'Poppett' and 'Babes'.

The above are just a few of many such terms noted by Hunt and Symonds(1995), who continue:

Two women said that they found the terminology both offensive and patronising. However most women seemed to accept that it was normal practice. One concluded: 'All midwives say things like that, don't they?'

It seems obvious that such terms, when used to address adults, may appear condescending, so why did so many midwives use them? This question is more complex than might at first appear, since it involves issues not only of culture, but also of status, power and control. The midwives may have merely become socialized into their professional subculture and adopted such language as part of that culture, while remaining unaware of its effect. However, in sociological terms, there are alternative theories that explain what Hunt and Symonds observed.

As already mentioned, culture includes the 'rules and regulations' by which individuals know how to behave if they are to remain part of their group or society.

Societies are usually structured, with certain members being afforded status, power and control. Language, being part of the culture and a method by which individuals recognize each other and the group, is also the way that individuals maintain and confirm each others' status within the group. Hence language is used to establish and maintain power over subordinates, and to assert control.

Hunt and Symonds use the analogy of a factory assembly line to describe the labour 'process':

As in the assembly-line process, there is constant flow, the emphasis is on the speedy and successful delivery of the product. In this case we have all the main actors in place; the labourers (mothers), the production area (labour ward), the product (the child), the line manager (midwife) and the final authority of the works manager (consultant). The midwife is in control of the day-to-day production line and need only get external support from the consultant when that line exhibits anomalies.

(Hunt and Symonds, 1995.)

In the above scenario, the midwife is clearly in control and uses language to assert, confirm and re-affirm her status. The use of 'obstetric' language, such as 'incompetent cervix' or 'failure to progress' has been criticized as having a negative effect on women and inducing feelings of failure (Leap, 1992). Midwives could develop an alternative midwifery language to empower rather than disempower women.

Transactional analysis (TA) is a method used by some psychologists to explain interactions between adults. Devised by Dr Eric Berne in the 1950s, transactional analysis (TA) is a sophisticated idea that is worth brief consideration here. It is based on the idea that in relationships people may behave and respond in the role of parent, adult or child (P–A–C). TA uses a model (**Figure 20.1**) to illustrate the many forms such interactions can take:

When stimulus and response on the P–A–C transactional diagrams make parallel lines, the transaction is complementary and can go on indefinitely.

(Berne, 1964.)

Using this model, the midwives in Hunt and Symonds' study could be said to be in the role of parents and the women in the role of child. Thomas Harris is a psychiatrist who uses TA extensively in his work. Harris (1973) describes the parent–child transaction (**Figure 20.2**) as a complementary transaction, in that both parties may conspire to the role play and derive satisfaction from the relationship. So if women are willing to

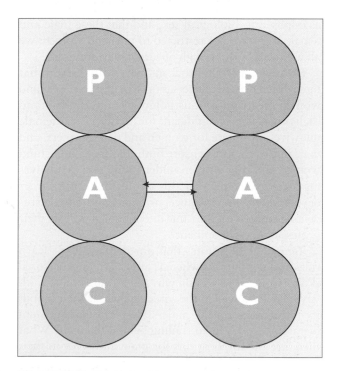

Figure 20.1 The P–A–C transactional analysis model – an adult–adult transaction.

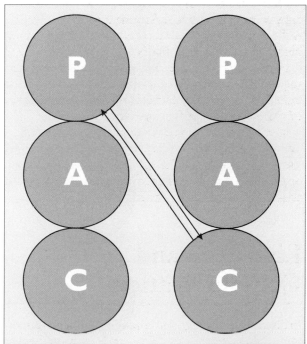

Figure 20.2 The P–A–C transactional analysis model – a parent–child transaction.

take on the child role and midwives willing to act as parent, the relationship can go on indefinitely with both parties happy with the arrangement. However, if a woman addresses her midwife as an adult, expecting an adult-to adult-transaction, yet the midwife responds as a parent to the child, this is termed a crossed transaction (**Figure 20.3**). Harris (1973) states:

> *If one or the other tires of the arrangement, the parallel relationship is disturbed, and trouble begins.*

It could also be argued that in adopting a parental stance the midwives Hunt and Symonds (1995) observed were hoping to elicit a 'child' response from women and thus re-assert their superior status in the relationship. Linguist Deborah Tannen conducted extensive research into the use of language, especially gender differences in conversational style and how conversations can send mixed messages when 'framed' within a power structure. Tannen (1993) concludes that there are male and female conversation styles and that mostly (though not always) men adopt a male style and women a female one. She explains that this is caused by differences in male and female cultures, so that men and women virtually grow up and live in different worlds. Though similarities can be found, she explains the difference as one of focus.

The male style is influenced by the view that the world is highly competitive and most interactions take place within the context of status and the struggle to be either 'one up' or 'one down'. This is a linear, asymmetrical view, because two people cannot both be 'one up', so out of any two people one must be higher and the other lower. Conversation is an opportunity to gain the upper hand. Tannen (1993) suggests this style is a result of men's desire for independence and autonomy, so their conversation sends the message: 'We're not the same, we're different.'

The female style is influenced by the view that the world is a community, and that in some ways people are all the same. This is a symmetrical view – all (wo)men are born equal. Conversation provides opportunities to 'connect', emphasize this 'sameness' and increase the strength of the community. Tannen (1993) suggests this style is a result of women's desire for intimacy and closeness, hence their conversation sends the message: 'We're close and the same.'

> *The essential element of connection is symmetry: People are the same, feeling equally close to each other. The essential element of status is asymmetry: People are not the same; they are differently placed in a hierarchy.*
>
> (Tannen, 1993.)

Tannen's analysis into gender difference in conversational style has some important implications for midwifery and is therefore worth closer examination. Note at this point the sociological view that gender is a social construction, as opposed to biological sex, and that these male and female styles are not restricted to men and women: we all use them both, though one style may dominate.

However, it is vital that midwives understand that these differences in conversation style between men and women create enormous potential to misunderstand each other. This is significant for midwives – as female midwives must care for women and their partners, and male midwives must ensure both that they understand women and that women understand them. Midwives may wish to remember this about their own career development. For instance, are male and female students starting with the same interpersonal skills in their professional development?

Tannen (1993) notes that during play, 'boys learn rules and regulations whereas girls learn interpersonal skills.' Could this explain why female nurses and midwives fare less well in the career stakes, as their inability to advance up the male-style NHS management hierarchy, leaves them trailing behind the men? What then, are the implications for male midwives in their interactions with women?

Let us return to the endearing terms used by the midwives who Hunt and Symonds (1995) observed, and

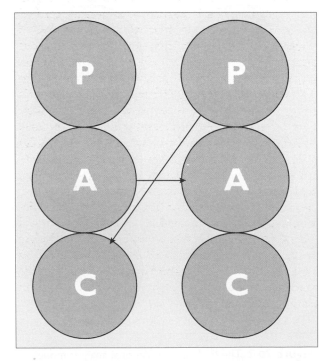

Figure 20.3 The P–A–C transactional analysis model – a parent–child transaction.

examine them again using Tannen's theory. It could be argued that the midwives were expressing a desire to be close to the women, so that by using a female conversation style they emphasized their 'sameness' to cement the relationship and bring them closer together. However, this ignores the reality that the midwives had, in the labour ward, higher status than the women.

Borrowing terminology from Bateson (1972), namely the terms messages and metamessages, Tannen (1993) illustrates how some communications may be ambiguous and the message that is received may not be the one that was intended:

There is always a paradox entailed in offering or giving help. Insofar as it serves the needs of the one helped, it is a generous move that shows caring and builds rapport. But insofar as it is asymmetrical, giving help puts one person in a superior position with respect to the other ... We may regard the help as the message – the obvious meaning of the act. But at the same time, the act of helping sends metamessages – that is information about the relations among the people involved, and their attitudes toward what they are saying or doing and the people they are saying or doing it to. In other words, the message of helping says, 'This is good for you.' But the fact of giving help may seem to send the metamessage 'I am more competent than you,' and in that sense it is good for the helper.

(Tannen, 1993.)

Here Tannen brings in the concept of framing, in that metamessages frame a conversation, placing it in context:

The conflicting metamessages inherent in giving help become especially apparent when people are in a hierarchical relationship to each other by virtue of their jobs. Just as parents are often frustrated in attempts to be their children's 'friends', so bosses who try to give friendly advice to subordinates may find that their words, intended symmetrically, are interpreted through an asymmetrical filter.

(Tannen, 1993.)

Thus, words intended to increase rapport may frame the speaker as condescending or patronizing. Again, this could explain the interaction between the midwives and their clients in Hunt and Symonds (1995) study.

Consider a recent situation in which you felt you were being patronized. Write down some of the conversation, and then review your own situation:

• Using transactional analysis.
• Considering Tannen's concept of framing.

Can you account for your feelings in that situation?

Later in this chapter, listening skills are discussed and counselling skills introduced. The importance of being nonjudgemental, genuine and sincere is stressed. In this section we have already explored the idea of body language and language sending confused or mixed messages, which seriously damage the speaker's appearance of genuineness and sincerity.

If you feel you are being patronized, do you feel that the speaker is sincere or genuine? The underlying issue is honesty. It is not enough to know that you are being honest with your clients. If you are sending mixed messages, your honesty may not be received, so you will be perceived as dishonest. Consider how would you decide whether someone was lying to you or telling the truth? Write down all the words, postures, behaviour, facial expressions and conversational style which may lead you to believe someone was lying to you.

We have examined culture in the context of language, but it must be pointed out here that aspects of culture, such as values and beliefs, shape our attitudes. This is examined in more detail later, but it is worth noting in this section that aspects of people's culture may lead to stereotyping. This can lead us to expect certain behaviours from particular individuals, and lead them to expect certain behaviour from us. These preconceived ideas and expectations can affect our interactions with others.

For instance, there is a tendency for society in general, and the media in particular, to portray 'medics' i.e. doctors, nurses and paramedics, as some kind of 'superbeing'. People who remain calm in the midst of disaster and devastation, performing heroic acts and sacrificing personal needs in their attempts to tend to the sick. Nurses in particular fall victim to the media image of 'angels', and are expected to maintain their saintly behaviour even when off duty. This is in stark contrast to the image of the 'sexy' nurse that is also propagated in the media. These 'good girl' versus 'bad girl' stereotypes deny the reality of nursing – that nurses are human and just as likely to be male! Midwives too, are subject to public image. The image of the gin-swigging Sairey Gamp, penned by Dickens in his novel *Martin Chuzzlewit* (1884), superseded previous images of the country midwife who dabbled in witchcraft as a matter of course. Both these images were in contrast to the realities. Such stereotypes exist and help to form peoples attitudes.

Professional Subculture

Midwives themselves have actions that may be specific to their own subculture – these are most apparent to the new student of midwifery. It may be useful to note any behaviour or language among midwives that seems strange or unfamiliar to you now, as a new student, and refer to this when you have absorbed the culture yourself. Reflect on the reactions of your friends and family to the news that you were becoming a midwife. What impression did they have of a midwife and how does this compare with actual midwives you have met?

In this section the issue of ethnicity has been deliberately avoided so far, as it is too easy to focus on language and culture merely in ethnic terms and avoid the wider issues. It must be acknowledged that Britain is a multiethnic, multilingual community and midwives, who work regularly with women whose language is not English, must understand that the language barrier is not the only difficulty – it may exacerbate the misunderstandings already discussed. Midwives should remember that smiling and genuineness are universal.

This chapter would be incomplete without mention of the language of the newborn. Exactly how do these tiny people interact with others, especially their mothers on whom they depend for survival?

The bonding theory (Klaus and Kennell, 1982) suggests that newborn babies are predisposed to 'bond' with their own mothers, much as a newly hatched duckling attaches itself to the first thing it sees upon hatching. The theory suggests that there is an optimal time around birth for this 'bonding' to take place and if this process is disrupted, for example when infants and mothers were separated for long periods after the birth, their relationship would be adversely affected. This theory remained fashionable for many years, gaining credence among psychologists. Despite sociologically based evidence to explain behaviour it was used as an excuse for all manner of human failings up to and including juvenile delinquency! (Bowlby, 1977).

The 'bonding' theory has now largely been displaced by more recent evidence. Richards (1986) suggests that human beings possess the ability to form relationships with one another throughout their lives, and that this ability is no greater in the newborn than in anyone else. The good news is that in cases where babies must be separated from their mothers, because of illness for example, they suffer no long-term effects, so mother and child can begin their relationship as soon as they are both able. This can be seen in the way that neonatal intensive-care units encourage communication between parents and baby, despite the barriers of the essential machinery.

It has also been suggested that newborn babies communicate with their mothers. On returning home from hospital with a new baby, many mothers discover that the baby wakes and cries out as soon as she places him/her in the new crib. This is because the baby is unused to being alone and is 'calling' to its' mother.

It is now known that the newborn infant possesses the ability to 'mimic' the actions of its mother. Slow-motion movies have demonstrated that infants watch their mothers facial expressions intently when talking to them, and make primitive attempts to copy the movements! Babies are thus active participants in their care, which contrasts with the previously held view of them being passive recipients.

Counselling Techniques

Counselling is a term that is used frequently in midwifery, yet most midwives are not trained counsellors. Midwives need to learn some basic counselling skills that will improve their ability to listen, enhance each interaction with a client, enable the midwife to receive a complete and accurate picture of what the woman is saying and ensure that the midwife's care is effective.

The term counselling, in this sense, is not in-depth psychotherapy, but rather a way of listening constructively and effectively. There is a growing awareness of the benefits of effective listening and counselling, demonstrated by the increasing role of counsellors in schools and other institutions. That someone can feel better and even find a solution by talking through their situation in a constructive way and exploring the issues involved is becoming increasingly recognized.

Midwives may have to incorporate the role of childbirth counsellor. There are many situations that arise during pregnancy and birth in which the mother has to make decisions and choices. To assist the mother, the midwife may not necessarily need to offer advice, but can facilitate the decision-making process by acting as a nondirective client-centred counsellor.

Midwives are facilitators of a process – the process of becoming a parent. This is a major life event for women, which involves change of lifestyle, increased stress and greater responsibility. Even a further child has to be accommodated into the family. Despite references to the 'new man', sociological research suggests that the primary responsibility for child care still rests with women (Oakley, 1976; Gavron, 1983).

Midwives are the key professionals involved with pregnancy and childbirth, and as such should recognize and value their potential as family counsellors during this period. Counselling can assist a person to acquire self-respect, inner strength and the confidence to accept personal responsibility. It can be a process of self-development, during which the client becomes autonomous – capable of making her his own decisions and taking responsibility for them. This may not be appropriate in some cultures or even subcultures, as 'personal responsibility' may not be an ideal to be striven for, so the midwife must guard against forcing her own ideals across. Also, by stressing that counselling can empower women, we are not underestimating women's role in society nor implying that women are responsible for the position in which they are placed within that society, or for everything that happens to them.

Egan (1994) refers to the counsellor as 'the skilled helper' who assists clients to solve their own problems. His model of counselling (**Box 20.1**) encompasses several aspects of Rogers' approach (*see* later). The key words associated with Egan are firstly *respect* for the client and, employing a *repertoire of skills*, the counsellor uses the *constructive* forces within individuals to enable them to handle their own problems in life more effectively. Egan's approach to counselling has been extended into determining *skills for living* and is not confined to the one-to one intensive exploration of problems.

Aims of Counselling

Mothers are expected to cope. They are supposed to know instinctively what to do with babies, and their own feelings are secondary to the task of being a good mother. They are expected to know immediately after delivery how to hold and suckle a baby. In some hospitals, staff watch for this as evidence of 'bonding'. If a woman does not understand immediately how to respond to her baby properly, she may be put on a secret 'at risk' list of women in danger of neglecting or maltreating their children. From the very beginning we are expected to put on a good performance ...

(Kitzinger, 1989.)

The benefits of counselling are not always immediately obvious, because they are not always visible or measurable. This may make it difficult for midwives to justify spending their time on counselling, especially to budget-conscious managers. Research demonstrates the benefit of extra support, such as the social studies by Oakley (1988). Consider a past issue in which you changed your mind, or thought differently after talking it over with someone. Write down your thoughts and feelings, and

Box 20.1

Application of Egan's (1994) Model

The midwife using Egan's model within a counselling situation first spends time exploring the client's own perspective of the problem or problems. At this stage the midwife helps the client to tell the complete story and to identify, if possible, significant aspects of it. In the counselling process the midwife demonstrates respect towards the individuality of the client and needs to draw on a wide repertoire of skills, including listening, acceptance, empathetic understanding and constructive challenge, to enable the client to fully define the problem from his/her own perspective.

The model leads on from problem definition to the determination of the best possible outcomes. The midwife enables the client to develop an awareness of the client's most preferred scenario. Again, this involves a variety of skills, including creative brainstorming balanced with the skills of evaluation and critique to ensure that the suggestions remain realistic. During this stage it may be helpful to the client to set goals on the path to achievement of the preferred outcomes – the midwife needs to facilitate the client to make his/her own choices and to demonstrate commitment to the decisions. The midwife should be aware of the difficulties that this may pose the client, who may not be ready to act at this stage and so may need to return to exploring the his/her own perspective of the problem (see above).

This commitment is greatly enhanced if the midwife enables the client to brainstorm the actions that could lead to the achievement of his/her identified goals. Again, the helper needs to demonstrate creativity balanced with critique. Gradually the skilled helper enables the client to plan and implement the action needed to meet the desired solution.

Although Egan's model tends to be described in linear terms with each stage running sequentially, it must be emphasized that it is a framework for counselling – sometimes it is necessary to modify the process, for example, it may be necessary to revert to the problem definition stage if the solutions are proving difficult for the client to attain.

Reflection

Reflect upon a recent situation in which you have fulfilled a counselling role, and apply Egan's model to that situation. Would you make any changes to the way in which you handled the situation?

reflect on how you came to alter your view.

Counselling involves a slow process of self-exploration and discovery. By talking about her feelings in a safe environment a mother may learn more about herself, why she responds to problems in certain ways, about the issues involved and any possible courses of action available whilst she receives support during her decision making.

Self-discovery can be a painful process, as people sometimes have to accept things they cannot change or discover aspects of themselves that they don't like. Rogers (1981) argues that some people do not complete the process but those that do lead more confident self-fulfilled lives, because they know themselves, they know what they want and are more responsible. The key is to take responsibility for your self and your own actions – in fact for your whole life.

Through this process the client becomes empowered, so able to take responsibility for herself. Women are faced with many choices that surround their pregnancy and birth, so supportive counselling enables them to make decisions and accept responsibility for their choices.

Rogers(1989) claims that counselling can create an empowered, autonomous, confident individual who accepts responsibility. Surely every parent can benefit from these qualities and midwives can recognize their potential as counsellors of childbearing women? As women are not wholly responsible for the organization of maternity services, empowering women only partly improves their autonomy. Social change is also required, such as recommended in *Changing Childbirth* (Department of Health, 1993), to shift some of the formal power to women and allow women true autonomy.

In a counselling relationship the woman is allowed to feel, she is allowed to explore issues in her own time and to discover her own responses. The counsellor respects the woman's right to her own opinions, though she/he does not have to agree with them, which gives value to the woman's feelings and attitudes. This is what Rogers calls *mutual positive regard* – in which client and counsellor have mutual respect for each other without necessarily having to agree on an issue. Though this appears straightforward, it can be difficult in practice. Consider the subject of clinical abortion or termination of pregnancy. This is a controversial area, upon which some midwives may have ethical objections. While the midwife has the right not to participate in the termination, she may still find herself in the position of having to counsel a woman on this matter in the antenatal period. This dilemma warrants closer examination.

You may conclude that if you counsel this woman you are condoning her actions, but this is precisely Rogers' point. You can respect her as an individual while not agreeing with her choice. If you allow your moral objection to transfer over into a judgement of the client then you are not holding her in positive regard. In other words, because her opinion differs from yours, this does not necessarily mean she is either a good or bad person.

Rogers insists that for counselling to be effective the counsellor must be nonjudgemental, though not necessarily *impartial*. If the woman in the above example feels she is being judged, she will not feel comfortable to explore her feelings and the possible actions available to her. The effectiveness of the counselling is diminished, so the result could be that the woman makes a poorly thought-through decision that she later comes to regret. The midwife must learn to accept the client's *feelings* without attaching a value judgement to them and realize that she is not responsible for the actions the client takes. It is therefore important in a counselling relationship that, while being nonjudgemental, the midwife remains honest and sincere. This is essential for building trust. If the client trusts the midwife she will feel safe and able to explore the issues that concern her. As the client's awareness and understanding of her own situation increases, she may identify her own strengths and weaknesses, make her own decisions and develop her own strategies. Remember Tannen's (1993) illustration of the paradox involved in helping? It is especially important that the counsellor appears genuine and avoids any tendency towards 'midwife knows best'.

Counselling may help people to identify their own wants and needs, to take responsibility for themselves, to allow mothers to express feelings and to facilitate the development of coping strategies and mechanisms in apparently hopeless situations like bereavement. Before going any further, write down your own feelings on the issue, and how you think you might proceed if you were in this situation. What are the issues for you?

Helpful Techniques

The following description of techniques is not intended to turn the midwife into an expert counsellor, but rather to help her use some of the skills of counselling during her everyday contact with clients and to improve her interpersonal skills. 'Practise makes perfect' and enables the midwife to develop her own style that feels comfortable to both midwife and client.

The environment

For counselling to be effective it is important to promote an emotionally 'safe' environment in which the mother is free to speak about her feelings, which means free from criticism or judgement. The woman's own home may not be quiet or private enough. Remember, it may be because of stresses in the home that she wishes to talk to you. A hospital or clinic is busy and plagued with interruptions, leaving the woman with the impression that the midwife has not fully committed herself to the counselling session.

The ideal setting is warm and quiet, with no interruptions. Seating should be comfortable – it is worth taking a little extra time to consider the seating arrangement. You may think that people don't care where they sit, but you would be wrong! When you first came into the classroom, where did you sit and why? Any waiter will tell you that the wall seats are always the first to fill up in a restaurant! People don't like to sit in the centre of the room because it makes them feel vulnerable. If you place yourself in a higher chair than your client, you could be signalling that you feel superior. Conversely, if you sit in a lower chair you are sending out signals of inferiority so your client may lose confidence in you! You may also want to give some thought to positioning the seats. If you are seated directly opposite each other the effect is confrontational and threatening; the least confrontational position is side by side, but this makes eye contact difficult so you may not be able to see facial expressions. It can also be interpreted as being overfamiliar. The ideal position for counselling is to place the seats at a 90° angle to each other, taking care not to put them too close together because if you invade your clients 'personal space' you will make her feel uncomfortable.

Avoid any physical barriers between you and your client, such as desks, as this may appear to the woman as a barrier to distance yourself from her; it is not consistent with the concepts of closeness and openness. It could also be argued that a uniform acts as a barrier in this fashion.

The Midwife as Counsellor

The counsellor attempts to create a friendly, non-judgemental atmosphere based on emotional honesty, empathy and genuineness, protecting confidentiality and promoting trust. Emotional honesty is being honest about your own feelings and emotions, although this may be difficult. During a counselling session you encourage the client to be honest with you. If you don't expect to have to return this honesty the relationship is asymmetrical so you may appear to be patronizing (Tannen, 1993). It is therefore important to be sincere with your clients, as this is a vital element in building trust and reduces the chance of you being perceived as condescending.

Eye contact is a form of body language that is very subtle, yet invariably linked to perceptions of honesty or dishonesty. One often relies on one's internal sense of timing to judge the appropriate time to look into someone's eyes! It is easy not to look long enough, but if one's eyes are fleeting from side to side and avoiding eye contact, this may be perceived as 'shifty' or dishonest. Most people regard looking directly into the eyes as a sign of honesty, yet look for too long and this may be interpreted as threatening, or as a sexual overture! In some cultures it may be considered impolite to look directly at the eyes, especially a woman to a man, or a child to an adult.

Adopting an 'open', relaxed posture conveys honesty. Politicians are aware that public speakers who adopt 'open' hand gestures are more likely to be believed and remembered.

We hear people speak of others as 'cold', 'stiff' or 'unfriendly'. These terms mean something to others, though it is not certain what the essential behaviour variables are that form the basis for such a perception.

(Rogers, 1990).

Being 'friendly' doesn't mean being over-nice and agreeing with everything the client says, as this does not appear genuine; nor does it mean being overfamiliar as that makes the client feel uncomfortable. Being friendly means being relaxed and informal enough to encourage openness (though not so laid-back that you appear disinterested!) while conveying warmth and empathy, as a friend would.

Empathy is different from sympathy, yet it is easy to confuse these terms. The *Concise Oxford Dictionary* (Allen, 1990) describes empathy as:

The power of identifying oneself mentally with (and so fully comprehending) a person ...

whereas sympathy is described as:

The state of being simultaneously affected with the same feeling as another ... the capacity for this ... the act of sharing or tendency to share (with a person etc.) in an emotion or sensation or condition of another person or thing ... compassion or commiseration; condolences ...

The difference is subtle, but it can be detected. Consider a woman whose baby was stillborn. It would be foolish, if not highly insulting, for you to proclaim: 'I know how you feel,' unless you have also experienced this tragedy. Most of us mean 'we can imagine how you must feel', yet even this falls short of the mark, because how can we possibly imagine how we would feel? Yet, with experience, counsellors can develop empathy. When midwives achieve a sophisticated balance between respect for the individual, recognition of their feelings, acceptance and understanding, the overall effect is empathy. It is easy to see how expressions of sympathy, such as the one above, can be rejected as patronizing, yet how does one develop the ability of empathetic experiencing?

Rogers (1989) states:

... it can come through literature, which can provide an entrance to the inner worlds of other persons. Perhaps it might come especially through the role-taking that goes with dramatic productions, though so few therapists have such a background that it is difficult to judge. It may come from psychology courses in which the approach is dynamically phenomenological. It can come simply through the process of living, when a sensitive person desires to understand the viewpoint and attitudes of another. It is a way of perceiving which can be learned in courses ...

Rogers' language may be unfamiliar to us, but he can be summed up thus: many of life's experiences can develop our *insight* and *understanding*, provided we desire them to do so.

Empathetic skills can be developed through reflection on personal experience and reflective practice. The more we reflect upon our interactions with others, clients and colleagues alike, the more understanding and empathetic we become. Hence the reflective practitioner continually evaluates and improves his/her empathetic skills.

It is important to be attentive and demonstrate that you are listening carefully. This gives the client respect and also grants the valuable gift of your time. If you are prepared to do this, you are sending the metamessage that the client has value.

Your own body language should indicate an alert posture, smiling, nodding and making appropriate use of eye contact, to show that that you are paying attention. Provided you smile and nod at the right moments, of course. Sometimes counsellors have been so overenthusiastic with their smiles and nods that they have demonstrated they were not listening, or perhaps the client thought they had a nervous twitch! It is impor-tant to use language appropriately; interjecting a 'yes ...' or 'mmm ...' at a well-timed moment shows that you are listening, but you must avoid interrupting or 'searching for gaps' in the client's speech in which you might 'jump in'. If you are gap searching, you must also be planning what you are going to say, so you are not listening effectively. Carefully reading and interpreting body language affords a greater insight into the situation.

Sometimes it is useful to use 'mirroring'. This refers to occasions where the counsellor 'mirrors' or 'reflects back' what the client has said; repeating the client's speech precisely, word for word, exactly as it was said. This serves a very important purpose. No-one can listen attentively to a speaker for prolonged periods of time, and still claim to be listening 100%. This is because our attention begins to wander after a short while. If this occurs during a counselling session it won't be long before the client senses that you are not listening.

Reflecting provides you with a short break in concentration, which enables you to check that you've heard and *understood* the client correctly. You may say something like: 'Now let me just check that I've got that right. You said ...' (repeat exactly as the client said it). As a result you will also be more likely to remember this part of the session. It also enables you to check your understanding of any unfamiliar language. You may say: 'You said ... (repeat the word or phrase) ....what does that mean?'

This is important if the client uses colloquialisms, as you need to be sure that you've taken the correct meaning. Reflecting also benefits the client as she can check that she really said what she meant. Finally, reflecting (or mirroring) is a very strong *positive reinforcer*. In psychological terms, this means it reinforces or strengthens positive feelings and attitudes and can improve self-esteem and confidence. Compliments are a common form of positive reinforcement. When the client realizes that someone really has listened carefully to everything she said, demonstrated by their ability to repeat it verbatim, it increases her sense of self-worth.

Another technique to clarify meaning is paraphrasing. This is where you repeat what the client has just said, but rephrased. In this case you would say: 'Do you mean ...' (then offer your interpretation of what the client said, in your own words). This enables you to clarify what the client intended to say and what you understood from it, but also that you are paying attention and care enough to want to *understand*. This shows your *empathy*. It also offers the client the chance to express herself differently if you misunderstood the first time.

Questioning or probing can be useful if you feel something could be achieved by asking the client to elaborate or be more specific. Care should be taken not to overuse this technique, or your client may end up feeling interrogated! Ideally, questions should be 'open' rather than 'closed'. Open questions, such as 'How do you feel?' generally invite a descriptive response and can be used to open a dialogue. 'Do you feel okay?' is a closed question that tends to generate one word answers, such as yes or no, so reducing the opportunity to open a dialogue.

Sometimes listening to the *intonation*, i.e. how the question was answered, may tempt you to probe further. Take the following example from an antenatal clinic:

Midwife:
'Hello Alison, how do you feel today?'
Alison:
'(sigh) ... Not bad ...'

With emphasis on 'bad' the client may be hinting at some problem that she thinks may appear trivial. The midwife could reply:

'Well that's good then!'
or
'Does that mean "not good" either?'

The first response closes the subject, but the second gives an opening for dialogue should the client wish to take it up. It is not easy to create open sentences. In the earlier example, 'How do you feel?', the client could just reply 'okay', and you'd have to think of another opening. With practice you can perfect your technique and keep a 'library' of open questions in your mind.

The concept of self-disclosure occurs when the counsellor discloses some piece of information about themselves. Its purpose is to increase rapport by emphasizing the 'sameness' between counsellor and client. Showing the counsellor to be human, with the same feelings, fears and failures we all possess, helps bring client and counsellor closer together.

This may prove difficult for midwives to achieve without appearing condescending. Refer to Tannen's (1993) theory of framing. Midwives must remember that their attempts to be symmetrical and convey sameness may be interpreted through the asymmetrical filter of their status. This can be minimized by choosing the right time to disclose information. Once the midwife–client relationship is established, the client may consider the midwife as a friend; self-disclosing in this situation is appropriate, strengthens the relationship and the influence of the midwife's status is minimized.

The technique of challenging refers to a situation in which the counsellor directly confronts the client on an issue. It is very threatening, and possibly disturbing to the client, as it may force them to confront feelings or emotions they have been trying to deny. It is used in psychotherapy when the counsellor feels that the counselling isn't leading anywhere and the client is not progressing because they are 'holding back' on something that is uncomfortable for them, but which may be essential for them to tackle if they are to move on.

Therapists carefully choose the right moment to confront the client with the suggestion that they may be hiding something of their true feelings. For example suicide may be hinted at, or joked about, as the client 'tests the water' to see how the therapist reacts. As overt confrontation may be perceived as aggressive and threatening to the client, it always takes place in the context of a very supportive, caring environment. It is not the midwife's role to attempt to psychoanalyse her clients. This could do more harm than good because people's emotions are complex, often taking psychologists many years to understand. Midwives are not in contact with their clients long enough to undertake this role and are not able to offer the necessary long-term support. However, it may be useful for midwives to have an awareness of this technique, as it can often highlight the severity or depth of the woman's feelings. Gentle probing, very rarely challenging, may enable the midwife to decide where expert referral is needed, as in cases of postnatal depression. Challenging can only take place in an established, 'safe', relationship. Midwives must be wary before attempting this, as it has the potential to unleash hidden emotions, recover unpleasant, long-forgotten memories and destroy trust. It can be a real 'Pandora's box' in the wrong hands.

Consider a case in which you have been providing antenatal care for Mrs X for some months. She is becoming increasingly anxious about the prospect of a vaginal examination, to the point where you feel it is having a deleterious effect on her mental state. Past conversations and half-suggestions lead you to suspect she may have been sexually abused. It is not appropriate for you to attempt therapeutic counselling, but what can you do? Under 'Further reading' some articles are listed that are relevant to this topic.

Midwives often have to give information to clients, ranging from parentcraft class times to test results. A recent television documentary (*The Decision*, Channel 4, January 30, 1996) followed women undergoing the 'triple test' at different hospitals. In this situation the midwife informs women of the results and provides nondirective counselling, so that the woman and her partner may make the decision that is right for them. The information given should be factual, and the counselling should be supportive and impartial. Yet some of these women felt that they were being coerced into make choices that would suit 'the hospital' or 'society'. Some felt they were being 'pressurized' to have an amniocentesis or termination rather than risk bringing a child with Down's syndrome into the world.

It could be that the midwives were not conscious of their power and status and that words intended to reassure were mistaken. The midwife must be conscious of this possibility, and ensure that information giving does not become advice giving or even coercion! Also midwives may sometimes retreat into information giving when counselling would be more appropriate, to save time or to avoid exploring wider issues. This can be a method which midwives use to maintain control and reinforce their status! Tannen (1993) explains how the person who has the information is in a superior position to the person who needs the information. It is also important not to resort to using professional language that the woman cannot understand.

Effective listening is equally important between midwives themselves, and in their interactions with students, doctors and other health care professionals.

Finally, a word to the wise. Midwives are not psychotherapists. Trained therapists may counsel people for years – exploring issues, untangling emotions and soothing bruised spirits. They must guard against dependency and encourage their clients to become independent. Midwives care for a woman for 10 months at the most during any one pregnancy. If she is lucky she may care for the same woman over subsequent pregnancies, though this rarely happens, and even then she is not around to give support between pregnancies. This is not long enough to repair damaged hearts, minds and souls. Regardless of how deeply they care, midwives should recognize their own limitations and beware of starting what they cannot finish.

Barriers to Communication

There are three main factors that may enhance or impede communications – environment (external factors), attitude (internal factors) and technique. We have already mentioned some environmental barriers, but other external factors may also impede communications.

Environment (external factors)

First we consider those which originate beyond the immediate sphere of the counselling relationship and beyond the control of either counsellor or client.

A pleasant and sunny day may make the atmosphere

comfortable and relaxed, but if it were stormy or icy both client and midwife may be preoccupied with concerns of family and the journey home.

Another example is the hospital environment. This may impede communications in several ways, as it may not be welcoming, private or conducive to a relaxed exploration of emotions, feelings and problems. There is also the issue of culture. Hospitals have their own rules, regulations and codes of behaviour to which the staff (including the midwives) must adhere, but which may make the client feel decidedly uncomfortable, as she is in the position of being the 'outsider' or cultural stranger. Language is an important part of culture and to this end the client is even excluded here. Hospital personnel invariably use a 'common' language; the repeated use of technical terminology and abbreviations serves to reinforce their rapport with each other and confirm their membership of the group. Language in this way is how members of a group recognize one another, but it is also how strangers or foreigners are identified. Continual exclusion from the language serves to reinforce the client's position as that of the foreigner.

Hospitals are hierarchical. They have a linear organizational structure with doctors at the top and clients at the bottom. The hospital staff, therefore, occupy positions in the organization in relation to one another. This is status, a social construction that is beyond the control of either midwife or client. It may be appropriate at this point to discuss the dynamics of power. With increasing status comes increasing power. So, being at the bottom of the hospital hierarchy, how much power can women realistically have? Midwives try to empower women, to increase their autonomy, but is women's autonomy real or illusory?

If midwives *allow* women autonomy, who has the real power? Indeed, if doctors *allow* midwives autonomy, who is in control? It can be seen that in discussing *empowerment* there are wider social and political considerations to be taken into account. The client only has as much power as the midwife and the organization allow her to have.

However, according to Barbara Johnstone:
Men live in a world where they see power as coming from an individual acting in opposition to others and to natural forces. For them, life is a contest in which they are constantly tested and must perform, in order to avoid the risk of failure. For women, the community is the source of power.
(cited by Tannen, 1993.)
From this point of view one could argue that women become disempowered when they are removed from

their communities and put into male-dominated hospitals.

Hunt and Symonds (1995) noted aspects of midwifery subculture, such as 'tea drinking', in which midwives were expected to participate to remain accepted within the group. The desire for acceptance is very strong in all human beings, and it is virtually impossible for someone to practise as a midwife if she is not accepted by other midwives. Midwives can make life difficult for 'deviants' from the accepted (midwifery) 'norm'. For example, midwives who encouraged alternative positions during labour, before this became accepted practice, may have been regarded as 'cranks' by their colleagues.

Attitudes (internal factors)

We all have attitudes towards others and opinions of others. Many factors can influence the formation of personal attitudes – culture, personal experience, mood, educational background, class, etc. Thus external factors, such as culture, religion, family, schools, our peers, role models and the media (especially television), all influence us and help to form our opinions; these manifest in our attitudes and behaviour. Some of our opinions may be accurate, but many others bear no relation to the truth. Culture is an example of how this can be. We are influenced by the cultural beliefs of the society we live in to the degree that we accept them as 'truth', yet what is true for one person may not be so for another. This idea has such an influence on our interactions with others that we feel it warrants further examination. As an example, we examine in detail the assertion that British culture *is* racist.

Some sociologists (Abercrombie and Warde, 1988) have claimed that British culture is inherently racist, in a generalized sense. It can be argued that this is a legacy of the British Empire. Taken in its historical context, the British Empire existed at the same time as the scientific revolution, colonialism, the Victorians' acceptance of Darwin's theory of evolution and a movement towards 'social' reform. The Victorians came to believe that mankind evolved from 'primitive' societies to 'advanced' scientific societies.

On this basis, the British came to view themselves as a superior 'advanced' race, who were destined to conquer the world, 'educating' primitive peoples. Hence racist attitudes came into being – they were even taught in schools at the time of the British Empire as a reason why working class children must attend school, 'You are part of a superior race and must behave accordingly.' Hence the emphasis on discipline rather than education.

Although this 'empire' no longer exists, the strong attitudes which were formed at the time about people from other cultures still remain.

Remember, though, in referring to 'culture' that we all belong to at least one culture, and during our lives may belong to several subcultures. For example, we may identify with the culture of Roman Catholicism, 'mainstream' British culture and the subculture of midwifery. Issues of culture are therefore not synonymous with issues of colour or race.

It is difficult to single out internal factors that affect us in isolation, as human beings are extremely complex creatures. Besides cultural aspects, our attitude and behaviour are heavily influenced by our own experiences and moods. Our memories of, and feelings from, those experiences can influence our current interactions since we tend to treat others as we have been, or are, treated. Suffice to say that if you feel cherished and nurtured you are able to do the same for others, but if you feel no-one cares for you, you are not likely to care for others. Why should you?

Studies of institutionalised bullying (MSF, 1994) have suggested that if managers are bullied by their seniors they are more likely to bully their subordinates, and so the phenomenon spreads throughout the organisation.

Similarly, women are likely to treat their baby as they imagine their mothers treated them, or as they've observed other mothers treating siblings. Such experiences and memories influence mothering skills.

In counselling or midwifery, certain attitudes are considered particularly unhelpful. The first example detracts from the client's feelings and devalues their experience: 'You think you've got problems? Wait 'till you hear about mine!' It may be that the midwife has failed to pick up cues and is unaware that the client requires someone to listen. The overall effect is akin to telling the client to go away and not bother you with their petty problems when yours are much more important. This effectively defuses the situation, closes the dialogue and denies the client support.

It is tempting for midwives to offer advice, as women often seek out their midwives in this capacity, but it is not always helpful. If you interject to offer a quick solution as soon as you think you have identified the 'problem', you may again defuse the situation, as in the above example. You deny the client the opportunity to soul-search, exploring feelings and possible options. You may also be encouraging the mother to be dependent upon you for all the answers, for you have deprived her of the decision-making process and the option to choose her own solution. This may also backfire on you: if she follows your advice and it goes wrong, she will blame you.

Offering quick reassurance can also be detrimental. In an emotionally charged atmosphere, such as the labour ward, it can be very tempting to reassure someone who appears distressed, but be conscious of the metamessages you may be sending. For example, the message 'Shh ... Don't cry' may be intended in the context of caring, but you may be sending the metamessage: 'Oh no! Don't start crying in front of everyone, it embarrasses me!' Promising that 'Everything will be all right' is often said because of a midwife's inability to cope with an emotionally charged atmosphere.

Unhelpful Techniques

Invading somebody's 'personal space' is unhelpful, as stated earlier, but the detrimental effects are exacerbated by external factors such as smelling of stale tobacco, overpowering perfume, body odour, last night's alcohol or garlic.

Midwives must resist 'taking over' as this robs the mother of the experiences of learning and problem-solving, and can reduce self-esteem. For example, the new mother who attempts to pacify her baby may feel inadequate when the midwife is able to achieve what she could not. Midwives must allow mothers the dignity of making mistakes sometimes. No baby has ever come to any harm by its mother failing to observe correct 'winding' procedure, yet many a new mother's confidence has been dented by observing a competent midwife.

New mothers need time to explore and discover their own ways of doing things. Even if the midwife stops short of virtually taking over, she may still damage a woman's confidence by offering unsolicited and unnecessary 'advice'.

> *Clack, clack, clack. The door opened. 'I've come to give Baby eye drops.' The midwife plucked my six-hour-old son from my arms. He cried out, startled. 'He doesn't like being handled, does he? Put him in his cot. It's time he got used to being alone.' Without further ado, she performed her task and swept out of the room, leaving me, my partner and our little son all feeling rather miserable. What had she done – and why?*
>
> (Holmes, 1990, p. 80.)

Another unhelpful technique is to 'control' the conversation by asking too many questions. This way the midwife either inadvertently or deliberately maintains control. She steers the conversation in the direction she wants it to go, decides how long to talk for and on which issues, and so may miss issues that are important to the woman.

Interrupting or finishing woman's sentences show impatience. It may be counter-productive as it closes the dialogue and you may not find out what troubles her. Filling silences is something we all tend to do, but it can be unhelpful in that it reduces thinking time. Sometimes silences allow the woman and midwife to reflect upon what has been said and if left unfilled the woman may enlarge on what has previously been said.

In some situations the midwife can be too 'problem-centred' or too 'solution-centred'. A woman may wish to talk about an issue that they don't perceive as a 'problem', and neither do they need or desire a 'solution'. Sometimes it is just good to talk and have someone listen. We can be too hasty with interpretations, forcing our insight through – 'You know what your problem is ...' springs to mind. We may decide what we think the 'problem' is, which is risky as it may seem to the client that you are right, but you may not be – the full picture may not yet have emerged. You may have made an inappropriate judgement based on incomplete information. Thus, the woman may make a 'wrong' decision or may leave your session feeling that you are unable to help.

Lastly, avoid psychoanalysing. When midwives are good listeners the care they provide is improved: but women will soon realize when you are out of your depth. They lose trust in you if they feel they are constantly being analysed.

Interpersonal Skills: Their Application to Midwifery

Interpersonal skills are necessary in every area of midwifery. The outcome of each interaction is dependent upon the effectiveness of your skills. We have seen that these skills are many and varied, incorporating linguistics, body language, counselling techniques and listening skills, and also they are influenced by culture and experience.

Although we concentrate here mainly on the special relationship and interaction between a midwife and her client, these skills are also needed in other parts of the midwife's role.

Teaching

The midwife is involved in teaching throughout her career. Many of the skills already discussed are just as important in the teaching role, and apply whether the midwife is teaching clients or students and whether this is by example or in a more formal situation.

Peoples' attention span is approximately 20 minutes, and may be less for some. People also tend to remember what they are told first and last, forgetting what came in the middle. This led to the old 'teaching' maxim: 'Tell them what you're going to tell them, tell them, then tell them you've told them!'

This is used by salesmen, vicars, politicians and midwives in teaching situations. It is based on the theory that you introduce your subject, present your subject, then sum-up at the end, which drives the message home.

Teaching skills are a further development of interpersonal skills, so the midwife should observe others teaching, incorporate effective techniques into her repertoire and make every effort to extend her skills in this area through further courses and reading. It is very easy to turn parent education sessions into a 'performance' and forget the two-way process of communication. The midwife as an educator should ensure that the information given is easily understood, allow time for questions and be aware of the nonverbal signals from the client that may indicate worry or lack of confidence. During classes or when teaching mothers on a one-to-one basis, the most important thing a midwife can do is to encourage self-confidence in the parent's own skills.

Teaching in most circumstances is enhanced by visual aids, as we remember 80% of what we see compared to approximately 30% of what we hear (Rogers, 1981). Many midwives use aids to teach, such as models, videos or posters. Some design and make their own models or games to stimulate interest and/or change the pace of the session. The techniques and aids used to teach parentcraft sessions can be used just as effectively when teaching in the home or hospital ward. Many women miss out on formal classes, but the midwife should ensure that all women benefit from her teaching skills whenever she gives her care.

Midwives may find it necessary to seek help to improve communication and teaching with their clients. They may need the assistance of a 'signer' if the client is deaf, for example. It is useful to make contact with people who offer such services before the need arises.

Some teaching aids may need to be simplified if the client has learning difficulties, to aid understanding. With clients who have difficulties the midwife must always remember who the client is and not fall into the trap of talking to the partner, parent or carer.

Midwives may find that they are caring for clients from different cultures than themselves, who may have difficulty understanding the midwifes' language. This is a wonderful opportunity for the midwife to learn more about another culture while giving care and teaching parenting skills by example or through an interpreter. Smiling is a universal language that is appreciated and is also infectious.

The midwife must be sensitive to cultural issues and respect for religious values will enhance communication.

(Khawaja, 1996.)

Language support workers, sometimes known as link workers, should be welcomed into the maternity services to enable both midwife and link worker to give the best possible service to the client and her family.

Telephone skills

Effective interpersonal skills are of prime importance when using the telephone. In this situation the midwife must use her voice alone to communicate caring, listening and information-giving, whether to clients or to other professionals. Both participants must identify each other as soon as possible and use the other person's name appropriately. The midwife must ensure that the caller knows she is talking to a professional person who takes responsibility for the call. This means that the midwife must give both her name and title to ensure that the caller knows she is speaking to a midwife. Active listening with encouraging sounds (instead of head nods) lets the caller know that you are giving him/her your full attention. We all know how frustrating it is to be put through to different people and have to repeat the same story. The midwife should take responsibility for the query, find out the answer or the person who can help and when they are available, and then call back with positive information. Of course, if promises of returned calls or further information are made they must be kept. These factors contribute to the perception that the caller has, not only of the midwife who answered, but of the team, the profession, the NHS Trust and the NHS in general. If the call is handled well the client's confidence in all these areas is boosted. Clearly, a poorly handled call can have the opposite and detrimental effect on the caller's impression of midwives.

Confidentiality

On the subject of telephone calls, it is important to note that confidentiality must be respected. Enquiries of a sensitive nature about any client should be made known to the client, who should also be asked whether she wishes information to be given and to whom. Although it may seem impolite, only the minimum information about a client should be given over the telephone and then only with her permission. During antenatal care it is wise to broach this subject with the woman, so that no-one is upset by the cautious information given over the telephone.

It is often necessary to use the telephone to communicate with other professionals. Before starting have all the relevant material ready so that you appear efficient. Ensure you are speaking to the correct person and identify yourself. It is helpful to repeat key elements back to the other person so that both parties know what action is to be taken and by whom. End the call with a positive statement, not just a slow fade-out.

Where possible follow up telephone calls in writing and don't forget to record the time, subject matter and agreed outcome of the call.

Although callers cannot see you, they form an impression of you. Smiling helps to put the caller at ease, as does a calm, helpful manner. This may be difficult at a hectic midwives' station during a busy shift, but the caller cannot appreciate this, and needs his/her queries answered efficiently, politely and sensibly. Remember all the points emphasized herein concerning genuineness and regard for the individual.

Written communication

Although we tend to think of interpersonal skills as those that occur during a physical meeting between people, communication also takes place by writing, whether this is in the form of letters or records. The importance of record-keeping cannot be stressed enough – all written communication must be legible, understandable, accurate, dated and signed. Good record-keeping safeguards you (the midwife) and your clients.

For busy midwives in the hospital and community it is easy to put off recording events, discussions and telephone calls until later and then forget to do so. Clause 2 of the UKCC *Code of Professional Conduct* (1992) states:

> *Ensure that no action or omission on your part or within your sphere of responsibility, is detrimental to the interests, condition or safety of patients and clients.*

Client records are the midwife's only support should an investigation become necessary. Records are confidential and should always be in folders and not left around for anyone to see.

Client-friendly records enable mothers and midwives to make easier decisions about planned care and mothers experience less anxiety about their care and gain more satisfaction.

Before we leave the subject of written communication just check that your handwriting is easy to read (legible), that your information is logical, timed and dated and above all that everything you have done for, or said to, the client is recorded, including making or receiving telephone calls to other professionals and the outcome of those calls.

The Reflective Practitioner

Midwives are now being encouraged to use reflective practice. In some units or teams reflection-on-action groups (Schon, 1987) are being used to highlight areas of good, effective practice and decision making and identify areas for improvement.

Clinical supervision groups can support the midwife in reflective practice. Communication and interpersonal skills can and should be discussed with colleagues in a nonthreatening and nonaccusatory manner. We can all ignore the effect that we may have on our clients and colleagues, imagining that they see us as we see ourselves.

A maxim to remember is that referred to in *The Water Babies* by Charles Kingsley when Tom meets Mrs 'Do-as-you-would-be-done-by', in that we should treat other people as we would like to be treated. It pays to step back from the hectic surroundings of work and consider our interpersonal skills and their effect on others.

Effects of Stress

Another point to remember when considering interpersonal skills in midwifery is that most of our clients are in a stressful situation – whether at antenatal clinic, through labour or learning to cope with parenthood. The effects of stress mean that people do not always behave as they normally would. There is more tendency to appear intense and sometimes angry, more likelihood of forgetting what is said; stress also makes people more emotional. Most of the clients and their partners, for most of the time during our care, feel under some stress, caused by worrying about the pregnancy outcome, coping with labour and becoming parents. They are usually on unfamiliar territory, speaking with midwives who are comfortable with their surroundings and the terminology being used. Pain may cause anger and fear may result in giggling – both give the midwife quite the wrong signals. It is the responsibility of the midwife to put the mother at her ease, establish a relationship and respect her particular and unique needs. In this respect the midwife must behave as a hostess, treating each client as though a guest in her home.

Effective Interpersonal Skills

Effective interpersonal skills assist the midwife to deliver good care and support her other midwifery skills. As with any other skill, practice and evaluation makes for improvement in the techniques involved and more expert use of these skills.

When midwives reflect on their practice and, in so doing, evaluate the effectiveness of their interpersonal skills in different circumstances, they often both enjoy increased job satisfaction and improve the care they give:

> *... there is no doubt that when specific attention was given to improving both interpersonal and communication skills, care was improved.*
>
> (Hunt and Symonds, 1995.)

Summary

Interpersonal skills are those skills which people use to communicate with each other. This chapter has discussed the complexity of human communication: from the basic concepts of language and body language, to the complex issue of how culture, attitudes and power permeate and influence every interaction. We have examined the implications of this for midwives and discussed how, with an awareness of these factors and their application to midwifery, midwives can become more effective in their encounters with women. This in turn can lead to a positive and satisfactory experience for women and their families during this period in their lives.

KEY CONCEPTS

- Effective midwifery care is reliant on good communication. Poor communication can have devastating effects on women and their families.
- Communication, facial expression and body language can maintain the power differential and make communication between mothers and midwives a hierarchical discourse.
- The sensitive midwife interprets the clients non-verbal communications and anticipates her needs.
- Differences of culture, status and gender influence conversational style and alter the context of communication.
- Midwives must be honest with clients and colleagues, and employ the counselling maxim of mutual positive regard.
- Empathy skills enable a midwife to be truly 'with woman'.
- The quality of care is affected by the quality of interpersonal skill.

References

Abercrombie N, Warde A: *Contemporary British society*, Cambridge, 1988, Polity Press.

Allen RE, editor: *The concise Oxford dictionary of current English*, 8th edn, Oxford, 1990, Clarendon.

Bateson G: *Steps to an ecology of mind*, New York, 1972, Balantine.

Bell SM, Ainsworth MDS: Infant crying and maternal responsiveness, *Child Development* 43:1171, 1972

Berne E: *Games people play*, New York, 1964, Grove Press.

Bowlby J: *Childcare and the growth of love*, New York, 1977, Penguin.

Department of Health, Expert Maternity Group: *Changing Childbirth. Part 1: Report of the Expert Maternity Group*, London, 1993, HMSO.

Egan G: *The skilled helper*, Monterey, 1994, Brooks/Cole.

Flint C: *Sensitive midwifery*, Oxford, 1986, Heinemann Medical Books.

Gavron H: *The captive wife*, London, 1983, Routledge and Kegan Paul.

Haralambos M: *Sociology: A new approach*, Ormskirk, 1987, Causeway Press.

Harris TA: *I'm OK – you're OK*, New York, 1973, Avon Books.

Holmes P. Listen to mother, *Nurs Times* 86(28): 80, 1990.

Hunt S, Symonds A: *The social meaning of midwifery*, London, 1995, Macmillan Publishers.

Khawaja R: Researching the needs of women from minority communities, In: Dodds R, Goofman M, Tyler S (editors): *Listen with mother*, Hale, 1996, Books for Midwives.

Kitzinger S. *The crying baby*, New York, 1989, Viking Penguin.

Klaus MH, Kennell JH: *Parent–infant bonding*, St Louis, 1982, CV Mosby.

Leap N: The power of words, *Nurs Times*, 88(21):60, 1992.

MSF Conference Report: *BULLYing at work: Confronting the problem*, London, 1994, MSF.

Morris D: *Manwatching: a field guide to human behaviour*, London, 1989, Grafton Books.

Oakley A: *Housewife*, Harmondsworth, 1976, Pelican.

Oakley A: Is social support good for the health of mothers and babies? *J Reprod Infant Psychol* 6(1):3, 1988.

Richards M: Psychological aspects of neonatal care. In Roberton NCR, editor: *Textbook of neonatology*, Edinburgh, 1986, Churchill Livingstone.

Rogers CR: *Freedom to learn, for the 80s*, London, 1981, Merrill.

Rogers CR: *On becoming a person*, London, 1989, Constable.

Rogers CR: *Client-centred Therapy*, London, 1990, Constable.

Schon D: *Educating the reflective practitioner*, San Francisco, 1987, Jossey Bass.

Tannen D. *You just don't understand: women and men in conversation*, London, 1993, Virago.

UKCC: *Code of professional conduct*, London, 1992, UKCC.

Further Reading

Bastian H: Confined, managed and delivered: the language of obstetrics, *Br J Obstet Gynaecol* 99:92, 1992.

This brief article demonstrates how terminology has been used to reinforce the divide between medical men and women patients to keep the latter as obedient recipients.

Egan G: *The skilled helper*, Monterey, 1994, Brooks/Cole.

Provides a good framework for the interactions in which nurses and midwifes are involved.

English National Board: *New dimensions in midwifery care, an open learning package. Book 1: Relationships in practice*, London, 1996, English National Board.

Considers issues central to interpersonal skills for the midwife. This is a valuable activity-based package.

Kirkham MJ: Communication in midwifery. In Alexander J, Lavy V, Roche S, editors: *Midwifery practice*, London, 1993, Macmillan.

An excellent review of the literature concerned with all aspects of communication in midwifery. This is a useful practice check that will help midwives enhance their communication skills.

Tschudin V: *Counselling skills for nurses*, 4th edn, London, 1995, Baillière Tindall.

A good, clearly presented basic introduction to counselling. The examples can be translated easily into midwifery practice.

21 | *Woman-Centred Care: The Way Forward*

LEARNING OUTCOMES

After studying this chapter you should be able to:

- Demonstrate knowledge of the reports, within the four countries of the UK, that relate to the maternity services, including the concepts common to all.
- Explore further some of the interactions and influences on the provision of a woman-centred service.
- Reflect on the implications of such a service to women, midwives and the organization.
- Identify some of the literature pertaining to woman-centred care and be aware of other sources to explore further.

Women, the Focus for Care

Putting those who use health services at the centre of care has become government policy in the past 10 years, partly caused by pressure from the public in the provision of all health care (Department of Health, 1989, 1990, 1991, 1992, 1993a, 1996). For the maternity services, the concern of women about the type of care received has gathered momentum since the 1960s, following the introduction of technology and more invasive techniques. The organization and pattern of care has become more complex, and services have becoming fragmented with disputes over who should manage childbirth and where (Currell, 1990; House of Commons Health Committee, 1992).

The criticism on behalf of women using the maternity services that their needs were not being met plus the fact that it had been over a decade since the previous inquiry into the maternity services led to the government's Health Select Committee (chaired by Sir Nicholas Winterton) to conduct a major inquiry in January 1991. The report was published in February 1992 – one of the main conclusions was that the woman and her baby should be central to care and that the maternity services should be geared around them:

> *We conclude that there is a widespread demand among women for greater choice in the type of maternity care they receive; and that the present structure of the maternity services frustrates, rather than facilitates, those who wish to exercise this choice.*

(House of Commons Health Committee, 1992, para 5.2.)

This inquiry, linked with other government initiatives, influenced inquiries conducted in all four countries of the UK, some of which were well into reviews of their maternity services – Scotland had already established an action group on the maternity services and the Welsh initiative had started. **Figure 21.1** identifies the reports that currently affect the maternity services in the UK and indicates common themes across all the countries.

What is significant is the shift towards the provision of a more sensitive service in which women are involved in the planning and monitoring of services, as well as being able to determine which elements of care they receive. Choice, continuity and control are the concepts that run through the documents. Improved communication is a key to a more sensitive and responsive service. Some documents include action plans with targets to be reached (Department of Health, 1994), whereas others have been followed up with published action plans or specific letters concerning the development of a strategy (NHSME, 1994). The ongoing monitoring systems within the four countries also differ, reflecting each country's particular policies relevant to their populations.

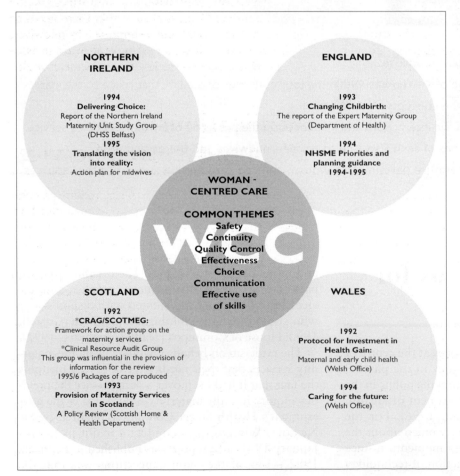

Figure 21.1 Reports produced within the four UK countries to influence the future direction of their maternity services. (Henderson, 1997).

Figure 21.2 Interactions and influences on the organization and type of care.
(Henderson, 1997).

Interactions	+	Influencing Factors	=	Effect
Women		Class / Values / Beliefs		Climate of organization
Midwives		Culture / Views of childbirth		Type of organization
Doctors		Gender / Tradition		Choices available
Others		Expectations Government Policy		Degree of woman-focused care

Influences on the Organization and Type of Care

There is no doubt that women will be able to have a voice on how maternity services are delivered, as this is clearly government policy; however, such statements are easy to make but often the reality is different. The interplay of factors that influence the system of care provided, choices available and level of participation are illustrated in **Figure 21.2**.

One important group of midwives who can make an enormous difference to the organization and quality of care are midwifery managers, particulary those designated Head of Midwifery Services. In an Action Research project undertaken in the 21 maternity units in the West Midlands (Henderson, 1997a) it was found that the importance of such a key role was not being recognised by some trusts and these posts were becoming extinct or downgraded in the move towards cost savings. The displacement of experienced managers was having a detrimental effect in some trusts and those left in more junior positions had an impossible task having to implement momentous change whilst at the same time having little authority with no control over the utilisation of resources. The value and role that midwives can play in strategic planning and priority setting is illustrated in a guide produced by the Royal College of Midwives (1997). Managers if allowed the responsibility and authority can create a cost-effective quality service for women. Organizations need to be supportive to staff creating a positive environment that fosters trust and facilitates change. One other powerful influence on maternity services that deserves mention concerns independent reviews and one just completed was that of the Audit Commission. The Commission is required to undertake studies to 'enable it to make recommendations for improving the economy, effi-

cency and effectiveness of the service provided in the NHS' (Audit Commission, 1997). Within the report recognition is given to the many good practices and effective changes being undertaken. Women generally are satisfied with the services but there are areas where progress needs to be made; for example, the development of clinical guidelines and protocols, improving information to women particulary antenatal screening and testing. Postnatal care was criticised: in particular, the hospital provision of these services. Recommendations include actions to be carried out by trusts, commissioning authorities and the NHS Executive. What is clear is that there needs to be a focused and collaborative approach by midwives, medics and others if we are to move forward in association with women – the key is involvement of all.

Implications of a Woman-Centred Service

Achieving a woman-centred service requires a commitment on behalf of everyone concerned, not least those who manage resources, those who act as carers (doctors, midwives and others), those who use the service and those who purchase services. General Practitioners are becoming more powerful (Henderson, 1997b) The interactions between the professionals themselves and the women using the services are a crucial part, but when determining care on whose values should we base our decisions? Inevitably, in a cost-conscious NHS, purchasers will ultimately have to decide. Their decision will be guided by the professionals and those using the service. However, the professionals' viewpoint may be considered the most relevant, regardless of the type of decision being made. The language spoken by those involved may also influence the situation, with the woman feeling disempowered (Leap, 1992; Shirley and Mander,

1996). Kirkham (1996) states that we are affected by our past and the process of professionalization has created dilemmas in three sets of relationships, with midwives, with women and with other professions. These relationships are fundamental to the way we practise and therefore they need to be developed.

Midwives have it within their power to help fashion the maternity service, to make it a woman-centred service. At the heart of midwifery is the concept of caring, so midwives need to be aware of their responsibilities to the women they care for. *A Philosophy for Midwifery*, published in 1991 by the Royal College of Midwives, reads as follows:

> *The aim of the midwifery profession is to provide a service which facilitates the safe and satisfying transition of women to motherhood. This is achieved principally by the processes of supporting, caring, guiding, monitoring and educating. The unique and personal needs of women in their childbearing years are central to this service.*

Does this reflect your own authorities philosophy? **Box 21.1** poses questions to reflect upon. Are the written statements a reality? Do midwives have the power to provide a flexible service? Gillen (1995) asks if midwives can practise autonomously or will they continue to provide a medically orientated service based on tradition? It is apparent that there exists, in many units, a conflict of interest between professionals that rotates around control, i.e. control of resources, knowledge, information giving and decision making. How can midwives empower women when they themselves do not have the power to affect how the services are provided (**Box 21.2**)?

It is recognized that if midwives are to move towards a truly woman-centred service, then it requires change within the structure of the organization and systems in operation, as well as preparation on behalf of individual practitioners. The NHS reforms affect midwifery management structures in different ways. For some comes the opportunity to develop, while for others change has become more difficult (Henderson, 1997a). The need to develop and update skills and the importance of building confidence is highlighted by a number of writers (Skinner and Roche, 1995; Kirkham, 1996; Henderson, 1997b). Skinner and Roche (1995) describe how midwives in one trust developed their own personal action plans using a skills inventory and a scale to help them assess their own philosophy of woman-centred care.

Many midwives say that 'woman-centred care' is something they have been doing and are continuing to do – it is part of practising as a midwife. To a degree we are all doing it, but some more successfully than others. As practice moves on, as our knowledge increases and new methods of care develop, it is vital to reassess and review continually how effective our care is.

The basis of such a service requires good communicators, a system which demonstrates choice and an information service that:

- Indicates exactly what the woman can expect.
- Enables women to have confidence in making choices by being provided with relevant information.
- Is involved in their care.

Ralston (1994) suggests that there is a reluctance, on behalf of midwives, to fully inform women of the choices available, sometimes through fear of the consequences. The system needs to allow midwives the flexibility, time and resources to enable such an approach. It takes time to develop a relationship, time

---

Box 21.1

Trust Policy, Midwives and the Users

Examine the trust business plans and annual report or or statements of the philosophy of care in your trust:

- How closely does this policy match yours and that of the midwives and other staff who practising within the trust where you practice?
- Does it match what users of the service want?
- Are all staff and users of the services given the opportunity to contribute to these documents?
- By what means does this happen?
- Is there a Maternity Service Liaison Committee (MSLC)?

Box 21.2

Which Services to Provide?

Consider the service being provided in your trust or area:

- Is it dictated by tradition or are there structures set up to enable midwives to deliver care that is tailored to the woman's needs?
- What proportion of births are normal or low risk and what proportion of the care is recognized officially as midwifery-led care?
- What mechanisms are in place for the trust and the commissioning authority to obtain user views?
- Do user views affect how and what services are provided?

to gain the trust and confidence of women and it takes time to find out what women really want. This relationship is vital. We need to listen actively to what it is that women need. Reid (1994), in her review of the research into consumer views, quite rightly points out that we need to ask the question 'Whose voice are we hearing?' and states that, 'We must not over generalize and be careful to listen to the silent minorities.'

There are a number of schemes that describe the benefits, successes and problems of woman-centred care. Some of the findings have been published (Changing Childbirth Update series, 1995/6; Turnbull *et al.*, 1995; Page, 1995; Hundley *et al.* 1994) and others are still being piloted. Some of the questions that you might ask about these schemes are identified in **Box 21.3**.

There is no doubt that when midwives and woman work together they are a powerful force for change. Perhaps the most important question is, 'Do midwives and women want change to happen?' Woman-centred care will only become a practical reality if midwives and women want it. Different women want different things, which has to be weighed up against the cost effectiveness of the care provided. There is a growing body of evidence that some pilot projects rated as more satisfying are more costly (Hundley *et al.* 1995; Turnbull, 1995; Spurgeon, 1996). These costings should be viewed with caution as they are in many ways imprecise, due to the complexity of the health service costing mechanism, and may not be comparable. However, this may be overlooked by those with the power to shape future services if a small proportion of women in pilot schemes are very satisfied, but the majority of women in trusts can be satisfied at no extra cost. The choice made could be to maintain the status quo. Commissioning authorities and provider units constantly have to make efficiency savings and always have to prioritize.

The Way Forward

The way forward must be to provide a service that is sensitive to the needs of those who use it; the skill is to reach all of those who use it and comply with their needs (Campbell and Garga, 1997). However, there will always be the dilemma of cost versus satisfaction in the provision of care within a market-driven health service. Successful change requires an empowered, developed and supported team of midwives who are confident and committed (**Figure 21.3**). They, in turn, need a visionary leader. However, change will not come about unless women feel confident, are empowered, developed and supported themselves. Part of empowerment concerns having good information about what is on offer and so being aware of choices available Knowledge is power but knowing how to use it is empowering. The government's support of the consumer campaign in the autumn of 1996 has raised the awareness of those who use the maternity services of their rights, access to information and

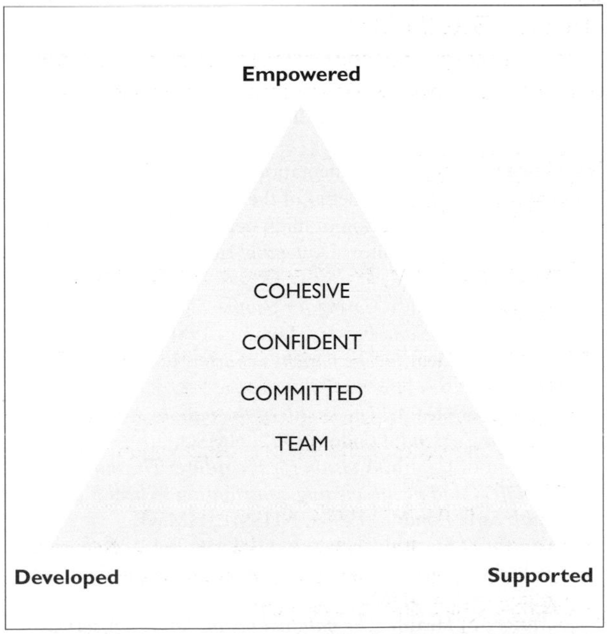

Box 21.3

Assessment of Schemes for Woman-Centred Care

• How is continuity of carer improved?
• What sorts of choices are given to women?
• How are midwives coping with the new patterns of work being introduced in the name of woman-centred care?
• What are the training and educational implications?
• Are interprofessional relations being affected and if so how?
• How is the scheme perceived by women?
• How much does the scheme cost and, perhaps more importantly, what exactly is costed and to what is it compared?

Figure 21.3 Successful change (Henderson, 1996b).

choices in care provision (DOH/CCIT, 1996). It is difficult to say the extent of the effect that the campaign has had as there are may other factors involved, but anecdotal evidence suggests that more women are questioning the organisation of maternity services and value of specific tests than ever before. Midwives in liaison with women have it in their power to make the service work both to the benefit of the profession and, more importantly, of the mother and her baby. As we approach the year 2000 perhaps there will be little need for pressure groups to fight the cause for women. Somehow I doubt it for there will always be those who are unable to speak out for themselves or are unsuccessful at making their voices heard.

Midwives and obstetricians (and others) need to be aware of this and must constantly monitor and evaluate their practice, ensuring that they are providing the type of care that is accessible, safe, beneficial and acceptable to women. The way forward must be in partnership, the midwife and obstetrician actively listening with women, hearing what they say to discover what they want and why, and taking heed. In the words of Proust, they need to see with new eyes:

The real voyage of discovery consists not in seeking new lands but in seeing with new eyes'

(Proust).

Childbirth does not change, it is midwives, obstetricians and women who change: that is why listening is so important.

References

Crag/Scotmeg Working Group on Maternity Services: Information pack of publications by the Scottish Office NHS, Scotland, 1996, HMSO.

Changing Childbirth Implementation Team: *Changing childbirth update*, quarterly newsletter of the CCIT, Cambridge

Currell R: The organisation of midwifery care. In Alexander J, Levy V, Roche S, editors: *Antenatal care*, London, 1990, Macmillan.

Department of Health: *Caring for people: Community care in the next decade and beyond*, London, 1989, HMSO.

Department of Health: *The patient's charter*, London, 1991, HMSO.

Department of Health: *The health of the nation: A strategy for health in England*, London, 1992, HMSO.

Department of Health: *A vision for the future: The nursing, midwifery and health visiting contribution to health and health care*, London, 1993a, NHSME, HMSO.

Department of Health: *Changing childbirth*, Vol. 1, Report of the Expert Maternity group (Chair, Baroness Cumberlege), London, 1993b, HMSO.

Department of Health: *The national health service. A service with ambitions*, London, 1996, The stationery office bookshoops.

DHSS, Belfast: *Delivering choice: Midwife and GP led maternity units*, Report of the Northern Ireland Maternity Units Study Group, 1994, Belfast.

DHSS: *Translating the vision, strategy for nursing midwifery, health visiting in Northern Ireland. Action plan for midwives*, Belfast, 1995, DHSS.

Gillen J: Can midwives practice autonomously? *Br J Midwifery* 3(5):245, 1995.

Henderson C: *Changing childbirth and the West Midlands 1995–1996*, Report of the Changing childbirth visiting scholar, London, 1997, RCM.

Henderson C: Choices and patterns of care. In Sweet, editor: *Mayes Midwifery*, 12th edn, 1997b, in press, Ballière Tindall.

Henderson C: *Midwifery managers and support in changing childbirth*, Scholarship report. Paper presented at the Department of Health Leadership in Midwifery Conferences, Coventry, Leeds, 1996b, unpublished.

House of Commons Health Committee: *Maternity services* (Chaired by Sir Nicholas Winterton), London, 1992, HMSO.

Hundley V, Cruikshank F, Lang G, Glazener C, Milne J, Turner M, Blyth D, Mollison J, Donaldson C: Midwife managed delivery unit: a randomised controlled comparison with consultant led care, *Br Med J* 309:1400, 1994.

Hundley V, Donaldson C, Lang G, Glazener C, Milne J, Mollison J: Costs of intrapartum care in a midwife managed delivery unit and a consultant led labour ward, *Midwifery* 11:103, 1995.

Kirkham M: Professionalization past and present. With women or with the powers that be? In Kroll D, editor: *Midwifery care for the future*, London, 1996, Ballière Tindall.

Leap N: The power of words, *Nurs Times* 88(21): 60, 1992.

NHSME: *Purchasing priorities 1994–1995*, EL 94 9, London, 1994, Department of Health.

Page L: *Effective group practice in midwifery: working with women*, Oxon, 1995, Blackwell Science.

Reid M: What are consumer views of maternity care? In Chamberlain G, Patel N, editors, *The future of the maternity services*, Ch 1, London, 1994, RCOG.

Ralston R: How much choice do women really have in relation to their care? *Br J Midwifery* 2(9):453, 1994.

Royal College of Midwives: *A philosophy for midwifery*, London, 1991, RCM.

Royal College of Midwives: *Woman centred care. The RCM view*, Position paper 4, London, 1995, Royal College of Midwives.

Scottish Office Home & Health Department: *Provision of maternity services in Scotland – a policy review*, Edinburgh, 1993, HMSO.

Shirley K, Mander R: The power of language, *Br J Midwifery* 4(6):298, 317, 1996.

Skinner G, Roche S: Creating confidence by building on experience, *Br J Midwifery* 3(5): 284, 1995.

Spurgeon P: *Report to the trust board of an evaluation of the Norton team pilot*, unpublished, Birmingham, 1996, Birmingham Women's Healthcare NHS Trust.

Turnbull D: *The establishment and evaluation of a midwifery development unit*, MDU Summary, Glasgow, 1995, Glasgow Royal Maternity Hospital.

Turnbull D, McGinley M, Fyvie H, Johnstone I, Holmes A, Shields N, Cheyne H, MacLennan B: Implementation and evaluation of a midwifery development unit, *Br J Midwifery* 3(9):465, 1995.

Welsh Office: The protocol for investment in health gain, Cardiff, 1991, HMSO.

Further Reading

Reports from all countries are useful document sources and can be used to influence change as can documents produced by your trust or health board.

Audit Commission: *First class delivery: Improving maternity services in England and Wales*, Oxon, 1997, Audit Commission.

The Commission collected information form 13 NHS trusts providing maternity services, 2375 recent mothers, 12 commissioning authorities and 300 GP's. It identified changes and suggested ways to progress.

English National Board: *New dimensions in midwifery care*, London, 1996, ENB.

A distance learning programme based on research into the education and training needs of midwives.

English National Board: *The challenge of 'Changing childbirth'*, Book 2 the context of care. Midwifery Educational Resource pack, London, 1995, ENB.

The purpose of the pack is to help midwives to reflect upon their practice. It explores many of the issues that face midwives in these challenging times. Of particular interest is book 1, 1.3 Using perinatal planning to meet the challenge of Changing Childbirth. Book 2 of the pack, sections 2.3 Communication and negotiation. The consumer's view; 2.6 Building partnerships with women and their families.

Campbell R, Garcia J, editors: *The organisation of maternity care*, Cheshire, 1997, Books for Midwives Press.

A comprehensive guide enabling those engaged in the management, provision or purchasing of maternity services to evaluate any aspect of the service organization.

Henderson C: *Woman centred care supplements*, edited by Tyler S, 1996, Royal College of Midwives.

A series of supplements highlighting issues surrounding the provision of woman-centred care. Commenced January 1996.

Midwifery Development Unit: *A resource manual*, Glasgow 1995, Glasgow Maternity Unit.

A manual produced by Glasgow supported by the Scotland Board of the Royal College of Midwives. The manual contains descriptions of the processes worked through in setting up and developing a midwifery led unit. Manuals have been distributed free of charge to all units and education institutions in Scotland. Others are obtainable from the Scottish RCM.

Royal College of Midwives: *Unlocking the door. A practical guide to purchasing for midwives*, London, 1997, RCM.

A guide to help midwives in the commissioning process, how to effectively represent the interests of midwifery and midwives. Also a companion smaller guide for purchasers.

Index